Vivienne Melyen 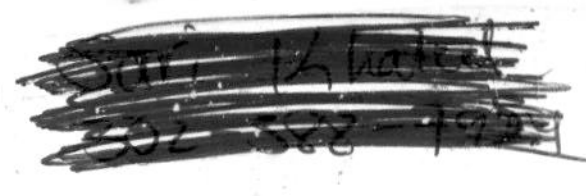
8026983413

Components of the AGPAR Score

	0	1	2
Activity/muscle tone	Limp	Some weak or inactive movements	Strong, active movements
Pulse/heart rate	Absent	Below 100 beats per min, slow	Over 100 beats per min, rapid
Grimace response	Absent	Grimace	Cry, cough, or sneeze (in response to catheter in nostril)
Appearance/skin color	Blue, pale	Body: pink; extremities: pink	Completely pink
Respiratory/breathing	Absent	Slow, irregular	Good

United States FDA Pharmaceutical Pregnancy Categories

Pregnancy Category A	Adequate and well-controlled studies have failed to demonstrate a risk to the fetus in the first trimester of pregnancy (and there is no evidence of risk in later trimesters).
Pregnancy Category B	Animal reproduction studies have failed to demonstrate a risk to the fetus and there are no adequate and well-controlled studies in pregnant women OR Animal studies which have shown an adverse effect, but adequate and well-controlled studies in pregnant women have failed to demonstrate a risk to the fetus in any trimester.
Pregnancy Category C	Animal reproduction studies have shown an adverse effect on the fetus and there are no adequate and well-controlled studies in humans, but potential benefits may warrant use of the drug in pregnant women despite potential risks.
Pregnancy Category D	There is positive evidence of human fetal risk based on adverse reaction data from investigational or marketing experience or studies in humans, but potential benefits may warrant use of the drug in pregnant women despite potential risks.
Pregnancy Category X	Studies in animals or humans have demonstrated fetal abnormalities and/or there is positive evidence of human fetal risk based on adverse reaction data from investigational or marketing experience, and the risks involved in use of the drug in pregnant women clearly outweigh potential benefits.

D1444640

Oxford American Handbook of

Obstetrics and Gynecology

ublished and forthcoming Oxford American Handbooks

Oxford American Handbook of Clinical Medicine
Oxford American Handbook of Anesthesia
Oxford American Handbook of Clinical Dentistry
Oxford American Handbook of Clinical Surgery
Oxford American Handbook of Critical Care
Oxford American Handbook of Emergency Medicine
Oxford American Handbook of ENT, Head and Neck Surgery
Oxford American Handbook of Nephrology and Hypertension
Oxford American Handbook of Obstetrics and Gynecology
Oxford American Handbook of Pediatrics
Oxford American Handbook of Psychiatry
Oxford American Handbook of Respiratory Medicine

Oxford American Handbook of
Obstetrics and Gynecology

Edited by

Errol R. Norwitz, MD, PhD
Associate Professor, Yale University School of Medicine
Director of Perinatal Research,
Co-Director, Division of Maternal–Fetal Medicine,
Department of Obstetrics, Gynecology & Reproductive Sciences,
Yale–New Haven Hospital, New Haven, CT, USA

with

S. Arulkumaran
Professor of Obstetrics and Gynaecology
St. George's Hospital Medical School,
University of London, UK

I. M. Symonds
Senior Lecturer and Honorary Consultant in Obstetrics and Gynaecology,
Derby City General Hospital, Derby, UK

A. Fowlie
Consultant in Obstetrics and Gynaecology
Derby City General Hospital, Derby, UK

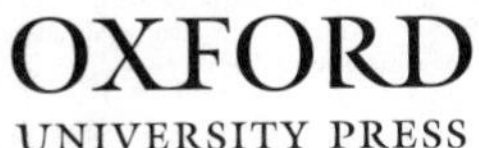

OXFORD
UNIVERSITY PRESS

OXFORD
UNIVERSITY PRESS

Great Clarendon Street, Oxford OX2 6DP

Oxford University Press is a department of the University of Oxford.
It furthers the University's objective of excellence in research, scholarship,
and education by publishing worldwide in

Oxford New York

Auckland Cape Town Dar es Salaam Hong Kong Karachi
Kuala Lumpur Madrid Melbourne Mexico City Nairobi
New Delhi Shanghai Taipei Toronto

With offices in

Argentina Austria Brazil Chile Czech Republic France Greece
Guatemala Hungary Italy Japan Poland Portugal Singapore
South Korea Switzerland Thailand Turkey Ukraine Vietnam

Oxford is a registered trade mark of Oxford University Press
in the UK and in certain other countries

Published in the United States
by Oxford University Press Inc., New York

© Oxford University Press, 2007

The moral rights of the author have been asserted
Database right Oxford University Press (maker)

First published 2007

All rights reserved. No part of this publication may be reproduced,
stored in a retrieval system, or transmitted, in any form or by any means,
without the prior permission in writing of Oxford University Press,
or as expressly permitted by law, or under terms agreed with the appropriate
reprographics rights organization. Enquiries concerning reproduction
outside the scope of the above should be sent to the Rights Department,
Oxford University Press, at the address above

You must not circulate this book in any other binding or cover
and you must impose the same condition on any acquirer

British Library Cataloguing in Publication Data
Data available

Library of Congress Cataloging in Publication Data

Oxford American handbook of obstetrics and gynecology/[edited by] Errol Norwitz.
p.; cm. – (Oxford American handbooks)

Based on: Oxford handbook of obstetrics and gynaecology/edited by S. Arulkumaran, I. Symonds, A. Fowlie. 2004.

Includes biblioraphical references.

ISBN-13: 978–0–19–518938–4 (flexicover : alk. paper)

1. Obstetrics–Handbooks, manuals, etc. 2. Gynecology–Handbooks, manuals, etc. I. Norwitz, Errol R. II. Oxford handbook of Obstetrics and gynaecology. III. Series. [DNLM: 1. Pregnancy Complications–Handbooks. 2. Genital Diseases, Female–Handbooks. 3. Pregnancy. WQ 39 O975 2007]

RG531.O94 2007 2007000564

618–dc22

Typeset by Newgen Imaging Systems (P) Ltd., Chennai, India
Printed in China
on acid-free paper by
Phoenix offset

ISBN 978–0–19–518938–4 (flexicover: alk.paper)

10 9 8 7 6 5 4 3 2 1

Oxford University Press makes no representation, express or implied, that the drug dosages in this book are correct. Readers must therefore always check the product information and clinical procedures with the most up-to-date published product information and data sheets provided by the manufacturers and the most recent codes of conduct and safety regulations. The authors and the publishers do not accept responsibility or legal liability for any errors in the text or for the misuse or misapplication of material in this work. Except where otherwise stated, drug dosages and recommendations are for the non-pregnant adult who is not breast-feeding.

Preface

Obstetrics and gynecology is often regarded as an orphan specialty, reaching out to the disciplines of general surgery, internal medicine, psychiatry, and family medicine in an attempt to define itself. More recently, the field has morphed into a broad-based specialty including all of women's health in which practitioners are equally comfortable performing complex pelvic surgery as they are delivering a second twin by internal podalic version or treating a vaginal discharge that 'Must have come from the toilet, Doctor'. To meet these burgeoning demands, obstetrics and gynecology care providers must keep up with new developments in the field and adapt their clinical practice style to meet the evolving recommendations.

This Oxford American Handbook is designed to provide the requisite depth and breadth of knowledge needed in *obstetrics and gynecology* to identify, investigate, diagnose, and manage clinical problems in the field. It will serve as a revision book for examinations as well as a quick reference guide for practitioners in the field of women's health. The editor has shifted through a vast array of topics and selected out those that can be regarded as fundamental to the discipline. In order to make this book useful for the medical student and the senior clinician, most chapters have been written by a multidisciplinary team of authors of varying seniority.

Clinical medicine continues to attract the brightest and most dedicated students to its ranks. The oppurtunity to nurture the talented young minds who will one day rise up to lead the medical community and deliver our grandchildren remains the single greatest privilege for the academic clinician. Nowhere is this privilege—and challenge—more apparent than in *obstetrics and gynecology*, a discipline that remains more art than science. Although clinicians in all disciplines aspire to practice rational evidenced-based medicine, many basic questions in the field remain unanswered. This text is written primarily as a handbook for medical students, doctors, and nurses. It is designed to give the reader a succinct yet comprehensive overview of *obstetrics and gynecology*. Special attention has been paid to incorporating an evidence-based approach to management while at the same time adhering to a uniform format to make it easy for the reader to navigate the text. It is the sincere hope of the authors that the readers will find this book interesting, easy to read, and informative. We hope that it will help you on a daily basis in the clinics and wards to diagnose and manage both simple and complex problems in *obstetrics and gynecology*. Not all questions can be answered in a formal text format. Students should be encouraged to question and challenge their clinical teachers. There are no mistakes in life, only lessons!

Errol R. Norwitz, MD, PhD

Acknowledgements

I would like to acknowledge the support of my family: my wife, Ann Giardina Hess, MD, PhD; my parents, Rollo and the late Marionne Norwitz; and my children, Nicholas, Gabriella, and Sam.

My sincere thanks to all the following for their valuable contribution: Mandy Abbett, Mrs R.A. Adekunle, MB BS MRCOG, Dr S. Ahuja, Professor S. Arulkumaran, J. Ashworth, MD MRCOG, Dr A. Bali, MD MRCOG, Mr A. Bunkheila, MBChB BSc M (ART) MD MRCOG, Mr Roger Chapman MB BS FRCOG, Mr M. Cust, Mr F.J. Darné, MD MRCOG, Dr Soo Downe, Miss Alison Fowlie, FRCOG, Dr David Guthrie PhD, FRCOG, FRCR, Mrs Hasiba Hamoud, MRCOG, Mr R. Hayman, MRCOG, M. Jackson, Mr H.M.L. Jenkins, DM FRCOG, Mr Olujimi Jibodu, MRCOG, Dr Devendra Kangalingam, Dr V.L. Keely, MA, MB, BS, PhD, DRCOG, MRCGP, Mrs Anne Meadows, Dr John McIntyre, Mr S. Mitra, MD DNB MRCOG, Dr M.P. Mohajer, FRCOG MD, Mr George E. Morgan, MB ChB MRCOG, Mrs Andrea Morris, RGN RM RHV BScHons, E.P. Morris, MD MRCOG, Mr S. Mukhopadhyay, MD DNB MRCOG, Karen Payne, RGN RM DPSM, Dr Suzie Peatman, MBBS, MRCOG, Mrs Lesley Roulstone, RM RGN DPPM, Dr W. Scott, Mr I. Symonds, MD BMedSci MRCOG ILTM, Mr Onnig Tamizian, BMBS BMedSci MRCOG, Dr S. Wallace, BA BM BCh.

Lastly, I would like to acknowledge the assistance and guidance I received from every member of the publishing team at Oxford University Press on both sides of the Atlantic, including, among others, Bill Lamsback, Kevin Kochanski, Dana Kasowitz, and Helen Hill.

E.R.N.

Acknowledgements

Contents

Detailed contents

Symbols and abbreviations

🕮	Cross-reference
5-FU	5-fluorouracil
5HIAA	5-hydroxyindoleacetic acid
5-HT	5-hydroxytryptamine (serotonin)
ABC	airway, breathing, and circulation (resuscitation protocol)
AC	abdominal circumference
ACA	anticardiolipin antibodies
ACE	angiotensin-converting enzyme
ACOG	American College of Obstetricians and Gynecologists
ACTH	adrenocorticotropic hormone
AFE	amniotic fluid embolism
AFI	amniotic fluid index
AFLP	acute fatty liver of pregnancy
AFP	α-fetoprotein
AFS	American Fertility Society
AGT	alanine glyoxalate transaminase
ALT	alanine transaminase
ANA	antinuclear antibodies
APLAS	antiphospholipid antibody syndrome
aPTT	activated partial thromboplastin time
ART	assisted reproduction techniques
ASCUS	abnormal squamous cells of undetermined significance
ASD	atrial septal defect
AST	aspartate transaminase
ATP	adenosine triphosphate
AZT	zidovudine
BCG	bacille Calmette–Guérin
BMI	body mass index
BP	blood pressure
BPD	biparietal diameter
BPP	biophysical profile
BSO	bilateral salpingo-oophorectomy
BV	bacterial vaginosis
CA-125	carcinoma antigen-125
CAH	congenital adrenal hyperplasia
CBC	complete blood count

CBZ	carbimazole
CCAM	congenital cystic adenomatous malformation
CF	cystic fibrosis
CGIN	cervical glandular intraepithelial neoplasia
CIN	cervical intraepithelial neoplasia
CMV	cytomegalovirus
CNS	central nervous system
CO_2	carbon dioxide
COCP	combined oral contraceptive pill
CP	cerebral palsy
CPA	cyproterone acetate
CPD	cephalopelvic disproportion
CPR	cardiopulmonary resuscitation
CPS	carbamyl phosphate synthetase
CRL	crown–rump length
CRP	C-reactive protein
CSE	combined spinal epidural
CSF	cerebrospial fluid
CT	computed tomography
CTG	cardiotocograph
CVA	cerebrovascular accident
CVP	central venous pressure
CVS	chorionic villus sampling
D&C	dilatation & curettage
D&E	dilatation and evacuation
DCT	direct Coombs' test
DES	diethylstilbestrol
DEXA	dual-energy X-ray absorptiometry
DHEAS	dehydroepiandrosterone sulfate
DHT	dihydrotestosterone
DI	donor insemination, diabetes insipidus
DIC	disseminated intravascular coagulation
DMT	dimethyltryptamine
DS	Down syndrome
dsDNA	double-stranded DNA
DUB	dysfunctional uterine bleeding
DVT	deep vein thrombosis
DZ	dizygotic
ECT	electroconvulsive therapy
ECV	external cephalic version
EDD	expected date of delivery
EE	ethinyl estradiol

EFM	electronic fetal momitoring
EKG	electrocardiograph, electrocardiography
ELISA	enzyme-linked immunosorbent assay
EOC	epithelial ovarian cancer
ESR	erythrocyte sedimentation rate
ET	embryo transfer
ETT	endotracheal tube
EUA	examination under anesthesia
FAS	fetal acoustic stimulation, fetal alcohol syndrome
FBS	fetal blood sampling
FDA	US Food and Drugs Administration
FDP	fibrin degradation product
fFN	fetal fibronectin
FFP	fresh frozen plasma
FHR	fetal heart rate
FIGO	International Federation of Gynecologists and Obstetricians
FISH	fluorescent *in situ* hybridization
FL	femur length
FSH	follicle-stimulating hormone
fT_3	free triiodothyronine
fT_4	free thyroxine
FTA	fluorescent treponemal antibody test
FTA-ABs	fluorescent treponemal antibody absorption
G6PD	glucose 6-phosphate dehydrogenase
GBS	group B β-hemolytic Streptococcus
GCSF	granulocyte colony-stimulating factor
GCT	glucose challenge test
GDM	gestational diabetes mellitus
GFR	glomerular filtration rate
GH	growth hormone
GIFT	gamete intrafallopian transfer
GLT	glucose load test
GnRH	gonadotropin-releasing hormone
GTT	glucose tolerance test
HAART	highly active antiretroviral therapy
Hb	hemoglobin
HB	hepatitis B
HbA_{1c}	hemoglobin A_{1c}
HBIg	hepatitis B immunoglobulin
HBsAg	hepatitis B surface antigen
HBV	hepatitis B virus
HC	head circumference

hCG	human chorionic gonadotropin
hCS	human chorionic somatotropin
HCT	hematocrit
HDL	high-density lipoprotein
HDL-C	high-density lipoprotein cholesterol
HDU	high-dependency unit
HELLP	hemolysis, elevated liver enzymes, low platelets
HIV	human immunodeficiency virus
HOCM	hypertrophic obstructive cardiomyopathy
hPL	human placental lactogen
HPV	human papillomavirus
HRT	hormone replacement therapy
HSG	hysterosalpingogram
HSV	herpes simplex virus (HSV1, HSV2)
IBS	irritable bowel syndrome
IC	interstitial cystitis
ICON	International Collaborative Ovarian Neoplasm (trial)
ICSI	intracytoplasmic sperm injection
ICU	intensive care unit
IDDM	insulin-dependent diabetes mellitus
Ig	immunoglobin
IM	intramuscular
INR	international normalized ratio
IOL	induction of labor
IU	international unit
IUCD	intrauterine contraceptive device
IUGR	intrauterine growth restriction
IUI	intrauterine insemination
IV	intravenous
IVF	*in vitro* fertilization
IVP	intravenous pyelogram
IVU	intravenous urogram
JVP	jugular venous pressure
L	liter
LAC	lupus anticoagulant
LATS	long-acting thyroid stimulator
LDH	lactic dehydrogenase
LDL	low-density lipoprotein
LDL-C	low-density lipoprotein cholesterol
LFT	liver function test
LH	luteinizing hormone
LLETZ	large loop excision of the transformation zone

LMP	last menstrual period
LMWH	low molecular weight heparin
LSD	lysergic acid diethylamine
MAC	minimum alveolar concentration
MAOI	monoamine oxidase inhibitor
MAS	meconium aspiration syndrome
MCA	middle cerebral artery
MCH	mean corpuscular hemoglobin
MCHC	mean corpuscular hemoglobin concentration
MCV	mean corpuscular volume
MDMA	3,4-methylenedioxymethamphetamine (ecstasy)
MG	myasthenia gravis
mmH_2O	millimeters of water
mmHg	millimeters of mercury
MoM	multiples of the median
MPA	medroxyprogesterone acetate
MRI	magnetic resonance imaging
MS	multiple sclerosis
MSAFP	maternal serum α-fetoprotein
MSU	midstream sample of urine
MVP	maximal vertical pocket
MZ	monozygotic
NET-EN	norethisterone enanthate
NIDDM	non-insulin-dependent diabetes mellitus
NSAID	nonsteroidal antiinflammatory drug
NST	nonstress test
NT	nuchal translucency
NTD	neural tube defect
NYHA	New York Heart Association
OCP	oral contraceptive pill
OCT	ornithine carbamyl transferase
OD	optical density
OHSS	ovarian hyperstimulation syndrome
OI	ovulation induction
p.r.n.	*pro re nata* (whenever needed)
$p\mathrm{aCO_2}$	partial arterial pressure of carbon dioxide
PAMG-1	placental α-microglobulin-1
$p\mathrm{aO_2}$	partial arterial pressure of oxygen
PAPP-A	pregnancy-associated plasma protein A
$p\mathrm{CO_2}$	partial carbon dioxide pressure
PCOS	polycystic ovary syndrome
PCP	phencyclidine, *Pneumocystis carinii* pneumonia

PCR	polymerase chain reaction
PCT	postcoital test
PCV	packed cell volume
PDA	patent ductus arteriosus
PE	pulmonary embolism
PESA	percutaneous epididymal sperm aspiration
PG	prostaglandin (PGE_1, PGE_2, $PGF_{2\alpha}$)
PGI_2	prostacycline
PID	pelvic inflammatory disease
PMS	premenstrual syndrome
PMT	premenstrual tension
POP	progestogen-only pill
PPH	postpartum hemorrhage
pPROM	preterm premature rupture of membranes
PROM	premature rupture of membranes
PTU	propylthiouracil
PUPP	pruritic urticarial papules and plaques of pregnancy
PZD	partial zonal dissection
RA	rheumatoid arthritis
Rh	rhesus
RPOC	retained products of conception
RPR	rapid plasma reagin
SAH	subarachnoid hemorrhage
SHBG	sex-hormone-binding globulin
SC	subcutaneous
SCJ	squamocolumnar junction
SD	standard deviation
SGA	small for gestational age
SIDS	sudden infant death syndrome
SLE	systemic lupus erythematosus
SOL	space-occupying lesion
SP-1	β_1 glycoprotein
SRY	sex-related Y (gene)
SSRI	selective serotonin-reuptake inhibitor
STD	sexually transmitted disease
SUZI	subzonal insemination
SVT	supraventricular tachycardia
T_3	triiodothyronine
T_4	thyroxine
TAH	total abdominal hysterectomy
TB	tuberculosis
TBG	thyroid-binding globulin

TENS	transcutaneous electrical nerve stimulation
TESA	testicular/epididymal sperm aspiration
TFT	thyroid function test
TIBC	total iron binding capacity
TOP	termination of pregnancy
TORCH	toxoplasmosis, rubella, cytomegalovirus, and herpes
TPHA	*Treponema pallidum* hemagglutination
TPI	*Treponema pallidum* immobilization
TSH	thyroid-stimulating hormone
TSIg	thyroid-stimulating immunoglobin
TV	transverse
TZ	transformation zone
uE_3	unconjugated estriol
UFH	unfractionated heparin
UR-NAP	urea-resistant neutrophil alkaline phosphatase
UTI	urinary tract infection
UV	ultraviolet
VBAC	vaginal birth after cesarean
VDRL	Venereal Disease Research Laboratory
VIN	vulval intraepithelial neoplasia
VMA	vanillylmandelic acid
VSD	ventricular septal defect
VT	ventricular tachycardia
VTE	venous thromboembolism
VZ	varicella zoster
VZIG	varicella zoster immunoglobulin
WHO	World Health Organization
ZIFT	zygote intrafallopian transfer

Chapter 1

Normal pregnancy: history, examination, anatomy, and physiology

Introduction and obstetric history

History-taking and physical examination are essential skills for good clinical practice. Competence in this area requires a sound clinical knowledge in order to direct questions that will help to shape the presentation appropriately. The basic framework to history-taking and physical examination can be readily acquired but the best result can only be achieved by improving these skills by practice and better knowledge.

The obstetric history

The obstetric history is both a synopsis of a woman's background risk and an account of the progress of her index pregnancy. A carefully taken history provides a clinical guide to the physical examination to follow. Further physical signs, which are not routinely elicited in a pregnant woman, may become necessary if the history warrants it. It is useful to have a template for taking the obstetric history. This allows the history to be taken and presented in a logical sequence and avoids inadvertent omission of important details, both positive and negative. The following is a guide to taking an obstetric history.

Current pregnancy

In presenting an obstetric case, it is appropriate to begin with a summary of the details to follow. This is especially so if the history that is to follow is complicated. It allows the listener to focus on the clinical issues in the pregnancy. The summary is best constructed by having some organization in history taking and is given below.

Personal and pregnancy details

A polite introduction followed by permission to take the history and examination is vital. Start with the enquiry of her name, age, gravidity (i.e. number of pregnancies including the current one) and parity (i.e. number of births beyond 20 weeks' gestation in the US or beyond 24 weeks' gestation in the UK). The expected date of delivery (EDD) can be calculated from the last menstrual period (LMP) by Naegele's rule (add 1 year and 7 days to the LMP and subtract 3 months).

Inquire about her health and that of her fetus (e.g. after 18–20 weeks, inquire about fetal movements). This should be followed by details of current problems, if there are any.

A chronological and concise account of the events in pregnancy is best obtained by inquiring about her pregnancy in the first, second, and third trimester. If she is in the postnatal period, details of labor and delivery are relevant.

This inquiry should include details of laboratory tests and ultrasound scans. The date the pregnancy was confirmed by a pregnancy test, results of the routine antenatal blood tests, and the date and details of the first scan (dating or nuchal translucency scan) are important. Subsequent antenatal check-ups and tests done including subsequent scans should be noted. The details of the results may be asked from the woman and, if necessary, can be cross-checked against the notes.

There should be an organizational logic of history-taking. At times it may be necessary to revisit an area of the history as the story unfolds further or during or after clinical examination.

- ***Menstrual history*** Determine the last menstrual period (LMP) and any details that may influence the validity of her EDD as calculated from the LMP, such as long cycles, irregular periods, or recent use of the oral contraceptive pill.
- ***Past obstetric history*** Outcome of previous pregnancies and any significant antenatal, intrapartum, or postpartum events may have influence in the management of the current pregnancy. Previous maternal complications, mode of delivery, birth weights, and the life and health of babies may be relevant.
- ***Past gynecological history*** Details of contraceptive history, previous surgical procedures, and cervical smears should be noted.
- ***Past medical/surgical history*** Some medical conditions may have a significant impact on the course of the pregnancy. Heart disease, seizure disorder, asthma, thyroid disorders, pregestational diabetes mellitus, and other medical conditions or the medications they take for these conditions may have significant impact on the pregnancy. Alternatively, pregnancy may have an impact on the medical condition. The condition may remain the same or get better or worse. These may be incorporated under 'current pregnancy' if it is of concern in this pregnancy. Outcome of medical consultations should be known and, if it has not been done, arrangements need to be made for looking after the mother in a multidisciplinary clinic or with the relevant physician.
- ***Drug history*** *History of allergies* should be highlighted and any use/abuse of drugs during pregnancy should be noted. Arrangements may have to be made to wean off the drug.
- ***Family/social history*** History of hereditary illnesses or congenital defects is important and may be of concern to the couple. Appropriate counseling and investigations may have to be organized. This will be a good opportunity to discuss stopping smoking or reducing excessive alcohol intake. Relevant social aspects such as childcare arrangements and plans for breast-feeding and contraception can be discussed at this point.
- ***Final summary*** This should include the salient details that will impact on the investigations to be carried out and the proposed plan of management.

It may be necessary to vary this template to suit different clinical situations. In a woman who has experienced many problems during her pregnancy, it may be better to provide details of each problem separately rather than a chronological account of the pregnancy.

Physical examination

Many aspects of the obstetric physical examination are unique. There are several necessary techniques and skills which are not required in other specialities.

General examination

The assessment should begin with a general examination. This is intended to provide the clinician with an overview of the woman's general physical condition upon which more specific examinations can be directed. The general examination should include the woman's height and weight. From these, the body mass index (BMI) can be calculated as follows:

$$\text{BMI} = \text{weight (kg)}/\text{height (m)}^2$$

Some antenatal and perinatal complications are associated with a BMI <20 or >30kg/m^2. The thyroid gland and breasts should be examined at a booking visit and auscultation of the heart sounds and lungs is essential. For many women, the obstetric booking visit will be their first visit to a doctor in many years. Hence it is not unusual for asymptomatic conditions such as a cardiac murmur from valvular heart disease, breast masses, or goiter to be detected at these visits. These conditions may have significant implications on the course of her pregnancy and, indeed, on her subsequent health. More detailed examinations are indicated when a sign is detected (e.g. multinodular goiter, bruit over a mass, ophthalmic signs, tremors, etc.) or in specific situations, e.g. examination of the eyes with an ophthalmoscope to look for retinopathy in a diabetic or hypertensive woman.

The measurement of maternal blood pressure is of great importance in pregnancy. It is not appropriate to measure this in the supine position as pressure from a gravid uterus >20 weeks on the inferior vena cava impedes venous return resulting in a falsely low blood pressure. This is often referred to as the 'supine hypotension syndrome'. The correct technique for blood pressure measurement in pregnancy is in the sitting position at rest for 5 minutes taken by auscultating the brachial artery at the level of the heart and using disappearance of audible pulsations (Korotkoff V) to denote the diastolic blood pressure. An appropriate size cuff should be utilized, with a larger cuff for those with a larger upper arm circumference; a smaller cuff in these women would give a falsely high reading.

Abdominal examination

The fundamental steps in abdominal examination, namely inspection, palpation, and auscultation, apply to the pregnant woman. Occasionally, the art of percussion will be needed to elicit a fluid thrill when polyhydramnios is suspected. The specific maneuvers and techniques vary in an obstetric examination. The clinician may be guided by the preceding history and general examination to conduct this more specific part of the physical examination. For instance, a history of abdominal pain should prompt a careful palpation for uterine contractions (suggestive of labor) or localized tenderness (associated with red degeneration of a fibroid, torsion of an adnexal mass, dehiscence of a previous scar, chorioamnionitis, or rarely placental abruption).

Inspection

- Note the distension of the abdomen that may indirectly indicate the shape and size of the uterus. For example, lateral distention of the uterus is often seen in a twin pregnancy. Any asymmetry of the abdomen and fetal movements should be recorded.
- It is important to note any surgical scars, particularly a low transverse Pfannenstiel incision that may be obscured by pubic hair and a laparoscopic scar within the umbilicus. The scars observed should be correlated with previous surgical and gynecological history.
- Cutaneous signs of pregnancy, such as linea nigra (dark pigmented line stretching from just below the xiphoid process of the sternum through the umbilicus to the suprapubic area) or striae gravidarum (recent striae are purplish in color), are often present, but are of no clinical significance. Old striae (striae albicans) are silvery-white and are evidence of previous parity. The umbilicus may be flat with the surface or everted due to increased intraabdominal pressure. Superficial veins may be seen, denoting alternate paths of venous drainage due to pressure on the inferior vena cava by the gravid uterus.

Abdominal examination: palpation

- *Uterine size* The uterine size is objectively measured and expressed as symphyseal–fundal height. First, the highest point of the fundus of the uterus should be palpated. The uterus is usually displaced to the right of the midline by the sigmoid colon. To accurately locate the uterine fundus, first correct for dextrorotation of the uterus with the right hand. Then use the ulnar border of the left hand, moving it down from below the xiphoid process of the sternum until the fundus is located. Once the highest point of the uterine fundus is identified, the symphyseal–fundal height can be measured with a tape measure. The upper margin of the bony pubic symphysis is located by palpating downwards in the midline starting from few centimeters above the pubic hair margin. The fundal height in centimeters ± 2 cm should approximate the gestation of the pregnancy in weeks from 20 until 36 weeks of gestation. From 36 to 40 weeks, this could be ± 3 cm and, at 40 weeks, it is ± 4 cm. The decrease in height after 36 weeks is due to reduction in the amniotic fluid volume and descent (engagement) of the fetal head into the pelvis. An increase in size after 36 weeks may be due to further growth of the fetus, increase of amniotic fluid, or non-descent of the fetal head. It is important that the number of fetuses is determined. Palpation of a larger uterus than expected for that gestation, two heads, three poles, multiple fetal parts, excessive amniotic fluid, and auscultation of two fetal heart rates with a difference of greater than 10 beats per minute suggests a multiple pregnancy.
- *Presentation* Presentation refers to that part of the fetus that overlies the pelvic brim, and is of importance especially after 37 weeks' gestation because of impending labor. This is determined by placing both hands on either side of the lower pole of the uterus while facing the woman's feet. Approximate the hands firmly but gently towards the midline to ascertain the presenting part. A hard rounded presenting part suggests a cephalic presentation, while a broader soft object suggests breech presentation. If the hands on the sides of the head converge above the pelvic brim, then the head is not engaged as more of the head is above, whilst if the hands diverge then it is suggestive of engagement i.e. more than half the head has descended below the pelvic brim. In cephalic presentation, the degree of engagement is typically reported as the number of fifths of the head palpable above the pelvic brim. This is a rough approximation of how many finger breadths are necessary to cover the head above the pelvic brim. As this step is performed, it is important to look at the woman's face as palpation of the fetal head may be tender. Pawlik's grip is a one-handed technique to feel for the presenting part. The cupped right hand is used to grasp the lower pole of the uterus, and it is possible to feel the hard rounded fetal head in nearly 95% of pregnancies at term. The left hand is often used to stabilize the uterine fundus. It can cause discomfort and is not a necessary part of the examination if the head can be palpated with ease by the two hands.

- *Lie of the fetus and location of the fetal back* Lie of the fetus describes the relationship of the longitudinal axis of the fetus to the longitudinal axis of the uterus. This is best done by facing the woman, placing one hand on each side of the uterus, and applying gentle pressure. One should be able to perceive the resistance of the firm fetal back and, on the opposite side, it may be possible to feel the fetal limbs. This can be confirmed by alternately palpating with one hand while using the opposite hand to steady the fetus. If the presentation is cephalic or breech (the buttocks of the fetus), it has to be a longitudinal lie as the lower pole of the longitudinal lie of the uterus is occupied by one pole of the longitudinal axis of the fetus. If no presenting part was palpable in the lower pole and if the head or a breech was in one of the iliac fossae, then it is an oblique lie. If the longitudinal axis of the fetus straddles right across the horizontal axis of the uterus, then it is a transverse lie. Once the fetal lie is determined, the anterior shoulder should be palpated as the fetal heart sounds are best heard over this area. A shallow groove palpable between the presenting part and the rest of the fetus helps to identify the prominent anterior shoulder in most cases.
- *Estimation of fetal weight and quantity of amniotic fluid* Assessing fetal weight can be difficult, but it is important to determine whether the fetus is small, average, or large for gestational age. It is usually assessed by placing one hand over each pole of the fetus and guessing the approximate weight. With experience and by checking the guessed weight with the actual weight after delivery, the clinician is able to improve his/her performance. Even with an experienced clinician, however, the error in estimated fetal weight is approximately ±20%, and is particularly inaccurate with very small and very large fetuses. The ease with which the fetal parts are palpable and the 'cystic' feeling of the fluid in the uterus should give some idea of the amniotic fluid volume.

Abdominal examination and reporting findings

Auscultation

The fetal (Pinard) stethoscope or an electronic device can be placed over the anterior shoulder and the fetal heart can be heard. The fetal heart rate should be determined by auscultation over a period of 1 minute.

Percussion

Percussion is generally not used in an obstetric examination. If the quantity of amniotic fluid is felt to be excessive (shining stretched abdomen with difficulty in feeling fetal parts), a fluid thrill may be elicited by tapping in the midpoint of the uterus on one side and trying to feel it with the hand placed on the opposite side at the same level. The passage of surface vibrations should be damped by an assistant or by the patient, keeping the ulnar border of the hand firmly in the midline on the abdominal wall.

Vaginal examination

Vaginal speculum and digital examinations are only performed when indicated, e.g. a speculum examination is indicated to confirm leaking amniotic fluid in cases of premature rupture of membranes or to carry out inspection and take swabs in cases with abnormal vaginal discharge. A speculum examination is often performed at the booking visit in order to perform a Pap smear (a screen for cervical cancer) and cervical cultures.

Reporting your history and examination findings

A concise, clear, and logical sequence of reporting the history and examination findings is essential to ensure that the rest of the medical team and the patient can understand the clinical condition. It should form the basis for further investigations, if needed, and help plan effective management.

A summary of the history should be followed by a summary of the examination findings. The general examination findings should be reported first, emphasizing any aspects that may influence management. Abdominal findings should be reported in the order that they were elicited, using the appropriate terminology (e.g. lie, presentation, engagement).

Anatomy of the bony pelvis

The bony pelvis

The pelvis is made up of three bones: the two innominate bones and the sacrum. When articulated they enclose a cavity. The sacrum is wedged between the two innominate bones. Each innominate bone is made up of three parts:
- ilium
- ischium
- pubis.

The innominate bones are joined anteriorly at the symphysis pubis.

Pelvic brim

The pelvic brim is formed by the pubic crest, the pectineal line of the pubis, the arcuate line of the ilium, the alae of the sacrum, and the promontory of the sacrum. The brim separates the false pelvis above from the true pelvis below. Inferiorly, it is separated from the perineum by the urogenital diaphragm. The plane of the pelvis is at an angle of 55° to the horizontal. In the anatomical position, the pelvic cavity projects backward from the pelvic brim. The upper border of the symphysis pubis, the ischial spines, the tip of the coccyx, the head of the femur, and the greater trochanter lie in the same plane.

The female pelvis

The female pelvis differs from the male pelvis. The basic differences are:
- The female pelvis is broader than the male pelvis and the female pelvic bones, including the neck of the femur, are more slender than those of the male.
- The outline of the male pelvic brim is heart-shaped and the brim is widest towards the back, whereas the female pelvic brim is transversely oval (widest further forwards) because of less prominence of the sacral promontory.
- The female pelvis has evolutionally developed for giving birth. Therefore it is roomier. The outlet is also wider than that of the male pelvis.
- The subpubic angle is acute (like a Gothic arch) in the male pelvis, whereas it is rounded (like a Roman arch) in a female pelvis.

The major obstetric interest in the bony pelvis is that it is not distensible. Only minor degrees of movement are possible at the symphysis pubis and sacroiliac joints. Therefore its dimensions are critical at childbirth. The diameters of the pelvis vary at different parts of the pelvis.

In addition, the shape of the pelvis determines the availability of pelvic diameters. There are four basic shapes:
- *Gynecoid type* (Fig. 1.1). The classical female pelvis with the inlet transversely oval and a roomier pelvic cavity.
- *Android type*. The inlet is heart-shaped. The cavity is funnel-shaped with a contracted outlet.

- *Anthropoid type*. This results from high assimilation, i.e. the sacral body assimilated to the fifth lumbar vertebra. It is long, narrow, and oval in shape.
- *Platypelloid type*. This is a wide pelvis flattened at the brim with the promontory of the sacrum pushed forward.

Pelvic walls

The inner aspect (cavity) of the pelvic bones is covered by muscles. Above the brim it is covered by iliacus and psoas. The sidewalls are clad with the obturator internus and its fascia. The curved posterior wall is covered by the pyriformis, which courses laterally to the greater sciatic foramen. The levator ani and coccygeus with their opposite counterparts constitute the pelvic floor.

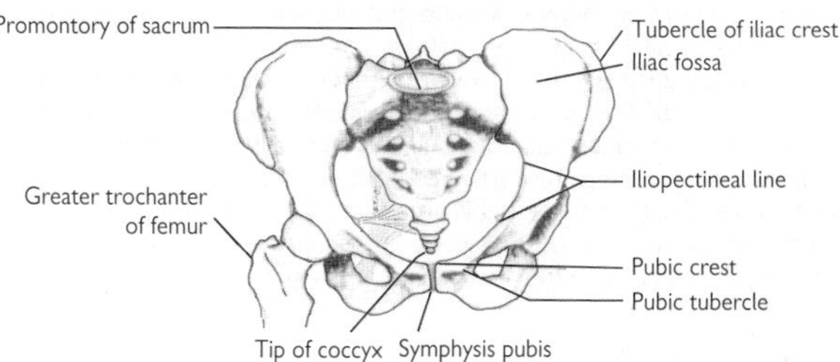

Fig. 1.1 A gynecoid pelvis. (Reproduced from *Last's Anatomy, Regional and Applied*, 9th edn (ed. RMH McMinn), p.395. © 1994 by permission of the publisher, Mosby.)

Adequacy of the pelvis to achieve vaginal delivery

This is best demonstrated using a model of a pelvis and a fetal head, but a description useful in understanding the mechanism of labor is given here.

The *true pelvis* is bounded anteriorly by the symphysis pubis (3.5 cm long) and posteriorly by the sacrum (12 cm long) (Fig. 1.2).

- The *zone of inlet* is made anteriorly by the upper border of the pubis, posteriorly by the sacral promontory, and laterally by the iliopectineal line. The transverse diameter is 13.5 cm and the anteroposterior (AP) diameter is 11.5 cm.
- The *zone of cavity* is most roomy just below the inlet zone and appears almost round with a transverse diameter of 13.5 cm and an AP diameter of 12.5 cm.
- The *zone of midpelvis* that follows is bounded by the apex of the pubic arch anteriorly, the tip of the sacrum posteriorly, and the ischial spines laterally (the interspinous distance should be >10 cm). This area is ovoid in shape and is the narrowest part of the pelvis.
- The *zone of outlet* has the pubic arch (desirable angle >90°) as its anterior border, whilst the sacrotuberous ligaments and ischial tuberosities delineate the posterolateral margins leading to the coccyx posteriorly.

The ideal female pelvis should be able to accommodate the head of a fetus at term. It has an oval brim, a shallow cavity, non-prominent ischial spines, a curved sacrum with large sciatic notches (>90°), and a sacrospinous ligament more than 3.5 cm long. The angle of the pelvic brim is 55° to the horizontal. The anterior–posterior diameter of the inlet is at least 12 cm and the transverse diameter is about 13.5 cm. The subpubic arch is rounded and is >90° and the ischial intertuberous distance is at least 10 cm. The pelvis is said to be clinically favorable if:

- The sacral promontory cannot be felt.
- The ischial spines are not prominent.
- The subpubic arch and base of the sacrospinous ligaments both accept two fingers and the intertuberous diameter accepts four knuckles on pelvic examination.

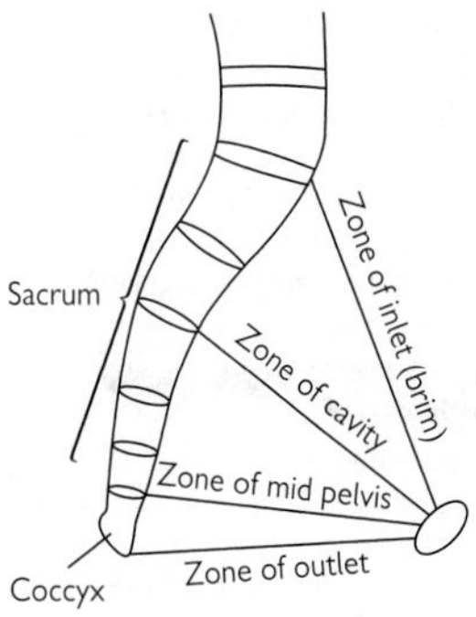

Fig. 1.2 Different zones of the pelvis. (Reproduced from *Oxford Handbook of Clinical Specialties*, 5th edn (ed. Collier J, Longmore M, Brown TD), p. 87. © 1997 by permission of the publisher, Oxford University Press.)

The fetal head

The fetal head is described using identifiable anatomical features:

- The *bregma* is the anterior fontanelle.
- The *brow* lies between the bregma and the root of the nose.
- The *face* lies below the root of the nose and the supraorbital ridges.
- The *occiput* is the bony prominence that lies behind the posterior fontanelle.
- The *vertex* is the diamond-shaped area between the anterior and posterior fontanelles and the parietal eminences.

Identification of the sutures and the fontanelles of the skull (Fig. 1.3) helps us to identify the position of the head in labor. The two frontal bones, the two parietal bones, the two temporal bones, the wings of the sphenoid, and the occipital bone form the skull. The area where the bones unite is not bony but is membranous and is called a *suture*.

- The *frontal suture* is situated between the frontal bones.
- The *sagittal suture* is situated between the parietal bones.
- The *coronal sutures* are between the parietal and frontal bones.
- The *lambdoid sutures* are between the parietal and occipital bones.
- The *temporal sutures* lie between the inferior margins of the parietal bones and the temporal bones. They cannot be felt because of the soft tissue covering them.

When two or more sutures meet, there is an irregular membranous area between them. This is called a *fontanelle*.

- The *anterior fontanelle* or *bregma* is a diamond-shaped space between the coronal and the sagittal sutures. This measures about 3 cm in the AP and transverse diameters and usually ossifies about 18 months after birth.
- The *posterior fontanelle* or *lambda* is a smaller triangle-shaped space that lies between the sagittal and the lambdoid sutures.
- The *temporal* or *casserian fontanelles* lie at the intersection of the lambdoid and the temporal sutures. They cannot be felt.

The position of the sutures and fontanelles plays a very important role in determining the position of the fetal head in labor.

The important diameters of the fetal head (Fig. 1.4) are as follows:

- *Biparietal* diameter (9.5 cm). The greatest transverse diameter of the head. It extends from one parietal eminence to the other.
- *Bitemporal* diameter (8.0 cm). The greatest distance between the two temporal sutures.
- *Bimastoid* diameter (7.5 cm). The distance between the tips of the mastoid processes. It is impossible to decrease this diameter by any obstetrical operation.
- *Suboccipitobregmatic* diameter (9.5 cm). The well-flexed vertex presents with this diameter, which extends from the middle of the bregma to the undersurface of the occipital bone where it joins the neck. The circumference of the fetal head at this plane is the smallest and measures 32 cm.
- *Suboccipitofrontal* diameter (10.5 cm). The partially flexed vertex presents with this diameter, which extends from a point just above the root of the nose to the undersurface of the occipital bone where it joins the neck.

- *Occipitofrontal* diameter (11.5 cm). A deflexed head presents with this diameter, which extends from a point just above the root of the nose to the most prominent point on the occipital bone. The circumference of the fetal head at this plane measures 34.5 cm.
- *Mentovertical* diameter (13.0 cm). A brow presentation: it has the largest AP diameter and extends from the chin to the most prominent point of the occiput.
- *Submentobregmatic* diameter (9.5 cm) A face presentation: it has a small diameter and extends from the chin to the middle of the bregma.

Molding of the head

With the descent of the head into the pelvis, the frontal bones slip under the parietal bones. In addition, one parietal bone can override the other and they in turn slip under the occipital bone, thereby reducing the head circumference. The degree of molding is assessed vaginally.

- Usually the suture lines are separate (molding 0).
- If the suture lines meet, the degree of molding is 1+.
- If they overlap but can be reduced with gentle digital pressure, the degree of molding is 2+.
- If the overlap is irreducible with gentle digital pressure, the degree of molding is 3+.

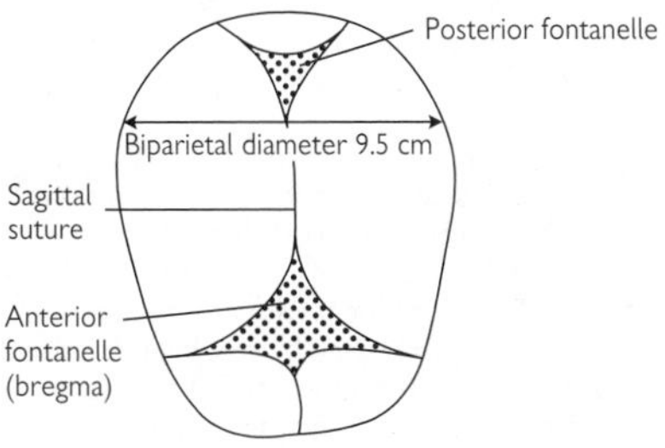

Fig. 1.3 Fontanelles, sagittal suture, and biparietal diameter. (Reproduced from *Oxford Handbook of Clinical Specialties*, 5th edn (ed. Collier J, Longmore M, Brown TD), p. 87. © 1999 by permission of the publisher, Oxford University Press.)

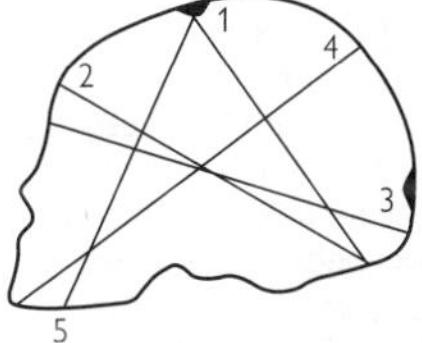

1 Suboccipitobregmatic 9.5 cm flexed vertex presentation
2 Suboccipitofrontal 10.5 cm partially deflexed vertex
3 Occipitofrontal 11.5 cm deflexed vertex
4 Mentovertical 13 cm brow
5 Submentobregmatic 9.5 cm face

Fig. 1.4 Different presenting diameters of the head. (Reproduced from *Oxford Handbook of Clinical Specialties*, 5th edn (ed. Collier J, Longmore M, Brown TD), p. 87. © 1999 by permission of the publisher, Oxford University Press.)

Placental development

The human placenta is discoid in shape, hemochorial, and deciduate. It is called hemochorial as the chorion is in direct contact with the maternal blood and deciduate as some of the maternal decidual tissue is shed at parturition. The placenta is attached to the uterine wall and is connected to the fetus via the umbilical cord. Placental tissue is fetal in origin, and the fact that maternal and fetal tissues come in direct contact with each other without rejection suggests some complex immunological mechanisms favoring acceptance of the fetus as a graft by the mother.

- Implantation occurs at the blastocyst stage. It usually starts at day 7 postconception and is completed on the 11th day. The inner cell mass within the blastocyst forms the embryo, yolk sac, and amniotic cavity, while the trophoblast will form the future placenta, chorion, and extraembryonic mesoderm.
- When the blastocyst embeds into the decidua, trophoblastic cells differentiate, and the syncytiotrophoblast and cytotrophoblast are defined. This is followed by the appearance of lacunar spaces in the syncytium. These cells advance into the surrounding tissues as early or primitive villi, each of which consists of cytotrophoblast surrounded by the syncytium. The lacunar spaces soon become filled with maternal blood.
- The villi subsequently mature to secondary and tertiary villi with the appearance of first the mesodermal core and then fetal blood vessels in the mesodermal core of the villi. This process is completed by day 21 postconception.
- At 16–17 days postconception, the surface of the blastocyst is covered by branching villi, which are best developed at the embryonic pole. The chorion here is known as chorionic frondosum and the future placenta is developed from this area.
- Simultaneously, lacunar spaces become confluent with one another and, by weeks 3–4, form a multilocular receptacle lined by syncytium and filled with maternal blood. This space becomes the future intervillous space.
- With the growth of the embryo, the decidua capsularis becomes thinner and both villi and the lacunar spaces in the decidua are obliterated, converting the chorion into chorionic laeve.
- The villi in the chorionic frondosum show exuberant division and subdivision and, with the accompanying proliferation of the decidua basalis, the future placenta is formed (Fig. 1.5). The process starts at 6 weeks and the definitive number of stem villi are established by 12 weeks' postconception.
- Thereafter, placental growth continues up to term and possibly beyond. Until the 16th week, the placenta grows in both thickness and circumference due to the growth of the chorionic villi with accompanying expansion of the intervillous space. Thereafter, growth occurs mainly circumferentially until term or beyond.

Stem villi and the placental barrier (Fig. 1.6)

Stem villi arise from the chorionic plate and extend to the basal plate. A major stem villus with its branching villi forms the fetal cotyledon or placentome. There are approximately 60 stem villi in the human placenta. Thus each cotyledon contains 3–4 major stem villi. The villi are the functional units of the placenta. Some of them anchor the placenta to the decidua, but the majority of them float freely in the intervillous space.

In the early placenta, the following structures are present, from outside inward:

- outer syncytiotrophoblast
- cytotrophoblast
- basement membrane
- stroma-containing mesenchymal cells and the endothelium and basement membrane of the fetal blood vessel.

This also constitutes the placental barrier (Fig. 1.6(b)). Despite close proximity, there is no mixing of the maternal and fetal blood. The barrier is about 0.025 mm thick. Near term, with the attenuation of the syncytial layer and sparse cytotrophoblast with marked distension of fetal capillaries, the placental membrane becomes thinner, down to 0.002 mm in places. However, all the constituent layers forming the placental membrane can be identified microscopically.

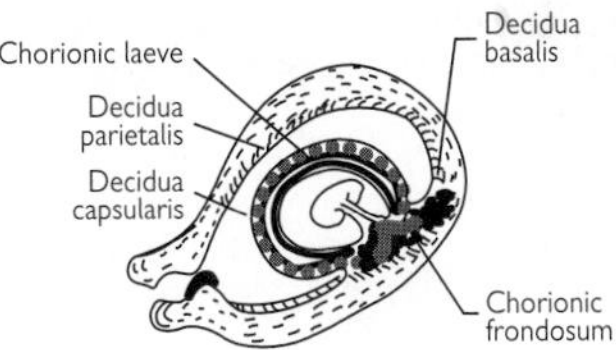

Fig. 1.5 Early development. Chorionic frondosum forms the future placenta.

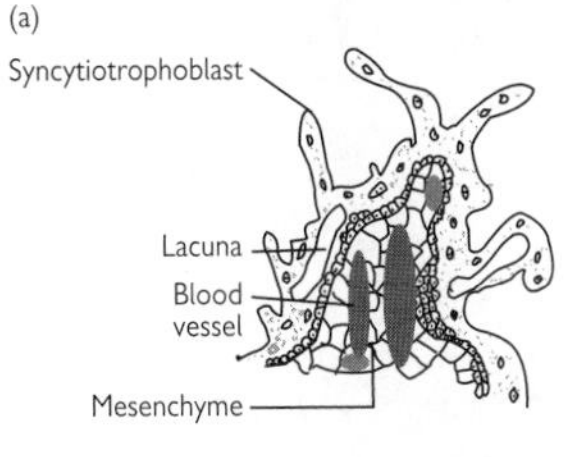

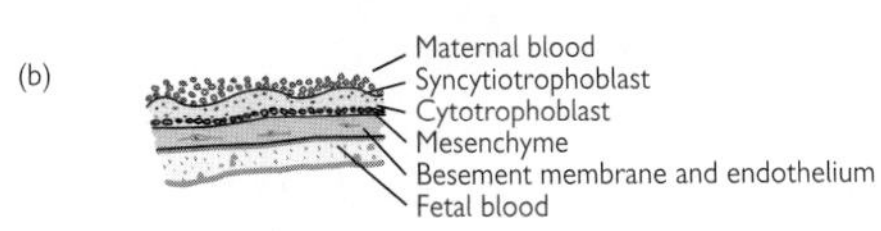

Fig. 1.6 (a) Structure of chorionic villi. (b) Simple line diagram showing cell layers of the placental barrier.

The placenta at term

The placenta at term is circular in shape and has a diameter of 15–20 cm. It is about 2.5 cm thick at the center and weighs approximately 500 g. The ratio of fetal to placental weight at term is about 6:1. Normally at term, the placenta occupies 30% of the uterine wall. It presents two surfaces:

- The *fetal surface* is covered by the smooth glistening amnion with the umbilical cord attached at or near to its center. The branches of umbilical blood vessels are visible beneath the amnion as they radiate from the insertion of the cord. The amnion can be peeled from the underlying chorion, except at the insertion of the cord.
- The *maternal surface* has a rough and spongy appearance. A shaggy layer may be visible on the maternal surface. This is the remnant of decidua basalis. The maternal surface is divided into several cotyledons (15–20) by septae arising from the maternal tissues. Each cotyledon may be supplied by its own spiral artery. Numerous small greyish spots may also be visible on the maternal surface. These are due to calcium deposition in the degenerated areas.

Placental circulation

The placental circulation consist of two distinctly different systems: the uteroplacental circulation and the fetoplacental circulation.

Uteroplacental circulation

This involves circulation of maternal blood through the intervillous space (Table 1.1). The intervillous blood flow at term is estimated to be 500–600 mL/minute and the blood in the intervillous space is replaced 3–4 times per minute. The pressure gradient between the fetal capillaries and the intervillous space favors placental transfer of oxygen and other nutrients to the fetus.

Arterial system

The spiral arteries respond to the increased demand of blood supply to the placental bed. They become more tortuous and less elastic by trophoblastic invasion. Trophoblastic invasion starts early in the pregnancy. It appears to occur in two stages:

- The decidual segments of the spiral arterioles are structurally modified during the first trimester.
- The second wave of trophoblastic invasion, occurring in the second trimester, begins to invade the inner third of the myometrium and the muscularis layer of the spiral arteries.

These morphological changes in the blood vessels create a low-pressure high-flow system in the placenta. The blood vessels become dilated, tortuous, and possibly less capable of responding to vasoactive amines. Failure of the second wave of trophoblastic invasion to remodel the myometrial segments of the spiral arteries of the placental bed (so-called shallow endovascular invasion) lays down the blueprint for the development of preeclampsia and intrauterine growth restriction in later pregnancy. See Chapter 2 📖 *p.68*

Venous system

Oxygenated blood from the spiral artery enters the intervillous space. Lateral dispersion occurs after the entering blood jet reaches the chorionic plate. Losing its original momentum, the blood then gradually flows towards the basal plate. This is facilitated by mild movement of the villi and uterine contractions. From the basal plate, deoxygenated blood drains into the uterine veins. Shunting of blood from the arterial circulation to the neighboring venous channel is prevented by the increased pressure of the endometrial spiral arteries driving the blood in jets towards the chorionic plate. Venous drainage only takes place during uterine relaxation and arterial flow is reduced during contraction. Spiral arteries are perpendicular and veins are parallel to the uterine wall. Therefore, larger volumes of blood are available for exchange at the intervillous space even though the rate of flow is decreased during contraction.

Fetoplacental circulation

The two umbilical arteries carry blood from the fetus to the placenta and enter the chorionic plate underneath the amnion. Each of them supplies half of the placenta. The arteries divide into small branches and enter the stem of the chorionic villi. Further division of vessels to arterioles and then to capillaries takes place within the villi. The blood then flows to the corresponding venous channel and subsequently to the umbilical vein. Maternal and fetal bloodstreams flow side by side in opposite directions. This countercurrent flow facilitates exchange between mother and fetus. The hemodynamics of the fetoplacental circulation are shown in Table 1.2.

Table 1.1 Hemodynamics of the uteroplacental circulation

Volume of blood in the intervillous space	150 mL
Blood flow in the intervillous space	500–600 mL/min
Pressure changes in the intervillous space	
Height of uterine contraction	30–50 mmHg
Uterine relaxation	10–15 mmHg
Pressure in the spiral artery	70–80 mmHg
Pressure in the uterine veins	8–10 mmHg

Table 1.2 Hemodynamics in the fetoplacental circulation

Fetal blood flow through the placenta	400 mL/min
Pressure	
In the umbilical artery	60–70 mmHg
In the umbilical vein	10 mmHg
Oxygen saturation	
In the umbilical artery	60%
In the umbilical vein	70–80%
Partial pressure of O_2	
In the umbilical artery	20–25 mmHg
In the umbilical vein	30–40 mmHg

Functions of the placenta

The placenta functions primarily as an organ responsible for the transfer of substances to and from the fetus. Far from acting as a simple filtering mechanism, it has many other important roles, some of which are not fully understood.

Placental transfer

The placenta acts as a relative barrier to most substances, but the speed of exchange and concentration of substance exchanged depends upon the concentration on each side of the placenta, the molecular size, lipid solubility, ionization, placental surface area, and maternofetal blood flow (Table 1.3). For example, a fast transfer to the fetus would be achieved by a low-molecular-weight lipid-soluble substance with a high concentration gradient across the placenta.

The placenta as a barrier

Infection

The placenta forms an effective barrier to the fetus against most maternal blood-borne bacterial infections. Other organisms such as syphilis, parvovirus, hepatitis B and C, rubella, human immunodeficiency virus (HIV), and cytomegalovirus (CMV) are able to infect the fetus during pregnancy.

Drugs

Almost all drugs administered to the pregnant woman can pass across the placenta into the fetus. They may have little effect on the fetus (e.g. acetaminophen) and be considered 'safe', but other drugs (e.g. warfarin and thalidomide) may significantly affect the development, structure, and function of the fetus—a process known as *teratogenesis*. Before giving any drug to a pregnant woman, it is the prescriber's obligation to ensure that it is considered safe for that stage of pregnancy.

The placenta as an endocrine organ

The placenta has been shown to be capable of producing most peptide and steroid hormones. The production of human chorionic gonadotropin (hCG), estrogens, and progesterone by the placenta is vital for the maintenance of pregnancy.

- hCG levels are detected from 6 days after fertilization and form the basis of modern pregnancy testing, being reliably measurable in urine and blood from at least 2 weeks post-fertilization. Concentrations of hCG reach a peak at 10–12 weeks' gestation and then plateau at a lower level for the remainder of the pregnancy.
- Progesterone and estrogen increase in concentration throughout pregnancy, with peaks reached prior to the onset of labor. Progesterone appears to antagonize uterine contractility, but the role of estrogen is unclear—possibly improving uterine blood flow, encouraging breast growth, and priming myometrial receptors to oxytocin.

- Human placental lactogen antagonizes the effects of insulin and enhances the passage of amino acids across the placenta. Prolactin concentrations also increase during pregnancy from both the placenta and pituitary, promoting breast development.

Table 1.3 Transfer mechanisms across the placenta for common anabolites and catabolites

Substance	Transfer mechanism	Direction of transfer
Oxygen	Simple diffusion	To fetus
Carbon dioxide	Simple diffusion	From fetus
Glucose	Simple and facilitated diffusion	To fetus
Amino acids	Facilitated diffusion	To fetus
Water	Simple diffusion	To and from fetus
Electrolytes	Counter-transport mechanisms	To and from fetus
Urea and creatinine	Simple diffusion	From fetus

Recommended further reading

1. Cross JC, Werb Z, Fisher SJ (1994). Implantation and the placenta: key pieces of the development puzzle. *Science* **266**, 1508–18.
2. Norwitz ER, Schust DJ, Fisher SJ (2001). Implantation and the survival of early pregnancy. *N Engl J Med* **345**, 1400–8.

Preparing for pregnancy

Introduction

Attention to reproductive health should start before conception, but expectations must be realistic. Not all poor obstetric outcomes can be anticipated or avoided. For general health education, a pre-pregnancy counselor needs to be informed, enthusiastic, dedicated, and skillful, but not necessarily medically qualified. Where specific risks and diseases are identified, specialists in those areas have to be involved as part of the multidisciplinary team required to provide adequate information for appropriate decision-making. The family physician is in an ideal position to identify obstetric risk preconception.

Couples preparing for pregnancy will probably need some time to develop a relationship by living together and to learn more about each other. On the other hand, once a woman is over 35 years old, her fertility starts to decline and by 40 years of age it drops very quickly. Age also carries with it an increased risk of chromosomal abnormalities in the baby—the most common abnormality being Down syndrome. Older mothers are also more likely to suffer from age-related illnesses, e.g. high blood pressure, diabetes mellitus, and uterine fibroids—all of which may affect the outcome of the pregnancy.

Preparing for pregnancy

Preparation for a baby should begin before conception because the development of the fetus begins from the third week after the last menstrual period (LMP). Any damaging effect, e.g. exposure to drugs, would have occurred even before the woman was aware that she was pregnant.

The intending mother should keep herself healthy by eating sensibly, as well as exercising moderately to improve her cardiovascular and muscular fitness in readiness for the challenging task of pregnancy and delivery. The best exercises are low-impact aerobics, swimming, brisk walking, and jogging.

Medication

Most drugs carry warnings about use in pregnancy. The pharmacist or a doctor should be consulted before using any over-the-counter drugs. Some conditions may not really need medication, e.g. tetracycline is sometimes used for the treatment of acne and long-term use may cause staining of baby's teeth and weakening of bones, even when tetracyclines were taken months before conception.

Relaxation and exercise

Relaxation is probably the most difficult and yet the most important guideline to follow whilst planning for pregnancy. The standard medical advice to men and women, almost regardless of age and complaint, is to exercise more since cardiorespiratory function will be improved, weight reduced, and blood pressure lowered. Exercise is associated with higher self-esteem and confidence. The intending mother should be encouraged to exercise.

Work

Some workplaces are more likely to present hazards for the pregnant woman, e.g. chemical factories, operating rooms, and X-ray departments. Health-care workers are at higher risk as they are exposed to anesthetic gases in the operating room and come into contact with toxic drugs, particularly those used in the treatment of cancer, ionizing agents in the diagnostic X-ray department, and infections such as hepatitis and AIDS. The intending mother must continually take precautions when coming into contact with these potential hazardous situations.

The computer terminal (video display unit or VDU) has been intensely scrutinized since the early 1980s when reports linked it to pregnancy problems. So far, however, no study has been able to prove a link between the low-level radiation emitted by VDUs and miscarriage.

Routine examination

- General examination including blood pressure, heart, and lungs.
- Family history of inherited disorders or congenital abnormalities.
- Routine urine examination for protein, sugar, and white blood cells.
- Blood tests for thalassemia, sickle cell disease, toxoplasmosis, and syphilis may be offered, if at risk.
- The presence or absence of immunity against hepatitis, rubella, and varicella should be ascertained and vaccination given preconception if not immune.
- HIV screening should be offered to all women attempting to conceive irrespective of the presence or absence of risk factors.
- Dental examination.

Recommended further reading

1. American Academy of Pediatrics and American College of Obstetricians and Gynecologists (1997). *Guidelines for Perinatal Care*. American Academy of Pediatrics and American College of Obstetricians and Gynecologists, Washington, DC.

Nutritional preparation for pregnancy

Women who are extremely underweight or obese are likely to have menstrual problems that may affect their fertility. These women are also more likely to have problems during pregnancy. Obesity is the most common nutritional disorder in the affluent industrialized world, with its attendant risks of gestational diabetes, hypertension, and monitoring/assessment difficulties for the mother during pregnancy, whereas malnutrition is a major life hazard for mother, fetus, and infant in the developing world. Malnutrition is a cause of anemia with its own attendant problems for the mother and with intrauterine growth restriction, a sequelae for the fetus.

Undernutrition in pregnant women of low socio-economic status is associated with the delivery of low-birthweight (less than 2500 g) infants. Therefore an improvement in nutritional status and maternal weight may have a positive effect on birth outcome.

- The intending mother should be made aware of the fact that a pregnant woman should consume an extra 350 kcal a day. This might comprise, for example:
  - two slices of whole wheat bread and butter/margarine
  - one carton (150 g/5 oz) yogurt
  - one apple.
- Food delicacies such as undercooked meats and eggs, patés, soft cheeses, shellfish and raw fish, and unpasteurized milk should be avoided as they are all potential sources of *Listeria monocytogenes. Listeriosis in pregnancy* is known to cause poor obstetric outcome with death of the fetus.
- Periconceptional multivitamin supplementation, including folic acid, has been shown to reduce the occurrence of neural tube defects (NTDs), not just for those at risk of recurrence but also for the first occurrence of NTD.
- Ingestion of preformed vitamin A in excess of 25 000–150 000 international units (IU) has been found to be associated with an increased incidence of fetal growth restriction and urinary tract abnormalities, but ingestion of vitamin A precursors (carotenoids), is not.
- Women with low serum zinc levels may be at increased risk of pre- and post-term labor and intrauterine growth restriction. Vegetarians should increase non-meat zinc sources such as leafy and root vegetables, whole grains, and nuts. Those who are able to take milk and dairy products will usually have an adequate zinc intake from their diet alone.
- Calcium metabolism may be adversely affected by smoking and alcohol consumption, and these should be avoided. Supplementation of calcium may be necessary if intake of calcium is low, but the ideal is increased calcium from dietary sources.
- Routine iron supplementation may not be necessary for all pregnant mothers. Iron should be prescribed only when medically indicated. In areas where the incidence of iron deficiency anemia is high, however, iron supplementation should be considered as a routine.

- Iodine deficiency is endemic in some parts of the world, resulting in neonatal hypothyroidism (cretinism). Where iodized salt is not available, iodized oil should be used. The maximum benefit will be achieved when iodized oil is given before conception.

Alcohol

Regular drinking of small amounts of alcohol has not been shown to be harmful, but excessive alcohol intake has been shown conclusively to be a cause of fetal malformations (fetal alcohol syndrome). The exact threshold of alcohol that will cause malformation in the fetus has not been established. For this reason, pregnant women should be told that there is no safe level of alcohol during pregnancy and should be encouraged to avoid alcohol whenever possible.

Recommended further reading

1. American Academy of Pediatrics and American College of Obstetricians and Gynecologists (1997). *Guidelines for Perinatal Care*. American Academy of Pediatrics and American College of Obstetricians and Gynecologists, Washington, DC.
2. Lumley J, Watson L, Watson M, Bower C (2001). Periconceptional supplementation with folate and/or multivitamins for preventing neural tube defects. *Cochrane Database Syst Rev* **3**, CD001056.
3. Reece EA, Eriksson UJ (1996). The pathogenesis of diabetes-associated congenital malformations. *Obstet Gynecol Clin North Am* **23**, 29–45.

Exacerbation of illness during pregnancy

Pre-existing illnesses may be made worse by pregnancy. The pregnancy effect may be transient and the condition may return to the pre-pregnancy state after the delivery, e.g. diabetes mellitus. Unfortunately, the deterioration may sometimes be permanent and progressive, and may result in permanent disability or death (e.g. severe kidney impairment). Where the risk is high, the intending mother may be advised not to attempt pregnancy at all. The advice of a specialist should be sought in cases of severe chronic illnesses, e.g. chronic renal failure and severe cardiac disease.

Pregnancy undertaken when the illness is in remission, stable, or cured will ensure a better outcome. For instance, good control of diabetes around the time of conception will minimize risks of miscarriage and congenital malformations in the baby.

Avoidance of pregnancy

Women should be advised about an effective method of contraception if they are not ready for parenthood or have just been given a vaccination. It is advisable to wait at least a month after immunization with rubella before attempting to conceive.

Hormonal and hemodynamic changes in pregnancy

Physiological changes occur in pregnancy to provide a suitable environment for the nutrition, growth, and development of the fetus and to prepare the mother for the process of parturition and subsequent support for the newborn infant.

Hormonal changes

- Progesterone is synthesized by the corpus luteum until 35 days postconception and mainly by the placenta thereafter. It decreases smooth muscle excitability (gut, ureters, uterus) and raises body temperature.
- Estrogens, mainly estradiol (90%), increase breast and nipple growth and pigmentation of the areola. With the progress of pregnancy, they make the uterus more sensitive to oxytocin by making uterine muscles more active and excitable by increasing the frequency of action potential of individual fibers. They also increase water retention and protein synthesis.
- Human somatomammotropin, also called chorionic growth hormone or human placental lactogen (hPL), is lactogenic and has some growth stimulating activity. It promotes growth and insulin secretion, but decreases insulin's peripheral effect, liberating maternal fatty acids (hence sparing maternal glucose use). These actions divert glucose to the fetus. It also stimulates mammary growth and maternal casein, lactalbumin, and lactoglobulin production.
- The maternal thyroid enlarges in 70% of pregnant women because of increased colloid production. Increased urinary excretion of iodine leads to a relative plasma iodide deficiency. The thyroid gland responds by tripling its iodide uptake from the blood—hence the hypertrophy. Thyroid-binding globulin (TBG) is doubled by the end of the first trimester. As a result total T_3 (triiodothyronine) and T_4 (thyroxine) rise early in pregnancy and then fall to remain within the normal non-pregnant range. Thyroid-stimulating hormone (TSH) may decrease slightly in early pregnancy, but tends to remain within the normal range. T_3 and T_4 do not cross the placental barrier and therefore there is no relationship between maternal and fetal thyroid function. However, iodine, anti-thyroid drugs, and long-acting thyroid stimulator (LATS) do cross the placenta.
- The pituitary gland enlarges in normal pregnancy mainly because of changes in the anterior lobe. Prolactin levels increase substantially probably because of estrogen stimulation of the lactotrophes. Gonadotrophin secretion is inhibited, whilst plasma adrenocorticotrophic hormone (ACTH) levels increase. Maternal plasma cortisone output increases but the unbound levels remain constant. The posterior pituitary releases oxytocin principally during the third stage of labor and during suckling.

Hemodynamic changes

The average weight gain for a nullipara throughout the whole pregnancy is 12.5 kg (27.5 lb) and is probably 0.9 kg (2 lb) less for multiparas. From 10 weeks, the plasma volume rises until 32 weeks when it is about 3.8 liters (L) (about 50% increase from nonpregnant state). Acute excessive weight gain is commonly associated with abnormal fluid retention. Failure to gain weight and sometimes slight weight loss may occur during the last 2 weeks of pregnancy.

- Red cell volume (sometimes called red cell mass) rises from 1.4 L in the nonpregnant state to 1.64 L at term if iron supplements are not taken (an increase of 18%). An increase of 30% has been reported with iron and folate supplements. The discrepancy between the rate of increase of plasma volume and that of red cell mass results in a decline in hemoglobin concentration, hematocrit, and red cell count during pregnancy and, in particular, in the second trimester, leading to 'physiological anemia'. Mean corpuscular hemoglobin concentration remains constant.
- Total white cell count rises during pregnancy, mainly because of the increase in neutrophil polymorphonuclear leukocytes, which reaches its peak at 32 weeks. A further massive neutrophilia occurs during labor. Eosinophils, basophils, and monocytes remain relatively constant during pregnancy, but there is a profound fall in eosinophils during labor and they are virtually absent at delivery. Although the lymphocyte count and the number of B and T cells remain constant, lymphocyte function and cell-mediated immunity are profoundly depressed by an as yet unidentified factor in maternal serum, giving rise to a lowered resistance to viral infection.
- Platelets, erythrocyte sedimentation rate (ESR) (up to fourfold), cholesterol, and fibrinogen are also raised.
- Albumin and gamma-globulin levels fall because of the dilution effect caused by the increase in plasma volume.

Cardiovascular and renal changes in pregnancy

Cardiovascular changes

Major cardiovascular changes occur in pregnancy, with the most significant taking place within the first 12 weeks.

- Cardiac output rises from 5 to 6.5 L/min by increasing stroke volume (10%) and pulse rate (by about 15 beats/min). During labor, contractions may increase cardiac output by 2 L/min probably due to injection of blood from the distended intervillous space. Pregnancy generally proceeds normally even when the mother has an artificial cardiac pacemaker—compensation occurs mainly from increased stroke volume.
- Secondary to hormonal changes, peripheral vascular resistance falls. Blood pressure (BP), particularly diastolic, falls during the first and second trimesters by 10–20 mmHg, rising to non-pregnant levels by term. The fall of peripheral vascular resistance to nearly 50% of the nonpregnant values is probably due to production of vasodilator prostaglandins and progesterone. The balance between vasodilator and vasoconstrictor factors regulating peripheral resistance may be the basis of blood pressure regulation in pregnancy and the development of pregnancy-induced hypertension. Vasodilatation and hypotension also stimulate renin-angiotensin release, which also plays a part in blood pressure regulation in pregnancy.
- The supine hypotension syndrome is due to compression of the inferior vena cava leading to reduced venous return and hence reduced cardiac output. Aortic compression may result in a conspicuous difference between brachial and femoral blood pressures, giving a pressure difference of 10–15% from the supine to the lateral position. This is rarely seen before 20 weeks of pregnancy.
- Progressive enlargement of the uterus results in upward displacement of the heart and the diaphragm.
- The heart enlarges during pregnancy by 70–80 mL in volume as a result of increased diastolic filling and concentric muscle hypertrophy.

Respiratory system changes

In pregnancy, the level of the diaphragm rises and the intercostal angle increases from 68° in early pregnancy to 103° in late pregnancy. Therefore breathing tends to be more diaphragmatic than intercostal.

- Tidal volume rises from 500 to 700 mL (increase of 40%); the increased depth of breathing is a progesterone effect. Inspiratory capacity (tidal volume plus inspiratory reserve volume) increases in late pregnancy.
- The respiratory rate changes slightly during pregnancy. Breathlessness is common as maternal pCO_2 (partial pressure of carbon dioxide) is set lower to allow the fetus to offload CO_2.

Renal function changes

Renal size increases by about 1 cm in length during pregnancy. There is a marked dilatation of the calyces and renal pelvis and of the ureters.

These changes appear in the first trimester and therefore are unlikely to be due to back pressure. Vesicoureteric reflux occurs sporadically. These changes are associated with a high incidence of urinary stasis and increased tendency to urinary tract infection (UTI).

- The bladder muscle relaxes, but residual urine after micturition is not normally present.
- Renal blood flow increases by 30–50% in the first trimester and remains elevated throughout pregnancy. Effective renal plasma flow and glomerular filtration rate (GFR) increase. Creatinine and urea production remain the same and therefore plasma levels fall during pregnancy. Uric acid clearance increases from 12 to 20 mmol/mL with a consequent reduction in plasma uric acid levels. With progression of pregnancy, the filtered load of uric acid increases while excretion remains constant, and therefore plasma levels return to nonpregnant values.
- The increased GFR plays an important role in the variable glycosuria and urinary frequency that occur in pregnancy.

Further physiological changes during pregnancy

Changes in the uterus

The nonpregnant uterus weighs 100 g. It undergoes a 10-fold increase in weight to weigh 1000 g at term. Muscle hypertrophy occurs up to 20 weeks with stretching after that.

- The uterus is divided functionally and morphologically into three sections: the cervix, the isthmus (later to develop into the lower uterine segment, becoming more clearly defined from 18 weeks), and the main body of the uterus (corpus uteri).
- Reduction in cervical collagen later in pregnancy enables its effacement and dilatation. Hypertrophy of cervical glands leads to the production of profuse cervical mucus and the formation of a thick mucous plug or operculum that acts as a barrier to infection.
- Vaginal discharge increases due to cervical ectopy and cell desquamation.
- The uterine body increases in size, shape, position, and consistency. The uterine cavity expands from 4 to 4000 mL.
- Uterine blood flow has been shown to increase from approximately 50 mL/min at 10 weeks' gestation to 500–700 mL/min at term. The vessels that supply the uterus, the uterine and ovarian arteries, and branches of the superior vesical arteries undergo massive hypertrophy.

Changes in the vagina

In pregnancy, the rich venous vascular network in the connective tissue surrounds the vaginal walls with blood and gives rise to the slightly bluish appearance of the vagina.

- High estrogen levels stimulate glycogen synthesis and deposition, and the action of lactobacilli on glycogen in vaginal cells produces lactic acid, which in turn lowers the vaginal pH to keep the vagina relatively free from any bacterial pathogens.

Changes in the alimentary system

Decreased esophageal sphincteric tone is responsible for the reflux esophagitis (heartburn) that occurs in pregnancy. An additional factor may be displacement of the esophageal sphincter through the diaphragm because of increased abdominal pressure.

- Gastric mobility is low and gastric secretion is reduced resulting in delayed gastric emptying. Gut motility is generally reduced resulting in constipation.

Skin changes

Pigmentations in the linear nigra, nipple, and areola, or as chloasma (brown patches of pigmentation seen especially on the face), are seen in pregnancy.

- Palmar erythema, spider nevi, and striae are also common. These changes vary in different women and in different populations. They represent the effect of disruption of collagen fibers in the subcuticular zone. They are probably related to the effect of increased production of adrenocortical hormones in pregnancy as well as to the actual stress in the skin folds associated with expansion of the abdomen.

Diagnosis and dating of pregnancy

The most common presenting symptom of pregnancy is cessation of periods (i.e. a period of amenorrhea) in a woman having regular menstruation. Other common symptoms of early pregnancy are as follows:

- *Nausea and vomiting* (morning sickness). This is common in the first 3 months of pregnancy. Thereafter it tends to disappear, although it may sometimes persist throughout pregnancy.
- *Frequency of micturition.* This is probably due to increased plasma volume and urine production and the pressure effect of the uterus on the bladder.
- Many women experience excessive lassitude in early pregnancy. This tends to disappear after 12 weeks' gestation.
- *Breast tenderness* and 'heaviness' are common and are particularly noticeable in the month after the first period is missed.
- *Fetal movements* or quickening are not usually noticed until 20 weeks' gestation in the nullipara and 18 weeks in the multipara. However, many women may experience fetal movements earlier than this and some may not be aware of them until term.
- *Pica.* An abnormal desire for a particular food may occur.

Clinical examination

The vagina and cervix have a bluish tinge because of blood congestion. Estimation of uterine size by vaginal examination is reasonably accurate in early pregnancy compared with later than 12 weeks' gestation.

Pregnancy test

The hormone β-hCG is secreted by the trophoblastic tissue or placenta. This increases in pregnancy and peaks at 10–12 weeks. The levels of this hormone can be measured by blood or urine. Test kits are available commercially to carry out the pregnancy test. Monoclonal antibodies have been raised against β-hCG and tagged with latex or red cells to carry out agglutination tests. The commercial kits can show a positive reaction with color change when the urinary hCG levels are >50 IU/L or with some kits >25 IU/L. The woman would be able to know about her pregnancy within 1 week of missing her period using this test.

Dating of pregnancy

Menstrual history

It is important to ascertain the date of the first day of the last menstrual period. This information may not be accurate because many women do not record the day on which they menstruate. In special circumstances such as *in vitro* fertilization (IVF) pregnancies, dating can be accurate as a record is always made of the day of embryo transfer. Gestational age is calculated from the first day of the last period. The length of the menstrual cycle is important. Ovulation usually occurs on the 14th day before the first day of the subsequent menstruation, but the duration of the proliferative phase may vary considerably.

- The length of the cycle, i.e. the interval from the first day of the period to the first day of the subsequent period, may vary from 21 to 42 days in normal women, although menstruation usually occurs every 28 days in most women.
- It is also important to ascertain the method of contraception employed prior to conception.
- The estimated date of delivery (EDD) can be calculated from the first day of the last period, especially if the cycle is 28 days. This can be obtained from Naegele's formula: add 1 year and 7 days and subtract 3 months from the date of the last menstrual period (LMP). Adjustments have to be made for long cycle lengths. This assumes a pregnancy duration of 40 weeks (280 days) with conception occurring 2 weeks after the first day of the last menstrual period. For example, if LMP = 7.9.02, EDD = LMP + 9 months + 7 days = 14.6.03. About 40% of women will deliver within 5 days of the estimated date of delivery and about two-thirds within 10 days.

Recommended further reading

1. American Academy of Pediatrics and American College of Obstetricians and Gynecologists (1997). *Guidelines for Perinatal Care*. American Academy of Pediatrics and American College of Obstetricians and Gynecologists, Washington, DC.
2. American College of Obstetricians and Gynecologists (2003). Clinical management guidelines for obstetrician-gynecologists. ACOG Practice Bulletin No. 44. *Obstet Gynecol* **102**, 203–13.
3. American College of Obstetricians and Gynecologists (2004). ACOG Committee Opinion No. 299. Guidelines for diagnostic imaging during pregnancy. *Obstet Gynecol*, **104**, 647–51.

Ultrasound verification of dates

- *Gestational sac.* The visualization of an intrauterine sac provides the first evidence of an intrauterine pregnancy. Vaginal ultrasonography can detect a gestation sac as early as 4 weeks from the last menstrual period.
- *Crown–rump length* (CRL). This is most useful in the first trimester. It measures a straight line from one fetal pole to the other along its longitudinal axis. Fetal flexion renders this of less value in the second trimester.
- *Biparietal diameter* (BPD). This measurement is useful from 14 weeks onwards. The ultrasound probe images the fetus longitudinally and then it is rotated 90° to obtain the transverse plane through the fetal head. Specific structures such as the thalami, septum cavum pellucidum, and the lateral ventricles with their anterior and posterior horns should be identified to make measurements valid. The BPD is measured between the leading edge of the echoes from the proximal and distal skull bones.
- *Head circumference* (HC) (Fig. 1.7). The measurements are made from the same section as for BPD. Electronic calipers measure the circumference around the head. The transcerebellar diameter in millimeters gives the gestational age in weeks.
- *Abdominal circumference* (AC) (Fig. 1.8). Abdominal circumference is a sensitive indicator of fetal growth. It is measured at a level where the image of the stomach and intrahepatic portion of the umbilical vein is seen.
- *Femur length* (FL) (Fig. 1.9). The fetal thigh is identified and the femur measured in the plane where the buttocks and the knee are included in the view. The femur image should be parallel to the transducer. FL can be underestimated if the correct plane is not obtained.

BPD and FL give assessment of gestational age. If this differs from the menstrual date by more than 1 week in the first trimester or 2 weeks in the second trimester, the ultrasound measurement should be accepted as the gestational age and the date of delivery should be adjusted accordingly.

Charts of measurements and nomograms are available for different population groups and should be used to obtain the best results (Fig. 1.10). Computer programs are typically incorporated into ultrasound machines to provide the gestation once a measurement is made.

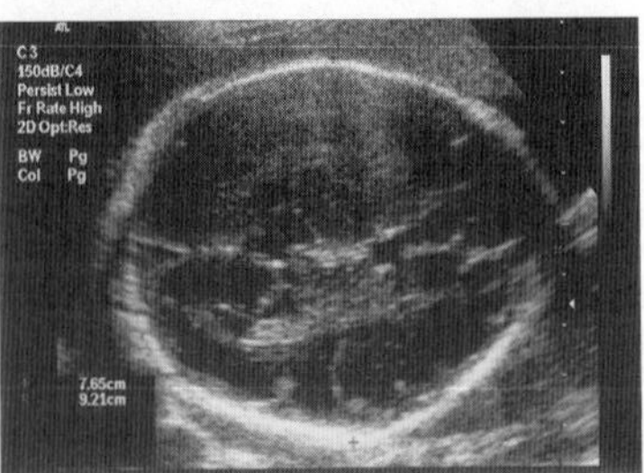

Fig. 1.7 Ultrasound measurement of the head circumference (HC).

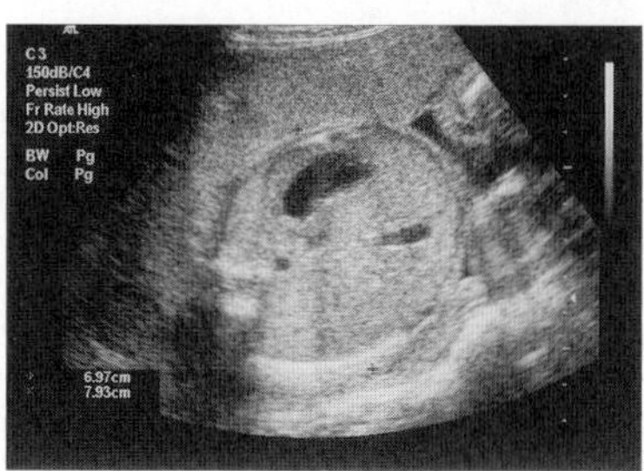

Fig. 1.8 Ultrasound measurement of abdominal circumference (AC).

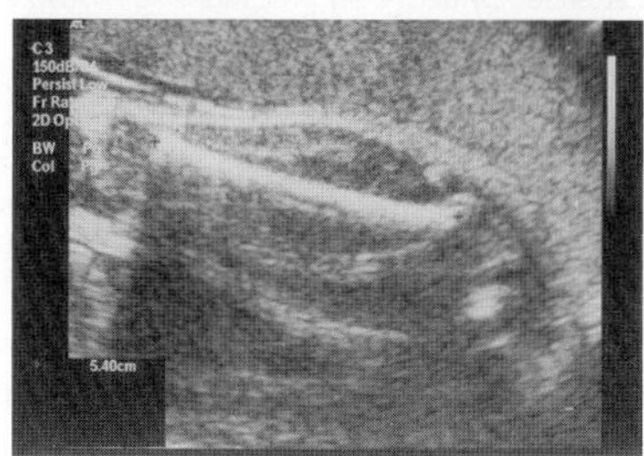

Fig. 1.9 Ultrasound measurement of femur length (FL).

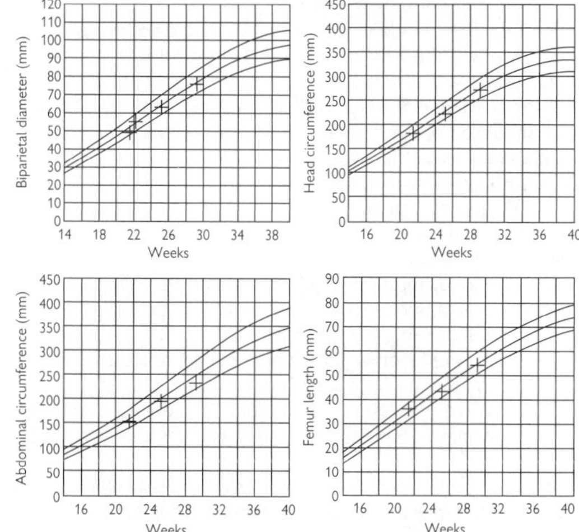

Fig. 1.10 Charts showing nomograms of various indices measured by ultrasound.

Booking visit

The purpose of the booking visit is to assess the mother and make a plan for her care in pregnancy. This should include a delivery plan. Increasingly, 'low-risk' women are cared for by their community midwives with medical staff involvement only if complications occur. However, certain risk factors make specialist visits necessary.

Only 1% of women deliver at home with a 5% chance of adverse maternal and fetal outcome even in low-risk pregnancy. As such, planned home births are not generally recommended. The birthing room concept probably is a good compromise as it offers a homely birth with congenial surroundings with labor ward facilities nearby if needed. In this case, the mother can be attended by her family practitioner or midwife in a hospital setting in a home environment.

Booking should normally be in the first trimester in order to take full advantage of antenatal care, but many women are seen for the first time in the second trimester. Children born to women who are late registrants for care, and especially to unregistered women, run the risk of higher perinatal mortality (4–5-fold) and morbidity with an attendant increase in maternal morbidity and mortality.

History

A comprehensive history should include the following headings: personal history, family history, and previous obstetric and medical/surgical history along with the history of the present pregnancy to the time of that visit.

- High-risk markers from past obstetric performance or from medical, surgical, and family history should be highlighted.
- An effort should be made to obtain past obstetric notes from institutions where the woman delivered before if it is thought that this information will change the course of management.
- History of inheritable diseases in close relatives of the woman and her partner should be sought as well as the history of migration and intercontinental travel. This may help to identify risk groups for diseases such as hemoglobinopathies, some forms of hepatitis, and HIV infection. With particular reference to HIV infection, intravenous (IV) drug injection and any high-risk sexual practices of the woman or her partner(s) are important.
- Histories of alcohol abuse, smoking, and/or addictive drug use are useful behavioral markers of other potential risks (e.g. fetal abnormalities, impaired growth, preterm labor).
- Early identification of women at risk of postnatal depressive illness or self-harm is important. Therefore history should be taken of maternal psychiatric disorder, severe social problems, and previous self-harm. Patients at risk should have appropriate psychiatric care and social support.
- Advice and support should be given on healthy lifestyles, including diet and exercise. Women should be told about the correct use of seat belts during pregnancy.

- Women should be made aware of symptoms and consequences associated with antepartum hemorrhage, preeclampsia, preterm labor, and premature rupture of membranes.

Examination

A complete physical examination of the pregnant woman must be undertaken. This should include the following:

- Height (very small stature may indicate a small pelvis), weight, and blood pressure in the sitting position to avoid compression of the inferior vena cava.
- Inspection of the mucosal surfaces (mouth, conjunctiva) for pallor and the general state of dentition (caries should be treated and appropriate advice given on dental hygiene).
- The thyroid gland tends to enlarge slightly in pregnancy but any abnormal enlargement, especially if associated with tachycardia and/or thyrotoxic symptoms or signs, should be investigated.
- The heart should be examined to exclude organic murmurs and, if needed, appropriate referral to the cardiologist should be made. Flow murmurs and mammary souffles are common in pregnancy. When in doubt, refer.
- The breasts are examined to exclude the presence of any masses, noting also the condition of the nipples.
- The limbs are examined for varicose veins and the presence of any shortening, and the vertebral column is examined for skeletal abnormalities such as kyphosis or lordosis.

Pelvic examination

This is not routinely done in many centers. It is argued that ultrasound gives more accurate information about the pregnancy and more certain detection of adnexal masses. However, it does not provide information on the state of the vagina or appearance of the cervix. Therefore it would be advisable to do a pelvic examination including a speculum examination if the patient has never been examined, has not had a recent Pap smear, or in cases of unusual vaginal discharge or bleeding.

If the woman has become pregnant with an intrauterine contraceptive device (IUCD) *in situ* (which is rare), it is best to remove the IUCD if the threads are visible. Retention of the device may lead to infection and abortion.

Recommended further reading

1. American Academy of Pediatrics and American College of Obstetricians and Gynecologists (1997). *Guidelines for Perinatal Care*. American Academy of Pediatrics and American College of Obstetricians and Gynecologists, Washington, DC.
2. American College of Obstetricians and Gynecologists (2003). *Clinical management guidelines for obstetrician-gynecologists*. ACOG Practice Bulletin No. 44. *Obstet Gynecol* **102**, 203–13.

Inspection, palpation, and presentation

The routine of inspection, palpation, percussion (although rarely employed, it may be useful in cases of polyhydramnios), and auscultation is used to examine the abdomen in pregnancy.

Inspection

Describe the enlarged abdomen giving suggestions as to the approximate gestational age. Describe signs of pregnancy such as linea nigra, striae gravidarum, and the presence of fetal movements. Note any superficial distended veins or scars: Pfannenstiel scars (i.e. transverse low abdominal scars usually used for cesarean deliveries) and laparoscopy, appendectomy, and cholecystectomy scars.

Fundal height measurements

The use of measurement of the fundal height from the top of the symphysis pubis to the fundus of the uterus (highest part of the uterus) is more objective than eyeballing. Measure this in centimeters. The mean fundal–symphyseal height measures approximately 20 cm at 20 weeks' gestation (up to the umbilicus) and increases to approximately 36 cm by 36 weeks' gestation (a centimeter per week roughly). Thereafter, the distance tends to plateau until term. Two centimeters either way of the gestation is acceptable up to 35 weeks, which becomes ± 3 cm at 36 weeks and ± 4 cm at 40 weeks because of such factors as increase in size of the baby, reduction of amniotic fluid volume, and engagement of the head.

- Using this technique, approximately 40–60% of all small-for-dates babies can be detected. The accuracy is considerably less if the measurement is made after 36 weeks' gestation.

The predictive value of this method is less for large-for-dates infants. Pregnancy factors such as large baby, polyhydramnios, twins, and uterine factors such as fibroids and pelvic tumors lead to fundal height greater than dates.

Oligohydramnios, leakage of amniotic fluid, intrauterine growth restriction (IUGR), presenting part deep in the pelvis, and abnormal lies may give rise to a uterus smaller than dates. The clinical diagnosis of uterus larger or smaller than dates needs to be investigated further by ultrasound examination.

Palpation for fetal parts

Fetal parts are not usually palpable before 24 weeks' gestation. The purpose of palpation is to describe the relationship of the fetus to the maternal trunk and pelvis.

- The lie describes the relationship of the long axis of the fetus to the long axis of the uterus. Palpate along the anterolateral sides of the abdomen and towards the midline to reveal either the firm resistance of the fetal back or the irregular projection of the fetal limbs.
  - The lie is longitudinal if the head or breech is palpable over the pelvic inlet.

    - The lie is oblique if the head or breech is in the iliac fossa.
    - The lie is transverse if the fetus lies at right angles to the uterine longitudinal axis and the poles of the fetus are palpable in the flanks.
- Feel for the head or breech by firm pressure with both hands, starting in the lower pole of the uterus as it is likely to be cephalic or breech in 96% of cases at term. The head is round, hard, and discrete. It can be 'bounced' or balloted between the examining hands. The buttocks are softer, more diffuse, and broad, and the breech is not ballotable.

Presentation

Presentation is the part of the fetus nearest to the pelvic inlet or in the lower uterine segment. Palpate with both hands over the lower uterine pole for presentation and degree of engagement. Pawlik's grip (examining the lower pole of the uterus between the thumb and the index finger of the right hand) can also be used to assess the engagement of the head. The presenting part may be the head (cephalic) or the breech (podalic) in a longitudinal lie.

Recommended further reading

1. American Academy of Pediatrics and American College of Obstetricians and Gynecologists (1997). *Guidelines for Perinatal Care*. American Academy of Pediatrics and American College of Obstetricians and Gynecologists, Washington, DC.

Engagement and fetal position

Engagement

This refers to the passage of maximal diameter of the presenting part beyond the pelvic inlet. The level of the head is assessed as engaged or in terms of the number of 'fifths' palpable abdominally above the pelvic brim (Fig. 1.11).

When the head is 'engaged', only two-fifths of the head can be felt abdominally. Conventionally, the palm width of the five fingers of the hand is used for this estimation. If five fingers are needed to cover the head above the pelvic brim, it is five-fifths palpable and, if no head is palpable, it is zero-fifths. Palpation of the occiput (most prominent lateral part of the head on the same side of the fetal back) and the sinciput or forehead (most lateral part on the opposite side of the occiput) gives the degree of flexion ('attitude') of the fetal head.

The baby normally engages in an attitude of flexion in the transverse diameter of the pelvic inlet, unless the pelvis is very roomy where it could engage in any diameter. Being able to palpate the sinciput and not the occiput (which is always ahead of the sinciput in a well-flexed head) suggests engagement. On palpating the head, if it is two-fifths palpable and the hands are diverging on palpating the lateral border of the head it is engaged.

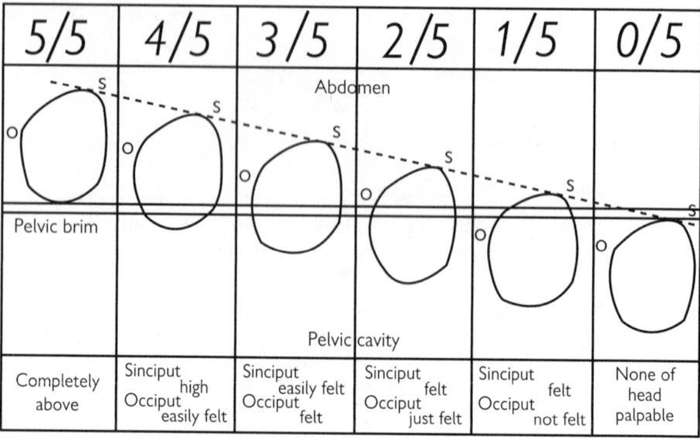

Fig. 1.11 Clinical estimation of descent of head.

In a nullipara, the head usually enters the pelvis by 36–37 weeks. However, nonengagement is not that uncommon at this gestation. Rare causes of nonengagement must be excluded, especially if the head is high (e.g. placenta previa or fetal abnormality). In multiparous women, the head may not engage until the onset of labor. Because of the exaggerated lumbar lordosis in the Black population, engagement in this population even in a primigravida may take place at the onset or during the course of labor.

Position

This describes the relationship of the denominator of the presenting part to fixed points on the maternal pelvis. These points are sacral promontory (posterior), symphysis pubis (anterior), sacroiliac joint (posterior lateral and may be right or left), and iliopectineal eminence (anterolateral and may be right or left). If the sagittal suture is lying in the transverse axis of the pelvis, then the denominator is in the right or left lateral position. The denominator is the most definable peripheral prominence in the presenting part. In a vertex presentation, it is the occiput. In face presentation, it is the chin (mentum), and in breech it is the sacrum.

Finally, note the amount of amniotic fluid present. Fetal parts are more easily palpable when the amniotic fluid is reduced (oligohydramnios) and are hardly palpable when the amniotic fluid is excessive (polyhydramnios). If there is clinical suspicion of polyhydramnios (shiny abdomen on inspection, tense to touch, fundal height greater than expected for period of gestation, and difficulty in feeling fetal parts), a fluid thrill should be demonstrated. Women can help by pressing the ulnar border of their hand on the midline of the abdomen along the linea nigra to avoid feeling the surface vibrations, whilst the fluid thrill is illustrated by the clinician.

Auscultation

The fetal heart may be heard by Doppler ultrasound from about 12 weeks' gestation and with a fetal (Pinard) stethoscope from about 24 weeks.

- The Doppler ultrasound or stethoscope is placed over the anterior shoulder detected by palpation. It can also be heard over the chest in the midline when the fetus is in the occipito-posterior position.
- With a cephalic presentation, when the vertex is in the occipito-anterior position, the fetal heart is best heard at the midpoint between the maternal umbilicus and the anterior superior iliac spine, where the fetal anterior shoulder could be palpated.
- In a breech presentation, the fetal heart is heard over the back of the baby and is at or above the level of the umbilicus of the mother.

The rate and rhythm of the fetal heartbeat should be noted.

Recommended further reading

1. American Academy of Pediatrics and American College of Obstetricians and Gynecologists (1997). *Guidelines for Perinatal Care*. American Academy of Pediatrics and American College of Obstetricians and Gynecologists, Washington, DC.

Plan for antenatal care

The aims of antenatal care can be defined as follows:

- Provision of education, reassurance, and support to the woman and her partner and family.
- Advice on minor problems and symptoms of pregnancy.
- Assessment of maternal and fetal risk factors at onset of pregnancy and as they develop throughout pregnancy.
- Provision of prenatal screening and management of abnormalities detected.
- Determination of timing and mode of delivery where complications arise.

Effective antenatal care needs to focus on what should be achieved at each key stage of the pregnancy rather than on the regularity of visits. Antenatal care needs to be provided as part of a broadly agreed and implemented program, but 'fine-tuned' to the individual requirements of the mother and fetus as assessed at booking and as these requirements evolve during the course of the pregnancy. The current emphasis is on provision of as much of the antenatal care as possible in the community and primary care team setting, and this is partly in response to what the patients would prefer themselves.

Preconception

In an ideal world, antenatal care would commence at the preconception stage where health education (general advice about nutrition, lifestyle, avoidance of teratogens, folic acid supplementation, etc.) and risk assessment can be focused towards a planned pregnancy. Preconception counseling is of much greater importance where there are underlying medical conditions (such as diabetes) which may be affected by or influence the outcome of a pregnancy.

First trimester

Antenatal care in the first trimester starts with a visit after a missed period and confirmation of pregnancy. The purpose of this initial visit is to obtain a comprehensive history, establish gestational age, and identify any maternal or fetal risk factors. It also provides an ideal opportunity for the woman to discuss any anxieties she may have.

- During this visit routine blood tests are performed: complete blood count (CBC); blood grouping and antibody screen; rubella, syphilis, hepatitis B, and HIV serology; and hemoglobin electrophoresis if appropriate. Urine is tested for glucose and protein, and a midstream specimen is sent for culture and sensitivity to detect asymptomatic bacteriuria.
- The hospital booking visit may be any time between 12 and 20 weeks of gestation, but there is an increasing tendency for earlier referral, especially in older women who may wish to have screening tests for chromosomal abnormalities in the first trimester.
- Many institutions now offer a first trimester ultrasound scan for pregnancy dating and measurement of nuchal translucency at the 11–14 week stage. Nuchal translucency measurements may be combined with measurements of serum markers such as free β-hCG

and PAPP-A (pregnancy-associated plasma protein A) as a sensitive screening test for trisomy 21. Prenatal diagnostic testing, such as chorionic villus sampling (CVS) may be performed toward the end of the first trimester (10–14 weeks) in selected groups of patients.

Second trimester

Early in the second trimester, at around 15 to 20 weeks, serum screening tests are performed for assessment of risk of open neural tube defect and Down syndrome. Prenatal diagnostic testing in the form of amniocentesis may be performed at around 16–18 weeks and a detailed ultrasound scan to assess fetal anatomy is usually performed at the 18–20 week stage by which time the results of serum screening should have been available and reviewed. Where fetal cardiac anomalies are suspected, a further ultrasound scan (fetal echocardiogram) may be required at the 20–22 week stage. After this stage of pregnancy, the patient is seen at 4-weekly intervals, and at each visit BP, urinalysis, and fundal height as well as maternal wellbeing are checked and fetal activity inquired about.

Third trimester

Monthly visits continue in the third trimester (>28 weeks). CBC is checked and antibody screen is repeated at 28–30 weeks, along with a repeat urinalysis and syphilis and HIV test, if indicated. A glucose load test (GLT) to screen for gestational diabetes should be offered to all women at 24–28 weeks. In women who are Rh(D)-negative, anti-D immunoglobulin (RhoGAM) prophylaxis is routinely administered at the 28–30 week visit. From 36 weeks onwards, in addition to BP, urinalysis, fundal height, maternal wellbeing, and fetal activity, fetal presentation is also assessed and, if not cephalic, the patient should be counseled about elective cesarean delivery at 39 weeks for persistent breech presentation and about the option of external cephalic version (ECV). During the third trimester, the mother and her partner need to be prepared for what to expect regarding onset and process of labor and delivery. At 35–36 weeks, a perineal/perianal culture should be sent to determine the patient's group B β-hemolytic Streptococcus (GBS) colonization status. Weekly antenatal visits are generally recommended after 35 weeks. The final routine antenatal visit is often timed between 40 and 41 weeks, where discussion takes place regarding induction of labor after 41 weeks. If the woman wishes to avoid induction after discussion of the rationale for induction and the risks involved in prolongation of pregnancy, a plan of increased surveillance with cardiotocograph (CTG) and ultrasound assessment of fetal growth and amniotic fluid volume can be individualized.

Recommended further reading

1. American Academy of Pediatrics and American College of Obstetricians and Gynecologists (1997). *Guidelines for Perinatal Care*. American Academy of Pediatrics and American College of Obstetricians and Gynecologists, Washington, DC.

Routine blood tests

A series of blood tests is performed in pregnancy. These tests are in general screening tests for potential maternal and fetal problems which, if identified, may affect the outcome of the pregnancy or give an opportunity, by adjusting antenatal care appropriately, to make a difference in pregnancy outcome.

Complete blood count (CBC)

This is the most commonly performed hematological investigation in pregnancy. Pregnancy is associated with a physiological dilutional anemia caused by a greater increase in plasma volume than red cell mass, and therefore the lower limit for a 'normal' hemoglobin (Hb) is 10.5 g/dL (hematocrit 30%) in pregnancy as opposed to 11.5 g/dL (hematocrit 35%) in the non-pregnant individual. Many women enter pregnancy with a low iron reserve, and therefore, if anemia is detected in pregnancy, it should be investigated by assessment of hematinic indices such as ferritin, total iron-binding capacity (TIBC), serum and red cell folate, and serum B_{12} levels. The most common cause of anemia in pregnancy is iron deficiency anemia. CBC estimation is performed at the first prenatal visit, at 28–30 weeks, and again in labor.

Blood grouping and screening for antibodies

Determining the blood group at the first prenatal visit makes it possible to identify those women who are rhesus-negative and therefore at risk of rhesus isoimmunization. The incidence of rhesus disease has dramatically fallen over the last 30 years following the introduction of anti-D immunoglobulin (RhoGAM) administration. Despite administration of prophylactic anti-D after screening at 28–30 weeks and after any potential sensitizing event, a small number of Rh (D)-negative women still develop anti-D antibodies because of small silent hemorrhages predominantly in the third trimester or because of failure of timely administration of anti-D immunoglobulin. Screening for red cell antibodies should be repeated in all women early in subsequent pregnancies even if they are rhesus-positive as there may be other clinically significant antibodies as a consequence of previous pregnancy or blood transfusion.

Infection screening

- All booking bloods are screened for evidence of immunity to rubella because of the devastating implications for the fetus of rubella in early pregnancy. The present data show that around 2% of primigravida and 1% of multigravida are nonimmune to rubella, and it is recommended that these women receive postpartum rubella vaccination. Since it is a live attenuated vaccine, vaccination in pregnancy is not recommended. To date, however, there have been no reports of adverse outcome where this has been performed inadvertently in pregnancy or within 1 month of conception.
- Screening for syphilis is also routinely performed. The rationale for screening for syphilis lies in the fact that early treatment of the disease can prevent congenital syphilis in the neonate.

- Hepatitis B screening is also universally performed on all antenatal booking bloods. A combined course of active and passive immunization can then be undertaken in the neonate at risk shortly after birth. The importance of preventing hepatitis B infection in the neonate lies in the fact that, while in the adult patient the virus is cleared within 6 months in 90% of infected individuals, 90% of infected neonates become chronic carriers with the risk of postinfective hepatic cirrhosis and hepatocellular carcinoma.
- The current recommendations are for universal screening for HIV at the initial antenatal visit and again at 28–30 weeks, if indicated. This has come about because of difficulties in effectively targeting affected women, even in areas of high prevalence. There is now clear evidence that the vertical transmission from mother to fetus can be significantly reduced (by at least two-thirds to a baseline of 0–2%) by treatment of the mother with antiretrovirals in pregnancy and labor and of the infant for 6 weeks postnatally. Furthermore, the risk of transmission can be further reduced by elective cesarean delivery at 38 weeks before labor and rupture of membranes in women with a high viral load (defined as >1000 copies/mL) and by avoidance of breast-feeding. It should also be borne in mind that HIV testing performed as part of routine antenatal screening is not used by insurance companies as a marker of high risk.

Recommended further reading

1. American Academy of Pediatrics and American College of Obstetricians and Gynecologists (1997). *Guidelines for Perinatal Care*. American Academy of Pediatrics and American College of Obstetricians and Gynecologists, Washington, DC.
2. American College of Obstetricians and Gynecologists (2003). Clinical management guidelines for obstetrician-gynecologists. ACOG Practice Bulletin No. 44. *Obstet Gynecol* **102**, 203–13.

Special blood tests

Screening for gestational diabetes mellitus (GDM)

There appears to be no consensus as to who, when, how, or even whether to screen for GDM. The only group of women for whom routine screening for GDM is not cost effective are women <25 years of age with no risk factors (which include previous GDM, family history of diabetes, previous macrosomic baby, previous unexplained stillbirth, obesity (BMI >26), glycosuria on more than one occasion, polyhydramnios, and large for gestational age infant in the current pregnancy), and who are not part of a high-risk ethnic group (Hispanic, Black, African American, or Asian). Since few women will meet these criteria, universal biochemical screening has been suggested. The glucose load test (GLT), also known as the glucose challenge test (GCT), involves the administration of a 50 g glucose load to all nonfasting pregnant women at 24–28 weeks' gestation and measurement of venous glucose levels 1 hour later. Using a cutoff of 140 mg/dL, this screening test will identify women with impaired glucose tolerance or GDM with a sensitivity of 78%, specificity of 90%, and false-positive rate of 15%. A cutoff of 130 mg/dL would pick up more women with GDM, but the false-positive rate would be 20–25%. All women with a positive GLT should have a definitive 3 hour 100 g glucose tolerance test (GTT) performed before a diagnosis of GDM can be made (see Chapter 15). A policy of selective screening using clinical risk factors (above) would identify only 50% of women with GDM. In women at high risk (above), an early GLT is recommended at 16–20 weeks. If this test is negative, it should be repeated at 24–28 weeks. The timing of testing is also controversial as, the later in pregnancy it is performed, the higher the detection rate since glucose tolerance progressively deteriorates. On the other hand, the earlier in pregnancy GDM is diagnosed and hyperglycemia treated, the greater the likelihood of influencing the outcome.

Screening for hemoglobinopathies

Hemoglobin electrophoresis should be routinely performed in women of ethnic or racial origins with a high incidence of hemoglobinopathies. These include women of Cypriot, Eastern Mediterranean, Middle Eastern, Indian, and Southeast Asian origin, where the incidence of thalassemia is greatest, and women of African or Afro-Caribbean origin who are at risk of sickle cell disease. If a patient herself is affected, then consideration should be given to testing her partner as this will have implications on counseling and prenatal testing. Persistent anemia where a cause cannot be identified may be an indication for hemoglobin electrophoresis in any woman irrespective of racial origin. It should be remembered that a diagnosis of α-thalassemia requires definitive DNA testing and can not be made on hemoglobin electrophoresis.

Miscellaneous tests

Other blood tests may be performed on an individual basis. Thus, if there is a history of thyroid disease, thyroid function tests may be required. In patients with hypertension or renal complications of diabetes, baseline urea, creatinine, and electrolytes would be advisable along with a baseline 24 hour urine collection for protein quantitation and estimation of creatinine clearance. Long-term diabetic control is monitored by means of serum HbA1c estimation. Where epilepsy is poorly controlled despite adequate doses of anticonvulsants, it may be useful to assess serum levels prior to further dose increases or as a means of confirming compliance. Patients with a family or personal history of coagulation disorders may need screening for bleeding disorders (such as antiphospholipid antibody syndrome or inherited thrombophilia) and checking of coagulation factor levels.

Recommended further reading

1. American Academy of Pediatrics and American College of Obstetricians and Gynecologists (1997). *Guidelines for Perinatal Care*. American Academy of Pediatrics and American College of Obstetricians and Gynecologists, Washington, DC.
2. American College of Obstetricians and Gynecologists (2003). Clinical management guidelines for obstetrician-gynecologists. ACOG Practice Bulletin No. 44. *Obstet Gynecol* **102**, 203–13.

Serum screening for fetal anomalies

Serum analyte screening

Triple/quadruple test

This refers to the estimation of serum-unconjugated estriol (uE3), α-fetoprotein (AFP), and β-hCG in the maternal blood at 15–20 weeks' gestation (triple test) or these three markers plus inhibin-A (quadruple test) as a screening test for trisomy 21 (Down syndrome) and other fetal aneuploidies (chromosomal abnormalities). The double test (AFP and β-hCG only) performs poorly and, as such, is no longer recommended. Down syndrome is the most common chromosomal condition, with an overall birth prevalence of 1 in 700, and has great clinical and societal significance in terms of severity and compatibility with life. Studies have shown that maternal serum AFP levels in pregnancies affected by Down syndrome are 25% lower than in women with chromosomally normal fetuses, and this is independent of maternal age. Similarly, the levels of another hormone produced by the fetoplacental unit, uE3, are also 27% lower in pregnancies affected by Down syndrome. However, the most effective marker to date appears to be the placental-specific product hCG, with levels being twice as high as normal in pregnancies affected by Down syndrome or other chromosomal abnormalities. While maternal serum AFP and uE3 rise between 14 and 21 weeks, hCG levels drop. Because maternal age is a major determinant of risk and is independent of these markers, it is used to define the *a priori* risk of fetal aneuploidy in a given pregnancy. Given that the three markers are not independent of each other, application of a trivariate Gaussian distribution allows calculation of individual risk with a commercially available software package assisting in the calculations. Different institutions define different cut-offs as high risk, with cutoff values ranging from 1 in 200 through to 1 in 300. As a general rule, if this screening test is regarded as positive, more definitive testing is recommended when the risk posed by the intervention (in this case amniocentesis, with a procedure-related pregnancy loss rate of approximately 1 in 270) is lower than the chance of finding an aneuploid fetus.

The management of a screen-positive result (i.e. an individual risk greater than the cutoff selected) involves confirmation of a singleton pregnancy and verification of gestational age and timing of the screening test. If these are correct, the patient and her partner need to be counseled about the options available to them, which include invasive diagnostic testing to obtain a karyotype. On the other hand, if such testing is unacceptable to them because of the risks involved for the pregnancy or because the outcome of diagnostic testing would not alter their attitude towards the pregnancy, the course of action chosen may be not to investigate further. As with all types of screening tests, there need to be agreed protocols on how abnormal results are managed, with adequate time set aside for pre- and post-test counseling and ongoing support.

Screening for neural tube defects (NTDs)

It is important at this stage to make the distinction between the triple/quadruple test for fetal aneuploidy and the role of maternal serum AFP (MSAFP) alone, which is used as a screening tool for open neural tube defect. AFP is produced first by the yolk sac and subsequently by the fetal liver, and enters the amniotic fluid by fetal urination. Its level continues to rise until 30–32 weeks after which it declines. During the period of screening (15–20 weeks' gestation), the levels of AFP rise at around 15% per week. A level greater than 2.5 multiples of the median (MoM) is considered elevated (MoM is calculated by dividing an individual MSAFP by the median for the gestational week). In addition to open NTD, a raised MSAFP may be a result of abdominal wall defects, congenital nephrosis, fetal bowel obstruction, placental or umbilical cord tumors, sacrococcygeal teratoma, multiple pregnancy, gestation more advanced than thought, and bleeding in early pregnancy, amongst other causes.

- Management of elevated MSAFP includes confirmation of gestation and exclusion of multiple pregnancy along with high-resolution ultrasound to exclude an anatomical cause.
- An unexplained elevation in MSAFP (i.e. an elevation in the absence of fetal aneuploidy or fetal structural malformation) should trigger a modification of prenatal care to provide enhanced fetal and maternal surveillance as it is a marker for adverse perinatal outcomes such as fetal death, intrauterine growth restriction (IUGR), early and late pregnancy bleeding, and preterm delivery. It may also be a marker for subsequent development of preeclampsia, but the data in this regard are conflicting. Interestingly, recent data suggest that it may also be a risk factor for unexplained death in the first year of life.

Recommended further reading

1. American Academy of Pediatrics and American College of Obstetricians and Gynecologists (1997). *Guidelines for Perinatal Care*. American Academy of Pediatrics and American College of Obstetricians and Gynecologists, Washington, DC.
2. American College of Obstetricians and Gynecologists (2003). Clinical management guidelines for obstetrician-gynecologists. ACOG Practice Bulletin No. 44. *Obstet Gynecol* **102**, 203–13.

Chapter 2

Pregnancy complications

First trimester symptoms of pregnancy

- Nausea and vomiting are the most common complaints of pregnant women in the first trimester, and these are collectively referred to as morning sickness. Morning sickness is believed to be due to high levels of pregnancy hormones secreted by the placenta. In women with multiple pregnancies or molar pregnancy, this symptom tends to be exaggerated. It becomes abnormal when vomiting is so severe that it prevents the pregnant woman from adequate fluid and food intake, causing severe dehydration, ketonuria, and electrolyte imbalance. This is referred to as hyperemesis gravidarum 📖 *p.66*.
  - *Treatment.* Women may need to be hospitalized for intravenous feeding and rehydration when vomiting causes ketonuria, dehydration, and electrolyte imbalance. Generally, morning sickness should diminish at about 14 weeks of pregnancy. Conditions such as urinary tract infection, molar and multiple pregnancies, and thyroid disease need to be excluded.
- Tiredness. Women in the early part of pregnancy may feel tired easily. In fact, this may be one of their first symptoms of pregnancy. This feeling will generally ease towards the second trimester but may return towards the end of pregnancy.
- Frequency of micturition. When the uterus enlarges in the first trimester of pregnancy, it presses on the bladder, resulting in decreased capacity and hence giving rise to urinary frequency. Also, urine production by the kidney increases during pregnancy and this in turn increases urinary volume and contributes to frequency. The pressure effect of the uterus eases off by the 14th week when the uterus rises out of the pelvis, and the symptom generally improves in the second trimester. Watch out for underlying urinary tract infection, which can also present with increased frequency.
  - *Treatment.* Advise not to drink before bedtime. Avoid caffeine-containing drinks, but have a sensible fluid intake throughout the day.
- Heartburn. Progesterone produced by the placenta in pregnancy causes relaxation of the esophageal sphincter producing reflux of gastric juices. This produces heartburn.
  - *Treatment.* Advise the wearing of loose clothing and sleeping on two pillows at night and prescribe antacids.
- Constipation. The relaxation effects of progesterone on the smooth muscles of the bowel cause less bowel activity during pregnancy. This may give rise to very troublesome constipation in some women which can continue throughout pregnancy.
  - *Treatment.* Adequate intake of fiber such as fruit and fluids is of help. Avoid powerful laxatives but bulk formula laxatives may be used.

Note. Iron supplements in pregnancy may cause constipation in some women.

- Breast changes. From the second month, under the influence of estrogen and progesterone produced by the placenta, the breasts start to enlarge because of increased fat deposition and glandular proliferation. There is also darkening and increase in size of the nipples and areola with elaboration of Montgomery's follicles scattered around the nipples.
  - *Treatment.* A good support maternity or athletic brassiere will help alleviate breast discomfort.
- Emotional lability. Some women will experience emotional lability and unusual food cravings.
  - *Treatment.* Emotional support and advice regarding diet.

Second trimester symptoms of pregnancy

- Aches and pains. The majority of these symptoms are benign but a small minority may require medical attention. Aches and pains begin in the second trimester and continue to the end of pregnancy. These are caused by the rapidly enlarging uterus and the increased levels of hormones such as progesterone and relaxin.
  - *Treatment.* Advise sufficient rest periods and the wearing of low-heeled shoes.
- Backache. Progesterone and relaxin produced by the placenta cause softening and relaxation of tendons and ligaments throughout the body. The weight of the womb and fetus in front causes the mother to compensate by arching her back to bring the center of gravity back between her legs. This imposes considerable strain on the joints on the back, resulting in backache. Excessive weight gain and previous back injury can aggravate the situation.
  - *Treatment.* Adopting a proper posture, having sufficient rest, avoiding wearing high-heeled shoes, avoiding lifting heavy objects, bending at the knees instead of the waist, and lifting by using the arms and legs instead of the back should all help to avoid backache. Avoid standing for too long; a foot on a low stool will offset some of the strain on the back. Sleeping on a firm mattress, massage, and using hot pads for the back also help to reduce the backache.
- Lower abdominal and groin pain. Some women may experience aching or sharp pain at the lower abdomen and groin. It may be felt on either side or both sides. This may be pain originating from the round ligaments because of the enlarging uterus pulling on the round ligaments. This pain is felt usually between 16 and 20 weeks and continues until about the 32nd week.
  - *Treatment.* Most abdominal pain during pregnancy is innocuous but any pain that develops suddenly and persists should be paid serious attention. Torsion of an ovarian cyst should be excluded.
- Headaches. Mild headaches are common in pregnancy. Persistent headaches after 20 weeks should raise the possibility of preeclampsia. Therefore blood pressure and urine must be checked.
  - *Treatment.* Prescribe simple analgesics like acetaminophen after ruling out a pathological cause.
- Calf pain. This is due to muscle spasm and tends to occur at night. Venous stasis due to poor circulation can give rise to dull discomfort. The possibility of deep vein thrombosis should be considered.
  - *Treatment.* Straighten the legs and flex the ankles and toes towards the face to reduce the discomfort. Gentle massage and application of hot pads should ease the pain. If calf pain persists and is associated with swelling of the lower limbs, investigate for deep vein thrombosis.

- Increased vaginal discharge. Leukorrhea is a clear white mucoid discharge from the vagina. This is secondary to increased blood flow to the vagina and increased cervical secretions. It becomes pathological when it is associated with an offensive odor or pruritus, or when it becomes colored, bloodstained, or 'watery', in which case it is suggestive of an infection.
  - *Treatment.* Reassurance if physiological. Identify and treat any underlying infection.
- Braxton–Hicks contractions. These are painless tightenings of the uterus which the pregnant woman experiences after the 20th week and which become more frequent and stronger towards the end of pregnancy. They originate from the top of the uterus and gradually fade off as they radiate downwards. They usually last for between 30 and 60 seconds. This could be confused with preterm labor, which usually occurs more than four times in an hour and is accompanied by abdominal pain or backache. Abdominal pain associated with vaginal bleeding or watery vaginal discharge may suggest an abruption or spontaneous rupture of the membranes.
- The first sensation of fetal movement or quickening can be felt as early as 17–20 weeks. Parous women tend to feel these earlier than primigravidas. It is perfectly normal for no movement to be felt for several days in the early part of pregnancy, but after 20 weeks absence of fetal movements should be investigated. Auscultation of the fetal heart sounds using a Doptone will allay maternal anxiety and a scan will reveal the growth and amniotic fluid volume in relation to the gestational period.

Third trimester symptoms of pregnancy

- Breathlessness. This symptom is felt when the diaphragm is pushed up by the expanding uterus, thereby decreasing lung capacity. Progesterone acts on the respiratory center of the brain causing deep breathing, which allows an increase in tidal volume and thus ensures an adequate oxygen supply to the baby.
    - *Treatment.* Improvement in posture; practicing sitting with the back straight and the shoulders relaxed and back and down. Lying on the side when sleeping. This symptom improves with the engagement of the head. *Caution.* Shortness of breath along with rapid pulse and rapid breathing and chest pain or discomfort may raise the possibility of pulmonary embolus.
- Sciatica. Pressure of the pregnant uterus against the two sciatic nerves or sciatica may cause pain, tingling, or numbness running down the buttocks, hip, and thighs.
    - *Treatment.* Adequate rest, warm baths, use of heating pads, change of sleeping positions. This symptom eases nearer the delivery date. More serious cases should be referred to the orthopedic surgeon or physiotherapist.
- Sleeplessness or insomnia. This may be due to a very active baby at night or discomfort due to the mother lying flat.
    - *Treatment.* A little exercise prior to going to bed and a drink of warm milk may help mothers to relax. Sleeping on the side with legs and knees bent is the ideal position. Cushions may be used to support the body, with additional pillows for the abdomen, upper body, and back. Avoid the use of sedatives.
- Itchy abdomen. This is due to stretching of the skin across the abdomen as pregnancy progresses.
    - *Treatment.* Use of lubricating lotion or moisturizers may help and an anti-itching cream may relieve the discomfort in intolerable cases. If itching continues and is generalized and unrelenting, investigate for possible cholestasis.
- Stretch marks. These are due to both the stretching of the abdomen and changes in tissues beneath the skin as a result of hormonal changes related to pregnancy.
    - *Treatment.* There is no proven treatment. Lubricant creams and ointments have been tried.
- Varicose veins. These may cause slight discomfort and may become worse towards the final stages of pregnancy.
    - *Treatment.* The blood venous circulation in the legs should be improved by regular exercise and the use of compression stockings. Varicose veins become less after delivery.
- Rashes. These are common in pregnancy, but are often not serious. While a few may require treatment, most will disappear after childbirth. PUPPP (pruritic urticarial papules and plaques of pregnancy) is a skin condition that occurs in about 1 in 150 pregnancies and is characterized by itchy reddish raised patches on the abdomen, arms, and legs.

    - *Treatment.* Simple rashes may respond to anti-itching creams. In the case of PUPPP, referral to a dermatologist may be useful. Topical steroids are recommended. Most skin conditions will disappear after delivery.
- Hemorrhoids. These occur in about one in every three women and may occur for the first time during pregnancy.
    - *Treatment.* Preventive measures such as avoidance of constipation by eating green leafy vegetables and high-fiber foods should be advised from early pregnancy. Increase in regular fluid intake, regular exercise, avoiding long hours of standing or sitting, and sleeping on the side may help. Suppositories or creams may be used for temporary relief. Refer to a surgeon if hemorrhoids increase in size or become very painful.
- Numbness of the hands. Carpal tunnel syndrome may occur as a result of tissue swelling during pregnancy.
    - *Treatment.* Avoid sleeping with the hands below the face or body. Increase circulation by hanging the affected hand over the side of the bed. Wearing of a wrist splint may be necessary in severe cases. Occasionally, referral to a surgeon may become necessary if there is evidence of neurological deficit.
- Urinary incontinence. This is due to the pregnant uterus pressing on the urinary bladder.
    - *Treatment.* Frequent emptying of the bladder and pelvic floor exercises are of value. UTI should be excluded. Stress incontinence persisting 6 months after delivery should be investigated.
- Weight gain. Women put on about 30% additional weight during pregnancy. Half of this may be during the third trimester. In heavier women, watch for diabetes, increased blood pressure, or thromboembolism.
    - *Treatment.* Weight gain is normal. Light exercise and a well-balanced diet are good for overall health. Rule out the possibility of diabetes or increased blood pressure if there is a sudden increase in weight.

Miscarriage

This section covers uterine bleeding with/without pain before viability. The pregnancy may remain viable (threatened miscarriage) despite the bleeding or it may be a feature of nonviability (missed abortion or blighted ovum). The pregnancy may also be expelled partly (inevitable/incomplete miscarriage) or completely (complete miscarriage). Miscarriage is very common, occurring in about 15% of confirmed pregnancies. It may cause significant psychological trauma, and therefore counseling and support are very important in management. The term 'miscarriage' is preferable to 'abortion', as the latter may be misunderstood as induced rather than spontaneous.

Threatened miscarriage

Vaginal bleeding is often minimal and may be associated with mild period-type pelvic pains. The volume of bleeding is usually less than the patient's usual menstrual blood loss. If the bleeding is light and resolves, the pregnancy, if viable, usually continues satisfactorily.

Diagnosis

The cervical os is closed, the uterine size corresponds to gestational period on pelvic examination, and ultrasound scan confirms viability of the pregnancy.

Management

- Reassurance that the pregnancy should continue satisfactorily once the bleeding settles. Advise avoidance of strenuous activity, but normal daily activities need not be restricted.
- If bleeding continues, repeat ultrasound scan (in about 7 days) to confirm viability. If ultrasound is doubtful, it is necessary to err on the side of caution and repeat after 1–2 weeks depending on the circumstances as an inconclusive scan may, for instance, be due to wrong dates.

Inevitable miscarriage

With an inevitable miscarriage, vaginal bleeding is associated with an open internal cervical os (the external os may seem 'open' in multiparous women). The bleeding is usually associated with 'crampy' pelvic pains which may vary from mild to severe.

Diagnosis

Usually clinical, based on bleeding and an open cervical os. Products of conception may be left in the canal. The bleeding usually continues until the uterus is emptied.

Management

- Expectant. Await spontaneous completion of miscarriage if the clinical condition permits and the patient wishes.
- Consider surgical evacuation if products of conception are protruding through the os.
- Medical management with prostaglandin analogues, e.g. vaginal misoprostol 200–600 μg orally, vaginally, or per rectum.
- Counseling and support should be given as needed.

Incomplete/complete miscarriage

With *incomplete miscarriage* some products of conception may be passed and some may be stuck in the cervical os or the uterus. The os remains open until miscarriage is spontaneously, medically, or surgically completed. It may be necessary to remove tissue stuck in the os or the uterus to prevent further hemorrhage.

- Oxytocin infusion should be given to maintain uterine contraction if the vaginal bleeding is heavy.
- Ultrasound scan, when appropriate, may show retained products of conception.
- Surgical evacuation is usually indicated for incomplete miscarriage.

With complete miscarriage, pelvic pains and vaginal bleeding reduce spontaneously, the cervical os closes, and ultrasound shows an empty uterus. In such cases in which no products of conception are available for pathologic examination, serum β-hCG levels should be followed until undetectable.

Recurrent miscarriage

This is defined as three or more unexplained first trimester pregnancy losses and affects 1% of all women.

Associated factors

A number of factors are implicated or associated with recurrent miscarriage including chromosomal abnormality (present in 3–5% of partners), congenital uterine abnormalities, cervical insufficiency, infection, inadequate secretion of progesterone in the luteal phase, polycystic ovary syndrome, subfertility and ovulatory defects, autoimmune conditions, and antiphospholipid antibody syndrome. However, no identifiable cause will be found in over 50% of couples with recurrent miscarriage.

Investigations

- Karyotyping of any fetal tissue.
- Pelvic ultrasound to assess ovaries and uterine cavity.
- Screening tests for antiphospholipid antibody syndrome and inherited thrombophilias (especially factor V Leiden mutation).
- Appropriate endocrine investigations (including thyroid function tests and prolactin levels).
- Karyotyping of both partners.

Further management

- Referral to geneticists if abnormal karyotype.
- Low-dose aspirin + heparin if positive for antiphospholipid antibody syndrome.

There are no other proven treatments but the problem is subject to considerable research.

Bleeding and/or pain in early pregnancy

Missed abortion/blighted ovum

Blighted ovum is failure to expel a non-viable fetus from the uterus. Abdominal pain and vaginal bleeding are usually minimal. Pregnancy symptoms have usually inexplicably resolved. The uterus is smaller than expected for dates. The ultrasound scan shows absence of fetal heart activity. Often, there is a misshapen gestation sac and the fetus may be smaller than expected for dates. With a blighted ovum, a gestation sac is seen on ultrasound but there is no fetal heart activity, yolk sac, or fetal pole.

Management

- Expectant. If very early, the pregnancy may resolve spontaneously. If the patient so wishes, it is reasonable to allow up to 2 weeks for resolution.
- Medical management using misoprostol as for inevitable miscarriage. (Mid-trimester missed abortion is best treated by medical means.)
- Surgical evacuation of uterus is usually necessary for missed abortion or blighted ovum.
- There is a risk of disseminated intravascular coagulation (DIC) with a long-standing missed abortion that has remained in the uterus for 3 weeks or more, especially in mid-trimester. Therefore it is necessary to check the coagulation status prior to any intervention.
- Diagnosis is usually unexpected by patient and so counseling/support may be required.

Hydatidiform mole

Hydatidiform mole usually presents as bleeding in early pregnancy. The bleeding may be profuse and accompanied by vaginal expulsion of grape-like tissues. The uterus is large for dates in 50% of cases.

Diagnosis may be incidental, with the finding of typical grape-like material during surgical evacuation of a non-viable pregnancy. More often, an ultrasound scan is requested because of a 'large for dates' uterus, hyperemesis, or slight vaginal bleeding and reveals the typical ultrasound 'snowstorm' appearance with the absence of a fetus (complete mole). β-hCG levels are very high and this may result in large bilateral ovarian (theca lutein) cysts. Pregnancy symptoms may be quite profound because of the high β-hCG levels.

Management

- The uterus is best evacuated surgically and tissue sent for histological confirmation.
- Clinical and biochemical follow-up is essential until serum β-hCG levels are undetectable as there is a risk of malignant trophoblastic disease.
- Advise barrier methods of contraception for a year to allow follow-up.

Hydatidiform mole may recur in future pregnancies with an overall risk of recurrence of 1% (tenfold higher than the general population).

Other causes of abdominal pain

For discussions of *fibroids* and *ectopic pregnancy* see 📖 *pp 388 and 486*, respectively.

Most of the coincidental causes of abdominal pain are related to the hormonal/physiological changes of pregnancy. The approach to management is to exclude a pathological cause and give symptomatic treatment. These conditions include:

- heartburn
- hyperemesis
- constipation.

However, more sinister conditions may occur in pregnancy. These are incidental to the pregnancy but diagnosis may be made more difficult because of displacement of abdominal viscera by the gravid uterus, leading to atypical location of pain compared with that of nonpregnant patients. When suspected, surgical opinion should be sought early. These conditions include:

- appendicitis
- cholecystitis
- pyelonephritis/UTI
- renal colic
- inflammatory bowel disease
- ovarian cyst accidents (torsion, hemorrhage)
- sickle cell crisis
- pancreatitis
- bowel obstruction.

Recommended further reading

1. James DK, Steer PJ, Weiner CP, Gonik B (eds) (1994). *High Risk Pregnancy: Management Options.* WB Saunders, London.
2. Neilson JP (2002). Ultrasound for fetal assessment in early pregnancy. *Cochrane Database Syst Rev* **2**, CD000182.

Hyperemesis gravidarum

Nausea and vomiting are both common in pregnancy. Persistent vomiting and severe nausea can progress to hyperemesis. The characteristics of hyperemesis are as follows:

- Prolonged and severe nausea and vomiting, dehydration, ketosis, and loss of body weight.
- Investigations may show hypernatremia, hypokalemia, low serum urea, metabolic hypochloremia, alkalosis and ketonuria, raised hematocrit, and increased specific gravity of the urine.
- There may be associated liver function test (LFT) abnormalities and abnormal thyroid function tests with biochemical thyrotoxicosis, i.e. raised free thyroxine levels and/or suppressed TSH levels.

Pathophysiology

Overall incidence is 1:1000. The pathophysiology is poorly understood. The risk is increased in youths, non-smokers, primiparas, those working outside the home, and those with multiple and molar pregnancy. A possible direct relationship between severity of hyperemesis, degree of biochemical hyperthyroidism, and the level of hCG has been postulated. Transient hyperthyroidism of hyperemesis gravidarum is a self-limiting hyperthyroidism. It typically resolves by 17–18 weeks of pregnancy without sequelae and no treatment is required.

Management

Hyperemesis gravidarum may be a result of an underlying disease. Differential diagnosis includes pyelonephritis, gestational trophoblastic neoplasia (hydatidiform mole), red degeneration of fibroids, increased intracranial pressure, an acute abdominal emergency, and hysterical vomiting. In the latter case, the patient is likely to complain of vomiting after every meal and of not being able to retain a drop of water. However, she manages to look well physically and her weight is appropriate. Both the patient and her partner are convinced that there is a physical explanation for her symptoms. Psychological explanation may not succeed because of denial of underlying emotional conflict.

Routine investigation should include:

- full blood count
- urea and electrolytes to help guide the IV fluid regime in addition to an input and output chart
- thyroid function tests (TFTs) may help to identify thyroid dysfunction
- exclude urinary tract infection by midstream urine for culture
- in protracted or severe cases, LFTs may be deranged
- ultrasound will be useful to confirm an intrauterine pregnancy, identify a multiple pregnancy, and exclude a molar pregnancy.

Treatment

- Development of ketonuria in a pregnant woman with severe vomiting should prompt admission to hospital.
- Time should be spent optimizing the woman's psychological wellbeing.

- IV fluid replacement in the form of normal saline or 5% dextrose saline is required until ketonuria clears and vomiting subsides.
- Potassium and other electrolytes should be replaced, guided by daily or twice daily urea and electrolyte measurements. Too rapid reversal of hypernatremia can cause fetal pontine myelinosis.
- Thiamine (vitamin B_1) supplementation may be required to prevent Wernicke's encephalopathy.

Most patients improve with the help of the above measures without long-term sequelae. Conventional antiemetics are not usually prescribed, especially before 12 weeks' gestation. The reluctance to use antiemetics relates to fears concerning their teratogenic effects. Antiemetic medication appears to reduce the frequency of nausea and vomiting in early pregnancy. There is some evidence of adverse effects, but there is little information on effects on fetal outcomes.

- Traditional antiemetics, such as metoclopramide 10 mg every 8 hours IV, may be tried safely followed by oral antiemetics.
- Treatment with pyridoxine (vitamin B_6) appears to be effective in reducing the severity of nausea.
- The results from trials of P6 acupressure and oral garlic supplementation are equivocal.
- Those resistant to conventional therapy may respond to steroid treatment. There is some evidence that a course of methylprednisolone is more effective than promethazine for treatment of hyperemesis.
- Placing a Dobbhoff nasogastric tube for enteral feeding has proponents. Isomolar feeds are recommended. Parenteral nutrition may be needed in rare instances and the advice of a dietitian would be valuable. This may need to be associated with regular aspiration of the stomach if there is continued vomiting due to delayed gastric emptying.
- When symptoms of hyperemesis gravidarum persist into the second trimester, active peptic ulcer disease from *Helicobacter pylori* should be included in the differential diagnosis.

Recommended further reading

1. Jewell D, Young G (2003). Interventions for nausea and vomiting in early pregnancy. *Cochrane Database Syst Rev* **4**, CD000145.
2. American College of Obstetricians and Gynecologists (2004). Nausea and vomiting of pregnancy. *Obstet Gynecol* **103**, 803–14.

Etiology, incidence, and prevention of preeclampsia and eclampsia

Introduction

Preeclampsia (gestational proteinuric hypertension) is defined as pregnancy-induced hypertension with a sustained elevation in BP ≥140/90 mmHg developing after 20 weeks' gestation in a previously normotensive woman in association with new-onset significant proteinuria (defined as ≥300 mg/24 hours or ≥1+ proteinuria in the absence of a urinary tract infection). Nondependent edema (swelling of the hands and face) is present in many such women, but is not a prerequisite for the diagnosis. The only effective treatment is delivery of the fetus and placenta. The condition resolves by 6 weeks postpartum (usually within 10 days).

Eclampsia (literally *flashing lights*) complicates approximately 1 in 2000 pregnancies and is characterized by the occurrence of generalized convulsions and/or coma in association with the signs and symptoms of preeclampsia and in the absence of other reasonable explanations (such as idiopathic epilepsy, subarachnoid hemorrhage, and meningitis).

Etiology and incidence

Preeclampsia/eclampsia is an idiopathic multisystem disorder specific to human pregnancy and the puerperium. It is a disease of the placenta. The primary defect is the consequence of a failure of the developing trophoblast to invade the spiral arteries during the second trimester. As the pregnancy continues and the demands of the fetoplacental unit increase, these arterial walls fail to distend to accommodate the required increase in blood flow. An increase in maternal BP likely serves as a compensatory mechanism to maintain uteroplacental perfusion. The maternal sequelae are a result of the abnormal behavior of the vascular endothelium likely resulting from the production of a circulating 'toxemia' factor from the dysfunctional placenta.

The incidence of preeclampsia is 5–7% of the pregnant population. There is an increased risk in the following cases:

- patient <20 or >35 years of age
- family history (first-degree relative)
- first pregnancy with a new partner
- hydatidiform mole
- multiple pregnancy.
- maternal obesity (BMI >32)
- fetal/placental hydrops (multiple causes)
- pregestational diabetes mellitus
- preexisting maternal hypertension and/or renal disease
- if multiparous, previous severe early-onset preeclampsia (<36 weeks' gestation).

There is a lower incidence in smokers (NB. Disease severity is often worsened in smokers because of preexisting vascular endothelial damage).

Prevention

Various strategies have been used to try to prevent the development of preeclampsia in both high- and low-risk populations but, despite initial promise, none have been shown to be effective. Since preeclampsia is a disease of implantation and placentation, it is not surprising that preventative strategies have not been successful. Preventative strategies that have been attempted to date include the following:

- Calcium supplementation (2000 mg elemental calcium daily): attempted in populations with deficiency, but no proven benefit.
- Sodium restriction and prophylactic diuretics: no benefit.
- Magnesium sulfate supplementation: preeclampsia is not associated with a deficiency of magnesium and dietary manipulation has no influence on the disease incidence.
- Low-dose aspirin (60–100 mg daily): initial small studies were promising, but larger prospective studies show no benefit. It is still possible that some subgroups of women may benefit, such as women with inherited thrombophilias or antiphospholipid antibody syndrome.
- Vitamin C and E supplementation: such antioxidants may lower the incidence of preeclampsia in some high-risk women, but the data are still too preliminary. Recent studies have suggested that vitamin C and E supplementation in pregnancy may be associated with fetal growth restriction.

Clinical features of preeclampsia and eclampsia

The clinical features of preeclampsia/eclampsia are variable and unpredictable. Preeclampsia is often asymptomatic (diagnosed through raised BP and proteinuria on routine antenatal screening), but clinical features can include nausea, vomiting, general malaise, headaches (frontal and occipital, may be hard to distinguish from migraine), visual disturbance (photophobia, fortification spectra, flashing lights), epigastric pain (due to liver edema and pericapsular swelling), and irritability and altered conscious state (due to cerebral edema). Eclampsia is characterized by generalized tonic–clonic seizures. Death may occur from intracerebral hemorrhage or hepatic, renal, or cardiovascular failure.

Examination

- A full obstetric examination should be performed, remembering that both mother and fetus are affected.
- A brief neurological examination, noting the presence or absence of hyperreflexia, clonus (more than two beats), focal neurological defects, and papilledema, plus an abdominal examination noting epigastric and/or hepatic tenderness.
- The findings from a vaginal examination yield important information concerning the suitability for induction of labor.

Hematological investigations

These should include CBC, urea and electrolytes and uric acid, LFTs, clotting studies, and blood type and screening.

- Hyperuricemia due to increased production and reduced renal excretion.
- Thrombocytopenia (typically regarded in pregnancy as <100 000 platelets/mm^3). A falling platelet count is a reflection of coagulopathy and is a sign of more severe disease.
- Abnormal LFTs. An increase in the enzymes lactic dehydrogenase (LDH), aspartate transaminase (AST), and alanine transaminase (ALT) may relate to alterations in liver perfusion or hepatic congestion. Note altered range in pregnancy in comparison with nonpregnant state.
- Consider cross-matching blood in case a cesarean delivery should prove necessary.

Recommended further reading

1. American College of Obstetricians and Gynecologists (2002). Diagnosis and management of preeclampsia and eclampsia. ACOG Practice Bulletin No. 33. *Obstet Gynecol* **99**, 159–67.

Management of mild preeclampsia

There are two patients: the mother and her fetus.

- The main risks to the mother are eclampsia, cerebral vascular damage, renal and liver failure, HELLP syndrome, and DIC.
  - HELLP (hemolysis, elevated liver enzymes, low platelets) syndrome is a variant of preeclampsia with a higher morbidity and mortality (complicates 4–12% of patients with severe preeclampsia).
  - DIC may be present in severe cases.
- The main risks to the fetus are intrauterine growth restriction, intrauterine death and iatrogenic preterm delivery.

Mild preeclampsia refers to all women in whom a diagnosis of preeclampsia has been made, but who do not have features of severe disease (see later). There is no category of moderate preeclampsia. In women with mild preeclampsia, BP is typically >140/90 mmHg but <160/110 mmHg and proteinuria >300 mg/24 hours but <5 g/24 hours. Such women are often asymptomatic; the diagnosis is made on routine antenatal BP and urine screening.

- If proteinuria is confirmed and the patient's condition permits, a 24 hour urine collection should be commenced.
- In such circumstances, BP measurements should be taken at hourly intervals and the trend observed over a period of 4–8 hours. There is no benefit to the mother or fetus of routinely treating the BP in women with mild preeclampsia. If the BP is >160/110 mmHg, consider control with antihypertensives (to prevent stroke) while moving towards delivery.
- Check hematological and biochemical parameters daily if the clinical condition is stable.
- Depending on the gestational age, a delay in delivery for even a few days may allow for the administration of antenatal corticosteroids and a reduction in the problems of prematurity after birth. However, if the fetus shows signs of compromise or if the risk of intrauterine demise exceeds the risk of prematurity, the pregnancy should be terminated as soon as possible.

Preeclampsia has an unpredictable clinical progression, and patients may become ill very quickly. There is no single sign, symptom, or investigation which predicts disease progression. In patient management, consideration of fetal maturity and disease progression is essential. It should be remembered that there is no benefit whatsoever to the mother remaining pregnant once a diagnosis of preeclampsia is made. It is always in her interest to be delivered.

However, in some circumstances remote from term, it may be reasonable (and safe) to delay delivery with a view to improving the perinatal outcome. Always involve the woman in formulating the management plan.

If the condition permits, consider the following.

- If the pregnancy needs to be terminated and is <34 weeks, promote fetal lung maturation by administration of antenatal corticosteroids (betamethazone 12 mg IM × 2 doses 24 hours apart or dexamethazone 6 mg IM x 4 doses 12 hours apart).
- Transfer care to a tertiary care unit with adequate neonatal facilities.

Fetal assessment

- Ultrasound to determine fetal growth, size, and presentation is vital for determining mode of delivery and counseling the parents regarding care of the neonate.
- Umbilical artery Doppler velocimetry: increased pulsatility index or persistent absence or reversed end-diastolic flow suggests fetal compromise, especially in the setting of IUGR.
- Biophysical profile scoring (CTG and sonographic assessment of amniotic fluid volume, fetal tone, fetal movements, and fetal breathing movements).

Antihypertensive therapy

There are only three reasons to administer antihypertensive therapy in pregnancy:

- Chronic hypertension.
- To prevent cerebrovascular accident (stroke) in women with preeclampsia while effecting delivery. Although it is not clear whether there is a threshold BP that should be treated to prevent stroke, most practitioners would recommend maintaining BP <160/110.
- Expectant management of severe preeclampsia by BP criteria only (i.e. BP >160/110 on two separate occasions at least 6 hours apart in the setting of preeclampsia) prior to 32 weeks' gestation. In this rare circumstance, there is precedent in the literature to treat the BP in such women and continue expectant inpatient management with a view to prolonging gestation and improving perinatal outcome. Since this approach offers no benefit to the mother and puts her at some risk of worsening preeclampsia, it should only be undertaken after extensive counseling and with patient consent.

Recommended further reading

1. Hallah, M. (1999). Hypertension in pregnancy. In: James DK, Steer PJ, Weiner CP, Gonik B, eds. *High Risk Pregnancy: Management Options*, (2nd edn), pp. 639–65 WB Saunders, London.
2. American College of Obstetricians and Gynecologists (2001). Chronic hypertension in pregnancy. *Obstet Gynecol* **98**, S177–85.
3. Norwitz ER, Robinson JN, Malone FD (2004). Pregnancy-induced physiologic alterations. In: Dildy GA, Belfort MA, Saade GR, Phelan JP, Hankins GDV, Clark SL eds. *Critical Care Obstetrics* (4th edn), pp. 19–42. Blackwell Science, Boston, MA.

Management of severe preeclampsia

Severe preeclampsia refers to all women with a diagnosis of preeclampsia who have one or more of the following features:

- Symptoms:
  - symptoms of central nervous system dysfunction (headache, blurred vision, scotomata, altered mental status)
  - symptoms of liver capsule distention or rupture (right upper quadrant and/or epigastric pain)
- Signs:
  - severe elevation in blood pressure (defined as ≥160/110 mmHg on two separate occasions at least 6 hours apart)
  - pulmonary edema
  - eclampsia (generalized seizures and/or unexplained coma in the setting of preeclampsia and in the absence of other neurologic conditions)
  - cerebrovascular accident
  - fetal IUGR
- Laboratory findings:
  - proteinuria >5g/24 hours
  - renal failure (rise in serum creatinine concentration by 1 mg/dL over baseline) or oliguria (<500 mL per 24 hours)
  - hepatocellular injury (serum transaminase levels ≥2 × normal)
  - thrombocytopenia (<100 000 platelets/mm^3)
  - coagulopathy
  - HELLP syndrome

Many women with severe preeclampsia are asymptomatic, but they may complain of epigastric pain, headache, or visual symptoms (flashes of light, blurred vision). Physical examination may reveal signs of abdominal tenderness, hyperreflexia, clonus, or altered conscious state. Progression of disease is unpredictable and the clinical condition may rapidly worsen. Liaise early with senior obstetricians, anesthesiologists, and pediatricians regarding management. Continuous fetal heart rate monitoring is essential.

Principles of management

- Delivery is the only cure. Induction of labor (IOL) or cesarean delivery are both reasonable options, provided that the mother and fetus are stable. However, since most women are nulliparous and remote from term, the likelihood of a successful vaginal delivery is only of the order of 15–20%.
- Close monitoring: consider one-to-one nursing care. Summon senior help when needed.

- Strict fluid balance (80–100 mL/hour total input). Site indwelling urinary catheter to monitor fluid status. NB. Fluid overload may lead to pulmonary edema. Stabilize the BP; aim to maintain sitting BP <160/110 mmHg. NB. BP control will prevent cerebrovascular accident (stroke), but does not prevent seizures (eclampsia) or change perinatal outcome. Many agents are available in the setting of hypertensive crisis. The most commonly employed is hydralazine 5 mg boluses every 10–15 minutes until the BP is controlled up to a maximum dose of 20 mg. Other agents include IV labetalol infusion 20 mg (maximum dose 220 mg) or nifedipine 10 mg orally (may exaggerate the hypotensive response in patients receiving concomitant magnesium sulfate).
- Magnesium sulfate should be given for seizure prophylaxis during labor and delivery and for 24–48 hours postpartum—MAGPIE (magnesium sulfate for prevention of eclampsia) trial.

Recommended further reading

1. Witlin AG, Sibai BM (1998). Magnesium sulphate therapy in pre-eclampsia. *Obstet Gynecol* **95**, 883–9.
2. Hallah M (1999). Hypertension in pregnancy. In: James DK, Steer PJ, Weiner CP, Gonik B, eds. *High Risk Pregnancy: Management Options* (2nd edn), pp. 639–65. WB Saunders, London.
3. American College of Obstetricians and Gynecologists (2001). Chronic hypertension in pregnancy. *Obstet Gynecol* **98**, S177–85.
4. Norwitz ER, Robinson JN, Malone FD (2004). Pregnancy-induced physiologic alterations. In: Dildy GA, Belfort MA, Saade GR, Phelan JP, Hankins GDV, Clark SL, eds. *Critical Care Obstetrics* (4th edn), pp. 19–42. Blackwell Science, Boston, MA.
5. Dudley L, Gulmezoglu AM, Henderson-Smart DJ (2003). Magnesium sulphate and other anticonvulsants for women with pre-eclampsia. *Cochrane Database Syst Rev* **2**, CD000025.

Management of eclampsia

Eclampsia has an incidence of 1:1600–2000 pregnancies. 50% of cases occur postpartum, and 25% after 48 hours, but eclampsia may occur up to several weeks after delivery. Call for help and protect the airway. Eclamptic seizures are usually self-limiting and resolve by themselves within 2–3 minutes.

Treatment

The initial seizure should be controlled by an IV loading dose of 4–6 g of magnesium sulfate ($MgSO_4$) to be infused over 20 minutes. $MgSO_4$ comes in a 50% weight/volume (w/v) solution, i.e. 1 g in 2 mL. Therefore the initial bolus should be 8–12 mL of 50% w/v $MgSO_4$ made up to 20 mL with 5% dextrose.

Thereafter, the maintenance dose is 2–3 g/hour, but may need to be adjusted in women with impaired renal function. The infusion volume needs to be deducted from hourly maintenance fluids. It is advisable to continue $MgSO_4$ for 24–48 hours after delivery or after the last seizure.

Magnesium sulfate

- *Contraindications.* Renal failure (give loading does but no maintenance infusion); cardiac disease.
- *Monitoring serum levels.* Therapeutic range 4–6 mEq/L (4.8–7.3 mg/dL; 2–3 mmol/L).
- *Monitor deep tendon reflexes* after loading dose and at hourly intervals whilst on maintenance. NB. Check arm reflexes in patients with working epidural.
- *Monitor respiration.* Consider pulse oximetry whilst on $MgSO_4$. Maintain respiratory rate >16/min and regular.
- *Dose alterations.* For oliguria (<0.5 mL/kg per hour over >2 hours) or for rising creatinine levels, use a maintenance dose of 1 g/hour and measure $MgSO_4$ levels every 6 hours.

$MgSO_4$ toxicity

- 8–10 mEq/L (9.7–12 mg/dL; 4–5 mmol/L): loss of patellar/biceps reflex, weakness, nausea, feeling of warmth, flushing, somnolence, double vision, slurred speech, hypotension, hypothermia.
- 12–15 mEq/L (14.5–18 mg/dL; 6–7.5 mmol/L): muscle paralysis, respiratory arrest.
- >24 mEq/L (>29 mg/dL; >12 mmol/L): cardiac arrest.

If toxicity occurs: stop magnesium infusion and give antidote—calcium gluconate 1 g in 10 mL 0.9% saline solution.

Important points to consider

- Delivery is the only cure: antihypertensives only lower the BP, potentially masking the signs, and do not prevent disease progression.
- Do not use ergometrine (Methergine) for management of the third stage. It may cause hypertensive stroke in the mother. Oxytocin 10–20 IU IV will suffice.

- If eclamptic seizures do not stop with $MgSO_4$ infusion, a bolus dose can be given or diazepam 10 mg IV can be given every 10–15 minutes. In status eclampticus, paralyse and ventilate.
- An eclamptic seizure is not an indication for emergent cesarean delivery. A fetal bradycardia lasting 6–8 minutes is common. The mother should be stabilized and the fetus resuscitated *in utero* before moving to delivery. If the bradycardia lasts longer than 10 minutes, consider the possibility of placental abruption and the need for emergent cesarean delivery.
- It is not necessary to perform head imaging of all women who have an eclamptic seizure. However, if the seizure lasts longer than 10 minutes, if there are focal neurologic signs, or if the patient seizes while on seizure prophylaxis, a head imaging study should be performed.
- Consider monitoring the patient on the labor floor for at least 24 hours after delivery—observations to be taken half-hourly to start with (BP, temperature, pulse, respiration; O_2 saturations; urine output; strict fluid regimens).
- Use intensive care unit (ICU) facilities when necessary. Consider invasive hemodynamic monitoring (central venous pressure (CVP)/Swann–Ganz catheter) if there is difficulty with maintaining fluid balance, especially if large-volume blood replacement becomes necessary. In the setting of preeclampsia, there is discordance between the left- and right-sided pressures in 20% of women. For this reason, if invasive hemodynamic monitoring is necessary, a Swann–Ganz catheter should be floated.

Recommended further reading

1. Hallah, M. (1999). Hypertension in pregnancy. In: James DK, Steer PJ, Weiner CP, Gonik B, eds. *High Risk Pregnancy: Management Options* (2nd edn), pp. 639–65. WB Saunders, London.
2. American College of Obstetricians and Gynecologists (2001). Chronic hypertension in pregnancy. *Obstet Gynecol* **98**, S177–85.
3. Norwitz ER, Robinson JN, Malone FD (2004). Pregnancy-induced physiologic alterations. In: Dildy GA, Belfort MA, Saade GR, Phelan JP, Hankins GDV, Clark SL, eds. *Critical Care Obstetrics* (4th edn), pp. 19–42. Blackwell Science, Boston, MA.

Multiple pregnancies

The incidence of spontaneous twins is approximately 11/1000 (or 1/80) pregnancies and that of triplets is 1/4000. The incidence of multiple pregnancies is increasing as a consequence of assisted reproductive technologies.

- Incidence following clomiphene treatment, 5–10%.
- Incidence at 20 weeks following three-embryo transfer:
  - IVF—zygote transfer, 32%
  - zygote intrafallopian transfer (ZIFT), 27%
  - gamete intrafallopian transfer (GIFT), 16%.

The incidence of triplets as a consequence of assisted reproductive technologies is:

- IVF—embryo transfer (ET), 4.1%
- GIFT, 4.3%.

The incidence of monozygous twins is 3.5/1000 (or 1 in 300 conceptions).

Predisposing factors and mechanisms

Dizygotic (DZ) twinning is caused by the duplication of the normal process of conception, implantation, and fetal development arising from the fertilization of two ova from the same or opposite ovaries during the same cycle. Each fetus has its own membrane, both chorion and amnion, and its own placenta (dichorionic, diamniotic).

Predisposing factors to dizygous twin pregnancy include the following:

- previous history of dizygous twins
- family history of twins
- increased maternal age (20 years, 6.4/1000; >25 years, 16.8/1000; >35 years, 19.1/1000).
- ovulation induction with or without IVF
- race (Japanese, 6.7/1000 pregnancies; Nigerian, 40/1000).

Monozygotic (MZ) twinning represents a random event occurring in approximately 1 in every 300 conceptions in which a single embryo divides into two. The only risk factor for monozygous twinning is ovulation induction and IVF (threefold increased risk). The arrangement of the membranes depends on the time after fertilization when the splitting occurs in the embryo.

- Less than 3 days (eight-cell stage): implantation at separate sites; however, same structural arrangements as in DZ pregnancies, but identical fetuses (MZ—dichorionic, diamniotic).
- 4–7 days (formation of inner cell mass): single placenta; however, since the amnion has not fully developed, each embryo will develop its own amniotic membrane (monochorionic, diamniotic).
- 8–12 days: prior to primitive streak formation; single amniotic cavity and chorion (monochorionic, monoamniotic).
- ≥13 days (*rare*): after primitive streak formation; conjoined twins.

Whenever there is a single chorion, vascular anastamoses inevitably connect the two circulations with frequent pathological sequelae.

Determination of zygosity at birth

- Twins of opposite sex are DZ.
- A single chorion on examination of the placenta and membranes suggests MZ twins.
- Dichorionic twins of like sex may be DZ (in 80% of cases) or MZ (20%), and genetic markers are required to distinguish DZ from MZ twins.

Recommended further reading

1. Walters W (1995). Multiple pregnancy. In: Chamberlain GVP, ed. *Turnbull's Obstetrics* (2nd edn), pp. 329–52. Churchill Livingstone, Edinburgh.
2. Neilson JP (1995). Multiple pregnancy. In: Whitefield C, ed. *Dewhurst's Textbook of Obstetrics and Gynaecology for Postgraduates* (5th edn) pp. 439–54. Blackwell Science, Oxford.
3. American College of Obstetricians and Gynecologists (2004). Multiple gestation: complicated twin, triplet, and high-order multifetal pregnancy. ACOG Practice Bulletin No. 56. *Obstet Gynecol* **104**, 869–83.
4. Norwitz ER (1998). Multiple pregnancies: trends past, present and future. In: Diamond M, DeCherney A, eds. *The Infertility and Reproductive Medicine Clinics of North America*, pp. 351–369. WB Saunders, Philadelphia, PA.

Diagnosis of multiple pregnancies

Suspect the diagnosis in the setting of hyperemesis gravidarum, large for dates, three or more fetal poles palpated, or two or more fetal heart sounds on auscultation. Definitive diagnosis is by ultrasound scanning. In current obstetric practice, multiple pregnancy is identified in the first trimester at the time of dating scan or when the scan for nuchal translucency is done.

Pregnancy

Maternal complications

Maternal complications are similar to those with singleton pregnancies, but there is an increased risk of minor and major complications at all stages. The following are increased: symptoms of early pregnancy; risk of miscarriage; anemia (greater iron and folate requirements); polyhydramnios (12% of multiple pregnancies); preeclampsia (5% singletons, 25% twins); musculoskeletal problems; antepartum hemorrhage; placenta previa; preterm labor; postpartum hemorrhage.

Fetal complications

- There is increased incidence of neural tube defects, bowel atresia, and cardiac anomalies. Congenital abnormalities are twice as common as in singletons, especially in MZ twins (conjoined 1:200; acardia 1:100).
- Vanishing twin syndrome (results from demise of one twin in the first trimester: prognosis is generally good for remaining DZ twin).
- Perinatal mortality 36.7/1000 (singletons 8/1000; triplets 73/1000). Especially high in monochorionic monoamniotic MZ twins because of cord entanglement and cord accident.
- IUGR (less than 10th centile, incidence of 25–33%).
- Antepartum fetal demise: psychological sequelae and risk of DIC (25% incidence after 3 weeks with demise of both twins).
- Acute polyhydramnios is more common in MZ pregnancies (10–15% of all twin pregnancies but 4–35% of monochorionic diamniotic pregnancies) and twin-to-twin transfusion syndrome with placental arteriovascular anastamoses with unequal vascular distribution of blood.
  - The donor twin becomes anemic, hypovolemic, oligohydramniotic, and growth-restricted, and may develop hydrops.
  - The recipient becomes polycythemic, hypervolemic, and polyuric with polyhydramnios. Ascites and pleural and pericardial effusions may result.
  - Mortality of ≥80% (preterm labor and preterm premature rupture of membranes (pPROM) contributing); cord accident and death of the co-twin are other causes.

Complications of labor

Intrapartum

- Preterm labor is more common (43.6% before 37 weeks compared with 5.6% for singletons). Mean duration of pregnancy decreases as number of fetuses *in utero* increases. It is estimated that 3.6 weeks of gestation are lost for every extra fetus in the uterus in the first trimester.

- Increased risk of pulmonary edema with tocolysis (especially β-sympathomimetics).
- Cord prolapse following pPROM.
- Cord entanglement and knotting in monzygotics (perinatal mortality up to 50%); mortality from asphyxia for a twin is 4–5 times that for a singleton.
- Malpresentation (cephalic/cephalic, 40%; cephalic/breech, 40%; breech/breech, 10%; cephalic/transverse (TV), 5%; breech/TV, 4%; TV/TV, 1%).
- Increased risk of operative delivery, either as an elective procedure or as an emergency before or after delivery of the first twin.
- Risk of bleeding from undiagnosed vasa previa.
- Intrapartum twin entrapment (1:817 twin pregnancies, typically with MZ twins in breech/cephalic presentation).
- Risk of postpartum hemorrhage (10% twin versus 5% singletons).

Postpartum

- There is a higher incidence of postnatal depression in mothers of twins.
- Breast-feeding twins is physically and psychologically demanding.
- There may be financial difficulties. Support groups may be helpful.

Recommended further reading

1. Walters W (1995). Multiple pregnancy. In: Chamberlain GVP, ed. *Turnbull's Obstetrics* (2nd edn), pp. 329–52. Churchill Livingstone, Edinburgh.
2. Neilson JP (1995). Multiple pregnancy. In: Whitfield C, ed. *Dewhurst's Textbook of Obstetrics and Gynaecology for Postgraduates* (5th edn), pp. 439–54. Blackwell Science, Oxford.
3. American College of Obstetricians and Gynecologists (2004). Multiple gestation: complicated twin, triplet, and high-order multifetal pregnancy. ACOG Practice Bulletin No. 56. *Obstet Gynecol* **104**, 869–83.
4. Norwitz ER (1998). Multiple pregnancies: trends past, present and future. In: Diamond M, DeCherney A, eds. *The Infertility and Reproductive Medicine Clinics of North America*, pp. 351–69. WB Saunders, Philadelphia, PA.

Management of multiple pregnancies

Antenatal care

Although a wide range of practices are seen and are acceptable, there are some general guidelines that should be followed for the management of twin pregnancy.

- Chorionicity should be documented by ultrasound scan in the first trimester in view of increased risks to monochorionic twins.
- Iron and folate supplements are useful from the second trimester onward.
- More frequent antenatal visits to detect complications such as preeclampsia.
- Detailed fetal anomaly scan at 18–20 weeks and cardiac anomaly scan (fetal echocardiogram) at 22–24 weeks. There is no proven benefit from routine bed rest.
- No place for prophylactic cervical cerclage. Consider following serial cervical length (every 2 weeks from 18 through 30 weeks) with or without fetal fibronectin testing of cervicovaginal discharge (every 2 weeks from 24 through 34 weeks) in twin pregnancies at risk of preterm birth.
- Routine screening for gestational diabetes at 24–28 weeks' gestation.
- Fetal assessment includes serial ultrasound scanning for growth and confirmation of fetal wellbeing at 24, 28, 32, 34, and 36 weeks.
- Increase in fetal surveillance if complications develop, such as IUGR, preterm labor, or growth or amniotic fluid discordance. In contrast with IUGR (defined as less than 10th centile for gestational age), growth discordance is defined as greater than 25% difference in estimated fetal weight (larger minus smaller divided by larger x 100).
- Laser ablation of aberrant placental vessels is useful in twin-to-twin transfusion syndrome. Although the rate of fetal loss is reduced to 40–50% by such treatment, neurologic, cardiac, and renal sequelae are common in survivors.
- Nuchal translucency (NT) measurements for Down syndrome screening may be performed (serum screening is of more limited use in multiple pregnancies), with amniocentesis for confirmatory diagnosis.
- It is uncommon for twin pregnancies to be allowed to progress beyond 40 completed weeks. Labor is often induced prior to this for fetal or maternal reasons.

Labor and delivery

- Consider induction of labor for pregnancy complications.
- IV access.
- CBC and blood type group and save (increased risk of operative delivery and postpartum hemorrhage (PPH)).
- Continuous fetal monitoring in labor. When feasible, consider placing a fetal scalp electrode on the first twin to facilitate monitoring.
- Epidural anesthesia minimizes the risks of pushing prior to full cervical dilatation and enables operative procedures (such as internal podalic version or cesarean delivery) without resorting to general anesthesia.

- Consider active intervention to aid delivery of the second twin if the time between the deliveries exceeds 30 minutes.
- Experienced staff should be present at delivery, including a senior obstetrician, an anesthesiologist, a pediatrician, and a neonatal nurse.
- Recommended route of delivery depends on gestational age, presentation, growth concordance, operator experience, and the preference of the couple.
  - Vertex/vertex presentation: aim for vaginal delivery.
  - Presenting twin is nonvertex: elective cesarean delivery prior to labor or PROM.
  - Vertex/non-vertex presentation: optimum mode of delivery is uncertain. Although vaginal delivery is preferred, there are no randomized trials to confirm whether elective cesarean or vaginal delivery is safer. In this setting, spontaneous vaginal delivery of the first twin is followed by either external cephalic version or, more commonly, internal podalic version and breech extraction of the second twin. Vaginal breech delivery of the second twin appears safe if the following guidelines are followed: greater than 32 weeks' gestation, estimated fetal weight greater than 1500 grams, concordant growth between twins (or presenting vertex twin is larger), adequate anesthesia, capacity to perform emergent cesarean delivery, and experienced operator.
- An oxytocin infusion is recommended if there is uterine inertia, especially after delivery of the first twin (10 IU in 1 L of 0.9% saline solution to run at 1–2 mIU/min, increasing in doubling doses every 15–30 minutes to restore adequate uterine activity (i.e. three to four contractions lasting 40 seconds per 10 minutes)).
- Active management of the third stage with uterotonic agents is recommended by some authorities as a prophylactic measure against uterine atony. Continued administration of uterotonic agents (such as 20–40 IU oxytocin in 500 mL 0.9% saline solution to run over 3–4 hours) may prevent early postpartum hemorrhage.

Higher-order multiple deliveries

- Defined as triplets and more.
- The recommendation is to deliver by elective cesarean as there is increased morbidity and mortality, and problems with adequate fetal monitoring in labor.

Postnatal

Persistence with and help in establishing breast-feeding. Ensure extra help is available in the community, if required.

Recommended further reading

1. Crowther CA (1999). Multiple pregnancy. In: James DK, Steer PJ, Weiner CP, Gonik B, eds. *High Risk Pregnancy: Management Options* (2nd edn), pp. 129–53. WB Saunders, London.
2. Dodd JM, Crowther CA (2003). Reduction of the number of fetuses for women with triplet and higher order multiple pregnancies. *Cochrane Database Syst Rev* **2**, CD003932.

Breech presentation

Breech presentation is the most common malpresentation. The incidence of breech presentation is higher in early pregnancy: 40% at 20 weeks, 25% at 32 weeks, and only 3–4% by term. It is normal in pregnancy for the buttocks and feet to come to lie in the fundus, perhaps because the fundus has more space and the heavier head gravitates to the lower pole.

Conditions predisposing towards breech presentation include contracted pelvis, uterine anomaly, fibroid uterus, placenta previa, multiple pregnancies, polyhydramnios, oligohydramnios, fetal spina bifida (baby cannot kick well), fetal goiter (baby cannot flex its head), or a hydrocephalic baby (the 'lower segment' is too small). Ultrasound may show the cause and influence the management, although in the vast majority of cases no cause can be identified.

Types of breech presentation

The breech may present in one of three ways.

- Extended (or frank) breech presentation is the most common, i.e. flexed at the hips but extended at the knees, with the buttocks presenting to the pelvic inlet.
- Flexed (or complete) breech presentation where the fetus sits with hips and knees both flexed so that the presenting part is a mixture of buttocks, external genitalia, and feet.
- Footling breeches are the least common. One thigh is flexed and one is extended so that the foot or knee would descend first through the cervical os into the vagina. This type has the greatest risk of cord prolapse (5–10%).

The position of the fetus is described by using the sacrum as the denominator (the occiput is the denominator for a vertex presentation).

Diagnosis

Diagnosis should be made antenatally. The mother may complain of pain under the ribs. On palpation, the lie is longitudinal, a broad pole is felt in the pelvis, and there is a smooth, round mass (the head) that can be palpated and balloted in the fundal area. The fetal heart is best heard at the level of the umbilicus or above. If the diagnosis is uncertain in late pregnancy, vaginal examination may resolve it, but, if doubt still remains, an ultrasound examination should be performed.

Management of breech presentation

Breech presentation is associated with an increased risk of perinatal mortality and morbidity caused principally by prematurity, congenital malformations, and birth asphyxia from cord compression or trauma. Recent evidence supports a policy of elective cesarean delivery prior to labor or rupture of membranes for all singleton breech fetuses as a way of reducing the associated neonatal problems. Despite the large Canadian trial recommending elective cesarean delivery as safest for the baby, some mothers may elect to have a vaginal breech delivery. Breech presentation, whatever the mode of delivery, is a signal for potential fetal handicap, and this should influence antenatal, intrapartum, and neonatal management.

This section deals with management of the singleton breech. Breech presentation in a second twin constitutes a unique clinical situation and is dealt with elsewhere.

Reducing the incidence of breech presentations

External cephalic version (ECV) of the fetus from breech to vertex can be offered after 36 weeks. The benefits and risks of ECV at term should be explained to women with an uncomplicated singleton breech presentation at term. ECV is best carried out with the mother awake and facilities for emergency delivery should be available nearby. Cardiotocography should be done prior to ECV. Use of tocolysis and regional anesthesia should be considered, as both have been shown to improve the success of ECV. The breech is maneuvered through a forward (less commonly a backward) somersault to become a cephalic presentation if vaginal delivery is planned. There is compelling evidence that ECV at term increases the chances of a cephalic birth. With ECV at 36 weeks, there is an 80% reduction in the odds of a noncephalic presentation at birth and a reduction of over 50% in the rate of cesarean delivery. Anti-D immunoglobulin should be administered to women who are rhesus-negative and a Kleihauer–Betke test (acid elution test on maternal blood to estimate volume of feto-maternal hemorrhage) should be considered to detect the 1% who may need additional anti-D immunoglobulin (300 µg anti-D immunoglobulin will cover 30 mL of fetal whole blood or 15 mL of packed red blood cells in the maternal circulation).

- The overall success rate of ECV is of the order of 50%. Factors that increase the success rate of ECV include an earlier gestational age, multiparity, flexed breech presentation with spine lateral, adequate amniotic fluid volume, and a station of the breech above the brim.
- Contraindications to ECV include placenta previa, multiple pregnancy, antepartum hemorrhage, small-for-dates babies, and mothers with uterine scars, preeclampsia, or hypertension (risk of abruption is increased).
- Theoretical risks of ECV include placental separation (abruption), cord entanglement, premature rupture of the membranes, precipitation of labor, and transplacental hemorrhage with rhesus sensitization if the mother is rhesus-negative with a rhesus-positive baby.

Planning the mode of delivery

In situations where ECV was contraindicated, was declined, or failed, the policy for term singleton breech pregnancy management should be based on available evidence and the choice of the woman. If assisted vaginal delivery is preferred, there should be a careful selection of patients and extensive antepartum counseling.

- A trial of singleton vaginal breech delivery is more likely to be successful if both mother and baby are of normal proportions. The size of the fetus should be estimated to be between 2000 and 3500 g and gestational age greater than 32 weeks.
- The presentation should be either frank (hips flexed, knees extended) or complete (hips flexed, knees flexed, but feet not below the fetal buttocks). Ultrasound examination after 36 weeks is useful in confirming the above.
- There should be no evidence of feto-pelvic disproportion with a 'clinically adequate' pelvis on pelvimetry (although there is little evidence that objective measurement of pelvic size correlates with the chance of vaginal delivery). If imaging pelvimetry is required, computed tomography (CT) scanning may be preferable to X-ray because the radiation dose is less.
- Vaginal delivery should probably only be allowed when labor is spontaneous. Cesarean delivery is preferable to induction of labor in this setting.
- Whatever the indication, the most important factor in determining whether or not a singleton vaginal delivery is achievable is the efficiency of uterine activity producing cervical dilatation and descent of the breech.

Recommended further reading

1. Hutton E, Hofmeyr G (2006). External cephalic version for breech presentation before term. *Cochrane Database Syst Rev* **1**, CD000084.
2. American College of Obstetricians and Gynecologists (2002). ACOG Committee Opinion No. 265. Mode of term singleton breech delivery. *Int J Gynaecol Obstet* **77**, 65–6.
3. Hofmeyr G, Hannah ME (2003). Planned caesarean section for term breech delivery. *Cochrane Database Syst Rev* **3**, CD000166.
4. Hannah ME, Hannah WJ, Hewson SA, Hodnett ED, Saigal S, Willan AR (2000). Planned caesarean section versus planned vaginal birth for breech presentation at term: a randomised multicentre trial. Term Breech Trial Collaborative Group. *Lancet* **356**, 1375–83.
5. Hannah ME, Hannah WJ, Hodnett ED, *et al.* for the Term Breech Trial 3-Month Follow-up Collaborative Group (2002). Outcomes at 3 months after planned cesarean vs planned vaginal delivery for breech presentation at term: the international randomized Term Breech Trial. *JAMA* **287**, 1822–31.

Intrapartum and preterm breech management

When singleton vaginal breech delivery is planned, the mother should be advised to present as soon as labor starts or the membranes rupture. Vaginal examination is performed at the time of admission to exclude cord presentation. The length of labor is the same as in a vertex presentation. Epidural anesthesia is recommended.

Delivery technique

- At full cervical dilatation, the mother is encouraged to bear down when the buttocks and anus of the baby come into view over the mother's perineum without retraction.
- After an episiotomy is performed (under local infiltration in cases without epidural), the mother is encouraged to push the child to the level of the umbilicus. Every effort should be made by the obstetric care provider to avoid 'pulling' on the breech. This will lead to extension of the head and difficulty affecting delivery.
- Abducting the baby's hip joint and flexing the knee helps to deliver the legs. It is important to keep the back sacro-anterior.
- Bearing-down efforts with contractions are encouraged to help descent until the scapulae are visible.
- The arms may be delivered by adduction at the shoulder and flexion at the elbow. If this is unsuccessful, the Lovset maneuver can be carried out by holding the baby with the thumbs on the sacrum and index fingers on the anterior superior iliac spines. The baby is turned in a clockwise direction (to deliver the posterior shoulder by rotating it below the symphysis pubis) and then in an anticlockwise direction to enable descent of the opposite shoulder.
- The trunk is allowed to hang until the nape of the neck becomes visible. The trunk is then swung upwards through 180° until the mouth comes into view or the delivery achieved by either the Mauriceau–Smellie–Viet maneuver (a finger is placed in the mouth and two fingers over the maxilla to flex the head and deliver) or the application of specialized forceps for the aftercoming head.
- The mouth, nose, and pharynx are cleared of secretions as they come into view.

Management of the preterm breech

Management of preterm (less than 37 weeks) breech delivery is an area of clinical controversy. The poor outcome for very low birth weight infants is mainly related to complications of prematurity and probably not the mode of delivery. Despite this comment, however, vaginal delivery of the singleton preterm breech is generally discouraged.

Recommended further reading

1 American College of Obstetricians and Gynecologists (2002). ACOG Committee Opinion No. 265. Mode of term singleton breech delivery. *Int J Gynaecol Obstet* **77**, 65–6.

2. Hannah ME, Hannah WJ, Hewson SA, Hodnett ED, Saigal S, Willan AR (2000). Planned caesarean section versus planned vaginal birth for breech presentation at term: a randomised multicentre trial. Term Breech Trial Collaborative Group. *Lancet* **356**, 1375–83.

3. Hannah ME, Hannah WJ, Hodnett ED, *et al.* for the Term Breech Trial 3-Month Follow-up Collaborative Group (2002). Outcomes at 3 months after planned cesarean vs planned vaginal delivery for breech presentation at term: the international randomized Term Breech Trial. *JAMA* **287**, 1822–31.

Antepartum hemorrhage

Antepartum hemorrhage is defined as bleeding from the genital tract after the 20th week of pregnancy. It complicates 2–5% of all pregnancies and is an important cause of fetal and maternal morbidity and mortality. Dangerous causes are placental abruption, placenta previa, and vasa previa. Other causes include additional bleeding associated with a 'show' (blood loss associated with the release of the mucous plug from the cervix that occurs prior to the onset of labor), cervicitis, lower genital tract trauma, vulvovaginal varicosities, genital tumors, and infections.

Management

Women with antepartum hemorrhage should be admitted to a hospital with adequate facilities for transfusion, emergent cesarean delivery, and neonatal resuscitation. Initial management depends upon the severity, the cause of bleeding, and gestational age. Rhesus-negative women will require anti-D immunoglobulin.

- Resuscitation with IV fluids and blood product transfusion is the first priority in women who are hemodynamically unstable. IV access should be secured in all patients with two large-bore (size 14) IV cannulae.
- History and examination are important to determine the likely cause of the bleeding and evaluate the patient's general condition.
  - Digital vaginal examination should be avoided until placenta previa has been excluded by ultrasound.
  - In those with minimal bleeding, speculum examination after an ultrasound examination to exclude placenta previa may help to identify local causes of bleeding.

Investigations

- Take blood for CBC, blood type and antibody screen, and blood cross-matching.
- If placental abruption is suspected, a coagulation profile and urea and electrolytes should also be performed.
- If the woman is rhesus-negative, send off a Kleihauer–Betke test (acid elution test on maternal blood to estimate the volume of feto-maternal hemorrhage).
- Arrange an ultrasound scan to exclude placenta previa. A major placental abruption with placental separation may be seen on ultrasound, but if seen on ultrasound, will usually be clinically obvious based on symptoms and signs. Ultrasound should only be done only when maternal and fetal conditions are stable.

Placenta previa

The placenta is partly or completely inserted in the lower uterine segment. This complicates 0.5% of pregnancies. The cause of placenta previa (PP) is unknown, but it is more common in older women, multipara, after a previous cesarean delivery, in smokers, and in women with a previous history of placenta previa (recurrence risk of 4–8%). Only 3–5% of women with a low-lying placenta seen on the midtrimester ultrasound scan will have placenta previa at term (the lower uterine segment develops in the second half of pregnancy). Placenta previa is classified as major (type III and IV) and minor (type I and II) (Fig. 2.1).

- In type I, the placenta is low but does not reach the cervical os.
- In type II, the placenta reaches the cervical os.
- In type III, the placenta partially covers the cervical os.
- In type IV, the placenta covers the os completely.

Maternal and fetal risks

- Placenta previa carries risks to the mother from massive obstetric hemorrhage (including postpartum hemorrhage), complications of surgery and anesthesia, air embolism, and postpartum sepsis.
- The major risk to the fetus is from iatrogenic preterm birth, but there is also an increased incidence of congenital malformation, malpresentation, fetal anemia, and cord complications. Placenta previa is not associated with IUGR.

Presentation and diagnosis

Presentation is usually as unprovoked painless vaginal bleeding or bleeding after sexual intercourse. Without routine scanning, one in six cases present for the first time in labor. Malpresentation is common. The uterus is soft and non-tender (although abruption can occur in women with placenta previa).

Diagnosis is as follows:

- Avoid vaginal examination as this may cause catastrophic bleeding.
- Ultrasound scanning is safe and generally reliable, although false-negative scans occur in 7% of cases. The latter are more common when the placenta is posterior, the bladder is full, the fetal head obscures the low edge of placenta, or the sonographer is inexperienced.
- Magnetic resonance imaging (MRI) may be useful to investigate the degree to which the placenta extends into the myometrium, especially in cases of posterior placenta previa.
- Where there is still doubt at term and bleeding has stopped, the diagnosis can be confirmed or excluded by performing a gentle pelvic examination in the operating room. This is known as a 'double set-up' examination, as a second surgical team should be scrubbed and prepared to perform an emergent cesarean delivery in the event of excessive bleeding.

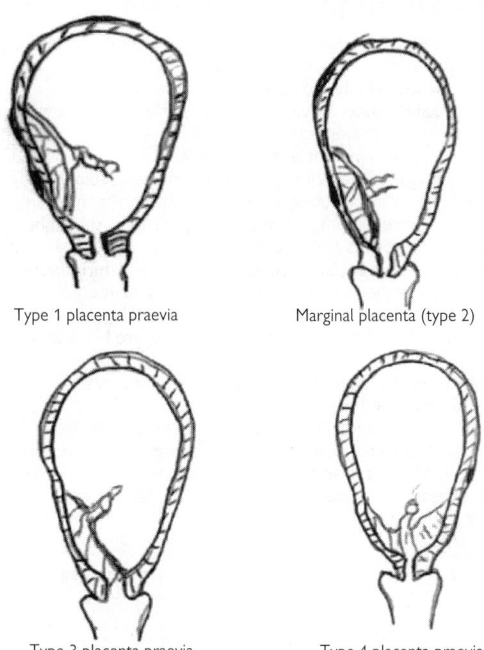

Fig. 2.1 Different types of placenta previa.

Management of placenta previa

Management depends on the clinical condition of the mother and fetus, the type of placenta previa, and gestational age.

- Antenatal corticosteroids should be given to women who are threatening to deliver under 34 weeks of gestation to help promote fetal lung maturity and prevent bleeding into the brain (intraventricular hemorrhage) and bowel (necrotizing enterocolitis).
- Immediate resuscitation and delivery is required if the bleeding does not settle down or is causing maternal or fetal compromise. In the absence of such conditions, elective cesarean delivery should be recommended at 36 weeks after confirmation of fetal lung maturity (or electively at 37 weeks if the patient declines fetal lung maturity testing).
- Hospitalization and expectant management is usually advised for patients with types III and IV placenta previa if the bleeding is not life-threatening and the fetus is not mature. A wide-bore IV cannula should be inserted and 4 units of blood made available for transfusion in the event that bleeding becomes excessive. This conservative management is continued until 36 weeks.
- Delivery for types III and IV placenta previa is always by elective cesarean, which should be performed by an experienced obstetrician. The woman should be counseled about the possibility of hysterectomy if placenta accreta is encountered or uncontrolled bleeding occurs. This is more likely when there has been a previous cesarean and the placenta is anterior.

Vaginal delivery may be possible in women with minor degrees of placenta previa.

Recommended further reading

1. Neilson JP (2003). Interventions for suspected placenta previa. *Cochrane Database Syst Rev* **2**, CD001998.

Placental abruption ('accidental hemorrhage')

Placental abruption is bleeding following premature separation of normally situated placenta. The incidence varies from 0.43% to 1.8%. It may be revealed (with vaginal bleeding (80%)) or concealed (with no bleeding (20%)). The cause is unknown in the majority of cases. It can be caused by direct trauma (such as a motor vehicle accident) or sudden decompression of the uterus after rupture of membranes in patients with polyhydramnios or multiple pregnancy. Abruption is more frequent where there is maternal hypertension or a history of placental abruption in the present or past pregnancies. It is more common in older women, those of high parity, cigarette smokers, substance abusers, and anemic patients.

Maternal and fetal risks

- Cases severe enough to produce coagulopathy are associated with a maternal mortality rate of 1%. Complications for the mother include hypovolemic shock, acute renal failure, DIC, postpartum hemorrhage, and feto-maternal hemorrhage.
- For the fetus, perinatal mortality varies from 4% to 68% depending on neonatal facilities and the size of abruption. IUGR and preterm delivery are common. Anemia and coagulopathy may occur as complications.

Presentation and diagnosis

Presentation is as abdominal pain with or without vaginal bleeding and uterine contractions, uterine tenderness, and non-reassuring fetal testing ('fetal distress'). The pain is typically sharp, severe, and sudden in onset. In severe cases, there may be signs of shock, increasing abdominal girth, or a rising fundal height, and the uterus is described as irritable and tender, which may later become woody and hard. Signs of shock may be out of proportion to the observed blood loss. Posterior abruptions may present as backache. The fetus may be difficult to palpate or monitor. Fetal compromise or death may follow. Up to 50% of cases are in labor at the time of presentation. If the membranes are ruptured, bloodstained ('port wine') amniotic fluid may be seen.

Diagnosis is usually made on clinical grounds. Ultrasonography is not an accurate diagnostic tool for placental abruption, because a minimum of 300 mL blood clot needs to be present before the retroperitoneal collection can be reliably visualized by ultrasound. However, ultrasound may be useful in cases of minor abruption for monitoring fetal wellbeing and amniotic fluid volume.

Management

Management depends on the severity, associated complications, maternal and fetal condition, and gestational age.

- Immediate delivery is required in severe cases, whether the fetus is alive or dead. Vaginal delivery (by induction or allowing labor to continue) is usually preferred if the fetus is already dead or where there is no evidence of maternal or fetal compromise. However, cesarean delivery is required in 15–25% of cases.
- DIC occurs in 5% of cases, and this must be diagnosed and aggressively treated before any operative procedures are undertaken.
- The prognosis for the fetus following a significant abruption is inversely proportional to the length of time from bleed to delivery, and the fetal condition may deteriorate with little warning. Gestational age is also an important determinant of perinatal outcome.
- Conservative management after 34 weeks' gestation should only be undertaken for minor degrees of bleeding. In such cases, the pregnancy should be regarded as high risk, followed with serial ultrasound scans to monitor growth, and delivery affected by 40 weeks.
- There is also an increased risk of postpartum hemorrhage in such cases.
- Postpartum management after a large abruption is supportive with regular monitoring of urine output, blood pressure and pulse, and coagulation profile.
- The recurrence rate of severe placental abruption in a subsequent pregnancy is of the order of 10%.

Acute abdominal pain related to pregnancy

Abdominal pain is a common complaint during pregnancy. The most common cause is the physiological onset of labor. Labor pain is intermittent and associated with uterine contractions. When these occur with cervical dilatation and descent of the presenting part, the diagnosis is usually straightforward, but this may be preceded by a latent phase of variable length. Remember that pathological causes of abdominal pain such as placental abruption may precipitate labor. Other physiological causes of abdominal pain during pregnancy include musculoskeletal pain from round ligament stretching and symphysis pubis pain.

Pathological condition related to pregnancy

- *Early pregnancy complications* such as ectopic pregnancy and miscarriage are discussed on 📖 *p.486* and *p.62*, respectively.
- *Placental abruption* occurs in 0.5–1% of all pregnancies. There is separation of the placenta and retroplacental and decidual bleeding. The patient usually presents with sudden onset of abdominal pain with or without vaginal bleeding and uterine irritability. If the placenta is posterior, symptoms of backache may predominate. On palpation, the uterus is tender and palpation of fetal parts may be difficult because of uterine irritability and increased uterine tone. Retroplacental bleeding may be seen on ultrasound, but is a late finding and the diagnosis in these cases has usually already been made clinically. The presence of a retroplacental collection on ultrasound suggests the presence of at least 300 mL blood. Abruption may lead to coagulopathy (33–50% of severe cases) and fetal death (up to 60%). PPH is also common.
- *Uterine leiomyoma.* Uterine fibroids may cause severe abdominal pain in pregnancy as a result of ischemia ('red degeneration') or when a pedunculated fibroid undergoes torsion. The mainstays of management are pain relief (parenteral if needed) and bed rest, as most cases are due to 'red degeneration' and will resolve with time. Rarely, the pain may be severe enough to require laparotomy for diagnosis and treatment.
- *Chorioamnionitis.* Although preterm rupture of the membranes (PROM) usually precedes chorioamnionitis, infection may be present without ruptured membranes and cause abdominal pain. Classic clinical signs include maternal tachycardia, maternal fever, fetal tachycardia, uterine contractions, and tenderness to palpation, and rarely a foul discharge emanating from the cervical os.
- *Uterine rupture.* Rupture of the gravid uterus is rare (overall risk approximately 1:1500 deliveries). It usually occurs during labor, but may precede it. It is associated with a high fetal mortality (30%) and significant maternal mortality (5%). Most cases are due to rupture of a prior cesarean scar, but it can also occur in cases of pregnancy developing in a rudimentary uterine horn, with excessive oxytocin use, in obstructed labor, with high parity, and following other surgical trauma (such as previous uterine perforation or transmural

myomectomy). Rupture of the uterus should be suspected in women at risk who present with constant abdominal pain, uterine tenderness, fresh vaginal bleeding, and nonreassuring fetal testing ('fetal distress') with or without maternal shock. The management should be aggressive fluid/blood product resuscitation followed by urgent cesarean delivery and repair of the uterus or hysterectomy.

- *Severe uterine torsion.* The uterus rotates axially by 30°–40° to the right in 80% of normal pregnancies (because of the location of the sigmoid colon in the left lower quadrant). Torsion may occur when this rotation extends beyond 90°, causing severe abdominal pain, shock, a tense uterus, and urinary retention. It typically occurs in the later half of pregnancy. In 80–90% of cases there is a predisposing factor such as a fibroid, congenital uterine anomaly, adnexal mass, or a history of pelvic adhesions. Maternal vasovagal shock and possible nonreassuring fetal testing ('fetal distress') are the main risks of severe uterine torsion. The diagnosis is suggested by a displaced urethra on catheterization. Conservative management is by analgesia and altering maternal position, but laparotomy and cesarean delivery may be required in cases that do not resolve with conservative management.
- *Ovarian tumors.* Ovarian cysts have the potential risk of torsion, rupture, or hemorrhage, which may cause severe abdominal pain, especially when torsion leads to infarction. Once ovarian torsion is diagnosed, a laparotomy should be carried out. If the adnexum appears necrotic, it should probably be removed, taking care not to 'untwist' it (because of the theoretical risk of a venous thromboembolic event). Ovarian cystectomy can be carried out if the adnexum appears viable.

Acute abdominal pain unrelated to pregnancy

- *Acute appendicitis* complicates about 1 in 1000 pregnancies. There is no increase in incidence during pregnancy but mortality is higher. During pregnancy, the cecum and appendix are displaced upwards and to the right with advancing gestation. The pain is less well localized and tenderness, rebound tenderness, and guarding are less obvious. This leads to delay in diagnosis and treatment and an increased incidence of perforation (15–20% of cases), peritonitis, and sepsis. When perforation occurs, maternal and fetal mortality reach 17% and 43%, respectively (compared with 5–10% for simple appendicitis). Ultrasound scan may be of value in excluding degenerating fibroids, twisted ovarian cysts, ureteric obstruction, and placental abruption. Early surgical referral and laparotomy by an experienced surgeon is essential.
    - In the first trimester, this can be through McBurney's (muscle splitting) incision; in the second and third trimester, a right paramedian incision at the site of maximum tenderness should be used. This incision can be extended if the appendix is displaced further upwards than expected or if a cesarean delivery is required.
- *Cholecystitis*. Gallstones grow rapidly during pregnancy because of biliary stasis. Acute cholecystitis complicates about 1 in 1000 pregnancies. Presentation is with sudden onset of right upper quadrant or epigastric colicky pain with associated nausea, vomiting, and fever. Jaundice is uncommon. It is important to differentiate cholecystitis from severe preeclampsia, acute fatty liver of pregnancy, and appendicitis. The diagnosis can be made on the basis of the clinical features, biochemical tests, and the presence of stones in the biliary tree on ultrasound scan. Treatment uses the appropriate antibiotics, adequate analgesia, and fluids. Where possible, cholecystectomy is deferred until after the puerperium.
- *Intestinal obstruction* occurs in 1 in 2500–3500 pregnancies. Sixty percent of cases are due to adhesions. Other causes include volvulus, intussception, hernia, and complications of inflammatory bowel disease. The presentation is usually in the second or third trimester with colicky abdominal pain, nausea, vomiting, constipation, and abdominal distension. The diagnosis can be made by observation of distended loops of bowel with fluid levels on erect and supine abdominal X-rays. Like appendicitis, delay in diagnosis is common and carries maternal and fetal mortality rates of 10–20% and 30–50%, respectively. Conservative management is by nasogastric suction, IV fluids, and analgesia but a midline laparotomy may be required to correct the cause of the obstruction. Cesarean delivery can be carried out at the same time if pregnancy is sufficiently advanced. Careful attention to fluid and electrolyte balance is essential.
- *Crohn's disease*. Patients complain of abdominal pain, diarrhea, anemia, and weight loss. Rectal bleeding and the passage of mucus may occur. Rectal bleeding by itself is more likely to be due to hemorrhoids in pregnancy. The diagnosis is confirmed by sigmoidoscopy and rectal biopsy. Treatment is as in nonpregnant patients, and sulfasalazine and steroids should be continued during pregnancy.

- *Peptic ulceration.* Pregnancy reduces the risk of peptic ulceration. However, acute upper abdominal/epigastric pain may rarely be caused by a perforated peptic ulcer. Management is by laparotomy and repair.
- *Acute pancreatitis.* Acute pancreatitis is rare in pregnancy (1 in 4000 pregnancies). The presentation is with upper abdominal pain radiating into the back and associated with vomiting. Raised serum concentrations of amylase (nonspecific) and lipase (specific) will confirm the diagnosis. Management is by IV fluid and electrolyte replacement, suppression of pancreatic activity, analgesia, antibiotics, and nasogastric suction. Laparotomy and definitive surgery are rarely indicated, but may be required if conservative treatment fails.
- *Acute pyelonephritis* occurs in 1–2% of pregnant women. Obstructive uropathy and stasis are predisposing factors. The diagnosis is made by clinical features (fever, flank tenderness, urinary frequency) and positive culture from midstream urine. Ultrasound findings may show hydronephrosis. Treatment should be as an inpatient with IV antibiotics, fluids, and adequate analgesia.
- *Urolithiasis* occurs in 0.03–0.5% of pregnancies. Urinary calculi in pregnancy normally present with sudden-onset abdominal pain that is severe enough to warrant hospital admission. Hematuria and evidence of a renal calculus on ultrasound will confirm the diagnosis. Ultrasound examination may also demonstrate hydronephrosis. An associated urinary tract infection should be excluded. IV urography for the purpose of diagnosis is not contraindicated at any stage of pregnancy. The management should be conservative with IV fluids, antibiotics, and effective analgesia. If a calculus is large enough to cause persistent ureteric obstruction, surgery may be required.
- *Acute fatty liver of pregnancy.* This occurs in 1 in 10 000–15 000 pregnancies. The symptoms are sudden abdominal pain, nausea, vomiting, and jaundice. The serum bilirubin is raised with abnormal liver enzymes and associated leukocytosis, thrombocytopenia, and coagulation defects. Profound hypoglycemia is a hallmark of this disease and is often resistant to treatment. The management is correction of fluid, electrolyte, and coagulation abnormalities and prompt delivery. This disorder carries a high maternal and perinatal mortality.
- *Severe preeclampsia* and HELLP syndrome may present with epigastric pain due to distension or hemorrhage stretching the liver capsule. This is discussed on 🕮 *p.74*.

Miscellaneous causes of abdominal pain unrelated to pregnancy

- Sickle cell crises in women who have homozygous SS or sickle cell disease can present with acute abdominal pain during crises.
- Porphyria and malaria may present with abdominal pain.
- Bleeding into the rectus muscle and subsequent rectus sheath hematoma formation following rupture of a branch of inferior epigastric vessels may be caused by coughing or trauma. This may cause sudden and severe abdominal pain.
- Rare conditions resulting in intraabdominal hemorrhage can cause acute abdominal pain in pregnancy. These include rupture of uteroovarian veins, rupture of aneurysms (splenic, hepatic, renal, aortic), and rupture of uterine veins requiring urgent laparotomy. These cases will present with clinical symptoms and signs suggestive of intraabdominal bleeding.

Preterm labor

Preterm labor is defined as the onset of labor prior to 37 weeks of gestation. The incidence of preterm delivery is around 7–10%, although a proportion of these deliveries (around 20%) will be iatrogenic.

Causes and prevention

Certain groups of women are at particular risk of preterm labor. Multiple pregnancies account for a growing proportion of such deliveries since the advent of modern methods of assisted conception. These pregnancies have their own particular determinants of risk, and are dealt with on 📖 *p.78*.

- Those with a *previous history of preterm labor* should be considered at risk of recurrence and the events surrounding their previous delivery should be carefully examined for any indicators of causation. At particular risk are those whose history suggests cervical insufficiency (cervical incompetence), in whom the risk of recurrence is of the order of 15–30%. Risk factors for cervical insufficiency include previous cervical surgery, *in utero* exposure to diethylstilbestrol (DES), recurrent late second trimester miscarriage, or a rapid painless progression to full dilatation. The use of elective cervical cerclage to reduce the risk of preterm delivery should be considered.
  - The MacDonald (without reflecting the bladder upwards) or Shirodkar (after dissecting the bladder upwards) techniques are the most commonly utilized cervical suture techniques, and are both performed transvaginally.
  - Abdominal cerclage is a reasonable option for women in whom a prior transvaginal cerclage has failed or is technically impossible to place. It is a more morbid procedure, requiring a laparotomy and elective cesarean delivery. As such, it is only used as a last resort.
  - All cerclage procedures carry risks, such as iatrogenic prelabor rupture of membranes or of inducing preterm labor or spontaneous abortion.
  - Clinical trials to assess the benefits of cervical cerclage are always confounded by the difficulties of differentiating cervical insufficiency from other precipitants of preterm delivery. However, the evidence suggests that, with careful case selection, prophylactic cervical cerclage can result in improved perinatal outcome in those with cervical insufficiency, but there is no evidence supporting the use of cervical cerclage in the presence of preterm labor.
- *Infection* is likely to play a significant part in the onset or promotion of preterm labor in many cases, and bacterial vaginosis is recognized as a contributory factor in a proportion of cases of preterm labor.
  - There is no evidence that screening for and treating bacterial vaginosis in asymptomatic high-risk women provides any reduction in the preterm delivery rate or any improvement in perinatal outcome.

- Pregnancies complicated by *polyhydramnios* are at risk of preterm labor. Women with this complication should be counseled accordingly and management tailored to take account of this risk. Amnioreduction (removal of several liters of amniotic fluid) may improve patient symptoms, but is associated with premature rupture of membranes and placental abruption. Moreover, the fluid tends to reaccumulate within a matter of days.
- *Placental abruption* may precipitate preterm labor. Significant placental abruption may result in acute fetal and/or maternal compromise necessitating precipitant delivery regardless of gestational age. Lesser clinically evident abruption may permit at least temporary conservative management to permit the promotion of fetal maturity. The only evidence of a silent abruption may be threatened preterm labor. Therefore this possibility should always be considered in women with spurious preterm labor, as the presence of placental abruption may result in isoimmunization of the rhesus-negative mother or in adverse pregnancy outcome (such as late intrauterine death or IUGR). Therefore appropriate investigation and follow-up is important in these women, even after the acute threat of preterm labor is over.
- The presence of *extrauterine irritants* may precipitate preterm labor, and signs of its onset should be anticipated and tocolysis considered if required. Relatively common precipitants may include intraabdominal surgery, appendicitis, or severe urinary tract infection.

Recommended further reading

1. Norwitz ER, Robinson JN, Challis JRG (1999). The control of labor. *N Eng J Med* **341**, 660–666.
2. Lockwood CJ, Kuczynski E (1999). Markers of risk for preterm delivery. *J Perinatal Medicine* **27**, 5–20.
3. Medical Research Council/Royal College of Obstetricians and Gynaecologists (1988). Multicentre randomized trial of cervical cerclage. Interim report. *Br J Obstet Gynaecol* **95**, 437–45.
4. Iams JD, Goldenberg RL, Meis PJ, *et al.* (1996). The length of the cervix and the risk of spontaneous premature delivery. *N Eng J Med* **334**, 567–72.
5. Medical Research Council/Royal College of Obstetricians and Gynaecologists (1988). Multicentre randomized trial of cervical cerclage. Interim report. *Br J of Obstet Gynaecol* **95**, 437–45.

Diagnosis and management of preterm labor

Preterm labor is diagnosed when regular uterine contractions and progressive cervical shortening and dilatation occur prior to 37 weeks of gestation.

- Contractions are typically regular and/or painful. Cervical dilatation in the absence of significant uterine contractions suggests cervical insufficiency. Conversely, contractions in the absence of cervical change constitute preterm contractions (or threatened preterm labor). The prediction of preterm labor would clearly provide benefits in the provision of appropriate care.
- The fetal fibronectin (fFN) test, which determines levels of fetal fibronectin in cervical mucus, may give some assistance in determining those most at risk of delivery within the next 7–14 days. A positive fFN test (>50 ng/mL) is associated with only a 23% risk of delivery prior to 35 weeks. However, the test has a high negative predictive value. More than 99% of women with a negative fFN (≤50 ng/mL) will still be pregnant in one week and 98% will still be pregnant in 2 weeks. Therefore this test can prevent unnecessary hospitalization and obstetric intervention.
- The assessment of cervical length at 18–32 weeks' gestation in women at high risk has been shown to be predictive of preterm birth. The shorter the residual cervical length on transvaginal ultrasound, the higher the risk of spontaneous preterm birth. Funneling of the internal os during a maternal Valsalva maneuver may also be a risk factor for preterm birth. Such measurements can be used alone or in conjunction with fFN testing.

Management

The mainstays of management of preterm labor involve the promotion of fetal maturity with consideration of causative factors endangering the mother or fetus. Prompt assessment of mother and fetus is required in the presence of preterm labor.

- Signs of acute fetal or maternal compromise may require immediate delivery regardless of the gestational age. Such situations would include maternal hemodynamic instability in the presence of placental abruption, clinical signs of established chorioamnionitis, or evidence of acute fetal compromise at a gestation compatible with neonatal viability (e.g. after 24–26 weeks, depending on neonatal facilities).
- In the absence of the above problems, attempts to arrest the progress of labor to improve fetal maturity may be appropriate, but tocolysis (see later) is unlikely to be successful in advanced labor with regular or painful contractions.

- Antenatal corticosteroid administration (betamethasone 12 mg IM every 24 hours x 2 doses or dexamethazone 6 mg IM every 12 hours x 4 doses) should be offered to all women at high risk of delivering prior to 34 weeks' gestation. Oral prednisone is not acceptable as it does not cross the placenta to any significant extent. Antenatal steroids have been shown to decrease the risks of respiratory distress syndrome, intraventricular hemorrhage, and necrotizing enterocolitis by 50% in infants born before 34 weeks. The effect is maximal 48 hours after the first dose and last for at least 7 days, but some effect is seen after just 4 hours exposure.

Recommended further reading

1. Norwitz ER, Robinson JN, Challis JRG (1999). The control of labor. *N Eng J Med* **341**, 660–6.
2. Lockwood, CJ, Kuczynski E (1999). Markers of risk for preterm delivery. *J Perinat Med* **27**, 5–20.
3. Iams JD, Goldenberg RL, Meis PJ, *et al.* (1996). The length of the cervix and the risk of spontaneous premature delivery. *N Eng J Med* **334**, 567–72.
4. Lockwood CJ, Senyei AE, Dische MR, *et al.* (1991). Fetal fibronectin in cervical and vaginal secretions as a predictor of preterm delivery. *N Eng J Med* **325**, 669–74.
5. National Institutes of Health (1994). Effect of antenatal steroids for fetal maturation on perinatal outcomes. *NIH Consensus Statement* **12**, pp. 1–24.
6. American College of Obstetricians and Gynecologists (2003). ACOG Practice Bulletin No. 43. Management of preterm labor. *Int J Gynaecol Obstet* **82**, 127–35.

Tocolysis and preterm labor

Tocolysis should be considered if there are no contraindications to its use and delivery is not imminent. The primary aim of tocolysis is to allow time for the antenatal corticosteroids to take effect. There is little evidence that outcome is further improved by prolonging tocolysis beyond 48 hours after steroid administration. Indeed, as most tocolytic drugs have significant side effects of varying severity (e.g. pulmonary edema with β-sympathomimetics), their prolonged use should generally be discouraged. Bed rest, while often recommended, has not been shown to prevent preterm birth.

The choice of optimal tocolytic drug remains the subject of much research. The most commonly used drugs and their complications are detailed below.

- *Magnesium sulfate*. This membrane stabilizer has long been used as a tocolytic. No advantages in efficacy have been demonstrated above those of ritodrine or nifedipine, and fetal and maternal nervous system suppression may occur. The therapeutic range of serum concentration is relatively narrow, and toxicity may occur at varying levels in different women. Magnesium has to be administered intravenously, as it is not absorbed orally (hence milk of magnesium to treat constipation).
- *Nifedipine*. In addition to its effect on vascular smooth muscle, this calcium-channel blocker also reduces myometrial contractility. There is good evidence for its effectiveness as a tocolytic, both in the acute phase of preterm labor and, more recently, in the further prolongation of pregnancy beyond 48 hours (maintenance tocolysis). Again, however, its use in either capacity has not been shown to definitively improve perinatal outcome. Its side effects are generally minimal and include headaches, flushing, and hypotension. It is administered orally, with a starting dose of 10 mg every 8 hours, switching to nifedipine XL 30 mg daily once control of contractions is achieved (various studies have used differing regimens, but the dosages have been broadly similar to this).
- *β-Sympathomimetics*. IV ritodrine hydrochloride is the only drug approved by the US Food and Drug Administration (FDA) for the treatment of preterm labor. However, because of its side-effect profile, it is no longer available in North America. Its use resulted in prolongation of pregnancy by up to 48 hours in a significant proportion of women with preterm labor, but it had not been shown to result in significant improvement in perinatal mortality or morbidity. Its complications included maternal tachycardia, arrhythmias, cardiac ischemia, hyperglycemia, hypokalemia, hyponatremia, tremor, and pulmonary edema. Hence it was poorly tolerated by many women. Relative contraindications to its use included multiple pregnancy, diabetes mellitus, antepartum hemorrhage, and preeclampsia. Another β-sympathomimetic agent, terbutaline, is still available and is commonly used. It too has not been shown to delay delivery by longer than 48 hours and has not been shown to significantly improve perinatal outcome. Its side effect profile is similar to that of ritodrine.

- *Glyceryl trinitrate patches.* These nitric oxide donors result in a reduction in uterine muscle contractility. Their efficacy is less well tested than that of other tocolytic agents, although a number of studies have demonstrated reasonable tocolysis with improved tolerance in comparison. They are rarely used as a first-line tocolytic agent. Their main side effects are severe headache, tachycardia, and flushing. A 5 mg patch may be replaced by a 10 mg patch if contractions are not controlled after 2 hours. Once effective control is achieved, the patch requires changing after 24 hours.
- *Indomethacin.* This nonselective cyclooxygenase inhibitor acts as an antiprostaglandin to reduce the stimulation and promotion of preterm labor. It may also help to reduce the threat of preterm labor in women with significant polyhydramnios by additionally reducing fetal renal output. Although effective, use of this agent is limited by adverse effects on the fetus. Its complications include premature closure of the fetal ductus arteriosus (with resultant persistent pulmonary hypertension) and oligohydramnios. It is administered orally or as rectal suppositories (1–3 mg/kg body weight of the mother). Use for greater than 48 hours in the latter half of pregnancy should be followed by serial fetal echocardiography looking for closure of the ductus arteriosus and pulmonary hypertension.
- *Oxytocin antagonist.* Atosiban, a selective oxytocin receptor antagonist, is a newer agent available for delay of labor. Clinical trials have suggested efficacy similar to that of β-sympathomimetics, but with fewer treatment discontinuations because of very much reduced side effects and no adverse events.

Progesterone supplementation starting at 16–24 weeks has been shown to prevent preterm birth in approximately one-third of women at risk of premature delivery by virtue of a prior preterm birth. Its efficacy has not yet been systematically tested in other high-risk subgroups or in women at low risk. The most common regimen is 17 α-hydroxy progesterone caproate 250 mg intramuscularly each week from 16–20 through 36 weeks. There is no evidence that progesterone administration can delay delivery in women presenting with acute preterm labor.

Recommended further reading

1. Gyetvai K, Hannah ME, Hodnett ED, Ohlsson A (1999). Tocolytics for preterm labour: a systematic review. *Obstet Gynecol* **94**, 869–77.
2. Smith P, Anthony J, Johanson R (2000). Nifedipine in pregnancy. *Br J Obstet Gynaecol* **107**, 299–307.
3. Gaunekar NN, Crowther CA (2004). Maintenance therapy with calcium channel blockers for preventing preterm birth after threatened preterm labour. *Cochrane Database Syst Rev* **3**, CD004071.
4. Sosa C, Althabe F, Belizan J, Bergel E (2004). Bed rest in singleton pregnancies for preventing preterm birth. *Cochrane Database Syst Rev* **1**, CD003581.
5. Kiong JF, Flenady VJ, Papatsonis DN, Dekker GA, Carbonne B (2003). Calcium channel blockers for inhibiting preterm labour. *Cochrane Database Syst Rev* **1**, CD002255.
6. Crowther CA, Hiller JE, Doyle LW (2002). Magnesium sulphate for preventing preterm birth in threatened preterm labour. *Cochrane Database Syst Rev* **4**, CD001060.

Diagnosis of preterm premature rupture of membranes

Premature rupture of membranes (PROM) refers to spontaneous rupture of the fetal membranes prior to the onset of labor, and can occur at any gestational age. Preterm PROM (pPROM) refers to PROM prior to 37 weeks' gestation.

Causes/risk groups

pPROM may be precipitated by a number of factors. An inflammatory process, particularly infective in origin, may alter the composition of the amnion or chorion or the intraamniotic pressure may be raised, e.g. in the presence of polyhydramnios or uterine irritability. Therefore the conditions that predispose to pPROM are as follows:

- Invasive procedures (such as amniocentesis).
- Uterine overdistention due to polyhydramnios or multiple pregnancy.
- A previous history of pPROM.
- Vaginal bleeding, even bleeding remote from presentation (which appears to weaken the membranes).
- Uterine anomaly.
- Lower genital tract infection with *Chlamydia* or bacterial vaginosis (particularly with a history of previous pPROM or preterm labor).
- Intraamniotic infection (chorioamnionitis).
- Chronic steroid therapy.

Women with these conditions should be considered at risk of pPROM and advised to self-present if they suspect that this has occurred. There is evidence that women with bacterial vaginosis and a previous history of preterm labor or pPROM may have their recurrence risk reduced by treatment of bacterial vaginosis (metronidazole is the drug of choice, with better results than clindamycin cream). Chlamydial infection should always be treated if it is detected, along with contact tracing.

Diagnosis

It is important that an accurate diagnosis is made as women with pPROM require careful surveillance until delivery to detect and treat infection or fetal compromise promptly. Conversely, it would be unfortunate to subject a woman to such close surveillance and potential prolonged hospitalization on the basis of a false-positive diagnosis.

- If the history is suggestive of pPROM (gush or trickling of fluid vaginally remote from micturition), a clean speculum examination should be performed looking for pooling of amniotic fluid in the upper vagina or trickling from the cervical os. (A digital examination should be avoided for fear of introducing infection.) This may be assisted by performing the examination when the woman has been semisupine for a period of time to allow pooling of amniotic fluid and by use of a maternal Valsalva maneuver to increase intraabdominal pressure.
- Cord prolapse should be excluded. High vaginal and endocervical swabs can be taken for detection of *Chlamydia* by ELISA (enzyme-linked immunosorbent assay) and culture.

Recommended further reading

1. Bengtson JM, Van Marter LJ, Barss VA, Greene MF, Tuomala RE, Epstein MF (1989). Pregnancy outcome after premature rupture of the membranes at or before 26 weeks' gestation. *Obstet Gynecol* **73**, 921–7.
2. Grieg PC (1998). The diagnosis of intrauterine infection in women with preterm premature rupture of the membranes (PPROM). *Clin Obstet Gynecol* **41**, 849–63.
3. American College of Obstetricians and Gynecologists (1998). ACOG Practice Bulletin No. 1. Premature rupture of membranes. *Int J Gynaecol Obstet* **63**, 75–84.

Management of preterm premature rupture of membranes

- *Tocolysis.* Once pPROM is confirmed, labor may intervene spontaneously. This is most likely in the first 48 hours. Tocolysis in the presence of ruptured membranes should only be undertaken with extreme caution and in the absence of any evidence of infection, and in cases of extreme prematurity or at the lower bounds of viability. Short-term (48 hours) tocolysis may allow for the administration of antenatal corticosteroids to diminish the risk of respiratory distress syndrome, intraventricular hemorrhage, and necrotizing enterocolitis.
- *Oligohydramnios.* The more severe the degree of oligohydramnios at presentation, the shorter the latency period (time from pPROM to delivery). In those in whom pPROM occurs very remote from term (e.g. in the latter part of the second trimester), the presence of significant and sustained oligohydramnios carries a poor prognosis, particularly being associated with pulmonary hypoplasia. Serial ultrasound scanning has a role to play in determining the persistence of severe oligohydramnios. In these patients, the offer of a termination of pregnancy may be considered, as even those fetuses that survive *in utero* may not be viable once delivered because of difficulties with effective ventilation. Serial transabdominal or transcervical amnio-infusion has been tried with variable success rates.
- *Chorioamnionitis.* If labor does not occur in the more mature fetus, then a balance needs to be found between avoiding the complications due to iatrogenic prematurity and those due to chorioamnionitis. At initial assessment, any signs of chorioamnionitis should be excluded (fetal or maternal tachycardia, maternal pyrexia, tender or irritable uterus, and/or offensive vaginal discharge), as should any signs of fetal compromise. Obstetric ultrasound scanning will again be useful to assess residual amniotic fluid volume and any obvious fetal or uterine abnormalities that may have contributed to rupture of membranes or that may influence the subsequent management.
- In those without evidence of infection or fetal compromise, conservative management to achieve improved fetal maturity is likely to be the optimal course. Close liaison with the neonatologists is essential, both in terms of informing and preparing the parents and to ensure that appropriate neonatal care is available from the moment of delivery. This may require *in utero* transfer to another unit if such facilities are not available.
- Careful ongoing surveillance for the onset of chorioamnionitis or fetal compromise is essential.
  - At least twice-daily fetal heart rate monitoring is important, as fetal tachycardia is commonly the first sign of chorioamnionitis. In the third trimester, CTG may be the optimal way to effect this, as signs of fetal compromise may be detected.
  - Eight-hourly observations of maternal pulse and temperature should be performed, and CBC should be checked twice weekly to detect leukocytes, or on any occasion where symptoms or signs suggest the onset of infection.

- Non-specific inflammatory markers, such as ESR or C-reactive protein (CRP), have been used in surveillance, but add little to improve infection detection rates.
- Equally, the value of repeated high vaginal swabs is dubious in the absence of any signs of infection, and the repeated examinations may, in fact, promote ascending infection.
- Perineal/perianal cultures for GBS colonization should be sent. If present, intrapartum (not antepartum) GBS chemoprophylaxis with penicillin should be administered. Cultures are predictive of perineal colonization for 5 weeks.

- *Care of the fetus.* During conservative management, placental function should be monitored with serial growth scans, amniotic fluid volume assessment, and CTG.
- *Labor and delivery.* Delivery should be effected at the onset of any signs of chorioamnionitis, excessive bleeding, fetal compromise, or unstoppable preterm labor. Delivery should also be effected when a favorable gestational age is attained. The weight of evidence in the literature suggests that the risks of ascending infection outweigh the risks of prematurity after 34 weeks. Delivery may be vaginal if there are no other contraindications and there is sufficient time to achieve this safely. Chorioamnionitis is an indication for delivery, but is not itself an indication for cesarean delivery.
- *Maternal complications.* The maternal effects of prolonged hospitalization should not be forgotten, in terms of both psychological and social effects (particularly if there are already children at home) and of the risk of thromboembolic disease. Risk factors for deep vein thrombosis (DVT) and thromboprophylaxis should be carefully considered.

Recommended further reading

1. Bengtson JM, Van Marter LJ, Barss VA, Greene MF, Tuomala RE, Epstein MF (1989). Pregnancy outcome after premature rupture of the membranes at or before 26 weeks' gestation. *Obstet Gynecol* **73**, 921–27.
2. Richards DS (1998). Complications of prolonged PROM and oligohydramnios. *Clin Obstet Gynecol* **41**, 817–26.
3. Mercer BM (1998). Management of preterm premature rupture of the membranes. *Clin Obstet Gynecol* **41**, 870–82.
4. Grieg PC (1998). The diagnosis of intrauterine infection in women with preterm premature rupture of the membranes (PPROM). *Clin Obstet Gynecol* **41**, 849–63.
5. Allen SR (1998). Tocolytic therapy in preterm PROM. *Clin Obstet Gynecol* **41**, 842–8.
6. Ernest JM (1998). Neonatal consequences of preterm PROM. *Clin Obstet Gynecol* **41**, 827–31.

Drug treatment for preterm premature rupture of membranes

- *Prophylactic broad-spectrum antibiotics* are commonly used in women with pPROM prior to 34 weeks' gestation with a view to prolonging the latency period. The most common protocol is IV ampicillin and erythromycin for 2 days followed by oral amoxycillin and erythromycin for an additional 5 days, although most broad-spectrum protocols appear to be effective in prolonging pregnancy and improving pregnancy outcome. The risks of allergic reaction with the antibiotics and increase in resistant strains should be kept in mind. In the presence of clinical infection (chorioamnionitis), the prompt use of appropriate intravenous antibiotics is essential.
- *Steroids.* The use of maternally administered intramuscular corticosteroids (betamethasone 12 mg every 12 hours for two doses or dexamethazone 6 mg every 12 hours for four doses) to promote fetal maturity has been widely credited with reduced mortality and morbidity in the premature neonate. However, their use in the presence of pPROM has been debated. There are arguments that steroids may facilitate the more rapid onset of infection by immune downregulation and that signs of infection may be masked by the steroids (antipyrogenic effects and leukocytes). However, if these effects are considered during surveillance of the patient and the above level of surveillance is closely adhered to, the benefits of steroids prior to 34 weeks' gestation far outweigh their disadvantages. Furthermore, the use of prophylactic antibiotics when steroids are used helps to counter the effects of any immune compromise.
- *GBS chemoprophylaxis.* Intrapartum (not antepartum) GBS chemoprophylaxis should be administered in women at high risk of GBS perineal colonization (prior GBS-infected infant, GBS bacteriuria in the index pregnancy) and in women with a positive GBS perineal culture within the past 5 weeks. In women whose GBS colonization status is unknown, GBS chemoprophylaxis should be administered if risk factors are present (premature labor, prolonged ROM >18 hours, or fever).

Recommended further reading

1. Kenyon S, Boulvain M, Neilson J (2003). Antibiotics for preterm rupture of membranes. *Cochrane Database Syst Rev* **2**, CD001058.
2. Kenyon SL, Taylor DJ, Tarnow-Mordi W, for the ORACLE Collaborative Group (2001). Broad-spectrum antibiotics for preterm, prelabor rupture of fetal membranes: The ORACLE I randomised trial. *Lancet* **357**, 979–88.

Intrauterine growth restriction and diagnosis

IUGR is a failure of the fetus to achieve the expected weight for a given gestational age. The term 'small for gestational age' (SGA) refers to any baby whose birthweight is below the 10th centile for any given gestational age in a given population. Many SGA babies will have reached their full growth potential and hence are not growth-restricted. Conversely, some babies with IUGR may have a birthweight well above the 10th centile for the population but have failed to achieve their optimum birthweight as a result of a pathological process. Hence the terms are not synonymous. In this section we examine how to identify the growth-restricted fetus in order to permit appropriate surveillance and intervention.

Causes of IUGR/SGA can be classified as: constitutional (i.e. SGA but not IUGR), chromosomal, uteroplacental, environmental (infection, drugs), or syndromic.

Available diagnostic tools

- The *history* should include: previous obstetric history (looking particularly for previous growth restriction, adverse outcomes, or maternal medical problems); medical history (connective tissue disease, thrombotic events, endocrine disorders); drug history (therapeutic and recreational); family history (congenital abnormalities, thrombophilias); antepartum hemorrhage/history suggesting abruptio placentae; personal or close family history of recent viral illness; fetal movements.
- *Palpation* is an important part of routine antenatal care, and each visit after 24 weeks should include a measurement of symphysis–fundal height. This measurement in centimeters should equate to the gestation in weeks. A measurement more than 2 cm different from that expected requires further assessment of the fetus. Gross oligo- or polyhydramnios may be evident on abdominal palpation.
- *Ultrasound scanning*
  - Biometry. Measurements of biparietal diameter, head circumference, abdominal circumference, and femur length may be valuable in the diagnosis, differential diagnosis, and surveillance of growth-restricted fetuses. Interpretation of an isolated set of measurements may be misleading. Thus serial measurements are more useful than a single set of measurements obtained at the same point in time.
  - Anatomy. Structural abnormalities may raise the suspicion of chromosomal abnormalities causing growth restriction.
  - Amniotic fluid volume. The amniotic fluid index (AFI) is the sum of the deepest pool in each quadrant and provides the most reproducible measure of amniotic fluid volume for the differential diagnosis or surveillance of IUGR.

- *Doppler waveform analysis.* The umbilical artery resistance index may be raised in the presence of raised placental resistance because of growth restriction of uteroplacental origin. Measurement of this parameter can aid in differential diagnosis (although abnormal umbilical artery Doppler waveforms can also occur in the presence of fetal aneuploidy) and in the surveillance of a growth-restricted fetus during conservative management. In IUGR of uteroplacental origin, a compensatory fall in resistance index of the fetal middle cerebral artery Doppler velocimetry may occur. The absence of uterine artery Doppler waveform notching at 20 weeks' gestation provides reassurance in a pregnancy with previous severe IUGR of uteroplacental origin (recurrence rate then only 2%).
- *Invasive fetal testing.* Amniocentesis can facilitate karyotyping if aneuploidy is suspected, and samples can be rapidly analyzed for the common trisomies using fluorescent *in situ* hybridization (FISH). Samples can also be cultured for more in-depth analysis. Amniotic fluid or fetal blood may be analyzed using molecular biology techniques if fetal viral infection is suspected as the cause of IUGR. All these sampling techniques carry risks of infection, premature rupture of membranes, and premature labor.
- *Retrospective tests.* Maternal blood testing for recent cytomegalovirus, rubella or toxoplasmosis infection; metabolic disorders (if suspected clinically), or thrombophilias may be carried out when IUGR is detected or retrospectively. The placenta should be sent for histopathological examination and, if fetal or neonatal death occurs, permission from the parents for post-mortem examination should be sought.

Recommended further reading

1. Kingdom J, Baker P, Blair E (2000). Definitions of intrauterine growth restriction. In: Kingdom J, Baker P, eds. *Intrauterine Growth Restriction, Aetiology and Management*, p. 1. Springer-Verlag, London.
2. Enkin M, Keirse MJNC, Renfrew M, Neilson J (eds) (1995). Assessment of fetal growth, size and well-being. In: *A Guide to Effective Care in Pregnancy and Childbirth* (2nd edn), pp. 61–72. Oxford University Press, Oxford.
3. Pollack RN, Divon MY (1992). Intrauterine growth retardation: definition, classification, and etiology. *Clin Obstet Gynecol* **35**, 99–107.
4. Warsof SL, Cooper DJ, Little D, Campbell S (1986). Routine ultrasound screening for antenatal detection of intrauterine growth retardation. *Obstet Gynecol* **67**, 33–9.
5. Yoshimura S, Masuzaki H, Miura K, Gotoh H, Ishimaru T (1998). Fetal blood flow redistribution in term intrauterine growth retardation (IUGR) and postnatal growth. *Int J Gynaecol Obstet* **60**, 3–8.
6. Pahal GS, Acharya G, Jauniaux E (2000). Biochemical markers of fetoplacental growth restriction. In: Kingdom J, Baker P, eds. *Intrauterine Growth Restriction*, pp. 239–56. Springer-Verlag, London.
7. Weiner CP (1994). Fetal growth deficiency and its evaluation. In: James DK, Steer PJ, Weiner CP, Gonik B, eds. *High Risk Pregnancy: Management Options*, pp. 759–70. WB Saunders, London.
8. Lin C-C, Santolaya-Forgas J (1998). Current concepts of fetal growth restriction. Part I: Causes, classification, and pathophysiology. *Obstet Gynecol* **92**, 1044–55.
9. Lin C-C, Santolaya-Forgas J (1999). Current concepts of fetal growth restriction. Part II: Diagnosis and management. *Obstet Gynecol* **93**, 140–6.

Fetal growth restriction

The constitutionally small baby

A fetus growing parallel to the lower centiles throughout the pregnancy that is anatomically normal and has normal amniotic fluid volume and umbilical artery Doppler velocimetry is most likely to be constitutionally small. This is particularly common in women of slight build. The use of population-specific growth charts for fetal ultrasound biometry has been explored, and these are utilized routinely in some units. Although a fetus persistently small to palpation may precipitate serial ultrasound biometry (every 3–4 weeks) to exclude decelerating growth, no deviation from normal antenatal or intrapartum management should be required provided that no additional concerns arise.

Fetal aneuploidy

The most common aneuploidies to cause fetal growth restriction are as follows, in order of descending frequency: triploidy, trisomies 18, 21, and 13, and deletion of 4p. Rearrangements may also result in IUGR.

- Findings that should prompt suspicion of trisomy in IUGR include symmetrical IUGR, increased amniotic fluid volume, abnormal Doppler studies, structural abnormalities and soft markers (these may occasionally be a confusing effect of starvation, e.g. echogenic bowel), advanced maternal age, and biochemical or nuchal translucency screening results.
- Triploidy, which most commonly presents prior to 26 weeks' gestation, may resemble IUGR of uteroplacental origin with asymmetry in the growth restriction, reduced amniotic fluid volume, and abnormal Doppler velocimetry. The mothers may also develop preeclampsia, encouraging the assumption that malplacentation accounts for the IUGR.
- If chromosomal abnormalities are suspected, karyotyping should be offered with appropriate counseling, as the diagnosis of aneuploidy may influence the approach of the parents to ongoing management of the pregnancy.

Causes of intrauterine growth restrictrion

Uteroplacental insufficiency

This is the most common cause of IUGR, and occurs because of abnormalities in placental development and trophoblast invasion. This may be idiopathic or due to one of a number of recognized causes. Growth restriction that is severe and of early onset may result in fetal cell hypoplasia such that, if the fetus survives to extrauterine life, it may never exhibit full catch-up growth.

Recognized causes of placental insufficiency include the following:

- *Connective tissue disorders* (e.g. systemic lupus erythematosis). Check history and autoantibodies, including antinuclear antibody and anti-double stranded DNA.
- *Preeclampsia.* Clinical diagnosis; see 📖 *p.70.*
- *Pregestational diabetes mellitus*, particularly when associated with peripheral vascular disease.
- *Placental abruption.* Check for history of antepartum hemorrhage or unexplained abdominal pains.
- *Placental infarction or thrombosis* (particularly associated with thrombophilias, especially antiphospholipid antibody syndrome, antithrombin III deficiency, and homozygous or compound heterozygous mutations in common inherited thormbophilias).
- *Chorioamnionitis* (bacterial or viral; see under 'Infection' below).
- *Chorionangioma* may be evident on ultrasound examination of the placenta.

Serial monitoring of the IUGR pregnancy thought to be due to placental insufficiency should involve regular (every 3–4 weeks) biometry. Amniotic fluid volume assessment and Doppler waveform analyses (umbilical artery ± middle cerebral artery) may be carried out fortnightly or weekly (or more frequently), dependent upon the clinical situation. Delivery should occur when the risk of continued exposure to a hostile intrauterine environment appears to outweigh the risks of prematurity.

Environmental causes of IUGR

Maternal drug usage

Therapeutic drugs

IUGR may occur as a result of the ingestion of some therapeutic drugs, particularly antihypertensive drugs.

- There is an established link with β-antagonists. The link with α and mixed α/β-receptor antagonists is less clear.
- Calcium-channel blockers and α-methyldopa have been weakly associated with IUGR.
- There is some evidence that cyclosporin (in transplant patients) may be associated with growth restriction in some cases, but no good evidence of a role for corticosteroids in causation of IUGR.

However, with all these therapeutic drugs, it must be remembered that the underlying maternal disease for which the drugs are being taken may cause a degree of IUGR.

Recreational drugs

- By far the most common and unequivocal recreational drug use implicated in IUGR is tobacco smoking. Cigarette smoking produces a twofold relative risk of having a growth-restricted fetus. The effects are dose and gestational age dependent, with the maximum growth-restrictive effects occurring in the third trimester, although it appears that those smoking in the first trimester undergo some degree of placental adaptation if the pregnancy is not lost. Although it is the nicotine in cigarettes that is addictive, it is the carbon monoxide and cyanide that exert adverse effects on the fetus. Carbon monoxide shifts the maternal oxyhemoglobin dissociation curve to the disadvantage of the fetus, and it is preferentially taken up by fetal erythrocytes. Therefore smokers should be strongly advised to stop. Nicotine patches are commonly used to aid their withdrawal from addiction, and appear to be safe for use in pregnancy.
- Alcohol to excess results in fetal alcohol syndrome (severe IUGR, central nervous system involvement, and facial dysmorphism). However, the safe daily dose of alcohol has not been determined, and even moderate or low alcohol intake in the third trimester may be associated with IUGR or mild central nervous system involvement. As such, women should be instructed that there is no safe level of alcohol consumption during pregnancy and they should be counseled to abstain completely from alcohol consumption throughout gestation.
- Of the illegal recreational drugs, cocaine and amphetamines are known to be associated with IUGR, and there is some evidence that opiates, inhaled solvents, and cannabis may also restrict fetal growth. IUGR as a result of ecstasy (MDMA) abuse appears rare, provided that its use is only sporadic. Management of patients using recreational drugs should be in conjunction with addiction services as sudden withdrawal of drugs of dependence may not be appropriate. The pediatricians should be involved, with careful surveillance of the neonate as withdrawal may be problematic.

Infection

- Congenital infection with cytomegalovirus, toxoplasmosis, or rubella may result in a number of problems, including IUGR. Serological evidence of infection in the mother may be sought and, if positive or if there are other indicators of fetal infection, invasive procedures may be used to determine fetal infection.
- Asymptomatic HIV infection does not appear to affect birthweight, but low birthweight may be encountered in advanced maternal disease. HIV-positive women on protease inhibitor therapy should be followed with serial ultrasound examination to monitor fetal growth.

Fetal syndromes

A variety of fetal syndromes may result in growth restriction. These include skeletal deformities, which are likely to be suspected or diagnosed ultrasonographically *in utero* (osteochondrodysplasias affecting the whole skeleton—thanetophoric dysplasias or osteogenesis imperfecta; dystoces affecting single bones—hemivertibrae or limb reduction defects), or chromosome or gene abnormalities resulting in general growth reduction (autosomal recessive disorders, such as Donohue's syndrome, confined placental mosaicism, uniparental disomy, and chromosome breakage syndromes, such as Fanconi's syndrome). An offer of pregnancy termination may be appropriate for some of these conditions, once the parents have been fully counseled. Should the fetus prove nonviable, a post-mortem should be recommended with careful directed chromosome analysis of the fetus, placenta, and parental blood wherever possible and acceptable. Genetic counseling should be offered.

Recommended further reading

1. Weiner CP (1994). Fetal growth deficiency and its evaluation. In: James DK, Steer PJ, Weiner CP, Gonik B, eds. *High Risk Pregnancy—Management Options*, pp. 759–70. WB Saunders, London.
2. Lin C-C, Santolaya-Forgas J (1998). Current concepts of fetal growth restriction. Part I: Causes, classification, and pathophysiology. *Obstet Gynecol* **92**, 1044–55.
3. Lin C-C, Santolaya-Forgas J (1999). Current concepts of fetal growth restriction: Part II: Diagnosis and management. *Obstet Gynecol* **93**, 140–6.

Chapter 3

Fetal medicine

Prenatal diagnosis and counseling

Introduction

Congenital abnormalities are common, contributing to 15% of all perinatal deaths and a further 10–15% of deaths in the first year of life in developed countries. Ninety-five percent of abnormalities are unexpected, occurring in pregnancies not considered at high risk of those conditions. Screening of whole populations aims to detect abnormalities in low-risk women. For women who have had a previous fetal abnormality, the risk of recurrence may be known and this will guide future testing. When screening test results show high risk or the recurrence risk of a previous abnormality is high, a diagnostic test is offered. There is a growing demand for prenatal screening and diagnosis, with families increasingly looking to obstetric and genetic services to assist in their quest for healthy offspring. Prenatal diagnosis is now a major part of antenatal care. It allows the following:

- Planning for place and method of delivery.
- Arrangements for repair of structural problems (preferable to deliver in a tertiary care center with pediatric surgery).
- *In utero* treatment where feasible.
- Preparation of parents to cope with a baby with a congenital abnormality.
- Termination of pregnancy (TOP) if requested.

Progress in ultrasound and laboratory techniques has produced an increasing number of conditions for which prenatal diagnosis is available. However, some abnormalities still cannot be diagnosed antenatally, and some physical and laboratory-detected abnormalities may be of minor or unknown significance. Even after diagnosis, some women may choose to continue with a pregnancy with a severe or lethal fetal abnormality. Provision of information and support, whatever the choices made by parents, is a major part of any prenatal diagnosis service.

Counseling

Counseling is a major aspect of prenatal diagnosis. Prospective parents may not perceive themselves as being at risk of congenital abnormalities or may not fully comprehend the concept of risk. Therefore the finding of a high-risk screening result or ultrasound abnormality is often not expected by them. Unlike other medical test results which are given as positive or negative, many screening tests in prenatal diagnosis are reported as a numerical risk. Although healthcare staff are advised to categorize these results as high or low risk, patients may become aware of the numerical risk and find it difficult to accept the imposition of a cutoff, which they perceive as arbitrary. Obstetric care providers need to be aware of this and other issues of communication and deal with the circumstances sensitively. Each unit should have a coordinator to serve as a reference point for inquiries on prenatal screening and diagnostic services. The services of a genetics unit, either locally or at a nearby tertiary center, should be utilized. Support groups of families with similar problems or experiences can be of value to patients.

Recommended further reading

1. Souka AP, Nicolaides KH (1997). Diagnosis of fetal abnormalities at the 10–14 week scan. *Ultrasound Obstet Gynecol* **10**, 429–42.

Screening

Screening tests identify pregnant women at increased risk or likelihood of a fetal abnormality in an apparently normal pregnancy. They have relatively low sensitivity and specificity but, because of their low physical risk, can be offered to whole populations. They are appropriate only when diagnostic tests are available for the specified condition. Screening modalities currently generally available include:

- genetic screening.
- biochemical screening.
- mid-trimester ultrasound scanning.
- first trimester nuchal translucency scanning.

Genetic screening

Genetic screening is not yet widely available for common congenital problems in most developed countries. In the USA, the American College of Obstetricians and Gynecologists (ACOG) recommend routine cystic fibrosis (CF) genetic screening for all Caucasian couples and couples at risk by virtue of a positive family history of CF. CF is an autosomal recessive condition with a gene frequency of 1 in 25 in Caucasians. Approximately 800 mutations in the single-copy CF gene have been described, and ACOG recommends that routine screening include at least the 25 most common mutations. Definitive prenatal diagnosis can be achieved by using DNA analysis from chorionic villus sampling (CVS) or amniotic cells. Advances in laboratory techniques are likely to make genetic screening and diagnosis more readily available in the future.

Biochemical screening

The most common problems screened for are Down syndrome (DS) and neural tube defects (NTDs). Screening for DS and NTDs is done on a maternal serum sample and the optimal time for taking a serum sample is at 15–20 weeks of gestation.

Down syndrome (trisomy 21, 46, XX + 21/46, XY + 21)

DS is the most common cause of congenital mental retardation, with a birth incidence of 1.5 in 1000. Associated structural anomalies include ventricular septal defects, anterior abdominal wall defects, and typical facies. Life expectancy is reduced (about 60 years) and patients are at increased risk of Alzheimer's disease and chronic myeloid leukemia. Biochemical screening for DS is based on a combination of maternal age, human chorionic gonadotrophin (hCG), α-fetoprotein (AFP), and unconjugated estriol (uE_3).

Advancing maternal age is the strongest single factor in the incidence of DS. The age-related risk of delivering a DS fetus is 1 in 1376 at 25, 1 in 424 at 35, 1 in 126 at 40, and 1 in 31 at 45 years. DS screening was previously based on maternal age alone, and women aged 35 years and over at the estimated date of delivery were offered amniocentesis. However, as a larger proportion of the child-bearing population was under 35 years of age, the maximum detection rate achievable was of the order of 30–35%. With the risks of amniocentesis, some women at risk by virtue of their age declined the procedure, making the eventual detection rate under 20%.

This led to the development of biochemical screening, which can be offered to all pregnant women irrespective of age. Currently available screening utilizes a minimum of three serum analytes (hCG, AFP, uE3) measured at 15–20 weeks' gestation in addition to maternal age (triple test), with a detection rate of up to 70% depending on the cutoff used. High hCG, low AFP, and low uE3 are associated with DS. The addition of inhibin A measurements to the triple test (the so-called quad test) is used by some institutions as it increases the DS detection rate by an additional 2–3%.

The duration of pregnancy must be confirmed by ultrasound, ideally before the test, to validate the result, as wrong dates significantly alter the results. The screening test result is used to recommend invasive/diagnostic procedure, e.g. amniocentesis or CVS for women with high-risk results.

Ultrasonography

Other placental products identified but not in routine clinical usage in the second trimester include pregnancy-associated plasma protein A (PAPP-A), pregnancy-specific β_1 glycoprotein (SP-1), and urea-resistant neutrophil alkaline phosphatase (UR-NAP).

More recently, first trimester fetal aneuploidy screening has been found to be as accurate as second trimester serum analyte screening. This testing includes maternal age, serum biochemical tests (specifically free β-hCG and PAPP-A), and sonographic nuchal translucency (NT) measurements at 11–14 weeks' gestation. The advantage of first trimester testing is that it makes CVS available to such women and allows the option of termination of pregnancy at an earlier gestational age.

Neural tube defects

The main abnormalities are spina bifida and anencephaly, each with a pregnancy incidence in the general population of about 1 in 1000. The widespread use of ultrasound, the option of termination, and the use of folic acid prophylaxis have resulted in very few anencephalic fetuses being born, except in instances when women have chosen to continue with the pregnancy in full knowledge of the diagnosis and prognosis.

Anencephaly and open spina bifida leak AFP into maternal serum leading to elevated levels. This forms the basis of NTD serum screening. The detection rates of NTDs from serum screening with AFP are 88%, 75%, and 68% for anencephaly, open spina bifida, and all spina bifida lesions, respectively. Raised AFP is also useful in highlighting fetuses with potential growth problems later in pregnancy.

Other causes of raised AFP include:

- exomphalos/gastroschisis (leakage of AFP).
- congenital nephroses (defective renal reabsorption).
- polycystic kidneys (defective renal reabsorption).
- fetal death (tissue autolysis).
- multiple pregnancy.
- fetal teratoma (synthesis of AFP in tumor).
- duodenal/esophageal atresia (defective fetal swallowing).

Ultrasonography is now the most common imaging test in prenatal diagnosis with over 90% of antenatal patients in developed countries having a 'routine' scan. It serves as a screening test by checking for soft markers of chromosomal defects and as a diagnostic test by revealing a structural abnormality. However, many women may not appreciate ultrasonography as a screening/diagnostic test, seeing it instead as a 'viewing' of a normal baby. Therefore the finding of an abnormality may be unexpected.

The mid-trimester anomaly scan

Currently, most units perform a scan for structural abnormality at 18–20 weeks, which is the optimal time to obtain the best views of all organ systems. However, it must be borne in mind that some abnormalities may not develop until after 20 weeks and some do not have a sonographic sign.

Although widely practiced, the clinical effectiveness and impact on perinatal mortality of routine scanning is still subject to debate. It is well established that the majority of fetal abnormalities occur in pregnancies with few or no risk factors. As prospective parents become more aware of the risk of fetal abnormality, the main benefit of ultrasound scanning for the majority is the reassurance of fetal physical normality. When abnormality is found, *in utero* treatment may be feasible, neonatal treatment can be arranged, or, when appropriate, pregnancy termination undertaken. When treatment is not available, acceptable, or appropriate, parents may value the foreknowledge of the condition and discussion of prognosis. A planned delivery at a tertiary care center may be appropriate.

The sensitivity of ultrasound in detecting abnormalities in various organ systems depends on several factors, including the skill and experience of personnel, gestational age at which the scanning is done, and the feasibility of verification of abnormalities. Ultrasound scanning programs in tertiary centers and centers with obstetricians and radiologists with ultrasound interest achieve higher detection rates than those in other centers. There is better visualization of fetal anatomy after 18 weeks than earlier in the second trimester, with resultant higher detection rates. Verification is easily achieved when pregnancy has been terminated for a significant abnormality and post-mortem examination undertaken. However, for some abnormalities, particularly mild ones of the heart and urinary tract, the lesion may be asymptomatic, even after birth, and may not be diagnosed early, making the collation of sensitivity data very difficult.

Technical difficulties during scanning may also influence detection rates. These include maternal obesity, fetal position, or multiple pregnancies. Structural abnormalities can be diagnosed in all systems in mid-trimester. Cardiovascular system, central nervous system, and urinary tract abnormalities are among the most common.

NTDs

Ultrasound in good centers detects up to 95% of *all* spina bifida compared with 75% detection of *open* lesions by AFP screening. The extent of the lesion can also be assessed by ultrasound to allow discussion of prognosis. Ninety-nine percent of all cases of anencephaly will be detected at the 18–20 week scan. The recognized association of intracerebral abnormalities, including frontal bone scalloping ('lemon' sign) and abnormally shaped cerebellum ('banana' sign), aids the detection of neural tube lesions. In a high-risk population, e.g. those with raised AFP, virtually all significant NTDs may be detected by 20 weeks.

Recommended further reading

1. Wald NJ, Cuckle H, Brock JH, *et al.* (1977). Maternal serum α-fetoprotein measurement in antenatal screening for anencephaly and spina bifida in early pregnancy. Report of the UK Collaborative Study on α-fetoprotein in Relation to Neural Tube Defects. *Lancet* **1**, 1323–32.

Abnormalities detected

Cardiac defects

These have a birth prevalence of 8–10 in 1000 of which 4 in 1000 are severe and life threatening. A four-chamber view of the heart may identify 60% of severe lesions and a complete fetal cardiac scan (including a four-chamber view and view of both outflow tracts) identifies 75% of all cardiac abnormalities. However, detection rates vary widely from 6% to 77%, with a mean of 39%. Much of the variation is due to mild lesions for which postnatal verification may be difficult.

It should be noted that a seemingly normal four-chamber view may be seen at the 18–20 week scan in some cases of serious cardiac abnormalities. This makes it necessary to repeat the scan and perform fetal echocardiography at a later date (typically 22–24 weeks) if risk factors, e.g. family, medical, or past history, and other ultrasound abnormalities are identified.

Urinary tract abnormalities

These are very common, accounting for 15% of abnormalities diagnosed in the prenatal period. Severe abnormalities include bilateral renal agenesis (Potter's syndrome), infantile polycystic kidneys, bilateral multicystic kidneys, and obstructive uropathies.

- *Potter's syndrome* has an incidence of 0.3 in 1000, over 90% of which may be detected at the mid-trimester scan. The main features are severe oligohydramnios/anhydramnios and nonvisualization of the bladder and kidneys. The condition is incompatible with life, with 40% of fetuses stillborn.
- *Infantile polycystic kidney disease* is an autosomal recessive condition, with an incidence of 1 in 6000. It has a variable spectrum of severity, such that it may not be apparent on the mid-trimester scan. Prognosis is poor.
- *Multicystic kidneys* have a poor prognosis when bilateral, but good prognosis if unilateral with a normal contralateral kidney.
- *Obstructive uropathies*, e.g. urethral stenosis or atresia and posterior urethral valves in male fetuses, may be very severe, leading to severe oligohydramnios, gross bladder distension with eventual rupture, and urinary ascites. Prognosis often depends on the degree of obstruction and the extent of the renal cortical injury.

The majority of abnormalities are relatively minor, e.g. isolated pelviureteric dilatation. These may carry a risk of neonatal urinary tract infection, but usually require no more antenatal intervention than ultrasound monitoring and pediatric notification. However, as they may remain asymptomatic or resolve spontaneously, diagnostic verification and assessment of the full impact of the lesions is difficult to undertake. Therefore long-term follow-up of these neonates may be necessary.

Gastrointestinal abnormalities

Detection rates for anterior abdominal wall defects (omphalocele and gastroschisis) at the mid-trimester scan are close to 100%. Isolated esophageal atresia will result in polyhydramnios and failure to visualize the stomach. However, in 95% a tracheal fistula coexists, amniotic fluid reaches the stomach, and a normal appearance is obtained. Intestinal atresia or obstruction is less detectable in mid-trimester as the effects of the pathology become more pronounced at a later stage. Obstruction or atresia is more often diagnosed in the late second trimester or the third trimester because of polyhydramnios or an incidental finding of dilated loops of bowel. The association between duodenal atresia/omphalocele and trisomies must be borne in mind.

Thoracic abnormalities

The main noncardiac abnormality in the thorax is congenital diaphragmatic hernia. This has a birth incidence of 1 in 2000–5000. It may be diagnosed in the second trimester but is usually more apparent in the third. The defect may be large and the herniation transient, making diagnosis more difficult. The defect is usually left-sided and the heart, although structurally normal, may be displaced to the right by abdominal visceral herniating into the left side of the chest. Normality of the displaced heart and great vessels may then be difficult to determine.

Severe skeletal dysplasias

The incidence is 0.2 in 1000. Because the femur is measured routinely, shortening of long bones is usually readily noted. Ultrasound detection of severe dysplasias is about 84% and that of musculoskeletal abnormalities in general is about 45%. Examination of the hands and feet is more difficult than that of the long bones. Deformities of the hands, e.g. clinodactyly, and feet, e.g. talipes equinovarus (clubfeet), are more difficult to diagnose but may be associated with chromosome abnormalities.

Abnormalities of the face and neck

The fetal face is routinely evaluated at the time of 18 week ultrasound examinations, with detection rates for facial abnormalities varying from 25% to 43% in a low-risk population. High-risk populations are more fully assessed and detection rates in this group are likely to be higher. Face and neck abnormalities amenable to ultrasound detection include clefts of lip/palate, Pierre–Robin syndrome, Treacher–Collins syndrome, holoprosencephaly, cyclopia, frontal and occipital encephaloceles, tumors, cystic hygromas, and fetal goiters. Many of these are associated with central nervous system and chromosome abnormalities and hence a full fetal assessment is necessary. Karyotyping may be indicated.

Recommended further reading

1. American College of Obstetricians and Gynecologists (2001). Prenatal diagnosis of fetal chromosomal abnormalities. *Obstet Gynecol* **97**, S1–12.

Mid-trimester markers

The mid-trimester scan may reveal markers of chromosomal abnormality. These markers are not of major significance on their own but may indicate an underlying problem. Significance increases when more than one marker is found or other risk factors coexist, e.g. maternal age or high risk on serum screening. When multiple abnormalities are seen, the overall risk of chromosome abnormality may be as high as 35%.

Markers and the conditions with which they may be associated include the following:

- Nuchal fold thickening, fetal hydrops, mild ventriculomegaly, duodenal atresia, sandal gap, clinodactyly, and renal pelves dilatation for trisomy 21.
- Echogenic bowel, mild shortening of femur, and cardiac defects for trisomies 18 and 21.
- Cystic hygroma for Turner's syndrome.
- Omphalocele and holoprosencephaly for trisomies 13 and 18.
- Early growth restriction for trisomies 13, 18, and 21.

First trimester scanning

Nuchal translucency

Edema of the fetal neck, detectable in the first trimester by ultrasound, is associated with cardiac defects, Down syndrome, and other trisomies (Fig. 3.1). NT screening is best performed between 11 and 14 weeks' gestation and, when related to maternal age, the detection rate for DS potentially increases to about 80% compared with 60% for maternal age and first trimester biochemical analytes. Introduction of NT screening into routine practice will have major implications in terms of training of personnel and scanning time. The benefits of large-scale first trimester screening need to be put in context, as many of the serious abnormalities diagnosed would have spontaneously aborted had they not been detected. Women may potentially be given the extra burden of choosing pregnancy termination for these conditions. Currently, most women are not referred for hospital antenatal care until the second trimester. Therefore the place of NT as a screening test is still being evaluated before its introduction into general use for low-risk populations.

Other abnormalities/limitations in first trimester

First trimester scanning may require a transvaginal probe to achieve optimal views. Abnormalities have been identified in the first trimester in the central nervous system, heart, gastrointestinal tract, urinary tract, and skeletal system. Care needs to be taken, however, as cranial vault ossification and the return of the intestines into the peritoneal cavity are not complete until about 12 weeks' gestation. Therefore anencephaly and omphalocele, for example, may not be confirmed until after 12 weeks. The natural history of some first trimester appearances may not be fully understood until large studies have been undertaken.

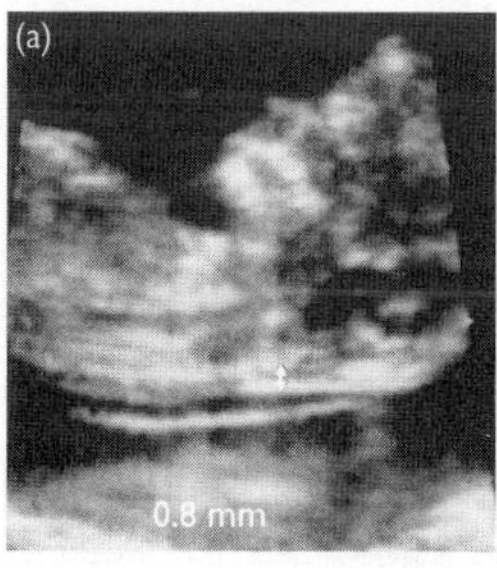

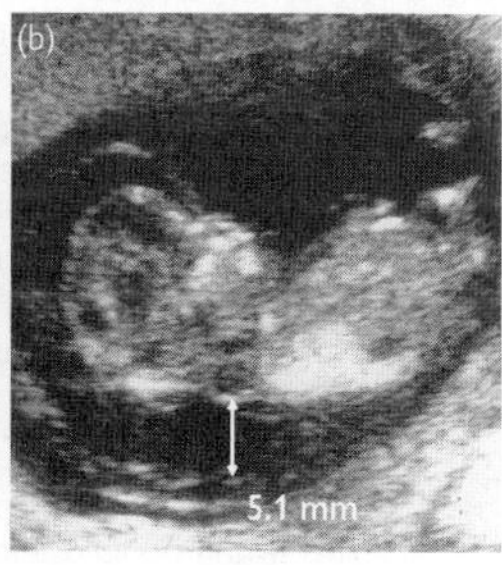

Fig. 3.1 First trimester scans of nuchal fold showing (a) a normal and (b) an abnormal nuchal translucency.

Recommended further reading

1. American College of Obstetricians and Gynecologists (2004). First-trimester screening for fetal aneuploidy. ACOG Committee Opinion No. 296. *Obstet Gynecol* **104**, 215–17.

Diagnostic tests

These are used to definitively confirm or exclude the existence of a fetal abnormality in pregnancies at increased risk of an abnormality on the basis of past history, family history, or a screening test result.

Ultrasound

Ultrasound confirmation of structural abnormality may follow the identification of specific risk factors, e.g. history or raised maternal serum AFP (MS-AFP). A suspicion of abnormality may be raised on the routine mid-trimester scan and confirmed by a more detailed examination. This is particularly relevant to abnormalities which may not be fully apparent at 18–20 weeks and need a repeat examination later to confirm. Some cardiac defects, e.g. hypoplastic left heart, are progressive and may become more apparent in late pregnancy. Microcephaly, bowel atresia, urinary tract obstruction, achondroplasia, and problems of amniotic fluid volume may not be confirmed until the third trimester.

The sensitivity and specificity of ultrasound increases with the level of skill of personnel. Specialist units with obstetricians/radiologists with ultrasound subspecialization achieve the highest detection rates, up to 76% overall, compared with up to 36% for smaller units. Management after diagnosis is also more appropriate in the specialist units. Smaller units are encouraged to refer to larger more specialized units.

Amniocentesis

Amniotic fluid contains fetal cells shed from the gut and skin. Important diagnoses can be made both from the cells and analysis of the amniotic fluid. Therefore the procedure is used for the following:

- Chromosome analysis: recommended in women at high risk for having a fetus with DS as identified by screening tests, including maternal age, serum analyte testing, and/or ultrasound markers.
- DNA analysis for genetic disease for which tests have been developed. The list of such conditions is rapidly expanding.
- Enzyme assays for inborn errors of metabolism.
- Amniotic fluid AFP and acetyl cholinesterase activity measurements to identify fetuses with NTD (although ultrasound is superior in diagnosing NTDs).
- Diagnosis of fetal infection, e.g. toxoplasmosis, cytomegalovirus (CMV).
- Investigation of fetal lung maturity.
- Bilirubin (to quantitate fetal risk in women with isoimmunization).

The main risk of amniocentesis is miscarriage (0.5% procedure-related risk). This risk is higher when the procedure is performed at 15 weeks or less (so-called 'early amniocentesis'). Risks of respiratory distress and postural abnormalities (clubfeet) have been reported in some studies but, in the absence of chronic amniotic fluid leakage, these are not significant. Needle injuries are rare, especially when real-time sonographic guidance is used.

- Culture failure is rare, with an overall rate of less than 0.5%. Maternal cell contamination occurs in less than 0.2%.

- Results of a full karyotype take about 2 weeks, but specific abnormalities such as trisomies, triploidy, and Turner's syndrome can be diagnosed using FISH with provisional results being available within 24 to 48 hours.
- 300 μg of anti-D globulin should routinely be given to Rh-negative women at the time of the procedure.

Chorionic villus sampling

The sampling of actively dividing trophoblast cells provides material that yields rapid karyotyping results in about 48 hours. This procedure also instantly provides material for DNA analysis, especially as the polymerase chain reaction (PCR) makes small amounts of tissue adequate for testing.

- CVS is performed in the first trimester by transabdominal or transcervical routes.
- First trimester diagnosis by CVS allows first trimester TOP, before pregnancy becomes physically apparent, when this option is taken because of fetal abnormality.
- Rh-negative women must be given anti-D globulin.

The most common indications for CVS are as follows:

- Karyotyping when ultrasound findings suggest fetal aneuploidy.
- DNA analysis, particularly for hemoglobinopathies and recessive or X-linked disorders, e.g. cystic fibrosis, Duchenne muscular dystrophy, and hemophilia.

However, with advances in laboratory techniques in the analysis of amniotic fluid, many conditions can now be diagnosed rapidly from simple amniocentesis with its well-established low pregnancy loss rates.

Complications of CVS include the following:

- Pregnancy loss: about 1–2%.
- Maternal cell contamination may lead to false-negative results, especially when PCR is used to increase the amount of DNA for analysis.
- Placental mosaicism: 1%, usually in direct preparation. Amniocentesis may be needed to clarify.
- Limb reduction deformities appear to be associated with CVS performed before 9 weeks' gestation.

Recommended further reading

1. Tabor A, Philip J, Madsen M, Bang J, Obel EB, Norgaard-Pedersen B (1986). Randomised controlled trial of genetic amniocentesis in 4606 low-risk women. *Lancet* **1**, 1287–2.
2. Hook EB, Cross PK, Schreinemachers DM (1983). Chromosomal abnormality rates at amniocentesis and in live-born infants. *JAMA* **249**, 2034–38.
3. Wald NJ, Cuckle H, Brock JH, *et al.* (1977). Maternal serum α-fetoprotein measurement in antenatal screening for anencephaly and spina bifida in early pregnancy. Report of the UK Collaborative Study on α-fetoprotein in Relation to Neural Tube Defects. *Lancet* **1**, 1323–32.
4. Souka AP, Nicolaides KH (1997). Diagnosis of fetal abnormalities at the 10–14 week scan. *Ultrasound in Obstet Gynecol* **10**, 429–42.
5. Alfirevic Z, Sundberg K, Brigham S (2003). Amniocentesis and chorionic villus sampling for prenatal diagnosis. *Cochrane Database Syst Rev* **3**, CD003252.

Fetal sampling

Antenatal fetal blood sampling

The risks of this procedure are considerably higher than those of amniocentesis or CVS. Therefore it is reserved for conditions in which the information required can only come from testing fetal blood, i.e. fetal Hb, white cells, or specific IgM. Such conditions include fetal hydrops or suspected fetal infection.

Fetal blood sampling (FBS) uses a transabdominal approach to obtain fetal blood for prenatal diagnosis. This is done under real-time ultrasound guidance from placental cord insertion, fetal intrahepatic vessels, or fetal heart.

- Anti-D globulin must be given to Rh-negative women.

Complications of FBS include the following:

- Bleeding from puncture site.
- Hematoma, leading to vascular compression at puncture site.
- Fetal bradycardia from umbilical artery vasospasm.
- Chorioamnionitis.
- Preterm premature rupture of membranes.
- Pregnancy loss (1–2.5%).

Fetal tissue sampling

Most prenatal diagnosis is done with ultrasound, CVS, or amniocentesis, but some very rare conditions require histological examination of skin or assay of enzymes restricted to the liver for diagnosis. Fetal tissue biopsies are done under real-time ultrasound guidance.

- Indications for fetal skin biopsy include harlequin ichthyosis, Sjögren–Larsson syndrome, epidermolysis bullosa letalis, epidermolysis bullosa dystrophica, oculocutaneous albinism.
- Indications for fetal liver biopsy include G6PD deficiency (von Gierke's disease), alanine glyoxalate transaminase (AGT) (primary hyperoxaluria type 1) deficiency, ornithine carbamyl transferase (OCT) deficiency, and carbamyl phosphate synthetase (CPS) deficiency.
- Fetal lung, kidney, and muscle have been biopsied, but the quality of currently available ultrasound and advances in DNA analysis make this rarely necessary.

Future trends

- *Pre-implantation diagnosis.* This is feasible in IVF with removal of a single cell from an eight-cell embryo or a trophoblast from the blastocyst before implantation.
  - Advantage. Diagnosis is done pre-pregnancy, thereby allowing for transfer of euploid embryos only and reducing the need for pregnancy termination for fetal aneuploidy.
- *Fetal nucleated cells or DNA in maternal circulation.* Fetal lymphocytes, erythrocytes, and trophoblast cells are present in the maternal circulation and harvesting them would provide prenatal diagnosis without a fetal-invasive procedure. Maternal cell contamination is the major obstacle. Recent studies suggest that isolation of free fetal DNA in the maternal circulation may be a more promising approach.
- *Three-dimensional ultrasound.* This is of value in defining structure, e.g. facial features/abnormalities (facial abnormalities may be associated with chromosome abnormalities), NTDs, and tumors. Availability and use are currently limited as most diagnoses can be made with conventional high-definition ultrasound.
- *MRI in pregnancy.* Severely limited by motion artefacts. This is a particular problem when trying to evaluate the fetal heart. At present, the only benefit over conventional ultrasound appears to be better resolution of the intracranial structures.

Rhesus isoimmunization

Introduction

Rhesus isoimmunization is the condition wherein incompatibility exists between the fetal and maternal blood group antigens such that an immune response occurs. If an exchange occurs between fetal and maternal blood (as at delivery, placental abruption, threatened miscarriage, or invasive procedures), the passage of fetal cells into the maternal system provokes in the mother an antibody response to the fetal red blood cell antigen. This primary response causes a production of IgM that does not cross the placenta. Therefore the fetus in the index pregnancy is not affected by this process. However, if the mother is exposed to the same red blood cell antigen in a subsequent pregnancy, her primed memory B cells swiftly produce IgG antibody. Maternal IgG antibodies are actively transported across the placenta and bind to the fetal red cell antigen causing red blood cell destruction and ultimately hemolytic anemia in the fetus.

If severe hemolytic anemia does develop, hydrops fetalis may occur. Hydrops fetalis is defined as an abnormal collection of fluid in two or more fetal body compartments, including ascites, pleural effusions, pericardial effusions, and skin edema.

There are five rhesus antigens: D, C, c, E, and e. There is no known d antigen. Rh(D) is the most prevalent and antigenic protein. There are also in addition atypical blood group antigens (e.g. Kell, Duffy, Kidd) which may occasionally give rise to hemolytic disease of the fetus and newborn. In this section, the discussion will be confined to Rh(D) disease.

Rhesus (anti-D) prophylaxis

Prophylaxis with anti-D immunoglobulin (RhoGAM) needs to be considered when an Rh(D)-negative mother is carrying a potentially Rh(D)-positive fetus. When a sensitizing event occurs, exogenous anti-D immunoglobulin should be administered within 72 hours. This binds to and destroys the antigenic fetal blood cells, thereby preventing the immunological response in the mother.

Anti-D immunoglobulin (RhoGAM) should be administered when a sensitizing event occurs, such as vaginal bleeding (threatened abortion) or invasive testing (amniocentesis). The protection is effective for 6–8 weeks. Despite this intervention, which was widely implemented in the 1970s, a significant number of cases of Rh(D) immunization still occurred each year. More recently, it has been shown that routine anti-D immunoglobulin prophylaxis given empirically to all Rh-negative women in pregnancy can dramatically decrease the incidence of isoimmunization. In the USA, anti-D immunoglobulin 300 μg by IM injection is now administered routinely to all Rh(D)-negative women at 28–30 weeks' gestation and again after delivery if the baby is Rh(D)-positive. In the UK, the most common protocol is anti-D immunoglobulin 500 IU by IM injection administered at 28 and 34 weeks' gestation and again after delivery if the baby is Rh(D)-positive.

Without a program of anti-D prophylaxis, 1% of Rh(D)-negative women will have antibodies by the end of the first pregnancy with an Rh(D)-positive baby, 7–9% will have antibodies 6 months postdelivery, and a further 7–9% after a second pregnancy. Therefore 17% of women will have Rh(D) antibodies by the end of their second pregnancy with an Rh-positive baby. With routine administration of anti-D prophylaxis after delivery if the baby is Rh(D)-positive, the incidence of Rh(D) isoimmunization can be decreased to 1.5%. With routine administration of Rh(D) prophylaxis in the second and third trimesters, the incidence of Rh(D) isoimmunization can be decreased even further to 0.1%.

Recommended further reading

1. Tovey LA, Townley A, Stevenson BJ, Taverner J (1983). The Yorkshire antenatal anti-D immunoglobulin trial in primigravidae. *Lancet* **2**, 244–6.
2. Rodeck CH, Deans A (1983). Red cell alloimmunization. In: Rodeck CH, Whittle MJ, eds. *Fetal Medicine: Basic Science and Clinical Practice*, pp. 785–804. Churchill Livingstone, Edinburgh.
3. American College of Obstetricians and Gynecologists (1999). Prevention of Rh-D alloimmunization. ACOG Practice Bulletin No. 4. *Int J Gynecol Obstet* **66**, 63–70.

Monitoring the pregnancy

Pregnant women should routinely have their blood group (ABO and Rh status) and antibody status tested at booking and again at 28–30 weeks' gestation and in labor.

- If anti-D autoantibodies are present, the paternal blood group should be checked. If the father is Rh(D)-negative and there is no doubt about paternity, it can be assumed that the fetus is Rh(D)-negative. Thus there is no requirement for further testing.
- If anti-D antibodies are present and if the father is Rh(D)-positive, it is necessary to determine whether he is homozygous or heterozygous for the D antigen. If he is homozygous, the fetus will be Rh(D)-positive. If he is heterozygous, there is a 50% likelihood that the fetus will be Rh(D)-positive.

Antibody titers

If anti-D antibodies are present, serial measurements of circulating antibody titers should be performed every 2–4 weeks.

- An anti-D antibody titer of 1:4 or less signifies no or very minimal risk of hemolytic disease in the fetus.
- If the antibody titer is above 1:4 at the beginning of the pregnancy or if it rises suddenly, the risk of fetal hemolytic anemia increases and further investigation of the pregnancy is mandatory.
- If the father is heterozygous for the Rh(D) antigen or the mother is known to be Rh(D) isoimmunized, amniocentesis should be considered to determine fetal Rh status. Several recent studies have suggested that the fetal Rh status can be determined from a maternal blood sample. Although this is an exciting new development, such tests remain investigational.

Recommended further reading

1. Queenan JJ (1982). Current management of the rhesus-sensitised patient. *Clin Obstet Gynecol* **25**, 293–301.
2. Liley AW (1961). Liquor amnii analysis in the management of the pregnancy complicated by rhesus sensitisation. *AM J Obstet Gynecol.* **82**, 1359–70.

Fetal surveillance and blood transfusion

Hydrops fetalis is a severe consequence of the hemolytic anemia due to Rh disease. This can be detected by ultrasound examination of the fetus. However, a fetus may be severely anemic and not have any evidence of hydrops. Hydrops is typically associated with a fetal hematocrit of less than 15% (compared with a normal hematocrit of 50%).

If anti-D antibody titers rise above 1:4, and the fetus is presumed to be Rh positive, fetal surveillance should commence weekly. Monitoring consists of the following:

- Ultrasound examination looking for signs of early hydrops fetalis, which may include visualization of both sides of the fetal bowel, pericardial effusions, or enlargement of the right atrium.
- The diagnosis of hydrops fetalis is made when there is sonographic evidence of abnormal collections of fluid in two or more fetal body compartments. This includes ascites, pleural effusions, pericardial effusions, or skin edema. In such cases, placental edema and polyhydramnios are also commonly seen.
- Doppler velocimetry to assess blood flow in the middle cerebral artery (MCA) of the fetus. Elevated peak MCA blood flow velocity for gestational age has been shown to be an accurate screening test for fetal anemia.

Invasive testing

If antibody titers continue to rise in the presence of an Rh(D)-positive fetus, invasive testing may be required.

Amniocentesis

This method was introduced into the management of rhesus disease by Liley in 1961.

- Bilirubin, the breakdown product of red blood cell hemolysis, is excreted into the amniotic fluid. A sample of amniotic fluid is taken and the bilirubin is estimated indirectly by measuring the optical density difference at 450 nm (difference in OD_{450} or ▲OD_{450}).
- The amniocentesis should be performed under direct ultrasound guidance with particular care to avoid the placenta.
- With the use of the Liley chart, a prediction can be made of when further interventions may be necessary, e.g. fetal blood sampling.
- This estimation of bilirubin production is less reliable before 27 weeks, and each invasive procedure may provoke a further rise in maternal antibody level.
- Measurements are no longer reliable after an intrauterine blood transfusion has been performed.

Fetal blood sampling

This method directly assesses the severity of the disease by measuring the fetal red blood cell parameters, but it is a morbid and invasive procedure. Therefore it is used only as a last resort. The procedure should be performed under direct ultrasound guidance.

- The umbilical cord is typically sampled at the placental insertion or at the intrahepatic portion of the umbilical vein. A sample of fetal blood is taken to measure hemoglobin (Hb), hematocrit (HCT), blood group, and direct Coombs' test (DCT).
- If the HCT is >2 SD below the mean for gestational age, an intrauterine fetal blood transfusion is indicated.
- If mild anemia is present (HCT >30%) and the reticulocyte count is high or DCT strongly positive, a repeat fetal blood sample is required in 1–2 weeks (fetus at high risk of fetal anemia).
- *Timing of fetal blood sample.* If a woman has had a severely affected fetus in a previous pregnancy (and the partner is homozygous for Rh(D) antigen), FBS should be planned for 10 weeks before earliest neonatal or fetal death, fetal transfusion, or birth of severely affected fetus.
  - The procedure should not generally be performed before 18 weeks' gestation unless fetal hydrops is already present.
  - If the father is heterozygous, amniocentesis at or after 15 weeks may be useful to determine fetal Rh status.

Intrauterine fetal blood transfusion

Intrauterine transfusion is indicated when the fetal HCT is >2 SD below the mean for gestational age or fetal hydrops is present.

- O-negative, CMV-negative blood is transfused either directly into the fetal vessel (intravascular transfusion) or directly into the fetal peritoneal cavity (intraperitoneal transfusion).
- The technique involves the ultrasound-guided insertion of a 20G needle into the placental insertion of the umbilical vein or intrahepatic vein.
  - Intravascular transfusion is more effective in the correction of anemia and reversal of hydrops, avoids trauma to intraabdominal organs, and allows the measurement of the post-transfusion hematocrit. Therefore it is regarded as the procedure of choice.
  - Intraperitoneal transfusion is useful under 18–20 weeks' gestation, when access to fetal vessels is hazardous, or when the position of the fetus poses difficulties in access to fetal vessels.
- A combination of both procedures allows increased blood volumes to be given (lengthening times between transfusions).
- Risks of the procedure include hemorrhage from the umbilical cord, non-reassuring fetal testing ('fetal distress') which may require emergent delivery, fetal demise (quoted at 3–5%), and the introduction of infection (rare, but a concern in women infected with hepatitis C or HIV).

Timing of delivery

Using the technique of intrauterine transfusion, treatment can proceed well into the third trimester. Once the fetus has reached 34 weeks, delivery is usually considered as risks of prematurity are likely to be less than the risks of further invasive procedures.

Hydrops fetalis: causes and clinical presentation

Introduction

Hydrops fetalis refers to the condition in which fluid has accumulated in two or more fetal body cavities or tissues. Fluid may not be seen in all compartments, but in its most severe form, the fetus has ascites, pleural effusions, pericardial effusions, and soft tissue edema. The placenta and cord may also be edematous. Hydrops is also frequently associated with polyhydramnios. Hydrops may occur at any gestation, but is not usually seen until 16–18 weeks. The earlier the presentation, the worse the prognosis.

Cystic hygroma is a specific condition that falls within the definition of hydrops. It is a collection of fluid behind the fetal neck, occasionally extending laterally to the sides of the neck. In its mildest form, it is termed nuchal thickening, nuchal edema, or nuchal translucency. In its most severe form, it can create a large septated sac of fluid around the fetal neck that can even extend down the fetal body.

Causes

Fetal hydrops can be divided into 'immune' causes (20% of cases) and 'nonimmune' causes (80%). Immune hydrops is due to feto-maternal blood group incompatibility and is dealt with on 📖 *p.140*.

Causes of nonimmune hydrops

There are a large number of maternal, fetal, and placental diseases that may result in hydrops unrelated to blood group incompatibility.

- *Chromosomal disorders.* When hydrops presents early in gestation, chromosomal disease is the likely diagnosis. Trisomy 21 (Down syndrome) and 46, X (Turner's syndrome) account for 75% of disorders, but other chromosomal disorders may also exist, including trisomies 18, 15, and 13, triploidy, tetraploidy, and partial chromosomal deletions or rearrangements.
- *Cardiovascular disorders* are the most frequent causes of non-immune hydrops. These may be either structural malformations or cardiac rhythm abnormalities. Hydrops may be associated with most major structural heart defects or cardiomyopathies, but the rhythm abnormalities are mainly due to supraventricular tachycardia or atrial flutter. Rarely, complete heart block may present with hydrops.
- *Thoracic malformations.* These mainly include:
  - diaphragmatic hernia.
  - pulmonary sequestration.
  - congenital cystic adenomatous malformation (CCAM) of the lung.
  - chylothorax.
- *Urinary tract abnormalities.* Obstruction at the lower end of the urinary tract (posterior urethral valves, urethral atresia) may lead to bladder overdistension and, ultimately, spillage of urine into the abdominal cavity, resulting in isolated fetal ascites (rather than generalized hydrops). In these cases, oligohydramnios is an important feature. Wilm's tumors may be associated with fetal ascites along with other rare disorders of the fetal kidney.

- *Meconium peritonitis.* Fetal ascites may result from intestinal perforation. Cystic fibrosis should be considered.
- *Skeletal dysplasias.* Many of the lethal skeletal dysplasias may be associated with hydrops.
- *Fetal anemia.* This is the mechanism leading to immune hydrops. However, there are other important causes of fetal anemia:
  - massive feto-maternal hemorrhage.
  - homozygous α-thalassemia (most common cause of hydrops worldwide).
  - G6PD deficiency.
  - Congenital infection with parvovirus B19.
- *Fetal infections.* In addition to parvovirus, other congenital infections may result in hydrops without fetal anemia:
  - CMV
  - rubella
  - varicella
  - cocksackie virus
  - respiratory syncytial virus
  - herpes simplex virus
  - hepatitis
  - toxoplasmosis.
- *Monochorionic twin gestation.* Hydrops may occur in the recipient twin in the twin-to-twin transfusion syndrome from overperfusion and congestive cardiac failure. The acardiac twin malformation may also result in the normal twin becoming hydropic.
- *Genetic conditions.* Many syndromes associated with multiple congenital malformations are associated with hydrops. Also, many metabolic and storage disorders may present with hydrops.

Clinical presentation

When a pregnancy is complicated by fetal hydrops, the woman may present with the following:

- Reduced fetal movement (a severely hydropic fetus often has poor activity).
- Large for dates (because of either associated polyhydramnios or a large grossly hydropic fetus).

When the fetus and placenta are grossly hydropic, the woman may present with preeclampsia (known as 'mirror syndrome').

Recommended further reading

1. Machin GA (1997). Hydrops, cystic hygroma, pericardial effusions and fetal ascites. In: Gilbert–Barness E, ed. *Potter's Pathology of the Fetus and Infant*, pp. 163–81. Mosby–Year Books St Louis, MO.
2. McCoy MC, Katz VI, Gould N, Kuller JA (1995). Non immune hydrops after 20 weeks gestation: review of 10 years experience with suggestions for management. *Obstet Gynecol* **85**, 578–82.

Diagnosis of hydrops

The diagnosis of hydrops is made by ultrasound examination of the fetus. Abnormal accumulation of fluid in the chest, peritoneal cavity, or fetal neck is easily identified and soft tissue edema can also be visualized.

Ultrasound assessment

Ultrasound examination of the fetus is also important in attempting to identify the underlying cause.

- Detailed examination of the fetal heart (including M mode ultrasound to detect cardiac dysrhythmias) must be performed to determine structural abnormalities or rhythm defects (in particular, supraventricular tachycardia).
- Tachydysrhythmias may be intermittent. Therefore it is important to check more than once.
- Careful examination of the intracranial structures and liver should be performed. Calcification may be suggestive of congenital infection (CMV, toxoplasmosis, etc.).
- Markers of chromosomal disease may be apparent.
  - Cystic hygroma *per se* carries a 70% chance of an associated chromosomal abnormality.
  - Other sonographic markers suggestive of chromosomal disease include choroid plexus cysts, ventriculomegaly, facial cleft, clinodactyly, sandal gap, pyelectasis (renal dilatation), echogenic intracardiac focus, and short femur length.
- A full skeletal survey will identify skeletal dysplasia as the underlying cause.
- The absence of amniotic fluid may suggest an obstructive uropathy.
- The placenta, cord, and fetus must be examined to exclude vascular abnormalities (e.g. chorioangioma of the placenta).

Maternal investigations

A careful enquiry should be made into any previously affected pregnancies, inherited genetic disease or metabolic disorders, and viral illness during the pregnancy. Investigations should include the following:

- Maternal blood taken for Kleihauer–Betke test (looking for feto-maternal hemorrhage), hemoglobin electrophoresis, blood group, and antibody screen.
- Viral serology (in particular, CMV, toxoplasmosis, parvovirus B19).

Fetal investigations

Further management should be directed at the likely etiology; in particular, the site of fluid accumulation may suggest the underlying cause. An invasive procedure is usually indicated as determination of the fetal karyotype is essential. Even if a cardiac malformation or rhythm abnormality is believed to have caused the hydrops, these malformations themselves may be associated with a chromosomal disorder.

- Invasive testing may be by amniocentesis, CVS, or FBS (cordocentesis). All these invasive procedures carry a risk to the pregnancy and, as the hydropic fetus is already compromised, this risk of complication is slightly higher than normal.
    - In the investigation of hydrops, FBS is a superior procedure as not only will a rapid and reliable karyotype be obtained, but hematological tests will also show whether fetal anemia is the underlying disorder and whether intrauterine blood transfusion is indicated (see 🕮 *p.144*).
- If a metabolic condition is suspected for which the gene sequence is known, CVS for DNA extraction may be appropriate.
- If a congenital infection is suspected, testing for a specific infection by PCR on amniotic fluid is the most reliable test.

Recommended further reading

1. Jones DC (1995). Non-immune fetal hydrops: diagnosis and obstetrical management. *Semin Perinatol* **19**, 447–61.
2. Nicolini U (1999). Fetal hydrops and tumours. In: Rodeck CH, Whittle MJ, eds. *Fetal Medicine: Basic Science and Clinical Practice*, pp. 737–54. Churchill Livingstone, Edinburgh.

Management and prognosis of hydrops

Fetal hydrops carries a very high perinatal mortality (81–95%). The mortality increases with decreasing gestational age at diagnosis. Treatment should be directed at the cause.

In utero treatment

- Fetal anemia is one of the more treatable conditions whether the anemia is due to maternal–fetal blood group incompatibility, viral infection, or hemorrhage. Intrauterine blood transfusions, in which blood is transfused directly into the umbilical vein (intravascular transfusion) or peritoneal cavity (intraperitoneal transfusion) are relatively safe (see 📖 *p.144*).
- Idiopathic tachydysrhythmias may respond to maternal administration of cardiac dysrhythmic agents (e.g. digoxin, verapamil, propranolol, flecanide). Some agents, although effective, do not cross the placenta to any large degree and therefore may need to be given by intraamniotic injection (e.g. adenosine).
- Isolated pleural effusions may be due to a benign condition (e.g. chylothorax), but prognosis is impaired because of fetal lung compression. *In utero* drainage and/or insertion of a pleuro-amniotic shunt may dramatically improve the outcome.
- If a lethal condition is diagnosed (e.g. chromosomal, skeletal dysplasia), the parents should be counseled and offered the option of termination of pregnancy.
- If maternal complications exist (e.g. preeclampsia), delivery of the fetus may be necessary for maternal health.

Prognosis

In general, the prognosis for fetal hydrops is poor. Fetal mortality has been reported as between 81% and 87%, and as high as 95% in cases diagnosed before 24 weeks' gestation. If the diagnosis is uncertain and a reasonable gestation has been reached, delivery may be considered to enable further investigation and treatment in the neonatal period.

Recommended further reading

1. Sebire NJ, Nicolaides KH (1996). Thoracoamniotic shunting for fetal pleural effusions. In: Chervenak FA, Kurjak A, eds. In *The fetus as a patient*, pp. 317–26. Parthenon, New York.
2. McCoy MC, Katz VI, Gould N, Kuller JA (1995). Non immune hydrops after 20 weeks gestation: review of 10 years experience with suggestions for management. *Obstet Gynecol* **85**, 578–82.

Origin, composition, and volume of the amniotic fluid

The precise origin of amniotic fluid in the third trimester still remains unresolved. It is largely derived from fetal urine and fetal lung secretions, although an additional contribution comes from amniotic membrane secretions. There is a continual exchange of fluid, most of which is swallowed and re-excreted by the fetus, and to a lesser extent it is exchanged through transfer of fluid to the mother through the membranes.

The composition of amniotic fluid is heterogeneous, consisting of proteins (albumins and globulins), lipids (phospholipids, cholesterol, and lecithin), carbohydrates (predominantly glucose), inorganic salts, and cells derived from fetal epithelium, amniotic membrane, and dermal fibroblasts. This latter cell type grows well in culture and is frequently used for karyotyping.

The volume of the amniotic fluid varies according to the gestational age of the fetus and is summarized in Fig. 3.2. The amniotic fluid index (AFI) is a quantitative ultrasonic assessment of amniotic fluid volume that is a summation of the deepest vertical pool depth in centimeters in each of four quadrants surrounding the fetus. An alternative objective measurement of amniotic fluid volume is the maximal vertical pocket (MVP) of fluid in centimeters. MVP is preferred to AFI when evaluating amniotic fluid volume in multiple pregnancies.

Underlying fetal or maternal conditions may alter the volume of fluid. Oligohydramnios and polyhydramnios are conditions associated with reduced and excessive amniotic fluid volume, respectively.

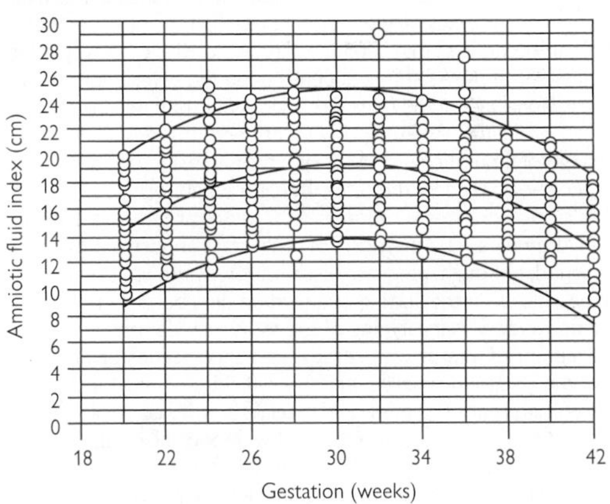

Fig. 3.2 Ultrasound four-quadrant assessment of AFI according to gestation. (Reprinted from Magowan B (1996). Oligohydramnios. In *Pocketbook of Obstetrics and Gynecology* (1st edn) (ed B Magowan), p. 50. © 1996 by permission of the publishers Churchill Livingstone, Edinburgh.)

Oligohydramnios

Oligohydramnios is commonly defined as an AFI of <5.0 cm in the third trimester (less than the 5th centile for gestational age). An alternative definitive is MVP ≤2 cm. The possible etiology of oligohydramnios is summarized in Table 3.1. An explanation for the reduction in amniotic fluid volume can be determined in over 85% of cases and therefore a careful history, thorough examination, and appropriate investigations are mandatory. The sequelae and management of oligohydramnios are dependent upon the cause. When oligohydramnios occurs early in pregnancy (<26 weeks) it can be associated with pulmonary hypoplasia and skeletal deformities (such as clubfeet). Of note, although maternal hydration status does affect amniotic fluid volume to some degree, maternal dehydration is never an adequate explanation for oligohydramnios.

Important causes and management

- *Premature rupture of the fetal membranes* (PROM) occurs in up to 15% of pregnancies and is defined as rupture of the membranes occurring prior to the onset of contractions. It can occur at any gestational age. The majority of patients with PROM are beyond 36 weeks, though an important minority present at an earlier gestational age. In most cases, the clinical history is diagnostic and is confirmed by visualizing pooling of amniotic fluid in the vagina. Management of term and preterm PROM is discussed in 📖 *p.268* and 📖 *p.112*. All patients with oligohydramnios should be regarded as having ruptured membranes until this diagnosis can be excluded.
- *Preeclampsia* is a complex multisystem disorder of uncertain etiology characterized by new-onset hypertension and proteinuria. It can affect any organ system, including the placenta itself. If the placenta is affected, IUGR can occur. This may often be associated with oligohydramnios. The management of preeclampsia depends upon the severity of illness and the gestational age of the fetus. Preeclampsia is discussed in 📖 *p.68*.
- *Fetal abnormalities.* As previously mentioned, there is a continual exchange of amniotic fluid, most of which is swallowed and subsequently re-excreted by the fetus. Renal tract abnormalities as listed in Table 3.1 prevent re-excretion and therefore are associated with oligohydramnios. The diagnosis of renal tract abnormalities is made by ultrasound, although adequate visualization of the fetal renal system may be difficult in the setting of anhydramnios because of lack of an acoustic window. Karyotyping of the fetus may be useful. The management of a fetus with renal tract abnormalities or Potter's syndrome (bilateral renal agenesis) is difficult and must include the input of maternal–fetal medicine specialists and neonatologists.
- *Prolonged pregnancy* can be associated with poor placental function. This can lead to redistribution of blood with selective perfusion for fetal brain and heart and reduced perfusion to the kidneys. As a consequence of diminished urine production, oligohydramnios occurs. Measurement of amniotic fluid volume forms an important part of assessing fetal wellbeing in prolonged pregnancy. Management options for prolonged pregnancy are discussed in the 📖 *p.270*.

Conclusions

Oligohydramnios can signify underlying fetal compromise. Detailed history, clinical examination, and ultrasound assessment of the fetus are necessary to determine the cause. Rupture of the fetal membranes should always be excluded. Severe oligohydramnios occurring at early gestation is associated with poor fetal prognosis. This is mainly due to skeletal deformities, prematurity, and underlying pulmonary hypoplasia. Reduced amniotic fluid volume is also associated with fetal heart rate abnormalities and an increased risk of cesarean delivery. The risk of hypoxia increases during labor, and passage of meconium is common. Labor should be regarded as high risk and continuous fetal monitoring should be employed.

Table 3.1 Causes of oligohydramnios

Iatrogenic causes
Following invasive testing (such as amniocentesis)
Maternal causes
Preeclampsia
Premature rupture of membranes (PROM)
Medications (such as ACE inhibitors)
Fetal causes
Fetal infections
IUGR
Renal tract anomalies
Bilateral renal agenesis (Potter's syndrome)
Renal dysplasia
Ureteric or urethral obstruction
Polycystic kidneys
Congenital abnormalities
Twin-to-twin transfusion syndrome
Placental causes
Postmaturity/prolonged pregnancy
Uteroplacental insufficiency (e.g. chronic hypertension)
Placental infection (e.g. malaria)
Thrombosis/placental abruption

Polyhydramnios

Polyhydramnios is defined as an AFI >20 cm (above the 95th centile for gestational age) or MVP ≥8 cm.

The causes of polyhydramnios are listed in Table 3.2. although in most cases the etiology is unknown. Polyhydramnios with IUGR should raise concerns about fetal aneuploidy. Polyhydramnios is diagnosed on the basis of a history of increasing abdominal distension beyond gestational age that is often accompanied by maternal discomfort, difficulty in palpating fetal parts, a symphyseal–fundal height greater than expected for gestational age, and a positive fluid thrill elicited on percussion. Measurement of the amniotic fluid by ultrasound confirms the diagnosis.

Risks and management

Polyhydramnios predisposes to preterm labor, PROM, malpresentation, cord prolapse, placental abruption following PROM, and postpartum hemorrhage. Therefore diagnosis is important for anticipation of the ensuing risks and management is largely dependent upon the degree of polyhydramnios.

When polyhydramnios is suspected clinically, an ultrasound examination should be carried out to quantify the degree of polyhydramnios and exclude multiple pregnancy or any fetal structural abnormality. A glucose tolerance test is useful in detecting gestational diabetes mellitus. Further management depends on the cause.

A severe degree of polyhydramnios gives rise to maternal discomfort and, in extreme cases, can cause respiratory embarrassment. Hospital admission may be indicated in such severe cases.

- If there is a threat of preterm delivery prior to 24 weeks, antenatal corticosteroids should be administered to reduce the risk of respiratory distress syndrome and other sequelae of prematurity.
- Indomethacin can be used for medical amnioreduction, but carries the risk of fetal anuria if used for a prolonged period. Therefore it is rarely used for this indication.
- Serial amnioreduction by amniocentesis is another therapeutic option. This is used most commonly in twin-to-twin transfusion syndrome in an attempt to reverse the imbalance in the shunting of blood within the placenta from the donor to the recipient twin. In some cases, this can result in complete resolution of the syndrome. The indication for serial amnioreduction is for patient comfort and in an attempt to prevent preterm labor. However, the fluid typically reaccumulates within 24–48 hours, and the amnioreduction procedure itself can result in PROM.
- Selective feticide of the growth-restricted twin and severing the vascular anastomosis by laser are some other invasive approaches used to manage severe polyhydramnios in twin-to-twin transfusion. They all carry considerable risks and should be performed only in centers with the requisite expertise and experience.

Conclusions

Severe polyhydramnios is rare and usually signifies some fetal abnormality or multiple pregnancy. A mild degree of polyhydramnios is often idiopathic and is usually managed expectantly with good prognosis. Increased vigilance is required during labor as the risks of cord prolapse, placental abruption, malpresentation, and postpartum hemorrhage are high.

Table 3.2 Causes of polyhydramnios

Idiopathic causes
Maternal causes
Diabetes mellitus
Fetal causes
Multiple pregnancy
Twin-to-twin transfusion syndrome (recipient twin)
Obstructive gastrointestinal abnormalities
Esophageal/duodenal atresia
Tracheo-esophageal fistula
Small intestine/colonic obstruction
Facial tumor interfering with fetal swallowing
Anencephaly (fetus unable to swallow)
Myotonic dystrophy and achalasia interfering with fetal swallowing
Macrosomia
Neural tube defects
Infections (e.g. parvovirus)
Uteroplacental causes
Chorioangioma
Placental tumors

Methods for antenatal surveillance of the fetus

Symphyseal–fundal height

Symphyseal–fundal height measurement provides a useful screening method for detection of the baby that is small or large for gestation. In the third trimester, this measurement (in centimeters) should approximate to the number of weeks of gestation. The variation is ±2 cm from 20–35 weeks, ±3 cm from 36–38 weeks, and ±4 cm after that due to engagement of the head and reduction in amniotic fluid volume. Inter- and intraobserver variation is small, but the measurement precludes the accurate differentiation of growth restriction from the constitutionally small baby. It is recommended that further investigation be instigated if the fundal height differs by more than expected for gestational age. The sensitivity of this screening method is further limited in the presence of multiple pregnancy, maternal obesity, uterine fibroids, or polyhydramnios. Its specificity is limited by ethnic origin. For example, women of Asian origin will commonly deliver healthy small babies. The use of customized population-specific growth charts for plotting fundal height has not been fully explored.

Fetal movement chart

The presence of fetal movement is a sign of fetal wellbeing and occurs in a cyclical pattern. A reduction or cessation in fetal movements may occur prior to fetal demise and may predate death by a number of days. Any marked decrease in movements or change in pattern may be significant and requires consideration and investigation. This should include a full assessment of the pregnancy utilizing clinical examination and ultrasound scanning (including fetal biometry and amniotic fluid volume and, if necessary, biophysical profile and umbilical artery Doppler velocimetry). The cardiotocograph (CTG) appears to be the main modality in many centers because of its ready availability. CTG alone may provide false reassurance, as the CTG carries no intermediate or long-term predictive value.

In high-risk pregnancies (previous poor obstetric outcome; maternal medical disorders, such as endocrine diseases, inherited thrombophilias, or drug dependency; pregnancies complicated by preeclampsia or antepartum hemorrhage) and those where a subjective reduction in movements has already been reported, the use of fetal movement charts ('kickcharts') may be of some benefit. Typically, women are asked to rest on their side after breakfast in the morning and after dinner in the evening and document the time it takes for the baby to move 10 times (or to document the number of movements in 2 hours). A significant change in baseline fetal movement or the absence of all movements over 6 hours requires further investigation. However, their use as a routine screening tool in low-risk pregnancies has demonstrated no benefits in improved obstetric outcome, and a high false-positive rate leads to increased testing and intervention.

Cardiotocography

The CTG provides a means of monitoring fluctuations in fetal heart rate (FHR) over time, and reflects the maturity of the fetal autonomic nervous system. In labor, FHR changes can be correlated with uterine activity. From 32 weeks, the fetal cardiograph can be categorized as reactive (reassuring), nonreactive (suspicious), or nonreassuring (pathological), and interpreted in light of the underlying clinical situation.

- A **reactive CTG** (nonstress test (NST)) should demonstrate an FHR with a normal baseline between 110 and 160 beats/minute with variability (exertions) around that baseline of 5–25 beats/minute (defined as moderate variability). At least two accelerations should occur within each 20 minutes (an acceleration being defined as a rise of at least 15 beats/minute from baseline lasting for at least 15 seconds). Ideally, there should be no decelerations from the baseline (a deceleration being defined as the converse of an acceleration), although some decelerations (such as early decelerations) can be normal.
- A **nonreactive CTG** is one in which the baseline is normal, but the variability is <5 beats/minute or accelerations are reduced or absent. Since accelerations often result from fetal movements, such a pattern may simply constitute a normal fetal resting trace, which may occur for up to 40 minutes. If the pattern continues, further assessment will be required.
- A **nonreassuring CTG** is one with a baseline outside the normal range, variability less than 5 beats/minute, and/or the presence of repetitive variable or late decelerations. Repetitive decelerations are decelerations that occur with more than 50% of contractions. The absence of uterine contractions, depending on the situation, will usually require additional testing by other modalities or delivery of the fetus.
- Prior to 32 weeks' gestation, interpretation of the antenatal CTG may be much more difficult. Incomplete development of the autonomic nervous system does not allow the predictable responses of the FHR to movement or stress that characterize the CTG of the more mature fetus.

The CTG provides a useful means of excluding current fetal hypoxia and acute compromise. The CTG may be nonreactive (show no accelerations) for reasons other than hypoxia, e.g. anemia, infection, medication, cerebral hemorrhage, maternal metabolic disturbance, and chromosomal or congenital malformation. It is part of the assessment following reported reduced fetal movements and is also employed in the assessment of many complications of pregnancy, namely antepartum hemorrhage, hypertensive disorders, and IUGR. It is rare to find an abnormal CTG in the presence of normal fetal movements. Therefore a reactive CTG is reassuring of fetal wellbeing. However, the converse is not true. A nonreactive CTG is a very poor predictor of a compromised fetus.

Ultrasound assessment of fetal growth

A fetus considered at risk of IUGR from maternal medical or obstetric history or thought to be small or large for gestational age clinically may be more accurately assessed by ultrasonic biometry. Various growth charts are used, all based upon cross-sectional (rather than longitudinal) population studies. The majority of centers will chart abdominal and head circumference, biparietal diameter, and femur length on charts with the 5th, 50th, and 95th centiles for gestational age defined. Some centers also plot AFI. However, the interpretation of fetal measurements is rarely straightforward, particularly when based upon a single scan, and overinterpretation frequently leads to unnecessary intervention.

- Dating of the pregnancy may be inaccurate and lead to the false diagnosis of a small or large baby.
- Precision of measurement is limited (error on ultrasound is ±20%) and may be further hampered by fetal position, maternal obesity, or oligohydramnios.
- A baby that appears small for gestational age may be constitutionally so and not subject to any pathological process, as the majority of centers use growth charts that are not customized for maternal size or ethnicity.

Serial growth scans are more useful than a single scan in the detection of a fetus with growth restriction. Growth scans are typically performed every 3–4 weeks (growth scans performed closer together are not reliable because of the inherent error in ultrasound measurements). Such growth restriction may be due to a number of possible causes, and determination of the cause may be essential to determine the optimal management of the pregnancy.

- For example, chromosomal abnormalities such as trisomies (e.g. trisomy 18) or triploidies may result in symmetrical growth restriction, where all parameters may show progressive descent through the centiles of the growth chart, sometimes from early in the pregnancy.
- In contrast, growth restriction due to uteroplacental insufficiency may demonstrate an asymmetrical pattern, with sparing of head measurements at the expense of abdominal circumference and amniotic fluid volume, and is more commonly manifest in the third trimester. Uteroplacental insufficiency may be idiopathic or related to an underlying problem, such as chronic hypertension, preeclampsia, maternal thrombophilia, or placental abruption.
- Other fetuses may demonstrate growth restriction that fits neither of these patterns and is caused by specific factors such as maternal alcohol or illicit drug abuse (particularly heroin, cocaine, and cannabis) or infection *in utero* (e.g. CMV).

The serial measurement of amniotic fluid volume, while contributing to fetal biophysical assessment and providing a useful indicator in fetal urinary tract disorders, has not been adequately independently evaluated in trials.

Serial ultrasonic growth assessment in low-risk women leads to increased intervention without a demonstrable improvement in perinatal outcome. Therfore it is not generally recommended.

Doppler ultrasonography

The Doppler waveform of a number of fetal and maternal vessels can be used to gain information about the wellbeing of the pregnancy. The Doppler signal indicates the directional velocity of flow of a liquid. Analysis of the difference between velocity of flow in the umbilical artery in fetal systole and diastole allows the calculation of the resistance or pulsatility indices.

- Decreasing umbilical artery diastolic flow velocity (often reported as increased systolic-to-diastolic ratio) is an indicator of increased placental resistance and hence of developing uteroplacental insufficiency.
- In pregnancies complicated by IUGR, the use of umbilical artery Doppler velocimetry has been demonstrated to reduce perinatal mortality by permitting timely delivery. Doppler waveform changes (increased systolic-to-diastolic ratio leading to persistent absent diastolic flow and finally to persistent reversed diastolic flow) may precede fetal demise by at least a week, permitting expediting delivery and giving time to introduce antenatal corticosteroids in the preterm infant. It is not clear how to interpret abnormal Doppler velocimetry studies in the setting of an appropriately grown fetus with normal amniotic fluid volume.
- The incidence of intrapartum signs of fetal compromise and of perinatal morbidity have not been shown to be significantly altered by the antenatal use of Doppler velocimetry.
- Umbilical artery Doppler velocimetry is of no demonstrated benefit as a screening tool in the low-risk population as the waveform varies with time, maternal positioning, hydration status, and distance from the cord insertion. Therefore it leads to false-positive results, resulting in unnecessary obstetric intervention. It is also not useful to document fetal wellbeing in post-term pregnancies.

The hypoxic infant with reduced, absent, or reversed end diastolic flow in the umbilical artery may demonstrate brain-sparing compensation with increased flow in the middle cerebral artery throughout the cardiac cycle, and particularly in diastole. The maternal uterine artery may demonstrate notching between the systolic and diastolic component, indicative of increased placental bed resistance secondary to poor spiral artery remodeling in response to trophoblast invasion. Such pathophysiological changes are thought to be pivotal in the development of preeclampsia and/or growth restriction later in the pregnancy. The presence of uterine artery waveform notching in women with a previous history of IUGR or preeclampsia is a strong predictor of recurrence, with absence of this sign in these women providing 98% reassurance for this pregnancy. However, this test is a poor screening tool in the low-risk population.

Recommended further reading

1. Goffinet F, Paris-Llado J, Nisand I, Breart G (1997). Umbilical artery Doppler velocimetry in unselected and low risk pregnancies: a review of randomized controlled trials. *Br J Obstet and Gynecol* **104**, 425–30.

Fetal biophysical profile and biochemical markers

Five parameters have been used together in an attempt to provide an assessment of fetal wellbeing that surpasses the CTG alone. These are:

- amniotic fluid volume
- fetal tone
- fetal movements
- fetal breathing movements
- the CTG.

Each parameter is given a score of 0 or 2. The lower the score, the further from normality the variable. A score of 8 or above out of 10 would be considered normal. A properly performed biophysical profile (BPP) assessment involves the evaluation of each parameter over a 30 minute period, and requires the time of a skilled obstetric sonographer. Originally developed to document fetal wellbeing in post-term pregnancies, its utility has subsequently been validated for term and preterm pregnancies. Of note, BPP is not useful for documenting fetal wellbeing in labor. Moreover, BPP has not definitively been shown by randomized controlled trial to provide any improvement in fetal outcome, although it is better at *predicting* outcome based on prospective descriptive studies involving large numbers.

Of the different components of the BPP, the single most important predictive parameter of perinatal deaths is amniotic fluid volume, and it has been suggested that this is as effective when used alone (so-called modified BPP). Amniotic fluid volume is commonly measured as AFI (the sum of the deepest pool in centimeters in each of the four quadrants of the uterus) or maximum vertical pocket (in centimeters).

Biochemical testing

A number of biochemical markers have been related to fetal compromise. The overlap of normal and abnormal ranges for most markers renders them poor screening tools, and most markers are no longer utilized in clinical practice. Two previously commonly used such markers were estriol and human placental lactogen (hPL).

Maternal serum α-fetoprotein (MS-AFP) is routinely measured in most centers during the second trimester (15–20 weeks' gestation) as a screening test for fetal abnormality (specifically, neural tube defects, abdominal wall defects, gastrointestinal tract obstruction) and, in conjunction with β-hCG, as part of screening for fetal aneuploidy. Raised MS-AFP may be due to increased placental permeability or to fetomaternal hemorrhage and, in the absence of fetal structural abnormality, is statistically significantly associated with poor obstetric outcome, particularly IUGR, low birth weight, increased perinatal mortality, preterm labor, and preeclampsia. Increasing the MS-AFP concentration by one multiple of the median (MoM) approximately doubles the risk of a pregnancy complication. For this reason, many clinicians will increase fetal testing in the third trimester and recommend routine induction of labor at 39 weeks in women with an unexplained elevation in MS-AFP. However, the sensitivity of MS-AFP as a predictor of obstetric complications remains too low to justify its use as a routine screening tool outside its use as an adjunct to the detection of congenital abnormality. More recently, an unexplained elevation in MS-AFP has also been shown to the associated with an increased risk of sudden infant death syndrome (SIDS) in the first year of life.

Summary

The low-risk pregnant population has long been well served by the use of simple clinical surveillance in antenatal care. More sophisticated methods of surveillance do not improve overall outcome in this group.

Suspicion raised by abdominal examination or by reported reduction in fetal movement, or the advent of other risk factors (such as antepartum hemorrhage or raised MS-AFP) that indicate that the fetus may be compromised, requires the use of appropriate testing to ascertain fetal wellbeing. The use of ultrasound scanning, with or without Doppler studies or biophysical profile, can improve the perinatal mortality rate when used to investigate this group if appropriate action is taken based on the results of these tests. Pregnancies considered to be high risk will require the tailoring of antenatal surveillance from the above techniques.

Recommended further reading

1. Manning FA (1990). The fetal biophysical profile score: current status. *Obstet Gynecol Clin North Am* **17**, 147–62.
2. Altman D, Hytten F, Grant A, Elbourne D (1995). Enkin M, Keirse M, Renfrew M, Neilson J, eds. Fetal biophysical profile. In: *A Guide to Effective Care in Pregnancy and Childbirth*, p. 68. Oxford University Press, Oxford.
3. Gardosi J, Francis A (1999). Controlled trial of fundal height measurement plotted on customized antenatal growth charts. *Br J Obstet Gynaecol* **106**, 309–17.
4. Grant A, Elbourne D, Valentin L, Alexander S (1989). Routine formal fetal movement counting and risk of antepartum late death in normally formed singletons. *Lancet* **ii**, 345–9.
5. Altman D, Hytten F, Grant A, Elbourne D (1995). Non-stress cardiotocography. In: Enkin M, Keirse M, Renfrew M, Neilson J, eds. *A Guide to Effective Care in Pregnancy and Childbirth*, pp. 63–4. Oxford University Press, Oxford.

Chapter 4

Infectious diseases in pregnancy

Syphilis

Introduction

There are a number of infections caused by viral, bacterial, and parasitic organisms that are known to cause clinically significant fetal infection resulting in miscarriage, preterm labor, intrauterine death, or long-term sequelae secondary to structural and neurodevelopmental abnormalities. The infections currently screened for routinely are syphilis, rubella, and hepatitis B.

Syphilis

Syphilis is a systemic chronic granulomatous infection caused by the spirochete *Treponema pallidum*. Infection occurs in three stages.

- The first stage of the disease, primary syphilis, is characterized by a painless genital ulcer 10–90 days postinfection which may pass unnoticed if on the cervix and which resolves spontaneously in 2–6 weeks.
- Secondary syphilis involves the widespread dissemination of spirochetes and is marked by lymphadenopathy, genital condyloma lata, and an extensive maculopapular rash, particularly involving the palms and soles, lasting for 2–6 weeks, followed by a latent phase of variable duration.
- In the absence of treatment, approximately one in three patients will progress to tertiary syphilis heralded by involvement of the cardiovascular (aortic aneurysms), central nervous (tabes dorsalis, paresis, optic atrophy), and musculoskeletal systems.

Obstetric significance

Treponema pallidum has the ability to cross the placenta and infect the fetus at all stages of the disease, although less commonly in late disease. Transmission of syphilis is more common with advancing gestation, especially after the 18–20 week stage, and adequate maternal treatment before 16 weeks' gestation will virtually eliminate the risk of infecting the fetus. It may well be appropriate to treat the mother in each subsequent pregnancy.

The risk in untreated maternal primary and secondary disease for development of congenital syphilis is of the order of 50% along with risks of prematurity and stillbirth. With early latent syphilis (disease duration <1 year) the risk is 40%, while with late latent disease (duration of disease >1 year) the risk is around 10%. The sequelae of congenital syphilis include stillbirth, hydrops, maculopapular rash, hepatosplenomegaly, lymphadenopathy, jaundice, chorioretinitis, and osteochondritis, along with characteristic findings of Hutchinson's teeth, mulberry molars, saddle nose, interstitial keratitis, saber shins, and eighth-nerve deafness. Thus treatment of syphilis in pregnancy aims to cure maternal disease and prevent congenital infection in the neonate.

Diagnosis

Diagnosis is possible using dark-ground microscopy of a smear from a lesion to detect spirochetes, but the most common method used for detection of syphilis is serological screening. This consists of an initial screening test involving detection of nontreponemal antibodies using the RPR (rapid plasma reagin) or VDRL (Venereal Disease Research Laboratory) tests, which are both positive in secondary and latent disease and frequently in primary disease. False-positive results may be associated with pregnancy, immunization, systemic lupus erythematosus (SLE), tuberculosis (TB), and leprosy. A positive screening test is confirmed with a specific antitreponemal antibody test, the most commonly used is the fluorescent treponemal antibody absorption (FTA-ABS) test, which remains positive throughout life even after cure.

Management

The treatment of choice is benzathine penicillin G as a single IM dose of 2.4 million units for primary, secondary, and early latent syphilis and the same dose repeated weekly for 3 consecutive weeks for late latent syphilis. Aqueous procaine penicillin may also be used, but requires a longer course of daily treatment (600 000–900 000 units for 10–21 days). Penicillin is the recommended first-line treatment in pregnancy as it offers a cure rate in excess of 98%, which is far higher than that of nonpenicillin alternatives such as erythromycin. Treatment failure may be associated with a failure to prevent congenital infection in the neonate. Given that about 90% of patients reported to be allergic to penicillin do not have true IgE-mediated hypersensitivity, there is a role for skin testing in such patients followed by inpatient temporary desensitization and penicillin therapy if a penicillin allergy is confirmed. Patients also need to be warned that after the first course of treatment, especially with secondary syphilis, there is a risk of Jarisch–Herxheimer reaction which may precipitate premature labor, so treatment after 20 weeks is best carried out in the hospital. By the third or fourth month post-treatment, quantitative nontreponemal antibody titers must drop at least fourfold. If this is not the case or if titers remain persistently high, the patient needs re-evaluation for neurosyphilis and retreatment. Contact tracing and treatment must be carried out together with counseling and testing for other sexually transmitted infections including HIV infection.

Recommended further reading

1. Adler MW (1997). *ABC of Sexually Transmitted Diseases* (3rd edn). BMJ Books, London.
2. Hurley R (1999). Infections in pregnancy. In: Chamberlain G, ed. *Turnbull's Obstetrics* (3rd edn), pp. 471–8. Churchill Livingstone, Edinburgh.
3. Yankowitz J, Pastorek JG (1999). Maternal and fetal viral infections. In: James DK, Steer PJ, Weiner CP, Gonik B, eds. *High Risk Pregnancy—Management Options* (2nd edn), pp. 525–58. WB Saunders, London.

Rubella

Rubella is also known as German measles. It is caused by RNA togavirus and acquired by respiratory droplet exposure. The affected individual is infectious for the last week of incubation and the first week after the rash appears. After a 2–3 week incubation, a rash with arthralgia, fever, and suboccipital and postauricular lymphadenopathy occurs, but clinical symptoms are present in only 50–75% of those infected. Thus many may have immunity in the absence of a history of symptomatic disease.

Obstetric significance

Rubella infection, though mild or even subclinical, has marked embryopathic consequences when acquired by the fetus *in utero*. Risk of transmission to the fetus with resultant congenital anomalies may be over 80% in the first trimester, dropping to approximately 50% by 13–14 weeks, and around 25% by late second trimester, compared with a less than 10% risk from rubella reinfection. Rubella reinfection may occur in up to 50% of cases of vaccine-induced immunity as opposed to 5% in cases of naturally acquired immunity.

Rubella-associated defects, which are generally attributed to vascular damage or reduced mitotic activity, are present in almost all infants infected before 11 weeks' gestation (mainly cardiac defects and sensorineural deafness) and in approximately 35% of those infected at 13–16 weeks (mainly deafness), with infection after 16 weeks rarely causing defects. Congenital anomalies, such as congenital cataracts, glaucoma, heart disease, deafness, microcephaly, and mental retardation, may be permanent, along with later development of diabetes, thyroid problems, precocious puberty, and progressive panencephalitis. Other features may be transient findings such as purpura, splenomegaly, jaundice, meningoencephalitis, and thrombocytopenia.

Diagnosis

Rubella is extremely difficult to diagnose because of nonspecific rash and commonly subclinical infection, and so serological assessment (latex agglutination, fluorescent immunoassay, or enzyme immunoassay) of paired acute and convalescent samples from women with suspect illness or exposure is the main method of diagnosis. During pregnancy, in cases of suspected exposure in a susceptible woman, it is important to confirm the diagnosis in the index case serologically whenever possible. Maternal infection is confirmed by the appearance of IgM antibodies or a fourfold rise in IgG antibody titers over a 4–6 week period. Assessment of fetal infection by amniotic fluid culture, IgM in fetal blood, or PCR has low accuracy, and so counseling is based on the gestation-age risk of congenital infection along with whether this was a primary maternal infection or a reinfection. If maternal seroconversion occurs in the first 12 weeks, a termination of pregnancy may be offered without invasive prenatal diagnosis. In cases of seroconversion between 12 and 18 weeks or reinfection in the first trimester or where termination of pregnancy is not an option, FBS may be offered to confirm fetal infection, but after 12 weeks the main risk is one of hearing defects. Children with no clinical manifestations but persistent antibodies need to be closely followed up as sensorineural deafness may be of late onset, bilateral, and progressive.

Immunization

All pregnant women should be tested prior to or in early pregnancy to confirm immunity, an expense justified by the significant risk of maternal rubella infection to the developing embryo. Prevention is through childhood vaccination, as well as assessment of the serological status of women pre-pregnancy or while undergoing fertility investigations and treatment. Immunity needs to be confirmed at the time of each subsequent pregnancy. The rubella vaccine is a live attenuated virus preparation and therefore should not be used in pregnancy or within 1 month of attempting conception. Despite these recommendations, there is no evidence that inadvertent use in pregnancy has been associated with congenital infection, and therefore parents can be reassured in such cases or in cases of pregnancy occurring soon after vaccination that the fetal risks are negligible.

Recommended further reading

1. Hurley R (1999). Infections in pregnancy. In: Chamberlain G, ed. *Turnbull's Obstetrics* (3rd edn), pp. 471–8. Churchill Livingstone, Edinburgh.
2. Yankowitz J, Pastorek JG (1999). Maternal and fetal viral infections. In: James DK, Steer PJ, Weiner CP, Gonik B, eds. *High Risk Pregnancy—Management Options* (2nd edn), pp. 525–58. WP Saunders, London.

Hepatitis B

This is a DNA virus that is hepatotropic, leading to viral liver disease with an incubation period of 2–6 months, though detectable in the circulation from 1 month post-infection. The carriage rate of hepatitis B virus (HBV) varies greatly throughout the world with rates ranging from a low in developed countries of around 1% to the Far East and tropical Africa where rates of 35% may be encountered. In developed countries, the major routes of transmission are through blood and blood products, sexual activity, and IV drug abuse, while vertical transmission at birth is the principal transmission route in developing countries. Approximately two-thirds of acute HBV infections are asymptomatic, subclinical, or associated with minimal influenza-like symptoms, but there may be upper gastrointestinal symptoms such as nausea, vomiting, anorexia, and occasionally right upper quadrant discomfort but with no evidence of jaundice in almost half the cases. HBV infection may be followed by a protracted period of malaise and anorexia, but in a previously healthy individual complete resolution occurs within 6 months in over 90% of cases. By definition, 10% become chronic carriers where hepatitis B surface antigen (HBsAg) persists beyond 6 months with presence of symptoms (chronic active hepatitis) or absent symptoms with deranged liver function tests (chronic persistent hepatitis). Rarely, the infection may progress to fulminant infection, hepatic failure, and death.

The severity of hepatitis B in pregnancy in the developed countries is similar to that in the nonpregnant state. However, vertical transmission from mother to neonate has major implications because, under such circumstances, chronic carriage is the norm with up to 90% of newborns developing chronic active or chronic persistent hepatitis. This has major implications because of risk of development of cirrhosis and hepatocellular carcinoma over a period of 20–30 years. The majority of infants are infected at birth from maternal blood and body fluids with a small minority infected *in utero* through transplacental bleeds.

Diagnosis

Laboratory diagnosis of HBV infections is based on the detection of a panel of viral-specific antibodies and antigens. HBsAg is a surface antigen from the viral capsule and signifies infectivity, while anti-HBs antibody (the antibody to the surface antigen) is a marker of immunological response and cure of infection. HBeAg is an antigen from the core of the virus and implies high infectivity (90% risk of transmission to fetus), while anti-Hbe (antibody to the core antigen) indicates a partial immune response (10% transmission risk).

Management

Treatment of acute HBV infection in pregnancy is symptomatic and supportive to control nausea and vomiting, monitor hydration and uterine activity, and perform LFTs as well as counseling, testing, and vaccinating family and sexual contacts as appropriate. There is no evidence of associated congenital syndrome or teratogenesis provided that the pregnancy survives the acute illness.

Obstetric significance

The impact of vertical transmission of HBV infection along with the low pickup rate of HBsAg carriers by risk assessment justifies universal antenatal screening for HBsAg carriage at antenatal booking. As the majority of cases of vertical transmission occur perinatally, preventative measures involving active and passive immunization at birth can be put into action in cases of HBsAg carriers identified by antenatal screening. This involves the newborn receiving hepatitis B immune globulin (HBIg) IM within 12 hours of birth along with the first of three doses of recombinant vaccine in the other thigh. The second and third doses of the recombinant vaccines are given at 1 and 6 months, and immunity confirmed at approximately 1 year. This policy relies on close cooperation between obstetrician, microbiologist, and neonatologist, and is effective in about 90% of cases. Clearly, repeated or additional testing may be required in further exposures/hepatitis-like illness in pregnancy or in high-risk individuals.

Recommended further reading

1. Adler MW (1997). *ABC of Sexually Transmitted Diseases* (3rd edn). BMJ Books, London.
2. Hurley R (1999). Infections in pregnancy. In: Chamberlain G, ed. Turnbull's Obstetrics (3rd edn), pp. 471–8. Churchill Livingstone, Edinburgh.
3. Yankowitz J, Pastorek JG (1999). Maternal and fetal viral infections. In: James DK, Steer PJ, Weiner CP, Gonik B, eds. *High Risk Pregnancy—Management Options*, (2nd edn), pp. 525–58. WB Saunders, London.

Toxoplasmosis

This is caused by the parasite *Toxoplasma gondii* which normally lives within the domestic cat. Infection is often asymptomatic or may produce a lymphadenopathy or present with a glandular-fever-like illness in the immunocompetent adult, but in immunocompromised individuals it may develop into a severe disseminated illness with chorioretinitis and encephalitis.

Obstetric significance

In the fetus and the neonate, toxoplasmosis leads to a syndrome comprising chorioretinitis, microcephaly/hydrocephaly, intracerebral calcification, and mental retardation as the predominant features. The earlier the infection occurs in pregnancy, the more serious the neonatal consequences with spontaneous miscarriage being common in first trimester infections. With primary maternal infection, the risk of transmission rises from 17% in the first trimester to 25% in the second and 65% in the third trimester of pregnancy, with overall 70% of babies born without any damage and a further 10% with chorioretinitis only.

Prevention

Prevention of maternal disease, and therefore fetal infection, is by avoidance of undercooked meat, unpasteurized milk, and contact with cat litter, as well as thorough washing of garden produce and hands after gardening activities and handling raw meat or vegetables soiled by earth.

Diagnosis

Routine serological testing is of no proven benefit. For this reason, serological testing should be carried out only in cases of clinical suspicion. A fourfold rise in IgG titers between acute and convalescent samples measured 4–6 weeks apart, concurrent high titers of IgG and IgM, or isolated very high IgM titers ELISA are indicative of acute infection or reinfection.

Management

If maternal infection is confirmed, maternal treatment with spiramycin 3 g/day should be commenced to reduce the risk of transplacental infection (this may reduce transmission by 60%), and consideration should be given to fetal testing and treatment. Fetal infection is confirmed by demonstrating specific IgM at amniocentesis and fetal blood sampling. If fetal infection is demonstrated, ultrasound scanning may be performed at around 22 weeks which may demonstrate ventricular dilatation. Further management depends on parental wishes. Termination of pregnancy is an option in the presence of structural abnormalities but, in cases of fetal infection without ultrasound evidence of fetal damage or where termination of pregnancy is unacceptable to the parents, treatment with 3-weekly cycles of pyrimethamine, sulfadiazine, and folinic acid alternating with spiramycin is recommended for the remainder of the pregnancy along with biophysical monitoring of the pregnancy (for IUGR, ventricular dilatation, and development of microcephaly).

Postnatally, it is important to carry out confirmatory tests (placenta, amniotic fluid, cord blood and maternal blood serology) and a thorough assessment of the neonate including ophthalmic review and cranial radiological assessment (ultrasound and X-ray). It is recommended to continue treatment for a year if toxoplasmosis is suspected. Long-term follow-up is recommended as children asymptomatic at birth may develop problems in later years. Future pregnancies should be delayed until toxoplasma IgM has been cleared, which may take up to 2 years.

Recommended further reading

1. Hurley R (1999). Infections in pregnancy. In: Chamberlain G, ed. *Turnbull's Obstetrics* (3rd edn), pp. 471–8. Churchill Livingstone, Edinburgh.
2. Yankowitz J, Pastorek JG (1999). Maternal and fetal viral infections. In: James DK, Steer PJ, Weiner CP, Gonik B, eds. *High Risk Pregnancy—Management Options* (2nd edn), pp. 525–58. WB Saunders, London.

Cytomegalovirus

The ability of CMV, which is a member of the herpesvirus family, to lie dormant in the host means that its most common manifestation is asymptomatic (95% of cases). Its clinical importance in pregnancy is due to intrauterine and neonatal infection. Congenital CMV infection may account for as much as 10% of mental retardation in children up to the age of 6. Primary infection in the adult may present with fever, malaise, atypical lymphocytosis, and lymphadenopathy, and rarely may lead to pneumonitis, myocarditis, thrombocytopenia, meningoencephalitis, and hepatitis. The virus can be cultured from urine, and excretion of virus may be prolonged from weeks to months and occasionally even longer. Reactivation and reinfection are common sequelae. CMV is transmitted by sexual intercourse, through transfused blood or marrow, and perinatally either transplacentally or by exposure to the virus from the cervix or birth canal. Neonates may acquire the virus through breast milk and, in childhood, transmission may occur through cross-contamination in nurseries as protracted viral shedding from the urine and respiratory secretions of infected children occurs. Viral shedding occurs more readily in pregnancy and with advancing gestation. Advanced gestation along with primary maternal infection increases the risk of neonatal disease. The incidence of primary infection in pregnancy is around 1–2%, and 50–80% of women are seropositive depending on race, parity, and socio-economic status.

Diagnosis

Diagnosis of primary infection is by detecting a significant rise in anti-CMV IgM titers, which may persist for 4–8 months after primary infection, while a recurrent infection may be confirmed by rise in IgG titers over a period of 4–6 weeks.

Management

The management of a patient with confirmed CMV infection in pregnancy will depend on careful counseling of the prospective parents about the risks to the fetus. Appropriate management may involve invasive procedures to determine fetal infection, regular biophysical assessment of fetal growth and health, or consideration of therapeutic termination of pregnancy. Congenital infection is three times more likely to occur after primary infection than after reinfection in the mother, with around 40% of fetuses infected following primary maternal infection in pregnancy. CMV is found in approximately 1% of newborns of whom 5–10% are clinically affected by one or more features of congenital CMV infection, the most common being hepatosplenomegaly, microcephaly, hyperbilirubinemia, petechiae, thrombocytopenia, and IUGR. A further 5–10% of infected infants, although asymptomatic at birth, will develop long-term sequelae such as sensorineural deafness, microcephaly, low IQ, or seizures, but over 85% of babies born to women with CMV in pregnancy, including 75% of infected infants, will have no CMV-related problems at birth or thereafter. Appropriate clinical and serological assessment and pediatric follow-up should be instituted if infection is confirmed postnatally.

Recommended further reading

1. Hurley R (1999). Infections in pregnancy. In: Chamberlain G, ed. *Turnbull's Obstetrics*, (3rd edn), pp. 471–8. Churchill Livingstone, Edinburgh.
2. Yankowitz J, Pastorek JG (1999). Maternal and fetal viral infections. In: James DK, Steer PJ, Weiner CP, Gonik B, eds. *High Risk Pregnancy—Management Options* (2nd edn), pp. 525–58. WB Saunders, London.

Chickenpox/herpes zoster infection

Varicella zoster (VZ) is a highly contagious DNA virus transmitted through respiratory droplets and close interpersonal contact with a 10–20 day incubation period. The patient is contagious for 48 hours prior to the appearance of the rash and until the vesicles crust over. The incidence of chickenpox (varicella) infection in pregnancy is of the order of 1 in 2000, with 85% of the adult population already seropositive for VZIg. Primary infection leads to chickenpox, while reactivation of the dormant virus leads to herpes zoster.

Obstetric significance

In pregnancy, VZ infection can have both maternal and fetal consequences. Maternal implications include pneumonia in up to 10% of infected adults, with a 6% mortality risk, with the risks of developing both pneumonia and respiratory complications being higher in pregnancy. Fetal consequences as a result of primary VZ infection in the first 20 weeks of pregnancy include spontaneous miscarriage in the first trimester and a 2% risk of congenital varicella syndrome. The latter is characterized by skin scarring in a dermatomal distribution, eye defects (chorioretinitis, cataracts, microophthalmia), hypoplasia of limbs, and neurological abnormalities (microcephaly, cortical atrophy, mental retardation, and dysfunction of bladder and bowel sphincters).

Transplacental passage of the virus increases with gestation age. Thus varicella infection may occur in up to 50% of fetuses whose mothers develop primary VZ infection in the last 1–4 weeks of pregnancy, with up to a third of the newborns developing clinical varicella despite high titers of passively acquired maternal antibodies. However, the main risk to the newborn is with maternal infection occurring up to 5 days prior to delivery or 2 days postdelivery, as there has been inadequate time for development and passage of maternal antibodies to the fetus and this leads a significant risk of disseminated VZ infection in the newborn with mortality risks of 20–30%. Finally, babies with no evidence of clinical VZ infection at birth may develop herpes zoster in childhood consistent with an *in utero* primary VZ infection.

Prevention

A live attenuated varicella vaccine has been shown to be effective in preventing chickenpox in adults, but is not approved for use in pregnancy. VZ Ig is known to be effective in preventing or reducing the severity of maternal infection or congenital varicella syndrome if given to a susceptible individual within 72 hours of contact, with some residual benefit if administered within 10 days. However, it is a blood product with the attendant risks and cost.

Management

The management of a pregnant woman with a suspected varicella contact involves review of the history (certainty of diagnosis in index case, the degree of infectivity, i.e. presence of rash or rash developing within 48 hours, degree of exposure) as well as the susceptibility of the pregnant woman (a history of VZ infection in the past and therefore immune but, even with no clear history, 85–95% of the adult population have antibodies to VZ). If there is any doubt regarding immunity, VZ Ig levels can be checked in the routine antenatal booking bloods. If immunity is confirmed, no further action is required. If the patient is nonimmune and is under 20 weeks pregnant then VZ Ig should be administered as soon as possible, preferably within 72 hours of contact, but for up to 10 days postcontact there may be some benefit.

In cases where VZ IgM is detected in the serum, the patient must be counseled regarding the 2% risk of congenital varicella syndrome. A specialist ultrasound assessment at 5 weeks postinfection or at 16–20 weeks (looking for polyhydramnios, microcephaly, hyperechogenic foci in the liver, hydrops fetalis) is recommended along with a neonatal ophthalmic examination at birth. In susceptible women who are beyond 20 weeks at time of exposure, congenital varicella does not occur and the only benefit of VZ Ig administration may be to reduce the severity of maternal infection and risk of VZ pneumonia, although this is not universally accepted.

Pregnant women presenting with VZ infection should be isolated from other pregnant patients or staff and neonates. If delivery occurs within 5 days of maternal infection or the mother develops VZ within 2 days of delivery, the high risk of neonatal VZ infection justifies administration of VZ Ig as soon as possible to the neonate, who should also receive acyclovir if there is any suggestion of neonatal infection. Maternal administration of acyclovir within 24 hours of development of VZ rash may reduce the duration and severity of the illness, but is not routinely recommended in the absence of complications. Pregnant women with primary VZ infection should be advised to look out for respiratory symptoms as this would be an indication for hospitalization and treatment with IV acyclovir. If, at around the time of discharge home of the mother and newborn, a sibling has chickenpox then, unless the mother is immune, both she and her newborn should be given VZ Ig.

Recommended further reading

1. Stirrat GM (1997). Maternal and fetal infections. In *Aids to Obstetrics and Gynecology* (4th edn). Churchill Livingstone, Edinburgh.
2. Yankowitz J, Pastorek JG (1999). Maternal and fetal viral infections. In: James DK, Steer PJ, Weiner CP, Gonik B, eds. *High Risk Pregnancy—Management Options* (2nd edn), pp. 525–58. WB Saunders, London.

Parvovirus infection

Parvovirus B19 is a DNA virus and the causative agent of a number of illnesses including aplastic crisis in conditions characterized by accelerated hemolysis such as sickle cell disease, a form of chronic arthropathy in adults, and an exanthematous illness in childhood known as fifth disease (erythema infectiosum). The latter presents with high fever and a rash giving the appearance of a 'slapped cheek'. Transmission is by respiratory droplets and the incubation period is 4–14 days. Although in children the infection may even be subclinical, the adult form is associated with lymphadenopathy and arthropathy as common sequelae as well as a postviral syndrome of fatigue and depression.

Obstetric significance

The obstetric implications of this condition are due to the transplacental passage of the virus in approximately one-third of cases of maternal infection. Parvovirus infection in early and mid-pregnancy carries a 10% risk of miscarriage. The interval between maternal infection and fetal loss is usually 4–5 weeks but it may be up to 11 weeks. The parvovirus has particular predilection for rapidly dividing bone marrow cells and erythrocytes, leading to hemolytic anemia and hemopoietic arrest, which in turn leads to high-output cardiac failure and nonimmune hydrops in some cases of maternal infection in the late second and third trimester. If the fetus survives the acute insult (fetal loss is uncommon) or is given supportive treatment, there is no evidence of a congenital syndrome postnatally.

Diagnosis

The diagnosis of the condition in adults is hampered by the variable presentation. Infection is confirmed by demonstrating seroconversion with acute and convalescent sera: IgM antibodies indicative of acute infection are present within a week in the majority of patients and persist for several months, while IgG antibodies appear at 10 days and persist for years. In a previously healthy individual the illness is self-limiting, but immunocompromised individuals are at risk of sudden hemolysis, and therefore they should be monitored and supportive treatment including blood transfusions given as appropriate.

Management

In pregnant patients with confirmed parvovirus B19 infection, treatment is symptomatic for the mother along with weekly ultrasonographic monitoring of the fetus for a minimum of 12–14 weeks looking for features of nonimmune hydrops, such as ascites and pericardial or pleural effusions, suggestive of fetal cardiac decompensation. In such cases, the options depend on the gestational age and include intrauterine transfusion or delivery and postnatal correction of anemia in the newborn, although there is now evidence that hydrops may resolve spontaneously *in utero*. Thus consultation with a subspecialist in maternal–fetal medicine is warranted.

Recommended further reading

1. Hurley R (1999). Infections in pregnancy. In: Chamberlain G, ed. *Turnbull's Obstetrics* (3rd edn), pp. 471–8. Churchill Livingstone, Edinburgh.
2. Yankowitz J, Pastorek JG (1999). Maternal and fetal viral infections. In: James DK, Steer PJ, Weiner CP, Gonik B, eds. *High Risk Pregnancy—Management Options* (2nd edn), pp. 525–58. WB Saunders, London.

Measles

This is an acute febrile illness caused by a paramyxovirus commonly attacking children and conferring lifelong immunity. Characteristic Koplik spots in the buccal epithelium along with fever, rash, rhinorrhea, and conjunctivitis are the most common findings. Rare but serious complications in adults are pneumonia and encephalitis, including subacute sclerosing panencephalitis.

Obstetric significance

As with any febrile illness, measles infection may precipitate uterine activity and premature delivery. There is no recognized syndrome of intrauterine measles infection although, if the mother has measles at the time of delivery, there is risk of neonatal measles.

Diagnosis

Diagnosis is clinical, based on rash and Koplik spots and serological confirmation through hemagglutination inhibition antibody assay or a complement fixation assay.

Prevention and management

Prevention is by childhood vaccination (which is also effective within 72 hours of exposure). Antenatal management is by treatment of upper respiratory symptoms and fever, with vigilance for uterine activity, whilst appropriate isolation/infection control measures are observed while in hospital.

Recommended further reading

1. Hurley R (1999). Infections in pregnancy. In: Chamberlain G, ed. *Turnbull's Obstetrics* (3rd edn), pp. 471–8. Churchill Livingstone, Edinburgh
2. Yankowitz J, Pastorek JG (1999). Maternal and fetal viral infections. In: James DK, Steer PJ, Weiner CP, Gonik B, eds. *High Risk Pregnancy—Management Options* (2nd edn), pp. 525–58. WB Saunders, London.

Listeriosis

This is caused by *Listeria monocytogenes*, a gram-positive non-spore-forming facultative anaerobe. The gastrointestinal tract is the major site of entry and preventive measures are centered around avoidance of soft cheese and pâtés, thorough cooking of raw food from animal sources, thorough washing of raw vegetables, and attention to hygiene in storage and preparation of food. Dissemination of the organism throughout the body is usually prevented by the immune system. For this reason listeriosis and some form of depression of cell-mediated immunity (pregnancy being an example) are often found together.

Obstetric significance

The incidence in pregnancy is around 1 in 10 000 and disease in early pregnancy may result in spontaneous miscarriage. Infection in the mother is usually in the form of a mild influenza-like pyrexial illness and is self-limiting. Transplacental passage of *L.monocytogenes* (which does not occur in all cases of maternal infection) gives rise to fetal infection with a spectrum of manifestations from spontaneous abortion, amnionitis with green-brown staining of amniotic fluid, through to premature delivery and early- or late-onset neonatal listeriosis. Fetal infection late in pregnancy may lead to multiorgan morbidity (intraventricular hemorrhage, pneumonitis, hepatitis, neurological handicap) and fetal mortality.

Early neonatal infection due to transplacental spread occurs within 2 days, with an appropriately grown premature infant suffering from congenital pneumonia, whereas late-onset disease acquired during passage through the birth canal presents mostly with meningitis. Diagnosis should be suspected in cases of an influenza-like illness with pyrexia, uterine irritability, and bloody vaginal discharge. Vaginal and blood cultures should be taken and the microbiologist warned regarding the clinical suspicion as *L.monocytogenes* can easily be confused with diptheroids. Pathological examination of the placenta may reveal mycotic abscesses, which are typical of intrauterine listeriosis.

Management

Infection is responsive to a wide range of antibiotics, including ampicillin, chloramphenicol, co-trimoxazole, and aminoglycosides such as gentamicin. Treatment should continue for 3–6 weeks to prevent relapses.

Recommended further reading

1. Hurley R (1999). Infections in pregnancy. In: Chamberlain G, ed. *Turnbull's Obstetrics* (3rd edn), pp. 471–8. Churchill Livingstone, Edinburgh.

Herpes simplex infection

Herpes simplex virus (HSV) is a DNA virus. HSV1 is predominantly responsible for orolabial lesions, while HSV2 is responsible for genital lesions, but there is considerable overlap between the two types. Genital herpes is usually acquired through sexual contact with an infected individual, who may well be asymptomatic, or by orogenital contact. Approximately 20–40% of the population have been infected by HSV at some time, but only one-third have ever had their infection diagnosed. The incubation period is around a week and the severity of the attack is dependent on the presence or not of anti-HSV antibodies in the patient from an earlier exposure. In the presence of antibodies, the attack tends to be of a shorter duration in terms of both lesions and viral shedding, with fewer constitutional symptoms and complications. Primary genital herpes infection may be quite severe with constitutional symptoms including fever, myalgias, and malaise along with lower motor neuron and autonomic neuropathy leading to bladder atony, urinary retention, and the need for hospitalization.

Obstetric significance

Primary HSV causing maternal systemic disease or fever may lead to miscarriage or preterm labor, while the relative immunosuppression in pregnancy may result in generalized viral dissemination. Although no congenital syndrome exists, neonatal concerns are centered around fetal acquisition of HSV in the perinatal period, as the neonatal immunological immaturity may be unable to control the spread of HSV. The majority of neonatal infections occur in women undergoing a primary attack of HSV and occur perinatally as the fetus emerges through an infected birth canal, with only about 5–10% occurring in the postnatal period. The risk in recurrent disease is low and estimated at less than 5% due to passive transfer of immunity. It should also be borne in mind that the majority of women whose babies are infected are in fact asymptomatic themselves. Neonatal HSV infection presents in the first 2 weeks of life, being limited to eyes and mouth in 25%, but with widespread dissemination to multiple organs in 75%. Presenting features include weight loss, poor feeding, fever with multiorgan involvement carrying a high mortality of 70–80% and long-term morbidity in survivors, including mental retardation and developmental delay.

Diagnosis and management

Laboratory diagnostic methods include tissue culture techniques with a fluorescent antibody test and serological testing.

The management of primary HSV infection in the first and second trimesters of pregnancy is based on symptomatic support with oral or intravenous acyclovir if the mother's condition warrants it. Provided that the pregnancy survives the acute episode, no complications are anticipated. A controversial suggestion in some quarters includes the use of continuous acyclovir in the last 4 weeks of pregnancy to suppress viral shedding or recurrence. It has been estimated that, with active primary genital herpes at the time of delivery, the risk of vertical transmission is around 40–50% and viral shedding may continue for 3–6 weeks. Therefore cesarean delivery to prevent vertical transmission would be recommended if the primary attack is within 6 weeks of labor or if visible genital lesions are present in labor, regardless of whether or not the membranes are ruptured. In cases of recurrent genital herpes, the risks and duration of viral shedding are less and a degree of protection will be conferred to the neonate by passive immunity. As such, cesarean delivery to prevent vertical transmission should be considered only if there are visible lesions or symptoms. There is no value of serial cervical cultures towards the end of pregnancy as there is no correlation between the culture result of the latest cervical swab and viral shedding at the onset of labor. In all cases, vigilance and observation of the neonate is imperative.

Recommended further reading

1. Adler MW (1997). *ABC of Sexually Transmitted Diseases* (3rd edn). BMJ Books, London.
2. Hurley R (1999). Infections in pregnancy. In: Chamberlain G, ed. *Turnbull's Obstetrics* (3rd edn), pp. 471–8. Churchill Livingstone, Edinburgh.
3. Stirrat GM (1997). Maternal and fetal infections. In *Aids to Obstetrics and Gynecology* (4th edn). Churchill Livingstone, Edinburgh.
4. Yankowitz J, Pastorek JG (1999). Maternal and fetal viral infections. In: James DK, Steer PJ, Weiner CP, Gonik B, eds. *High Risk Pregnancy—Management Options* (2nd edn), pp. 525–58. WB Saunders, London.

Human papillomavirus infection

Human Papilloma Virus (HPV) is a double-stranded DNA virus with over 70 subtypes identified so far. It is the most common sexually transmitted infection. Subtypes 6 and 11 are associated with condylomata acuminata (genital warts) and juvenile laryngeal papillomatosis, while subtypes 16, 18, 31, 33, and 35 are associated with cervical intraepithelial neoplasia (CIN), cervical carcinoma, and other lower genital tract precancers and cancers.

Obstetric significance

The significance of HPV infection in pregnancy is related to its association with CIN, the tendency of genital warts to grow rapidly in pregnancy on occasion causing obstruction in labor, and the risks of perinatal exposure to HPV with the development of juvenile laryngeal papillomatosis. The severity of juvenile laryngeal papillomatosis may range from minor hoarseness in voice to complete obstruction of the upper airways, but a positive maternal history for genital warts is present in only half of cases. The overall risk of developing juvenile laryngeal papillomatosis following perinatal exposure is minimal and estimated at approximately 0.25%. Thus elective cesarean delivery is justifiable only where mechanical obstruction of the birth canal by warts is evident.

Management

In the majority of cases, HPV infections are subclinical. The presence of HPV infection may be suspected from characteristic cytological features on cervical screening smears or at colposcopy and is straightforward in cases of genital warts presenting as pale pink or white papillary growths. In general, treatment of genital warts involves excision or destruction of visible lesions by pharmacological, physical, or surgical methods, but warts tend to recur because of the presence of latent provirus in epithelial cells. Warts in pregnancy are not treated routinely unless symptomatic. Methods that can be used in pregnancy include application of 80% trichloroacetic acid, which may have to be repeated weekly, and liquid nitrogen cryotherapy as first-line treatments. In refractory cases or for patients with multiple or extensive lesions, treatment under a general anesthetic with laser or diathermy destruction of warts is an alternative. Use of podophyllin, 5-fluouracil, and interferon intradermally are not suitable in pregnancy. Excision of the lesion at time of delivery is not recommended, as warts tend to shrink in size following pregnancy and may be very vascular in pregnancy risking significant hemorrhage.

Recommended further reading

1. Adler MW (1997). *ABC of Sexually Transmitted Diseases* (3rd edn). BMJ Books, London.
2. Hurley R (1999). Infections in pregnancy. In: Chamberlain G, ed. *Turnbull's Obstetrics* (3rd edn), pp. 471–8. Churchill Livingstone, Edinburgh.
3. Stirrat GM (1997). Maternal and fetal infections. In *Aids to Obstetrics and Gynecology* (4th edn). Churchill Livingstone, Edinburgh.
4. Yankowitz J, Pastorek JG (1999). Maternal and fetal viral infections. In: James DK, Steer PJ, Weiner CP, Gonik B, eds. *High Risk Pregnancy—Management Options* (2nd edn), pp. 525–58. WB Saunders, London.

Chlamydia trachomatis

This obligate intracellular organism is responsible for one of the most common sexually transmitted infections in the world and is a significant cause of subfertility. Among the 15 serotypes identified, subtypes D and K are responsible for genital infections, while others lead to blindness and lymphogranuloma inguinale. The majority of patients with genital chlamydia infection are asymptomatic, but in pregnancy may present with mucopurulent cervicitis, endometritis, acute salpingitis, and acute urethral syndrome. The long-term consequences of chlamydial pelvic inflammatory disease may include subfertility, adhesions, pain, and ectopic pregnancies. Diagnosis is based on culture-independent immunoassay by either PCR detection of DNA or ELISA techniques. Culture of the organism is possible but, because of its intracellular nature, is labor intensive and very costly and therefore is not widely used.

Obstetric significance

The obstetric significance of chlamydia infection is twofold.

- There appears to be a modest association (especially of recently acquired infection) with preterm delivery, preterm premature rupture of the fetal membranes, low birthweight, and postpartum endometritis (all of which can be reduced by maternal therapy to eliminate the infection).
- Of neonates born to mothers with maternal chlamydial cervicitis, 50–60% will be colonized, leading to inclusion conjunctivitis in about one-third within the first 2 weeks of life (which is why prophylactic 0.5% erythromycin or 1% tetracycline ointment is routinely applied to the eyes of the newborn within 1 hour of birth) and to pneumonia in approximately 15% of neonates within the first 4 months of life.

Management

Treatment of chlamydial infection in pregnancy is limited to erythromycin 500 mg 6-hourly for 1 week. In the non-pregnant adult, a single 1 g dose of azithromycin or a 1-week course of doxycycline, tetracycline, or ofloxacin can be used. If erythromycin is not tolerated, alternatives in pregnancy include amoxicillin or clindamycin, but these have lower cure rates of 98% and 93%, respectively. Contact tracing for the past 30 days and appropriate counseling and treatment is essential.

Recommended further reading

1. Adler MW (1997). *ABC of Sexually Transmitted Diseases* (3rd edn). BMJ Books, London.
2. Hurley R (1999). Infections in pregnancy. In: Chamberlain G, ed. *Turnbull's Obstetrics* (3rd edn), pp. 471–8. Churchill Livingstone, Edinburgh.
3. Stirrat GM (1997). Maternal and fetal infections. In *Aids to Obstetrics and Gynecology* (4th edn). Churchill Livingstone, Edinburgh.
4. Yankowitz J, Pastorek JG (1999). Maternal and fetal viral infections. In: James DK, Steer PJ, Weiner CP, Gonik B, eds. *High Risk Pregnancy—Management Options* (2nd edn), pp. 525–58. WB Saunders, London.

Gonorrhea

This is a common sexually transmitted infection caused by *Neisseria gonorrhea*, a gram-negative intracellular diplococcus. It may cause acute cervicitis, urethritis, bartholinitis, proctitis, pharyngitis, and disseminated systemic infection (more common in pregnancy, with malaise, fever, rash, and septic arthritis). The most common presentation in pregnancy is asymptomatic infection of the cervix.

Obstetric significance

- The obstetric significance of gonococcal cervical infection in pregnancy is the association with premature rupture of membranes, preterm delivery, chorioamnionitis, and postpartum endometritis.
- Acute salpingitis is rare in the first trimester and even less likely thereafter because the endometrial cavity is obliterated by the conceptus.
- Although gonococcal infection in pregnancy is not associated with an intrauterine syndrome, 40–50% of babies born to mothers with such infection develop ophthalmia neonatarum—hence the importance of diagnosis and treatment of the mother and prophylactic treatment to the newborn.

Diagnosis and management

Diagnosis is based on the presence of gram-negative diplococci within leukocytes from the infected exudate or discharge and culture of endocervical swabs inoculated in Thayer Martin or other selective medium soon after obtaining the specimen.

Treatment depends on the severity of the infection and sensitivities need to be obtained as penicillin-resistant strains, though uncommon, may be responsible. Test of cure, contact tracing, and screening for other sexually transmitted infections are also important. For uncomplicated genital infection a single dose of ciprofloxacin may be adequate, but this is not suitable in pregnancy because of potential adverse effects on the fetus. In pregnancy the recommended regimens include spectinomycin 2 g IM or a combination of probenecid 1 g orally with either aqueous procaine penicillin G 4.8 million units IM or amoxicillin 3g orally followed by a 7-day course of erythromycin 500mg four times a day. For disseminated infections, hospital admission and IV cephalosporins may be required. There is no contraindication to breast-feeding.

Recommended further reading

1. Adler MW (1997). *ABC of Sexually Transmitted Diseases* (3rd edn). BMJ Books, London.
2. Hurley R (1999). Infections in pregnancy. In: Chamberlain G, ed. *Turnbull's Obstetrics* (3rd edn), pp. 471–8. Churchill Livingstone, Edinburgh
3. Stirrat GM (1997). Maternal and fetal infections. In *Aids to Obstetrics and Gynecology*, (4th edn). Churchill Livingstone, Edinburgh.

Group B streptococcal infection

Group B β-hemolytic streptococcal infection (GBS) is one of the most important causes of neonatal bacterial infection and of maternal intrapartum and postpartum infective morbidity. GBS forms part of the normal vaginal flora in about 20% of women of childbearing age. Of infants born to colonized mothers, 60–70% will become colonized with approximately 1% developing invasive disease (sepsis), the latter group carrying a 20% mortality.

Obstetric significance

A positive perineal culture for GBS at 35–36 weeks confers a 90–95% chance of carriage at term, but eradication prior to delivery is not possible despite multiple courses of antibiotics.

- Women colonized with GBS may present with obstetric complications such as preterm labor, preterm premature rupture of the fetal membranes, or intrapartum fever.
- Neonatal infection may take the form of early-onset disease within the first 4 days of life, presenting with pneumonia or septicemia and occasionally with concurrent meningitis, especially in low-birth-weight babies (<2.5 kg).
- The late-onset form of neonatal disease occurs after the first week of life, with 80% presenting with meningitis, and carries a 20% mortality risk and a 50% risk of sequelae including cortical blindness and deafness in survivors. Late-onset neonatal GBS sepsis is regarded as a nosocomial (hospital-acquired) infection and cannot be prevented by intrapartum antibiotic chemoprophylaxis.

Diagnosis and management

- Diagnosis of GBS colonization is by perineal/perianal (not cervical) swabbing and overnight culture in selective media. The culture result is predictive of perineal colonization for 5 weeks.
- Routine perineal culture for GBS is recommended for all pregnant women at 35–36 weeks of gestation.
- Given that eradication of GBS colonization by antepartum antibiotic therapy is not effective and universal chemoprophylaxis to all women is not practical because of the cost and risk of anaphylaxis, together with development of resistance in the community, management involves selective chemoprophylaxis to women deemed to be at high risk. The risk factors identified are based on the observation that the majority of early-onset disease and fatalities occur in low-birth-weight and premature infants, those with prolonged rupture of membranes, and especially in the presence of intrapartum fever.
- The presence of GBS on perineal/perianal culture within the past 5 weeks, GBS bacteriuria at any stage in the pregnancy, or a history of a previous infant with GBS sepsis are significant risk factors. Such women should all receive intrapartum antibiotic chemoprophylaxis. Evidence of GBS colonization in a prior pregnancy should not be regarded as a significant risk factor.

- If the GBS colonization status of the patient is unknown, the decision of whether to administer intrapartum antibiotic chemoprophylaxis should be determined by the presence of additional risk factors, specifically prematurity, prolonged rupture of membranes (defined as >18 hours), or fever in labor (which should also prompt broad-spectrum antibiotic treatment for intrauterine infection).
- The antibiotic of choice is benzylpenicillin IV 3 g immediately and 1.5 g 4-hourly until delivery. A minimum of 4 hours of intrapartum treatment is recommended. Ampicillin 2 g immediately followed by 1 g 4-hourly until delivery is often used, but is not the first-line agent of choice as it is too broad spectrum. In patients allergic to penicillin, clindamycin 900 mg 8-hourly or erythromycin 500 mg 6-hourly are acceptable alternatives, but are associated with significant failure rates because of increasing resistance.
- The presence of GBS on a perineal/perianal swab in the setting of preterm premature rupture of membranes without evidence of chorioamnionitis should not be regarded as an indication for delivery.
- The neonatal pediatricians need to be informed at delivery and the clinical condition of the neonate should be monitored closely.

Recommended further reading

1. Hurley R (1999). Infections in pregnancy. In: Chamberlain G, ed. *Turnbull's Obstetrics* (3rd edn), pp. 471–8. Churchill Livingstone.
2. Stirrat GM (1997). Maternal and fetal infections. In *Aids to Obstetrics and Gynecology* (4th edn). Churchill Livingstone, Edinburgh.

Bacterial vaginosis

Bacterial vaginosis (BV), which is present in about 20% of pregnant women is one of the most common vaginal infections. It is due to an alteration of vaginal microflora with overgrowth of facultative and anaerobic bacteria which normally form part of the vaginal microflora along with a 1000-fold reduction in *Lactobacillus* species. The organisms that are greatly increased in concentration include *Peptostreptococcus* spp., *Mobiluncus* spp., *Bacteroides* spp., *Gardnerella vaginalis*, and *Mycoplasma hominis* amongst others. A thin greyish watery non-pruritic discharge with a fishy odor is the most common presenting feature, but half the patients are asymptomatic.

Obstetric significance

Numerous studies have shown an epidemiological association between BV and preterm labor/delivery, chorioamnionitis, and postpartum endometritis. However, routine screening and treatment of asymptomatic high-risk parturients has not been shown to decrease the incidence of these complications, and therefore is not recommended.

Diagnosis

A clinical diagnosis is made on the basis of the presence of three of the following four well-established criteria:

- The presence of a thin homogeneous discharge that adheres to the vaginal walls.
- The presence of clue cells on wet prep microscopy.
- A vaginal pH > 4.5.
- The release of a fishy odor on addition of 10% potassium hydroxide to the discharge.

Management

The treatment of choice for BV in pregnancy is metronidazole 200 mg three times daily or 400 mg twice daily for a week, achieving cure rates of >90%. Clindamycin 300 mg twice daily for a week is a reasonable alternative. There are theoretical concerns about the use of metronidazole in the first trimester. Although it crosses the placenta, there is no increase in the risk of congenital anomalies. Alternative treatment regimens (such as a single dose of 2 g oral metronidazole, metronidazole gel 0.75% vaginally once daily for 5 days, or 2% clindamycin gel vaginally once daily for 7 days), while effective in nonpregnant women, are associated with a higher failure rate in pregnancy and therefore are not generally recommended.

Recommended further reading

1. Hurley R (1999). Infections in pregnancy. In: Chamberlain G, ed. *Turnbull's Obstetrics* (3rd edn), pp. 471–8. Churchill Livingstone, Edinburgh.
2. Stirrat GM (1997). Maternal and fetal infections. In *Aids to Obstetrics and Gynecology* (4th edn). Churchill Livingstone, Edinburgh.

Candidiasis

Candidiasis can be caused by a variety of species of *Candida* but almost 90% of cases are caused by *C. albicans*. *Candida* are saprophytic fungi and can be recovered from the vagina of 30–40% of asymptomatic women. *Candida* accounts for 25% of cases of vaginitis in the nonpregnant population, and this proportion rises to 45% in pregnancy. The altered vaginal microflora in pregnancy, along with depressed cellular immunity and increased glycogen availability, make for more favorable conditions for *Candida* in pregnancy. Patients present with vulvovaginal pruritus, external dysuria, and a non-malodorous flocculent discharge like cottage cheese.

Diagnosis and management

- *Diagnosis.* Vaginal pH < 4.5; microscopy in 10% potassium hydroxide reveals pseudohyphae and mycelial forms.
- The mainstay of *treatment* is with the antifungal imidazoles such as clotrimazole, miconazole, etc. These may be administered as creams or pessaries as a single dose or a 3–7 day course. Topical imidazoles are not absorbed systemically and are safe in pregnancy.

Recommended further reading

1. Hurley R (1999). Infections in pregnancy. In: Chamberlain G, ed. *Turnbull's Obstetrics* (3rd edn), pp. 471–8. Churchill Livingstone, Edinburgh.
2. Stirrat GM (1997). Maternal and fetal infections. In *Aids to Obstetrics and Gynecology* (4th edn). Churchill Livingstone, Edinburgh.

HIV in gynecology

Introduction

HIV is a retrovirus transmitted via contact with blood or other bodily fluids. HIV infects CD4 lymphocytes, causing their gradual depletion and thus leading to immunosuppression. Carriage of HIV can be asymptomatic but, as CD4 levels fall, symptoms associated with opportunistic infections, tumors, or neurological states can result. Monitoring of HIV is by CD4 levels and viral load. Highly active antiretroviral therapy (HAART) can be given either when symptoms occur or to slow disease progression. Prophylaxis against opportunistic infection is also an important part of treatment.

Premalignant change and malignancy

- HIV-positive women are at higher risk of developing lower genital tract neoplasia. The association is thought to be due not only to immunosuppression but also to sexual behavioral risks and the interaction of HIV and HPV at a molecular level.
  - As a result of this known increased risk, HIV-positive women are advised to have annual cytological surveillance and possibly regular colposcopy.
- CIN in HIV-positive women (prevalence 30–63%) is more likely to be extensive, recurrent, rapidly progressive, and nonresponsive to standard treatment. Invasive cervical cancer is characteristically high grade, aggressive, and recurrent. In 1993 cervical cancer was included as an AIDS-defining diagnosis. Cervical disease is more likely to develop with increasing immunosuppression.
- Vulvovaginal lesions are also more common in HIV-positive women. Careful assessment of the whole lower genital tract is necessary in HIV-positive women referred for colposcopy. Ideally, vulvoscopy to look for the presence of vulval intraepithelial neoplasia (VIN) should also be performed.

Opportunistic infections

HIV-positive women are at risk of opportunistic infections in the lower genital tract as they are elsewhere. Infection with *Candida* can be a particular problem. Microbiological assessment of *Candida* species and sensitivity to antifungals may be required if the problem is persistent or recurrent. Advice regarding skin care and avoidance of allergens is an essential element of management, as well as appropriate antifungals.

Contraception

Contraceptive discussions must include the need to reduce the risk of HIV transmission and also provide effective protection against unwanted pregnancy. Barrier contraception is essential. In addition, another contraceptive may be used to increase contraceptive efficacy. There is no evidence that use of the combined oral contraceptive pill, intrauterine contraceptive device, levonorgestrel intrauterine system, or Depo-Provera alters the risk of transmission.

Fertility

- Couples with HIV wishing to conceive should be counseled preconception regarding the risk of vertical transmission.
- For couples with subfertility, HIV should not be regarded as an absolute contraindication to fertility services.
- In HIV-discordant couples, either artificial insemination (with an HIV-negative male partner) or sperm washing and artificial insemination (with an HIV-negative female partner) can be considered.

Recommended further reading

1. American College of Obstetricians and Gynecologists (2004). Prenatal and perinatal human immunodeficiency virus testing: expanded recommendations. ACOG Committee Opinion No. 304. *Obstet Gynecol* **104**, 1119–24.

HIV in obstetrics

Introduction

Unlike other viral infections, HIV infection has not been associated with a specific fetal syndrome. Vertical transmission is the predominant concern. The rate of vertical transmission without intervention ranges from 15% to 35%. Risk of transmission is increased with a higher viral load, lower CD4 count, or clinically advanced disease. In developed countries with appropriate interventions, vertical transmission rate can be reduced to less than 2%. The key to reducing vertical transmission is early detection. Universal screening for HIV should be offered to all pregnant women.

General antenatal care

- Management of pregnant women with HIV should be by a multidisciplinary team including obstetrician, genitourinary medicine or infectious disease physician, and pediatrician.
- Invasive tests such as amniocentesis are generally avoided to reduce the risk of vertical transmission.
- It may be appropriate to consider testing for other blood-borne viruses, such as hepatitis B and C.

Antiretrovirals

- Zidovudine (AZT) monotherapy from the second trimester has been shown to decrease vertical transmission by two-thirds. The standard regime involves oral therapy antenatally, IV therapy during delivery, then oral therapy to the neonate for 6 weeks. However, because of the rapid development of resistance, AZT monotherapy is not generally recommended for pregnant women.
- For women with relatively advanced disease, triple therapy may be more appropriate, aiming to reduce viral load and improve CD4 count.
- For women conceiving on treatment, this is often continued with AZT added in if not already included.
- If the CD4 count is <200 cells/mm^3, chemoprophylaxis against *pneumocystis carinii* pneumonia (PCP) should routinely be given. Similarly, if the CD4 count is <50 cells/mm^3, tuberculosis chemoprophylaxis should be given.

Delivery

- Elective cesarean delivery in women with a viral load >1000 copies/mL reduces the risk of vertical transmission compared with that of planned vaginal delivery by 50%, independent of antiretroviral therapy or clinical stage of disease. When combined with antiretroviral therapy, the risk is lowered by 87%. Whether this is also true of women with a low viral load is not known. This is thought to result from avoidance of microtranfusions of maternal blood during contractions and avoidance of contact of the fetus with maternal genital secretions or blood. Cesarean delivery should be performed at 38 weeks before the onset of labor and rupture of membranes.

- It should be remembered that, in some countries, the risks of surgical delivery to the mother may outweigh the advantage of reducing the risk of vertical transmission.

Breast-feeding

Breast-feeding significantly increases the risk of vertical transmission and therefore should not be encouraged unless there is no access to safe bottle-feeding.

Surveillance of infant

- Previously, serial testing of infants using ELISA screening tests was required until 18 months of age as results could be confused because of passive acquisition of maternal IgG antibody.
- More recently, PCR detection of DNA or RNA of HIV antigen has led to much earlier diagnosis.
- Infants who have been exposed to antiretrovirals during pregnancies should be reported to the Antiretroviral Pregnancy Register.

Recommended further reading

1. Johnson MA, Olaitan A (1998). Human immunodeficiency virus in obstetrics. In: Studd J, *Progress in Obstetrics and Gynecology*, Vol. 13, pp. 27–42. Churchill Livingstone, Edinburgh.
2. Connor EM, Sperling RS, Gelber R, *et al.* (1994). Reduction of maternal–infant transmission of human immunodeficiency virus type 1 with zidovudine treatment. Pediatric AIDS Clinical Trials Group Protocol 076 Study Group. *N Engl J Med*, **331**, 1173–80.
3. Sperling RS, Shapiro DE, Coombs RW, *et al.* (1996). Maternal viral load, zidovudine treatment, and the risk of transmission of human immunodeficiency virus type 1 from mother to infant. Pediatric AIDS Clinical Trials Group Protocol 076 Study Group. *N Engl J Med* **335**, 1621–9.
4. Read J, Newell M, Read JM (2005). Efficacy and safety of cesarean delivery for prevention of mother-to-child transmission of HIV-1. *Cochrane Database Syst Rev* **4**, CD005479.
5. Brocklehurst P, Volmink J (2002). Antiretrovirals for reducing the risk of mother-to-child transmission of HIV infection. *Cochrane Database Syst* Rev **2**, CD003510.
6. Brocklehurst P (2002). Interventions for reducing the risk of mother-to-child transmission of HIV infection. *Cochrane Database Syst* Rev **1**, CD000102.
7. American College of Obstetricians and Gynecologists (2004). Prenatal and perinatal human immunodeficiency virus testing: expanded recommendations. ACOG Committee Opinion No. 304. *Obstet Gynecol* **104**, 1119–24.

Immunization in pregnancy

Introduction

Immunization may be indicated for short-term (passive) or long-term (active) protection against maternal and or fetal infection.

- Active immunization uses attenuated live organisms, inactivated organisms, or components of the organisms for which immunization is being performed.
- Live attenuated vaccines include poliomyelitis, measles, mumps, rubella, varicella, and bacille Calmette–Guérin (BCG). These are generally contraindicated in pregnancy, although these vaccines have not been shown to be associated with adverse fetal outcomes.
- Active immunization produces an antibody response, IgM initially and IgG later.
- Passive immunization utilizes human immunoglobulin to achieve rapid protection, but this only lasts a few weeks. Immunoglobulin specific for a condition is obtained from pooled plasma containing the required antibody.
- Except when there is a specific risk of infection, e.g. travel to an endemic area, vaccines containing attenuated or inactivated organisms are avoided in pregnancy.
- The main conditions for which immunization may be required in pregnancy are varicella zoster and hepatitis B virus infections.

Rubella

Rubella vaccination is a live attenuated vaccine and, therefore is not recommended in pregnancy. However, active surveillance in many countries has failed to reveal any case of congenital rubella syndrome in cases of inadvertent vaccination of nonimmune women shortly before pregnancy or in early pregnancy. There is no evidence that the vaccine is teratogenic, and the pregnancy need not be terminated because of such inadvertent vaccination. Nonimmune antenatal patients should be vaccinated after delivery.

Varicella zoster virus (VZV, chickenpox)

VZV is highly infectious and is common in childhood, where it is a mild illness. Over 90% of adults are immune and 80–90% of persons with no history of varicella infection are found to be seropositive.

- However, primary infection in adults can be severe, leading to pneumonia, myocarditis, pericarditis, encephalitis, and adrenal insufficiency.
- Pregnant women are more susceptible to severe illness from primary infection, with pulmonary complications occurring in about 10%.
- Severe illness may precipitate premature labor.
- Fetal infection may occur with a risk of 2–9% if maternal infection occurs before 20 weeks' gestation. This may result in the congenital varicella syndrome, comprising of skin scarring, limb hypoplasia, microcephaly, cataracts, neural damage, and growth restriction.
- Primary maternal infection within 4 days of delivery (before or after) carries a 30% risk of disseminated zoster infection in the newborn as transplacental transmission of IgG antibodies would not have been established.

Maternal infection following exposure in pregnancy can be confirmed by the presence of IgM antibodies or a fourfold rise in IgG antibody titers over a 4–6 week period. The pregnant woman should be observed for signs of severe illness.

Varicella zoster immune globulin (VZIG) may be given to exposed non-immune high-risk pregnant women to prevent or reduce the clinical manifestations. VZIG is expensive and therefore is used only when strongly indicated.

- Antiviral agents, e.g. acyclovir, should also be considered, either alone or with VZIG.
- Neither VZIG nor antiviral drugs remove the risk of congenital malformations in the fetus.

Hepatitis B

Parenteral drug abuse, sexual activity, and transfusion of blood/blood products are the main modes of transmission of hepatitis B, although vertical transmission from an infected mother to the fetus is a major factor in developing countries. Without immunization, up to 90% of fetuses of infected women may become infected. Of these, 5% are infected *in utero*, while the rest acquire their infection from maternal blood and body fluids during delivery. Chronic carriage is more common when infection has been acquired perinatally or in childhood.

There are two immunization products for hepatitis B.

- Hepatitis B immunoglobulin (HBIG) provides immediate temporary passive immunity after accidental inoculation or contamination with an infected product.
- HBIG is given in doses of 500 IU for adults and 200 IU for the newborn.
- Hepatitis B (HB) vaccine produces an immune response.
- Antibody levels of 100 mU/mL are considered protective, and <10 mU/mL is considered a non-response to the vaccine. A level of 10–100 mU/mL is a poor response and requires a booster dose.
- HB vaccine is typically given into the deltoid muscle as vaccine efficacy may be reduced when given into the buttocks.
- The dosage for HB vaccine is specified by the manufacturers. Pregnant women who are negative for HBsAg and considered to be at risk of acquiring hepatitis B infection should be offered vaccination with HBIG and HB vaccine during pregnancy.
- HBIG does not suppress the immune response to HB vaccine and neither product is known to cause any fetal abnormality.
- As most fetal infection is postpartum, neonates of carrier mothers or mothers infected during pregnancy should be vaccinated with HBIG within 12 hours of birth, followed by HB vaccine within 7 days and again at 1 and 6 months.

Tetanus and travel vaccination

Tetanus

Tetanus toxoid and tetanus immunoglobulin are safe in pregnancy and may be used when the risk of acquiring tetanus infection is high for inducing active or passive immunity, respectively. In parts of the world where neonatal tetanus is a major health problem, vaccinating the mother in pregnancy induces transplacental passive immunity in the fetus.

Travel vaccination

Information regarding vaccination when traveling to regions of the world where specific conditions may be endemic and the risk of infection high can be obtained from the US Centers for Disease Control and Prevention (www.cdc.gov/travel) or from obstetric care providers, travel agencies, or embassies.

- *Hepatitis A* is transmitted by the feco-oral route and risk of infection comes from traveling to endemic areas. Travelers to areas of moderate to high endemic activity are advised to be vaccinated, especially if sanitation and food hygiene are likely to be poor. Hepatitis A vaccine is a formaldehyde inactivated vaccine and the risks of congenital malformation are low. However, its use in pregnancy has not been fully assessed and it should only be given if there is a definite risk of infection.
    - Human normal immunoglobulin (HNIG) offers short-term immunity against hepatitis A infection and may be a more suitable prophylactic measure for pregnant women traveling for short periods to endemic areas.
- *Typhoid* is also transmitted by the feco-oral route and therefore is a disease of areas where sanitation and food hygiene are poor. Three typhoid vaccines are available: monovalent whole cell typhoid vaccine, typhoid Vi polysaccharide antigen vaccine, and oral typhoid vaccine.
- *Yellow fever* vaccination is required for travel into highly endemic areas. The immunity conferred lasts for at least 10 years and is probably lifelong.
- *Cholera* vaccination is no longer a prerequisite for travel as it only gives limited personal protection and does not prevent spread of the disease.
- *Rabies* vaccination should only be used in pregnancy if the woman is traveling to a high-risk area and the risk of exposure is high. The appropriate globulin may be used for postexposure prophylaxis.
- *Meningococcal* vaccine may be used when unavoidable, e.g. during an epidemic or when traveling for long periods to high-risk areas.

Recommended further reading

1. Centers for Disease Control and Prevention in the United States and American College of Obstetricians and Gynecologists (1997). Vaccination during pregnancy. *EPI Newsl* **19**, 6.
2. James DK, Steer PJ, Weiner CP, Gonik B, (eds) (1999). *High Risk Pregnancy—Management Options*. WB Saunders, London.
3. American College of Obstetricians and Gynecologists (2003). Immunization during pregnancy. *Obstet Gynecol* **101**, 207–12.

Chapter 5

Medical disorders

Anemia

Plasma volume expansion in pregnancy exceeds the increase in red cell mass, thus leading to a fall in hemoglobin concentration, hematocrit, and red cell count. The hemodilution does not affect the mean corpuscular volume (MCV) or the mean corpuscular hemoglobin concentration (MCHC). During pregnancy, there is a two- to threefold increase in iron requirements to meet the demands of hemoglobin synthesis as well as synthesis of enzymes, and to meet the demands of the fetus. Pregnancy is also accompanied by a 10–20-fold increase in folate requirements. Platelet count falls in pregnancy, with 5–10% of patients falling in the range 100–150 × 10^6/mL. Thus, for practical purposes, a count below 100 × 10^6/mL is considered to indicate thrombocytopenia.

In pregnancy, a hemoglobin concentration <10.5 g/dL should be considered abnormal. In the majority of cases, anemia presents in the latter third of pregnancy when demands reach their peak, but some women start pregnancy with poor reserves (poor social circumstances and poor nutrition, repeated pregnancies in quick succession), while other situations such as multiple pregnancy are associated with a greater drain on maternal reserves and may result in earlier development of anemia. Routine screening in pregnancy picks up the majority of cases, although occasionally women may present with classical symptoms of lethargy, fatigue, shortness of breath, dizziness, or fainting.

Iron deficiency anemia

The most common cause of anemia in pregnancy is iron deficiency resulting from an increased requirement of iron during pregnancy in combination with poor maternal reserves. The increased demands for iron are partly met from increased absorption from the gastrointestinal tract but, if there is no iron supplementation, the shortfall is made up by mobilizing iron stores. The diagnosis of iron deficiency is confirmed by demonstrating a fall in the red cell indices (MCV, MCHC, and mean corpuscular hemoglobin (MCH)). Depletion of iron stores is reflected by a fall in serum ferritin levels.

Management

- Iron deficiency anemia is treated by oral iron supplementation.
- In certain situations, such as multiple pregnancy or where there is a higher risk due to poor maternal reserves, prophylactic supplementation prior to the development of anemia may be advisable.
- Parenteral iron preparations are only of value in patients who do not tolerate oral supplementation. These preparations do not correct anemia any more rapidly than do oral supplements.
- The expected improvement in hemoglobin on maximal iron supplementation is around 1 g/dL/week.
- In cases where iron deficiency is diagnosed very near term and correction by iron supplementation is not feasible, blood transfusion may be an alternative option if the anemia is severe (<7 g/dL).

Folate deficiency

Folate deficiency is also a common cause of anemia in pregnancy. Inadequate dietary folate leads to megaloblastic anemia. Nutritional status, along with conditions such as epilepsy (through the use of anticonvulsants) and hematological problems that predispose to rapid turnover of blood cells (hemolytic anemia, thalassemia, hereditary spherocytosis), may all predispose to folate deficiency. A raised MCV along with reduced serum and red cell folate confirms a diagnosis of folate deficiency. Folate supplementation at 0.4 mg/day is recommended preconception and in early pregnancy as prophylaxis against neural tube defects (NTDs), with the dose being increased to 4–5 mg/day if the patient is on anticonvulsants or where there is a history of a previous child affected by NTD or the patient is at higher risk of folate deficiency through hematological disorders such as hemoglobinopathies or hemolytic anemia.

Vitamin B_{12} deficiency

Vitamin B_{12} deficiency is uncommon in pregnancy and presents in the form of pernicious anemia that predates pregnancy. Therefore, treatment should be continued in pregnancy. Vitamin B_{12} deficiency is associated with subfertility and therefore, will often have been corrected before pregnancy can be achieved. Rarely, strict vegans and chronic tropical sprue sufferers may present with vitamin B_{12} deficiency. Oral supplementation should be considered with strict vegans and women with diets deficient in animal protein. Anemia due to hemoglobinopathies is discussed in the section on 'Hemoglobinopathies'.

Epilepsy

Introduction

Epilepsy is the most common neurological disorder encountered in obstetrics given that 1% of the general population suffer with it. In the majority of cases, epilepsy is idiopathic but, in rare cases, it may be a result of an insult to the brain (trauma, surgery, space-occupying lesion) or a manifestation of a more generalized metabolic disorder. Idiopathic epilepsy can be broadly classified into generalized seizures (tonic–clonic, absence seizures), partial or focal seizures (complex if associated with loss of consciousness), and special epileptic syndromes such as myoclonic epilepsy. The majority of patients with epilepsy in pregnancy have already been diagnosed. In cases where the first seizure occurs in pregnancy, the differential diagnosis includes eclampsia, cerebral vein thrombosis, thrombotic thrombocytopenic purpura, cerebral infarction, drug and alcohol withdrawal, hypoglycemia, and electrolyte imbalances such as hypernatremia or hypocalcemia.

Effect of pregnancy on epilepsy

One-third of women experience an increase in seizure frequency, while the remaining two-thirds experience no change or a fall in seizure frequency. Women who have been seizure free for many years are unlikely to have a seizure in pregnancy unless they discontinue their medication, while the poorly controlled epileptics are the most likely to deteriorate in pregnancy. The majority of women who have one or more seizures a month are likely to deteriorate. Deterioration of epilepsy in pregnancy may be a result of poor compliance with medication because of fear of its teratogenic effects, decreased drug levels because of nausea and vomiting, and reduced gastrointestinal absorbance with increased hepatic and renal clearance. There is also increased volume of distribution along with alteration in free drug levels because of a fall in albumin levels. Lack of sleep towards term and in labor may also be a contributory factor.

Effect of epilepsy on pregnancy

In general, the fetus is resistant to short episodes of hypoxia and there is no evidence that isolated seizures have a detrimental effect. However, status epilepticus is dangerous for both mother and fetus and needs to be vigorously treated. The risks from seizures to the fetus are due to maternal abdominal trauma, while maternal risks are due to loss of consciousness and injuries sustained during epileptic seizures. Partners or other family members should be aware of how to manage a seizure and, in particular, should be aware of the importance of the left lateral ('recovery') position. The women themselves should be advised against taking a bath unattended.

There may well be a genetic predisposition to epilepsy as, even when there is no parental history of anticonvulsant use, children of epileptic parents have a 4% risk of congenital anomalies as opposed to a 2–3% risk in the general population. If either of the parents have epilepsy, the chances of the child of having epilepsy are of the order of 4%. This figure rises to 15–20% if both parents have epilepsy, and 10% with a previously affected sibling.

One of the main concerns regarding the effect of epilepsy on pregnancy stems from the teratogenic potential of anticonvulsant drugs. Phenytoin, primidone, carbamazepine, phenobarbitone, and sodium valproate all cross the placenta and are associated with increased risks of congenital abnormalities. The risk of malformations with any one drug is around three times the background risk and is about 6–7%, increasing to 15% for those taking two or more drugs.

- Sodium valproate is associated with NTDs (1–2%) and congenital heart defects.
- Phenytoin is associated with orofacial clefts and congenital heart defects, while carbamazepine is associated with neural tube defects.
- Phenytoin, phenobarbitone, and to a lesser extent carbamazepine and valproate all interfere with folate metabolism and this is thought to be a possible mechanism of teratogenesis.
- There is limited data on newer drugs (such as gabapentin). Lamotrigine appears to be safe, while there are some animal studies suggesting a risk for vigabatrin.

Management of epilepsy

Preconception management

Preconception counseling would be the ideal management and should be part of educating the female patient of reproductive age about her condition. The aim of preconception care is to optimize treatment and achieve control of the epilepsy with a single drug using the lowest effective dose, taking into account its teratogenic potential.

- All women on anticonvulsants should be advised to take folic acid at a dose of 4 mg/day for 12 weeks preconception and throughout pregnancy.
- If seizure free for several years, a further option may be to discontinue medication preconception and for the first trimester after full counseling concerning the implications of a seizure and, in particular, the implications for driving.

Antenatal management

- Provided the woman is well controlled on single-agent therapy there is no need to change medication, but it is important to stress the significance of complying with it.
- General advice should be given regarding adequate sleep and the avoidance of precipitating factors.
- Prenatal screening should include maternal serum α-fetoprotein (MS-AFP) and detailed ultrasound focusing on the detection of congenital anomalies, in particular, NTDs and cardiac malformations. If the latter is suspected, a further scan (fetal echocardiogram) at 22–24 weeks may be helpful.
- The monitoring of serum levels of anticonvulsants is limited to women who continue to have regular seizures on high doses or where compliance is an issue. There is no role for routine monitoring of drug levels in seizure-free women.
- Coagulopathies due to deficiency of vitamin-K-dependent clotting factors have been reported in babies of some women on hepatic-enzyme-inducing drugs and therefore some practitioners recommend vitamin K 10 mg/day orally from 36 weeks' gestation.

Postnatal management

- Postnatally, the baby needs to receive vitamin K to reduce the risk of hemorrhagic disease of the newborn.
- There are no contraindications to breast-feeding and, in some cases, breast-feeding may facilitate drug withdrawal in the babies.
  - Neonates who are being breast-fed and whose mothers are on phenobarbitone, primidone, or ethosuximide, need to be watched for signs of sedation and poor feeding.
- If the anticonvulsant dose had been increased in pregnancy, this needs to be done gradually over 2–3 months.
- Prior to discharge from hospital, contraception should be addressed. If the woman is on a hepatic-enzyme-inducing anticonvulsant (phenytoin, primidone, carbamzepine, or phenobarbitone), a higher dose of estrogen will be required to achieve reliable contraception. Similarly, higher doses of the progestogen-only pill or a more frequent dosing regimen for Depo-Provera will be required.

Heart disease: general management

Introduction

The pattern of heart disease in pregnancy has changed over the last quarter of a century with a reversal in the ratio of rheumatic heart disease to congenital heart disease. This phenomenon is a result, on the one hand, of the dramatic fall in rheumatic heart disease while, on the other hand, a significant improvement in medical and surgical management of congenital heart disease has enabled such patients to live to adulthood and reproductive age. Pregnancy leads to marked hemodynamic changes such as increased blood volume, increase in cardiac output, fall in systemic vascular resistance, and hypercoagulability, to name just a few. These physiological changes of pregnancy are well handled in the healthy woman, but carry the risk of cardiovascular decompensation in those with heart disease. Therefore it is not surprising that heart disease in pregnancy can result in significant morbidity and mortality, and remains the second most frequent cause of all maternal deaths.

General management

Successful management of the pregnant woman with heart disease requires a multidisciplinary approach involving an obstetrician, a cardiologist/obstetric physician, an anesthesiologist, and, occasionally, a cardiothoracic surgeon. Ideally, preconception counseling of women with heart disease would enable discussion of maternal and fetal risks as well as optimization of maternal cardiovascular health, including modifying any medical treatment, prior to embarking on pregnancy.

- The risk of the fetus having congenital heart disease is higher if the mother rather than the father has congenital heart disease, with the overall risk being 3–5%, twice that of the general population.
- The risk of an affected offspring varies with the type of lesion being highest with aortic stenosis (18–20%) and around 5–10% with atrial septal defect (ASD).
- Other conditions such as Marfan's syndrome and hypertrophic obstructive cardiomyopathy (HOCM) have a known pattern of inheritance (autosomal dominant).

Unfortunately many pregnancies are unplanned despite patients' knowledge of their underlying problems. Furthermore, there are increasing numbers of immigrant patients who may never have had a medical examination and thus present in pregnancy with previously undiagnosed cardiac disease. The ability to tolerate pregnancy will broadly depend on the functional reserve of the patient (which can be evaluated using the New York Heart Association (NYHA) heart functional classification), the presence of pulmonary hypertension, and the presence of cyanosis. Although the majority of patients (90%) would fall in NYHA classes 1 or 2 (no breathlessness or limitation of physical activity/breathlessness on severe exertion, slight limitation of physical activity), 85% of maternal deaths occur in NYHA classes 3 or 4 (breathlessness on mild exertion or marked limitation of activity/breathlessness at rest, inability to carry out physical activity without discomfort). Chest X-ray can be safely performed with appropriate shielding if deemed appropriate, and echocardiography is an invaluable tool to assess not only cardiac anatomy but also ventricular function and to estimate intracardiac pressure gradients.

- Every effort should be made to avoid and correct factors that may contribute to cardiac decompensation such as anemia, infections, arrhythmias, and hypertension.
- During the antenatal period, the patient should be routinely questioned about symptoms and examined for signs of heart failure.
- Fetal growth assessment should be regularly performed in patients at risk of IUGR.
- During labor, it is important to monitor fluid balance and avoid aortocaval compression by use of a wedge or maintaining the patient in the left or right lateral position.
- The nature of cardiac monitoring in labor (ECG, invasive monitoring, oximetry) will depend on the nature of the underlying cardiac condition and its severity, and a plan for intrapartum care should have been made and documented in the patient's records.
- Close fetal surveillance throughout labor is recommended.
- Cesarean delivery should be performed for obstetric indications. Operative vaginal delivery to shorten the second stage and avoid blood pressure changes with pushing may be wise in certain patients. Blood loss during delivery should be minimized and promptly replaced.
- Epidural analgesia minimizes changes in heart rate and blood pressure due to pain and, although well tolerated in those with adequate cardiac reserve, should be administered with extreme caution in those with restricted cardiac outputs and right to left shunts.
- Significant fluid shifts occur during the first 24–72 hours of the postpartum period, and may lead to congestive heart failure. Therefore close surveillance of fluid balance and oxygen saturations (by pulse oximetry) is advisable to enable early detection of pulmonary edema.
- Prior to discharge, it is essential to discuss and implement plans for effective contraception.

Endocarditis prophylaxis

The American Heart Association classifies cardiac conditions into high- and moderate-risk categories with respect to endocarditis prophylaxis, which is recommended in both these categories.

- Cardiac conditions considered high-risk include prosthetic cardiac valves (including bioprosthetic and homograft), previous history of bacterial endocarditis, complex cyanotic congenital heart disease (uncorrected tetralogy of Fallot, transposition of great vessels, single ventricle states), and surgically constructed systemic pulmonary shunts or conduits.
- Moderate risk of endocarditis is encountered with acquired valvular lesions, hypertrophic cardiomyopathy, mitral valve prolapse with regurgitation, or thickened leaflets.
- Prophylaxis is not warranted for the following groups where the risk does not exceed that of the general population: surgical repair of atrial or ventricular septal defects or patent ductus arteriosus without residual defect beyond 6 months so long as no graft materials were used in the repair; cardiac pacemakers and implantable defibrillators; physiological or functional heart murmurs; previous rheumatic fever with no valvular dysfunction; mitral valve prolapse without valvular regurgitation.

The current recommendations for treatment are amoxycillin 1 g IV or IM plus 120 mg gentamicin at the onset of labor or at rupture of membranes. If the patient is allergic to penicillin, vancomycin 1 g IV (run in slowly over 30 minutes) or teicoplanin 400 mg IV can be substituted for amoxicillin.

Conditions associated with minimal/ moderate risk of maternal complications

Minimal risk

These conditions carry a very small risk of maternal mortality (<1%):

- Atrial (ASD) and ventricular septal defects (VSD) are generally well tolerated in pregnancy.
- Most cases of patent ductus arteriosus (PDA) have had surgical correction and pose no problems in pregnancy. Although uncorrected cases of PDA also do well, there is a risk of congestive cardiac failure.
- Similarly, corrected Fallot's tetralogy, porcine valve prosthesis, and pulmonary/tricuspid valve disease also carry low risk of complications.
- In cases of mitral stenosis, the outlook depends on cardiac reserve with a good prognosis anticipated with NYHA class 1 or 2 patients.
- Benign arrhythmias are relatively common in pregnancy and include sinus bradycardias, sinus tachycardias, and premature atrial and ventricular contractions. After underlying pathology has been excluded as a cause, the management in healthy asymptomatic patients is observation.
- After investigation, symptomatic and sustained arrhythmias such as supraventricular tachycardia (SVT), ventricular tachycardia (VT), and atrial fibrillation require appropriate anti-arrhythmic treatment using drugs such as digoxin, β-blockers, adenosine, quinidine, etc. depending on the underlying arrhythmia.

Moderate risk

These conditions carry a maternal mortality risk of 5–15%:

- Patients with mitral stenosis and NYHA class 3 or 4 may deteriorate rapidly in pregnancy, developing pulmonary edema. Tachycardia (due to exercise, infection, etc.) in the presence of mitral stenosis leads to reduced diastolic filling of the left ventricle and hence a fall in stroke volume, leading to a rise in left atrial pressures and precipitating pulmonary edema. Management involves treating the pulmonary edema with diuretics and reducing heart rate with β-blockers to improve ventricular filling and atrial emptying, after treating any underlying cause for the tachycardia.
- The severity of aortic stenosis determines the risk it poses in pregnancy; provided that the gradient across the valve is less than 100 mmHg in the nonpregnant state, it is unlikely to cause problems. In cases of moderate to severe disease, symptoms of angina, syncopal attacks, hypertension, cardiac failure, and sudden death may be encountered. β-Blockers can help to control hypertension and symptoms of angina, dyspnea, and syncopal attacks. Early signs of emerging left ventricular failure may be a subtle resting tachycardia.

- Patients with mechanical heart valves require lifelong anticoagulation to minimize the risks of valve thrombosis. Anticoagulation of choice with mechanical valves is warfarin and this carries risks of teratogenesis and hemorrhage. Subcutaneous (SC) therapeutic unfractionated heparin is a reasonable option for anticoagulation in the presence of mechanical valve prosthesis in pregnancy.
- Although grafted tissue valves do not routinely require anticoagulation, there is a more rapid deterioration of such valves in pregnancy.
- Patients with corrected Fallot's tetralogy are generally at minimal risk of complications.
- Those with uncorrected Fallot's tetralogy but no pulmonary hypertension have a moderate risk of complications. The main maternal consideration is one of paradoxical embolization causing cerebrovascular accidents from right to left shunting; the risks are reduced by SC heparin prophylaxis. The principal fetal problems are secondary to maternal hypoxemia and can be summarized as IUGR, increased risk of miscarriage, and prematurity (spontaneous or iatrogenic). Maternal oxygen saturations may be improved by reducing physical activity in the latter half of pregnancy—hence the rationale for bed rest.
- Coarctation of the aorta is usually diagnosed and corrected prior to pregnancy. The main considerations with an uncorrected coarctation include hypertension, congestive cardiac failure, and angina. Tight control of blood pressure through the use of β-blockers helps to reduce the associated risks of aortic rupture or aortic dissection.
- A risk of aortic root dissection and rupture also exists with Marfan's syndrome, an autosomal dominant condition characterized by clinical features such as high arched palate, arachnodactyly, joint laxity, tall stature, and dislocatable lens of the eye. The risk of complications in Marfan's syndrome is related to family history of aortic rupture and to the degree of pre-existing aortic root dilatation; if the latter is greater than 4–4.5 cm, pregnancy would be contraindicated until after aortic root replacement. β-Blockers have been shown to reduce progression of aortic root dilatation and also reduce the rate of complications in patients with Marfan's syndrome. In labor, an early epidural, a shortened second stage, and avoidance of hypertension are recommended along with at least 8-week postnatal vigilance for aortic root dissection.

Conditions associated with high risk of maternal complications and mortality

A significant risk of maternal mortality (25–50%) may be encountered with conditions such as pulmonary hypertension, complicated aortic coarctation, and Marfan's syndrome with aortic root involvement.

Pulmonary hypertension associated with pregnancy carries a risk of maternal death of up to 50%, with labor, delivery, and early postpartum periods being the most hazardous times.

- Primary pulmonary hypertension is an idiopathic abnormality of pulmonary vasculature seen primarily in women, whereas secondary pulmonary hypertension is usually a result of long-standing rises in pulmonary pressures due to underlying cardiac causes.
- Eisenmenger's syndrome is an example of the latter where pulmonary hypertension is secondary to an uncorrected left to right shunt of a VSD, ASD, or PDA with subsequent shunt reversal and cyanosis. The increase in blood volume and the fall in systemic vascular resistance can lead to right ventricular failure, with fall in cardiac output and sudden death.
- In both primary pulmonary hypertension and Eisenmenger's complex, the maternal risks justify consideration of termination of pregnancy, and this issue should be addressed along with long-term contraceptive plans.
- Where pregnancy is to continue, joint obstetric and cardiological input with early involvement by specialist anesthesiologists is likely to offer the best chance for a favorable outcome.
  - The antenatal care needs to address thromboprophylaxis, maternal surveillance, including hospital admission and oxygen saturation monitoring, and fetal surveillance—IUGR is the main fetal concern.
  - Labor and delivery will need to be in a high-dependency setting with invasive monitoring planned during the antenatal period. Supplementary oxygen and tight control of blood pressure and fluid balance are imperative.
  - In the postpartum period, high-dependency care with monitoring of oxygen saturations, thromboprophylaxis, and vigilance for fluid retention and cardiac decompensation should be among the priorities.

Puerperal cardiomyopathy

This is a rare condition limited to pregnancy. It can occur between the sixth month of gestation and 6 months postnatally, although the most common presentation is in the first month after delivery. Risk factors for this condition include increasing maternal age, hypertension in pregnancy, multiple pregnancies, African American ethnicity, and a multiparous patient.

- The presentation is usually with shortness of breath, poor exercise tolerance, palpitations, peripheral and pulmonary edema, and embolic phenomena.
- The diagnosis is based on detection of global dilatation (involving all four chambers of the heart) with marked reduction in ventricular contractility.

- Prognosis is variable with 50% spontaneous recovery with supportive treatment.
- Management is supportive with anticoagulants and angiotensin-converting enzyme (ACE) inhibitors and, where there is evidence that the condition follows myocarditis, immunosuppressive therapy may be of some value.
- In cases of antenatal presentation, elective delivery is recommended.
- In cases that fail to respond, cardiac transplantation may be an option.
- Where the condition resolves, further pregnancy should be discouraged due to risks of recurrence.

Asthma

Physiological changes in pregnancy

During pregnancy, there is an increased metabolic rate and therefore increased consumption of oxygen. In order to cope with this increased oxygen consumption and carbon dioxide production, there is a 20–50% increase in ventilation (mainly by increased tidal volume) from the end of the first trimester, and this change is maintained throughout pregnancy. The increase in ventilation is thought to be stimulated by the effect of circulating progesterone on the respiratory center. This leads to a fall in arterial pCO_2 and a compensatory fall in serum bicarbonate resulting in a compensated respiratory acidosis.

Asthma

Asthma is the most common respiratory disease encountered in pregnancy. Asthma is caused by reversible bronchoconstriction due to smooth muscle spasm in the airway walls with inflammation, swelling, and excess production of mucus. There is often a diurnal variation in severity of symptoms, with exacerbations in early morning and at night. Possible provoking triggers include pollen, exercise, emotion, and upper respiratory tract infections. The effect of pregnancy on asthma is variable.

- Patients with mild disease are generally unaffected while those at the severe end of the spectrum are most likely to deteriorate late in pregnancy. Deterioration may also result from cessation of maintenance therapy because of anxiety about taking medication in pregnancy.
- Any improvement during pregnancy may be followed by postnatal deterioration.

In general, asthma does not appear to have adverse effects on pregnancy unless it is severe and poorly controlled.

- Although there are theoretical concerns about IUGR with severe poorly controlled asthma, they do not pose a major problem in clinical practice.
- Other risks that have been associated with asthma in pregnancy are preterm delivery and hypertension (not preeclampsia), but these risks have not been demonstrated consistently.
- The risk of the child developing asthma in later life is around 6–30% and depends on whether the mother is atopic and whether or not the father is atopic and has asthma.

The emphasis on the management of asthma is prevention rather than treatment of attacks. Thus medication needs to be adjusted to control symptomatology. It is essential to educate and reassure patients regarding the safety of asthma medications in pregnancy, including systemic and inhaled steroids.

- Inhaled steroids such as budesonide (Pulmicort), beclomethasone (Becotide), and fluticasone propionate (Flixotide) all appear safe, though more information is available for the first than for the latter two.

- Oral corticosteroids such as prednisone are safe and, since prednisone is metabolized by the placenta, less than 10% of the active drug crosses to the fetus. Oral steroids do increase the risk of gestational diabetes and cause deterioration of blood sugar control if there is already impaired glucose tolerance, but this can be managed by dietary modifications and, if required, by insulin administration.
- Other drugs used in the management of asthma include inhaled β_2-agonists such as salbutamol, terbutaline, and the longer-acting salmeterol, all of which reach the systemic circulation in minute amounts and appear to be safe in pregnancy. Similarly, inhaled sodium chromoglycate and inhaled anticholinergic drugs are safe and should not be withheld in pregnancy.
- Methyl xanthines such as theophylline and aminophylline are not used in first-line management of asthma. They readily cross the placenta and, although large studies have shown no significant increase in congenital abnormalities in women receiving theophylline, aminophylline has been shown to be a cardiovascular teratogen in animals. In the relatively small number of women dependent on theophylline, the dose may have to be increased in pregnancy, guided by drug levels.

Management of both chronic and acute severe asthma should be no different from that in the nonpregnant state, including performing chest radiography where indicated.

- During labor, there is no contraindication to the use of inhaled β_2-agonists as there is no evidence that they interfere with uterine activity.
- If patients are on long-term corticosteroids (i.e. >7.5 mg/day for >2 weeks), additional cover with parenteral hydrocortisone should be administered during periods of stress such as labor ('stress dose' steroids).
- Prostaglandin E_2 used for induction of labor is safe as it is a bronchodilator, but caution is required if prostaglandin F_{2a} is needed for intractable postpartum hemorrhage as it can lead to bronchospasm.
- Narcotic analgesia, nitrous oxide, and epidurals are safe and appropriate in asthma.

Cystic fibrosis

Cystic fibrosis (CF) is an autosomal recessive multisystem genetic disease caused by defective function of the CF transmembrane conductance regulation (CFTR) chloride channel. The lungs, gastrointestinal tract, pancreas, hepatobiliary systems, and reproductive organs are affected. It is one of the most common genetic diseases, affecting 1 in 2000 Caucasians. A cycle of recurrent respiratory tract infections leads to bronchial damage, with eventual respiratory failure and death. Advances in the management of CF have led to a marked improvement in life expectancy, with patients born now having the potential to reach their thirties and early forties. Therefore they also have the potential of presenting with pregnancy.

- The effect of pregnancy on CF and the risk of developing complications depends in large part on underlying lung function.
  - Where lung function is >50% of the predicted value, pregnancy is likely to be well tolerated.
  - As lung function deteriorates, so does prognosis.
- Low body weights, dyspnea, and cyanosis are all associated with a poorer outcome and, in one-third of pregnancies, pulmonary exacerbations occur that require hospital admission and treatment with IV antibiotics.
- The main maternal morbidity is through poor maternal weight gain (even in those without pancreatic insufficiency), pulmonary infective exacerbations, deterioration of lung function with reduced exercise tolerance, cyanosis and dyspnea, and congestive cardiac failure.
- The most common complications due to CF in pregnancy are prematurity (30% less than 37 weeks) and IUGR secondary to chronic maternal hypoxemia.
- Factors predicting poor obstetric outcome include pulmonary hypertension, cyanosis, arterial hypoxemia, moderate to severe lung disease, and poor maternal nutrition.

Counseling of women with CF needs to cover a number of aspects.

- There is an obvious risk of the child inheriting CF, and this will depend on the genotype of the father. If the genotype of the father is unknown, assuming that the carrier rate in Caucasian men is 1 in 25, the risk is approximately 2–2.5%, while if the father is a known carrier, the risk of an affected offspring will be 50%.
- Another issue that needs to be addressed as part of preconception counseling is the shortened life expectancy of CF patients and the harsh reality that they may not be alive to bring up their child.

The cornerstone of management of pregnancy in CF patients involves a multidisciplinary approach with particular attention to maternal nutrition, control of pulmonary infection, avoidance of hypoxia, and fetal surveillance.

- CF patients require a high calorie intake with pancreatic enzyme supplements.

- It is important to bear in mind that 20% of adults with CF have diabetes and a further 15% have impaired glucose tolerance. The latter may deteriorate to gestational diabetes, while insulin requirements are likely to rise in the former.
- Physiotherapy regimes need to be as strictly adhered to as in the nonpregnant state.
- Any pulmonary infections must be aggressively treated with antibiotics, which can be modified according to sputum cultures.
- Towards the latter half of the third trimester, breathlessness may become an increasing problem even in the absence of infective exacerbations. If oxygen saturations fall to the low nineties or less at rest, hospital admission for bed rest and supplemental oxygen may be required. This should also prompt fetal growth assessment.
- The aim should be vaginal delivery, but an operative vaginal delivery may be indicated to shorten the second stage as CF patients are particularly prone to pneumothoraces especially with repeated and prolonged Valsalva maneuvers.
- Breast-feeding should be encouraged.

Sarcoidosis and tuberculosis

Sarcoidosis

Sarcoidosis is a chronic multisystem granulomatous disease affecting around 5 in 10 000 pregnancies a year. The patient is often asymptomatic or may present with chest and/or extrapulmonary manifestations.

- The most common extrapulmonary manifestations include anterior uveitis, hypercalcemia, fever, and central nervous system (CNS) involvement.
- Pulmonary infiltration may gradually progress to pulmonary fibrosis.
- Chest X-ray may be diagnostic with bilateral hilar lymphadenopathy.
- Where the lung parenchyma is involved with no obvious infiltration in the lung fields, the diagnosis is made by broncheo-alveolar lavage and transbronchial biopsy.
- Serum ACE inhibitor levels may help in the diagnosis and monitoring of disease activity, but should not be used in pregnancy.

Pregnancy does not seem to affect the course of the disease. Any improvement in radiological findings of the disease in pregnancy is often followed by relapse in the puerperium. There appear to be no specific fetal risks. Management of sarcoidosis is as in the nonpregnant state, with extrapulmonary and CNS involvement, along with respiratory impairment, being the main indications for steroid treatment. Women need to be reassured about the safety of steroids in pregnancy and, if on long-term steroids, need to receive parenteral cover in labor. Vitamin D supplementation is not generally advisable as it may precipitate hypercalcemia.

Tuberculosis

The rates of tuberculosis (TB) appear to have been rising over the past two decades. The main causes of the increased prevalence appears to be the influx of individuals from areas where TB is endemic (Asian and West Indian immigrants) and the increasing numbers of HIV-positive individuals. The onset of the disease is often insidious with cough, hemoptysis, weight loss, and night sweats. The causative organism in the general population is *Mycobacterium tuberculosis*, while, in patients with AIDS, *Mycobacterium avium intracellulare* is an important cause of pulmonary disease. The diagnosis is based on the characteristic chest X-ray appearances as the disease most commonly affects the upper lobes. Culture of *M. tuberculosis* takes 6 weeks, but the diagnosis can be confirmed by microscopic examination of sputum (or bronchoscopic washings) for acid-fast bacilli (Ziehl–Nielsen stain).

There is no evidence that TB has a detrimental effect on pregnancy or that pregnancy adversely affects disease progression. The principles of treatment are similar to those in the nonpregnant patient. Untreated TB poses a greater risk to the mother and her fetus than treatment. A multidisciplinary approach with joint care from a respiratory physician with an interest in management of TB is recommended, and chest X-ray should not be withheld where required for diagnosis or management.

Treatment is usually with more than one of the drugs to which the organism is sensitive. The course of treatment needs to be prolonged and supervised to encourage and confirm compliance. The drugs most commonly used in the management of TB in the nonpregnant individual include rifampicin, isoniazid, ethambutol, pyrazinamide, and streptomycin.

- Streptomycin is associated with a high incidence of eighth nerve damage, and therefore is best avoided in pregnancy.
- With regard to rifampicin, there have been concerns about teratogenesis, but no adverse fetal effects have been proven. Some authorities would recommend avoidance in the first trimester.
- Ethambutol and isoniazid appear to be safe throughout pregnancy, but all patients on isoniazid should take pyridoxine 50 mg/day to reduce the risk of peripheral neuritis.
- There is little information about pyrazinamide and therefore avoidance during organogenesis is recommended unless warranted to treat severe disease.

The treatment needs to be carried on for 6–9 months and is usually modified once sensitivities are available.

During labor and delivery, infection precautions need to be taken with active disease, but it should be borne in mind that the mother becomes non-infectious within 2 weeks of beginning treatment.

- The neonate should be given BCG vaccination.
- Prophylactic treatment with isoniazid is recommended for the baby if the mother's sputum is positive.
- Breast-feeding is permissible when the mother is taking antituberculous drugs as the amounts of drugs excreted in breast milk are negligible.

Pneumonia

Bacterial pneumonia

The incidence of pneumonia in pregnancy is 1.5–2.5 episodes per 1000 pregnancies, and bacterial pneumonia appears to be no more common than in the nonpregnant population.

- The most common bacterial pathogens are *Streptococcus pneumoniae* (in over 50% of cases), *Haemophilus influenzae* (more common with pre-existing lung disease), spp. *Staphylococcus* (associated with influenza), and spp. *Klebsiella*. Atypical organisms include *Mycoplasma pneumoniae* and *Pneumocystis carinii* pneumonia (PCP) found in association with HIV infection.
- Signs and symptoms of the disease are as in the nonpregnant individual, although reluctance to perform a chest X-ray may delay diagnosis unnecessarily. Other investigations include sputum culture, white cell count, C-reactive protein (CRP), and arterial gases in the breathless patient.
- Maternal and fetal morbidity remain serious complications of pneumonia and therefore it is important that it is promptly treated.

The principles of management are adequate oxygenation, hydration, and physiotherapy to clear secretion, accompanied by appropriate chemotherapy.

- The community-acquired pneumonias (*Strep. pneumoniae, H.influenzae*) are best treated with amoxycillin (or erythromycin in the penicillin-allergic patient).
- Cephalosporins are a better choice for hospital-acquired infections, while atypical organisms such as *Chlamydia psittaci*, *M. pneumoniae*, and *Legionella pneumoniae* are all sensitive to erythromycin.
- Flucloxacillin is the agent of choice for staphylococcal pneumonia (erythromycin if allergic to penicillin).
- Tetracyclines are best avoided as they can cause discoloration and weakening of teeth and bones.

PCP is the most common opportunistic infection in patients with AIDS and is associated with adverse obstetric outcome, especially if the diagnosis is not suspected. If conventional treatment fails or where there is profound hypoxia out of proportion to the radiographic findings, the diagnosis should be considered. Confirmation may require bronchoscopy.

- The treatment of choice for PCP is high-dose Bactrim with or without pentamidine.
- There is a theoretical risk of kernicterus or hemolysis from sulfonamides given at term but, in practice, only long-acting sulfonamides such as sulfadimidine have been implicated in this.
- In women known to be HIV-positive and who have a CD4 count <200 cells/μL, PCP prophylaxis with either Bactrim or nebulized pentamidine is recommended.

Viral pneumonia

Viral pneumonia such as influenza pneumonia is more severe in pregnancy. Pregnant women appear to be more susceptible to varicella zoster (VZ) pneumonia. VZ infection occurs in 0.05–0.07% of pregnancies and, of these women, 10–20% develop varicella pneumonia. The condition carries a mortality ranging from 6 to 40%.

- Pregnant women not immune to VZ in whom the infection occurs before 20 weeks' gestation should be given VZ IgG as soon as possible after the contact.
- If the infection occurs after 20 weeks' gestation there is little risk of congenital varicella, but the risk of maternal varicella remains and administration of VZ IgG should be considered.
- Varicella pneumonia at a later gestation appears to be associated with a higher maternal mortality, possibly through increased immunosuppression.
- Women who develop clinical varicella should be treated with acyclovir. Oral acyclovir is safe in pregnancy, but caution is needed when using IV acyclovir in pregnancy as it readily crosses the placenta.
- If respiratory symptoms develop in a patient with VZ, hospitalization is recommended.
- Maternal and neonatal morbidity and mortality in cases of maternal varicella pneumonia may be improved by the use of IV acyclovir and, if required, by mechanical ventilation.

Inflammatory bowel disease

The incidence of Inflammatory bowel disease (IBD) (ulcerative colitis, Crohn's disease, nonspecific colitis, and proctitis) has been on the rise over the last 40 years. The annual prevalence rates for ulcerative colitis are 40–100 per 100 000 population and the prevalence rate for Crohn's disease is 4–6 per 100 000 population. The cause of IBD remains unknown, but a multifactorial element involving infection, genetic factors, autoimmunity, and environmental toxins may be implicated.

Clinical features

- Ulcerative colitis is usually confined to the colon and causes liquid diarrhea, lower abdominal pain, urgency of defecation, and passage of blood or mucus per rectum. Potential complications in ulcerative colitis include colonic dilatation/toxic megacolon, perforation, and malignancy.
- In Crohn's disease, the terminal ileum alone is affected in 30% of cases, the colon alone in 20% of cases, and both ileum and colon are affected in 50% of cases. Colonic involvement presents with symptoms similar to those of ulcerative colitis, while involvement of the terminal ileum is manifest by cramping mid-abdominal pain, diarrhea, and weight loss. Potential complications in Crohn's disease include perforation, stricture formation, perianal problems, fistulae, and abscess formation.

Effects of pregnancy on disease

In general, pregnancy has little adverse effect on the course of IBD.

- Patients with Crohn's disease limited to the terminal ileum fare better in pregnancy and postpartum than those with colonic Crohn's disease or ulcerative colitis.
- Relapses are frequent in pregnancy, especially in the first two trimesters in ulcerative colitis (50% relapse rate—similar to that in the non-pregnant population) and in the first trimester in Crohn's disease, although in about three-quarters of patients Crohn's remains quiescent in pregnancy.

Effects of disease on pregnancy

Female fertility may appear to be reduced as a result of voluntary infertility of the couple, nutritional status, and effects of chronic disease, along with psychological problems with sexual dysfunction especially after resective surgery.

- In ulcerative colitis, fertility is affected adversely only in severely active disease with no impairment for quiescent or well-controlled disease.
- In Crohn's disease, amenorrhea and involuntary infertility correlate with disease activity, and normal fertility can be anticipated in well-controlled disease including after resection.

Medical therapy

- Drug treatment in the form of salazopyrine and corticosteroids has no detrimental effect on female fertility (salazopyrine causes reduction in sperm count and increase in abnormal forms, but is a reversible cause of male infertility and therefore a change to 5-aminosalicylic acid alone may be an alternative).
- Earlier reports had suggested a detrimental effect of IBD on rates of spontaneous miscarriage. Recent data show rates of spontaneous miscarriage that are not significantly different from those in the normal population. With quiescent disease around the time of conception, good fetal outcome is anticipated in 80% of cases.
- In contrast, active disease at conception, first presentation in pregnancy, colonic rather than small bowel disease alone, active disease after resection, and severe disease being treated by surgery are all associated with increased fetal loss and prematurity.
- Women with IBD should be encouraged to aim for pregnancy during clinically quiescent disease and whilst taking minimum medication.

Management

Management of acute attacks and chronic disease is not substantially different from that in the nonpregnant situation. Exacerbation of disease should be investigated by CBC, serum albumin (falls in pregnancy), and flexible sigmoidoscopy or rigid proctoscopy to assess activity of colitis. Fresh stool should be sent for culture of pathogenic microorganisms and analysis of their toxins, along with screening to exclude parasites.

- Sulfasalazine appears to be safe in pregnancy and breast-feeding and is used for maintenance and induction of remission in women with ulcerative colitis and colonic Crohn's disease, but it interferes with folate metabolism and therefore supplemental folic acid is required.
- Supplementation with vitamin B_{12} should be considered, especially with involvement of the terminal ileum. Corticosteroids, orally and rectally, are safe in pregnancy, and oral doses of 20–40 mg/day may be required.
- Use of metronidazole in early pregnancy is controversial and, although no definitive evidence of adverse effects has been confirmed, its use is generally avoided in the first trimester.
- During pregnancy, constipation should be avoided by high fluid intake, a high-fiber diet, and bulking agents.
- Surgical intervention may be required for obstruction, toxic megacolon, hemorrhage, or perforation, and should be performed for the same indications as in the nonpregnant patient.
- Vaginal delivery is the preferred option unless there are obstetric indications for a cesarean delivery.
  - Elective cesarean delivery should be considered if there is severe scarring and inelasticity of the perineum secondary to severe perianal Crohn's or where there is active perianal Crohn's that may delay healing of a perineal laceration or episiotomy.
  - If abdominal delivery is required, it is wise to anticipate difficulties due to peritoneal adhesions.

Thyrotoxicosis

Thyrotoxicosis

The most common cause of thyrotoxicosis is Graves' disease, an autoimmune disorder associated with the presence of thyroid-stimulating immunoglobulins. Other rarer etiologies for thyrotoxicosis include autonomous nodules and pregnancy itself, the latter because of the similarity of the β-subunits of TSH (thyrotrophin) and β-hCG. Diagnosis of thyrotoxicosis depends on the demonstration of suppressed pituitary TSH and elevated free thyroxine (fT_4) and free triiodothyronine (fT_3). The use of radioactive iodine or technetium is contraindicated in pregnancy.

- Graves' disease accounts for 95% of cases of hyperthyroidism in pregnancy. Thyrotoxicosis may be caused by autonomous thyroid nodules, while other rarer causes of hyperthyroidism include subacute thyroiditis and amiodarone or lithium therapy.
- Hyperthyroidism may lead to amenorrhea and anovulation secondary to associated weight loss, but pregnancy may still occur despite thyrotoxicosis. During pregnancy, the disease frequently ameliorates with postpartum flare-up. There have been suggestions that thyrotoxicosis may itself be associated with fetal malformations and that the risk could be reduced by antithyroid treatment.
- Perinatal mortality is higher, along with higher incidence of premature delivery and IUGR, all of which can be reduced to the normal range with appropriate treatment.
- Fetal hypothyroidism is a risk with all antithyroid medication, and so the lowest possible dose to maintain biochemical euthyroidism in the mother should be used with bimonthly checks on free thyroid hormone and TSH concentrations throughout pregnancy.
- Poorly controlled or undiagnosed hyperthyroidism in conjunction with the stress of infection, labor, or operative delivery may precipitate 'thyroid storm'—a medical emergency characterized by hyperthermia, mental disorientation, and cardiac decompensation. Transplacental passage of thyroid-stimulating immunoglobulin (TSIg) may result in fetal/neonatal thyrotoxicosis in 1–10% of babies of mothers with current or previous history of thyrotoxicosis (including women who have had thyroid ablation) and, in these cases, serial scans to assess fetal growth, heart rate, and neck are advisable. Management in such cases involves treatment of the mother with antithyroid drugs (and with additional thyroxine if mother is euthyroid), using the fetal heart rate as a guide to adjusting therapy.
- Carbimazole (CBZ) and propylthiouracil (PTU) are the drugs most commonly used for the management of hyperthyroidism.
  - Both drugs cross the placenta, but PTU less so than CBZ. Also, both drugs have the potential, when used in high doses, to cause fetal hypothyroisim and goiter.
  - Neither drug is grossly teratogenic, although CBZ occasionally causes aplasia cutis—a scalp defect.

    - The aim of treatment is to achieve clinical euthyroidism, with free T_4 at the upper end of the normal range. In newly diagnosed cases, initial treatment is with high doses to achieve control and then reducing to lowest possible maintenance doses by 4–6 weeks.
    - PTU is preferable in newly diagnosed cases in pregnancy (less transfer across the placenta and excretion into breast milk), but patients stable on CBZ need not be changed to PTU.
    - The appearance of a rash or urticaria following the commencement of treatment should prompt changing to an alternative antithyroid agent.
- Women should be seen monthly in cases of newly diagnosed hyperthyroidism, but less frequent thyroid function tests (TFTs) are required if they are on stable doses of antithyroid medication.
- Doses of PTU <150 mg/day and CBZ <15 mg/day are unlikely to cause problems with the fetus and do not preclude breast-feeding, but TFTs should be checked at regular intervals in the neonate if the mother is breast-feeding and on higher doses of antithyroid medication.
- Thyrotoxicosis due to toxic thyroid nodules is more difficult to treat in pregnancy as antithyroid drugs will suppress both fetal and maternal thyroid, but there are no TSIgs to counteract their effect on the fetal thyroid.
    - β-Blockers are used instead to control symptoms until the pregnancy is completed or, alternatively, hemithyroidectomy can be considered in the second trimester.
- Other indications for surgical treatment include dysphagia, stridor, suspected carcinoma, and allergy to antithyroid medication.

Recommended further reading

1. American College of Obstetricians and Gynecologists (2001). Thyroid disease in pregnancy. ACOG Practice Bulletin No. 32. *Obstet Gynecol* **98**, 879–88.
2. Norwitz ER (2003). Endocrine disease in pregnancy. In: Yen SSC, Jaffe RB, Barbieri RL, Strauss J III, eds. *Reproductive Endocrinology: Physiology, Pathophysiology, and Clinical Management* (5th edn). WB Saunders, Philadelphia, PA.

Other thyroid complications of pregnancy

Hypothyroidism

This complicates 1% of pregnancies, but has often been diagnosed and treated prior to pregnancy. The etiology may be autoimmune thyroiditis (Hashimoto's disease), viral thyroiditis, congenital absence of thyroid, or iatrogenic following thyroid ablation for hyperthyroidism.

- Autoimmune hypothyroidism ameliorates in pregnancy, but recurs after delivery.
- Untreated hypothyroidism leads to anovulatory infertility.
- Poorly controlled hypothyroidism in pregnancy is associated with higher risks of miscarriage, fetal loss, preeclampsia, preterm labor, low birthweight, and subnormal neurological development.
- For patients on adequate replacement therapy at the outset of pregnancy who are therefore euthyroid, the maternal and fetal outcomes are good.

Management

The mainstay of management is thyroxine replacement.

- Most patients require 100–150 μg/day and often this requirement is unchanged during pregnancy. In newly diagnosed cases in pregnancy in the absence of cardiac disease, a dose of 100 μg/day may be an appropriate starting dose.
- Only trace amounts of thyroxine cross the placenta and therefore the fetus is not at risk of hyperthyroidism from maternal replacement therapy.
- TFTs need to be checked each trimester, unless there has been a dose adjustment in which case TFTs should be repeated in 4–6 weeks.

Postpartum thyroiditis

This presents with vague symptoms of fatigue, lethargy, palpitations, or depression, often attributed to the postpartum state. Its incidence is 5–11% and it is more common in women with a family history of hypothyroidism. The condition is due to destructive autoimmune thyroiditis causing release of preformed thyroxine from the thyroid (accounting for the transient phase of hyperthyroidism) followed by hypothyroidism when the thyroid reserve is depleted. Thus patients may present with transient hyperthyroidism in the first 6–12 weeks postpartum and then develop hypothyroidism 4–8 months postpartum.

Treatment should be tailored to symptoms and the majority of patients recover spontaneously.

- In the hyperthyroid phase, treatment is with β-blockers as antithyroid drugs are of no value where the problem is one of release rather than synthesis.
- The hypothyroid phase is more likely to require treatment with thyroxine, but this should be withdrawn at 6 months to determine whether the patient has recovered.

- Of the women who develop postpartum thyroiditis, 3–4% will remain permanently hypothyroid while 20–30% of them who are thyroid peroxidase antibody positive will develop permanent hypothyrodism over the next few years, and so annual screening with TFTs is recommended.

Thyroid nodules

These are present in approximately 1% of women of reproductive age and almost 1 in 3 of those discovered in pregnancy may be malignant. Features suggestive of malignancy include a history of growth of the thyroid and radiation to the neck or chest, rapid growth of a painless nodule, a fixed lump associated with lymphadenopathy, voice change, and neurological involvement such as Horner's syndrome. The differential diagnosis may be a toxic solitary nodule, subacute thyroiditis, or a bleed into a cystic lesion.

- Diagnosis involves biochemical assessment of thyroid function and thyroid antibodies and ultrasound to distinguish solid from cystic lesions.
- A raised thyroglobulin level (>100 μg/L) may elicit suspicion of malignancy.
- Histological diagnosis may be obtained by fine-needle aspiration cytology or biopsy of a solid lesion.

Malignancy needs to be treated surgically, postponing any radioiodine treatment until after the end of the pregnancy. Pregnancy has no detrimental effect on previously treated thyroid malignancy.

Recommended further reading

1. American College of Obstetricians and Gynecologists (2001). Thyroid disease in pregnancy. ACOG Practice Bulletin No. 32. *Obstet Gynecol* **98**, 879–88.
2. Norwitz ER. Endocrine disease in pregnancy. In Yen SSC, Jaffe RB, Barbieri RL, Strauss J III, eds. *Reproductive Endocrinology: Physiology, Pathophysiology, and Clinical Management* (5th edn). WB Saunders, Philadelphia, PA.

Jaundice

Jaundice complicates about 1 in 2000 pregnancies, although there is a much higher frequency in countries where the general incidence of hepatitis is increased.

- Viral hepatitis is the most common cause and may account for up to 40% of cases.
- Other conditions include hemolytic jaundice, recurrent intrahepatic cholestasis of pregnancy (up to 25%), and gallstones (6%).
- Hyperemesis, acute fatty liver, and hypertensive disease of pregnancy are responsible for less than 10% of cases.
- Jaundice may also occur in association with treatment with drugs such as chlorpromazine and, rarely, in severe cases of excessive vomiting.

Diagnosis and management

- A detailed history should be obtained, especially with regard to recent travel abroad, past and current medical or surgical illnesses, drugs, substance abuse, and blood product transfusion.
- Enquiries should be made into family history of jaundice or liver disease, symptoms of pruritus, pain, nausea, vomiting, fever, and color and consistency of stools.
- Gestational age and estimation of fetal weight and fetal movement and viability should be established.
- Cutaneous manifestations of liver disease, e.g. palmar erythema and spider nevi, are present in 60% of normal pregnant women. Clinical assessment includes degree of jaundice, hydration status, level of consciousness and cardiovascular stability, and the presence of flapping tremor. Evidence of ecchymoses, ascites, hepatic tenderness, and uterine irritability should be sought and a rectal examination should be performed to observe the color of the stool.

Hospitalization for investigation and monitoring may be required.

- CBC, urea and electrolytes, LFTs, clotting studies, viral hepatitis screen, and urine analysis should be preformed.
- An ultrasound scan of the biliary tract may be useful in the diagnosis.
- Liver biopsy, if indicated at all, should only be performed after correction of any clotting dysfunction.
- Joint management with a physician or surgeon would be useful to identify the etiology and carry out supportive therapy with maintenance of hydration, nutrition, correction of electrolyte disturbances, correction of coagulopathy, and control of blood glucose levels.
- Intensive care with ventilatory support may be necessary in some cases depending on the etiology and severity of the disease. It may be necessary to expedite delivery even though the fetus may be premature.

Viral hepatitis

This does not appear to occur more frequently in pregnancy than at other times, nor is it significantly different in its cause or management as far as the mother is concerned. Management of the patient is not influenced by pregnancy and treatment similar to that in the nonpregnant should be given.

Prematurity and stillbirths are more common if the disease occurs later in pregnancy. However, if jaundice occurs earlier, it appears to be less harmful. Neither hepatitis B nor hepatitis A virus causes congenital abnormalities, and so an infection during pregnancy is not an indication for termination. Jaundice due to gallstones is rare in pregnancy but, if it does occur, removal of the stone(s) would be indicated.

Liver diseases peculiar to pregnancy

- Hyperemesis gravidarum.
- Hypertensive disease of pregnancy.
  - Vascular changes lead to liver infarction and subcapsular hemorrhage.
  - Overt jaundice is uncommon; the patient presents with epigastric pain, vomiting, and hepatic tenderness.
  - Its association with HELLP syndrome is well recognized and regular platelet counts should be done.
  - Treatment is by delivery of the fetus.
- Intrahepatic cholestasis of pregnancy.
  - This presents with pruritus and jaundice.
  - It usually resolves within 48 hours of delivery and up to 45% of cases recur in subsequent pregnancies and also with the use of the combined oral contraceptive pill.
  - The most consistent abnormalities on LFTs are slightly raised serum bilirubin and significantly raised alkaline phosphatase and bile acids.
  - The jaundice is obstructive in origin and is due to intrahepatic cholestasis.
  - There is a recognized fetal mortality associated with this condition, especially in late pregnancy.
  - Cholestyramine reduces pruritus.
  - Fetal assessment in the form of frequent cardiotocographs (CTGs) and biophysical profiles is indicated, especially in late pregnancy. However, it is not clear that frequent antepartum testing can prevent the adverse outcomes in pregnancies complicated by intrahepatic cholestasis.
- Acute fatty liver and acute hepatic failure.
  - Rarely, in late pregnancy, a patient will develop vomiting, upper abdominal pain, and jaundice. This may quickly be followed by headaches, mental confusion, and death. The whole duration of the disease may be merely a few days.
  - The urine is bile-stained and the stools are pale, indicating that the jaundice is obstructive in type. Acute liver failure of this type may arise at other times following drugs or various poisons.
  - The most prominent histological feature is fatty degeneration in the center of the liver lobules.
  - The progress of the condition is so rapid that effective treatment may be almost impossible. Early delivery is indicated at the first appearance of jaundice if the diagnosis is not in doubt.

Systemic lupus erythematosus

Systemic lupus erythematosus (SLE) is a systemic connective tissue disorder affecting women nine times more commonly than men. It has an incidence of 1 in 1000 women and is most common during the childbearing years; the average age at diagnosis is 31. SLE is an idiopathic chronic inflammatory disease which affects skin, joints, kidneys, lungs, serous membranes, nervous system, liver, and other body organs. It is characterized by periods of remission and relapse.

The pathogenesis is unknown, but is thought to be multifactorial, involving a genetic predisposition and environmental triggers such as viral infection and ultraviolet (UV) radiation. Inappropriate or excess immune activation leads to immune complex formation and deposition of immune complexes causes vasculitis and glomerulonephritis.

The most common clinical complaints are fatigue, fever, weight loss, myalgia, and arthralgia, but the symptomatology will vary according to the organ systems that are affected. Joint involvement occurs in 90% of cases, while skin involvement occurs in 80% of patients and 6% have other autoimmune disorders.

The suspicion of a diagnosis of SLE is confirmed by demonstrating the presence of circulating autoantibodies and, in particular, antinuclear antibodies (ANA) which are present in 96% of SLE patients.

- Antibodies to double-stranded DNA (anti-dsDNA) are the most specific for SLE and the titer of anti-dsDNA is also related to disease activity.
- Patients with SLE may also have antibodies to RNA–protein conjugates, which are referred to as soluble or extractable antigens since they can be separated from tissue extracts.
- Of the extractable nuclear antigens, anti-Ro and anti-La are of particular importance in obstetrics as they are associated with neonatal lupus syndromes including cardiac lesions such as congenital complete heart block and endocardial fibroelastosis.

Effect of pregnancy on SLE

There is controversy as to whether pregnancy exacerbates SLE and increases the number of flare-ups both antenatally and in the postpartum period. When flare-ups do occur, they tend to be in the first two trimesters, but diagnosis of a flare-up is hindered as many features of the condition (hair loss, edema, facial erythema, fatigue, anemia, raised ESR, and musculoskeletal pain) also occur in normal pregnancy. Where there is lupus nephritis, pregnancy does not jeopardize renal function in the long term. Even though women with moderate renal impairment usually have uncomplicated pregnancies, the risk of deterioration of renal function is greater the higher the baseline serum creatinine.

Effect of SLE on pregnancy

- SLE is associated with increased risks of spontaneous miscarriage, fetal death, preeclampsia, prematurity, and IUGR. Pregnancy outcome is particularly affected by the degree of renal involvement.

- Lupus nephritis in particular is associated with fetal loss, preeclampsia, and IUGR, especially if hypertension or proteinuria predate the pregnancy.
- Other indicators of increased risk of complications in pregnancy are the presence of anticardiolipin antibodies, lupus anticoagulant, active disease at time of conception, or first presentation in pregnancy.

Management

- Ideally, a woman with SLE should seek *preconception* counseling where a full discussion regarding potential obstetric and medical complications can take place, questions can be answered, and a management plan can be formulated.
  - The patient should be in remission and ideally have discontinued cytotoxic medication and nonsteroidal anti-inflammatory drugs (NSAIDs).
  - Assessment to document baseline renal function (urinalysis, serum creatinine, and 24-hour urine for creatinine clearance and total protein), along with CBC (to exclude anemia and thrombocytopenia) and screening for antiphospholipid antibodies (lupus anticoagulant and anticardiolipin antibodies) should be performed.
- Antenatal care should be undertaken in a combined medical–obstetric clinic. Close follow-up is recommended with fortnightly visits in the first and second trimesters and weekly visits in the third.
  - Disease activity needs to be regularly monitored along with fetal welfare by regular fetal biometry combined with umbilical artery Doppler blood flow examination.
  - There is a need to watch for superimposed pregnancy-induced hypertension and fetal growth restriction.
  - In patients with renal involvement, monthly 24-hour urine collections for total protein and creatinine clearance is recommended.
- Disease exacerbation needs to be actively managed and corticosteroids are the drugs of choice.
  - If the patient is on hydroxychloroquine, this needs to be continued since discontinuation may lead to disease flare-up.
  - Azathioprine appears to be safe in pregnancy, although there are theoretical concerns that it may cause chromosomal aberrations in germ cells.
  - NSAIDs are associated with oligohydramnios through their action on the fetal kidneys and may also lead to premature closure of the ductus arteriosus. Both effects may be reversible with early discontinuation of NSAIDs. Under special circumstances it may be warranted to use NSAIDs for pain control, but this should be avoided in the third trimester and especially after 32 weeks.
  - The antihypertensive agent of choice is methyldopa with nifedipine and hydrallazine as agents of second choice. Consideration should be given to thromboprophylaxis.
- Delivery at term is recommended in the absence of complications, avoiding postmaturity.
  - In labor, continuous electronic fetal monitoring (EFM) should be instituted along with IV steroids for patients on chronic steroid therapy and the pediatricians need to be alerted.
- Postnatally, restart maintenance therapy, consider thromboprophylaxis, and watch for exacerbations of SLE.

Antiphospholipid antibody syndrome

The diagnosis of antiphospholipid antibody syndrome (APLAS) requires the combination of antiphospholipid antibodies (anticardiolipin antibody (ACA) and/or lupus anticoagulant (LAC)) with one or more of a series of recognized clinical features, the most common being a history of thrombosis (arterial or venous), recurrent pregnancy loss (usually late first and second trimester), and autoimmune thrombocytopenia.

- Other clinical features associated with APLAS include hypertension, pulmonary hypertension, heart valve disease, and cerebral involvement (epilepsy, cerebral infarction, chorea, and migraine).
- The prevalence of antiphospholipid antibodies in the general population is around 2%. The diagnosis of APLAS requires positive readings for ACA and/or LAC on two occasions at least 3 months apart, and there is considerable variation in results between different laboratories.

Management

APLAS is associated with increased risks of pregnancy loss, thromboembolic disease, and stroke. There is also significant risk of severe early-onset preeclampsia, fetal growth impairment, and non-reassuring fetal testing ('fetal distress'), all of which contribute to increased risk of prematurity. Ideally, these issues should be discussed as part of preconception counseling.

- Antenatal management should be in a joint medical–obstetric clinic.
- Low-dose aspirin is now generally recommended early in pregnancy (even preconception) to prevent failure of placentation in the belief that placental damage occurs in early gestation.
- Controversy surrounds the use of low molecular weight heparin (LMWH). In women with a history of previous thromboembolism and APLAS, the very high risk of further thromboembolism during pregnancy and in the puerperium justifies thromboprophylaxis with SC LMWH in the antenatal and postpartum period. However, opinion is divided about the use of prophylactic heparin where there is no previous history of thrombosis. The benefits of heparin need to be balanced against the risks of heparin-induced osteoporosis.
- The use of steroids in combination with aspirin is no longer recommended.
- There needs to be close surveillance of fetal wellbeing and growth by serial biometry and Doppler studies of umbilical artery waveform as well as fetal activity monitoring.
- Maternal surveillance needs to concentrate on screening for preeclampsia and detection of signs/symptoms of thromboembolic disease.
- Postnatal thromboprophylaxis should not be forgotten.

Rheumatoid arthritis

Introduction

Rheumatoid arthritis (RA) is a chronic inflammatory disease affecting synovial joints. It has a 3:1 predilection for females and affects 1 in 1000–2000 pregnancies. The characteristic symptoms are joint pains and morning stiffness. RA is a systemic disorder with extra-articular manifestations including fatigue, vasculitis, and pulmonary and subcutaneous nodules as well as affecting the eyes. It is an autoimmune disorder involving immune complexes in the circulation and synovial fluid, leading to progressive damage and destruction of joints. Of RA patients, 80–90% are positive for rheumatoid factor while 30% are positive for antinuclear antibodies.

- *Effect of pregnancy on RA*. Up to 75% of women experience improvement of symptoms in pregnancy, beginning in the first trimester. Unfortunately, 90% of those who experience remission suffer postpartum exacerbations.
- *Effect of RA on pregnancy*. The main concerns relate to the safety of medication used in the treatment of RA during pregnancy and breast-feeding. In women with anti-Ro antibodies, the infants are at risk of neonatal lupus. Rare complications include atlanto-axial subluxation with general anesthesia and, in cases of severe limitations of hip abduction, interference with vaginal delivery.

Management

Pre-pregnancy management should concentrate on stabilization of underlying disease at the lowest maintenance doses possible and avoiding teratogenic agents. During pregnancy, increased rest and physiotherapy for symptomatic relief and maintenance of mobility are advisable.

- Acetaminophen should be used as the first-line analgesic.
- NSAIDs should, in general, be avoided (see under SLE), but in certain circumstances may be used to control arthritic pain. If they are used, their use should be discontinued after 32 weeks' gestation.
- Corticosteroids such as prednisone should be the first-line medication for worsening disease and are safe in pregnancy, but increase the risk of gestational diabetes. Thus blood glucose should be monitored. If patients are on long-term maintenance steroids, parenteral steroids should be administered to cover labor and delivery.
- Sulfasalazine is safe in pregnancy.
- Antimalarials and azathioprine can be used in pregnancy if required for disease control.
- Other disease-modifying agents such as chlorambucil, methotrexate, cyclophosphamide, and gold salts are generally contraindicated in pregnancy.

Myasthenia gravis

Introduction

Myasthenia gravis (MG) is an autoimmune disorder characterized by variable weakness and fatiguability of skeletal muscle (not myometrium). It is an uncommon disorder with an incidence of 2–10 in 100 000, affecting women more than men. The immediate cause of the disease is an autoimmune attack on the acetylcholine receptor complex at the neuromuscular junction, with autoantibodies to the human acetylcholine receptor complex present in the serum of three-quarters of patients with MG.

- Ocular muscle weakness resulting in diplopia (double vision) or eyelid ptosis is the usual presenting symptom, while some patients present with difficulty talking or chewing.
- MG progresses from ocular to generalized skeletal muscle involvement over 1–2 years. Muscle weakness varies throughout the day, but tends to be worse towards the end of the day. The long-term course of the disease is variable with periodic fluctuations in severity.
- The diagnosis rests on clinical presentation, physical examination, and confirmatory tests including restoration of muscle vigor after intravenous injection of short-acting anticholinesterase drugs such as endrophonium. Other more sophisticated tests include single-fiber myography and repetitive nerve stimulation studies.
- MG is treatable, but not curable. The agent of choice is pyridostigmine, an anticholinesterase that impedes degradation of acetylcholine, thus improving muscle function.

Management

Preconception counseling is important to discuss risks of pregnancy and formulate a management plan. There may be a need to adjust medication in pregnancy because of reduced gastrointestinal absorption, increased plasma volume, and increased renal clearance. Patients need to be counseled about the increase in fatigue, especially during the second and third trimester, with the potential of respiratory compromise in late pregnancy.

- Pregnancy should be postponed in women recently diagnosed with MG as this time period represents the greatest risk. There is a high risk of premature delivery (up to 60%).
- Weakness due to MG can be increased by the exertion required in the course of labor and delivery, especially in the second stage of labor.

Treatment of MG in pregnancy does not differ significantly from that in the non-pregnant state.

- The quaternary ammonium compound pyridostigmine is the most popular long-acting medication with anticholinesterase activity.
- Prednisone in high doses is effective in most patients, with slow tapering of dose over many months after improvement.

- Unfortunately, remission appears to be maintained only while the patient is on steroids. Hence, pregnant patients with MG on glucocorticoids should be maintained on them throughout pregnancy and the postpartum period.
- It is worthwhile limiting exercise and work and minimizing emotional and physical stress—all factors that may exacerbate MG.
- Any infections should be promptly identified and treated.
- Poor fetal movements and polyhydramnios may raise the possibility of fetal involvement, but may be difficult to differentiate from reduced fetal activity due to hypoxemia—hence the need for regular biometry and biophysical scoring to confirm fetal wellbeing.
- During labor and delivery, anticholinesterase drugs may have to be administered parenterally together with steroid cover if on long-term steroids.
    - Certain drugs such as magnesium sulfate are *absolutely contraindicated* and hypokalemia (as may occur with β-sympathomimetics) should be carefully avoided.
- Regional anesthesia and analgesia is preferable as it limits fatigue and anxiety and is ideal for assisted instrumental deliveries.
- In the postpartum period, drug dosages may need to be rapidly adjusted downwards as the effect of volume expansion of pregnancy clears.
- Special care and surveillance of the newborn may be required to detect transient neonatal MG, which is easily treatable with endrophonium and usually resolves by 4 weeks postnatally.
  It is caused by transport of maternal antibodies across the placenta.

Autoimmune thrombocytopenia (idiopathic thrombocytopenia)

Introduction

The incidence is 1 in 1000 pregnancies. If a low maternal platelet count is diagnosed in the first half of pregnancy, it is likely to be due to immune thrombocytopenia. The presence of antiplatelet antibodies in the maternal serum is diagnostic.

- The major risks to the mother in this condition usually occur during labor or postpartum and include hemorrhage, particularly from lacerations or from episiotomies, but not usually from the placental site. The incidence is 5–26% and is correlated with the degree of thrombocytopenia. Insertion of an epidural cannula may result in epidural hematoma. These manifestations usually occur when the platelet count is less than 50×10^6/mL and clotting characteristics are abnormal. With regards to neonatal thrombocytopenia, which occurs as a result of IgG antibodies crossing the placenta, maternal platelet count is a poor predictor.
- About 10–15% of babies of affected mothers will have platelet counts of less than 50×10^6/mL at delivery, although this is not associated with significant morbidity. The perinatal mortality for a baby with ITP is about 5%. Intracranial hemorrhage occurs in less than 1% of all cases and this occurs mostly in the 3% of severely affected babies with platelet counts of less than 50×10^6/mL. Cesarean delivery is not necessarily preventive. The practice of establishing the degree of severity with a fetal blood sampling antenatally or in early labor to decide on the mode of delivery is debated.

Management of idiopathic thrombocytopenia (ITP)

- As long as the booking platelet count is more than 100×10^6/mL, regular repeat counts are not necessary until about 26–28 weeks. Thereafter, the platelet counts should be monitored at monthly intervals until delivery.
- Platelet counts at booking of less than 100×10^6/mL would need weekly measurement. If the platelet count is less than 50×10^6/mL, a coagulation screen is necessary to exclude any additional coagulation defect.
- Steroids in the form of prednisone are indicated for maternal platelet counts $<20 \times 10^6$/mL and are preferable in those with counts $<50 \times 10^6$/mL (prednisone 60–80 mg per day). This usually increases the platelet count $>50 \times 10^6$/mL within 3 weeks. Thereafter, the dose of prednisone can be reduced to maintain the platelet count at $>70 \times 10^6$/mL.
- An alternative therapy is immunoglobulin at 400 mg/kg/day. Given intravenously, it would give a rapid rise in maternal platelet count that lasts for about 2 weeks.
- During delivery, it may be necessary to cover labor and delivery with a platelet transfusion if the platelet count is $<30 \times 10^6$/mL. Each unit raises the platelet count by approximately $5–10 \times 10^6$/mL.

Pregnancy is associated with changes in all aspects of the hemostatic mechanism (platelets, vessels, coagulation factors, natural anticoagulants, and fibrinolytic system) such that, towards the end of pregnancy, the overall balance shifts towards hypercoagulability.

- *Hemophilia.* The prevalence of hemophilia is reported to be 13–18 in 100 000 male population with a ratio of 4:1 between hemophilia A (factor VIII deficiency) and hemophilia B (factor IX deficiency), both of which are X-linked recessive disorders.
  - Female carriers have a second normal gene and therefore do not have significant bleeding problems. Troublesome bleeding may occur in a minority of carriers, especially in those with very low clotting factor levels (5–10 IU/dL) which may be a result of extreme lyonization or coinheritance of another bleeding disorder or where another chromosomal abnormality affects the X chromosome.
  - Male offspring of an affected father will always be affected, while male offspring of a carrier mother may either be affected or normal.
  - Female offspring of an affected male will always be carriers.
  - Hemophilia centers actively seek to educate families and promote the significance of carrier testing, which should ideally be performed ahead of puberty when a girl is old enough to understand the implications but before she is sexually active and certainly before her first pregnancy.
- *von Willebrand's disease* is the most common clinically significant hereditary coagulation abnormality affecting women, but it is a milder disorder than hemophilia. Its prevalence in the general population is estimated at 1%. Synthesis of von Willebrand factor is controlled by a gene on the short arm of chromosome 12.
  - Three major types of von Willebrand's disease are described with both autosomally recessive and dominant forms. Thus both male and female offspring may be carriers or be affected by the condition.
  - von Willebrand factor is essential for normal platelet activity and acts as a carrier for clotting factor VIII in the circulation.
  - Type III von Willebrand disease is the most severe.
- *Factor XIc deficiency* is an autosomal disorder most prevalent amongst Ashkenazi Jews and other families of European extraction. Bleeding is most common amongst individuals with significantly reduced levels of factor XIc. Bleeding problems such as menorrhagia and postpartum bleeds are reported among women with a factor XIc activity around 50% of normal values.

Prenatal diagnosis and pregnancy care in autoimmune diseases

Prenatal diagnosis

Chorionic villus sampling (CVS) in conjunction with fetal genotype analysis by mutation detection or linked polymorphism is the main method of prenatal diagnosis. Where the mother's DNA analysis is noninformative or there is inadequate information on the family, diagnosis of clotting factor deficiency in the fetal blood obtained by cordocentesis is used. The uptake of prenatal diagnosis for hemophilia is low at 30–35%, the reason often given being that hemophilia is not considered a serious enough disease to justify termination of pregnancy.

Antenatal care

- This should start with preconception counseling where the options for prenatal diagnosis and other aspects of the management of the pregnancy should be reviewed.
- Where blood products may be required, it may be appropriate to ensure immunity to hepatitis B. If this is not the case, it may be appropriate to complete a course of hepatitis B (and hepatitis A) vaccination prior to embarking on pregnancy.
- The pregnancy should be managed jointly by an obstetrician and a hematologist with interest in hemophilia.
- Maternal coagulation factor activity along with von Willebrand factor antigen and activity should be checked at booking.
- Invasive procedures in pregnancy may cause maternal, fetal, or placental bleeding, and this includes prenatal diagnostic procedures such as CVS. Thus full discussion of the risks as well as the perceived benefits of each course of action is essential.
- In the majority of cases of carriers or potential carriers of hemophilia where prenatal diagnosis has not been performed, fetal gender determination is possible by visualization of the external genitalia from 18–20 weeks.
- Maternal coagulation factor activity and (if appropriate) von Willebrand factor levels should be rechecked at 28 and 34 weeks and at any stage where there is a possibility of surgery or invasive procedures and with miscarriage or accidental bleeding.

Labor and delivery

- In the absence of obstetric contraindications, vaginal delivery at term is the preferred option with early recourse to cesarean delivery if labor fails to progress.
- On admission in labor, maternal von Willebrand factors should be checked, aiming for levels greater than 40 IU/L if an uncomplicated delivery is anticipated, but levels of at least 50 IU/L if operative delivery becomes necessary. If the maternal levels are below these thresholds, prophylactic treatment should be given.

- Invasive monitoring, scalp blood sampling, vacuum extraction, and mid-cavity rotational deliveries should be avoided in cases of von Willebrand's disease or other autosomally inherited disorders or where the fetus is known to be an affected male or the sex is unknown in cases of hemophilia carriers.
- Low forceps delivery is considered less traumatic than trying to deliver a deeply engaged head at cesarean, but should be used with caution.
- Epidural anesthesia is not contraindicated in patients with a normal coagulation screen, provided that their clotting factor levels are >50 IU/dL, their platelet count is $>100 \times 10^6$/mL, and their bleeding time is normal.

Postnatal care

- In all patients with hereditary bleeding disorders, it is important to ensure that clotting factor activity and von Willebrand activity is maintained above 40–50 IU/dL for at least 4–5 days after delivery to reduce the risk of postpartum hemorrhage.
- A blood sample needs to be collected from the neonate at delivery, but sometimes repeat testing at 3–6 months is required for definitive exclusion of some disorders such as mild to moderate hemophilia B or von Willebrand's disease.
- IM injections must be avoided in neonates with possible inherited bleeding disorders, giving oral prophylactic vitamin K instead along with SC or intradermal administration of routine immunizations.
- Immunization against hepatitis B should be considered in affected neonates, who should also be registered with a hemophilia center.

Sickle cell disease

Introduction

The sickle cell disorders are a group of inherited abnormalities of hemoglobin synthesis. Although these disorders are more commonly seen in Black people of African origin, they are also seen in Saudi Arabians, Indians, and Mediterraneans. There are in excess of 40 different hemoglobinopathies in this group, all sharing an abnormal form of hemoglobin due to substitution of the glutamic acid residue by the valine residue at position 6 of the β-globin chain of the hemoglobin molecule.

- The most commonly found variants are sickle cell anemia (HbSS, homozygous for sickle cell gene), sickle cell hemoglobin C disease (HbSC, heterozygous for sickle cell and hemoglobin C), and sickle cell β-thalassemia (HbS B thal, heterozygous for sickle cell and β-thalassemia).
- Sickle cell trait (Hb AS) is much more common but does not affect pregnancy in the same way as sickle cell disease. However, it does have implications for genetic counseling.

The pathophysiological basis of the condition involves distortion of the shape of the red cell into a rigid sickle shape occurring as a result of hemoglobin S forming fibrous precipitates under conditions of deoxygenation. The distorted erythrocytes lead to microvascular blockage and stasis leading to further sickling, stasis, and infarction that may affect any organ in the body (bones, kidneys, lungs, and spleen).

- The sickle crises can be precipitated by cold, infection, dehydration, and pregnancy in addition to hypoxia.
- Their clinical presentation is with hemolytic anemia and vaso-occlusive symptoms.
- Clinical features include anemia, infections, acute chest syndrome (fever, chest pain, tachypnea, leukocytosis, and pulmonary infiltrates), retinopathy, leg ulcers, stroke, avascular necrosis of bone, renal papillary necrosis, and splenic sequestration.

Effect of pregnancy on disease

Complications of sickle cell disease are more common during pregnancy especially in the form of acute chest syndrome. Sickle crises may affect up to 35% of pregnancies and there is an increased risk of urinary tract infections (UTIs), pyelonephritis, pneumonia, puerperal sepsis, and anemia. Pulmonary embolism may be difficult to distinguish from acute chest syndrome. Maternal mortality is estimated at around 2%.

Effect of disease on pregnancy

As there is a risk of the fetus having sickle cell disease, the couple needs to be counseled as to whether prenatal diagnosis is appropriate or acceptable to them as it may lead to further ethical and religious dilemmas. These dilemmas are complicated by different variants of the disease and the wide diversity of the clinical course with sickle cell disease both between individuals with the same genotype and any individual during the course of their life. Women with sickle cell disease in pregnancy have a higher risk of miscarriage, IUGR, premature labor, and early onset and accelerated preeclampsia resulting in higher incidence of nonreassuring fetal testing ('fetal distress') and delivery by cesarean. There is a four- to sixfold increase in perinatal mortality.

Management

Ideally, preconception counseling with a discussion of risks and a plan for antenatal care along with screening of partner should be undertaken. However, most commonly, the antenatal booking visit is the first opportunity to address issues such as screening the partner, prenatal diagnosis, assessment of maternal health with respect to hematological parameters, and complications associated with sickle cell disease.

- The booking investigations should include quantitative hemoglobin electrophoresis, blood group and antibody screen, liver function tests, antibodies to hepatitis B and C, syphilis and rubella serology, and urine culture.
- A multidisciplinary approach with combined obstetric and hematological input is required, setting out a clear management plan.
- Folic acid should be prescribed to aid hemopoiesis, and hemoglobin (Hb) level should be checked on a regular basis throughout pregnancy along with estimation of the HbS percentage to consider the need for blood transfusion.
- Urine should be regularly screened for infection.
- Fetal surveillance with ultrasound biometry and umbilical artery Doppler velocimetry should be performed from 24 weeks.
- Iron supplementation is indicated only where there is biochemical evidence of iron deficiency as iron may have accrued from previous transfusions.
- Sickle crises should be managed aggressively with IV hydration, antibiotics, adequate analgesia, warmth, and maintaining the patient well oxygenated.
- During labor and delivery and during the first 24 hours postnatally it is essential to ensure adequate hydration and avoid hypoxia.
- Continuous EFM in labor is recommended.
- The use of prophylactic antibiotics in the peripartum period is controversial, but careful consideration should be given to thromboprophylaxis.
- Prior to discharge, the issue of contraception should be addressed.

Thalassemias

The thalassemia syndromes are the most common of the genetic blood disorders, the basic defect being a reduced rate of globin synthesis through deletion of one or more of the α-globin genes or the presence of defective β-globin genes. As a result, the red cells formed have inadequate hemoglobin content. α-Thalassemia is more common in Southeast Asia, whereas β-thalassemia is more common in Cypriots, Asians, and a broad band of peoples around the Mediterranean.

- In α-thalassemia trait, there may be three normal genes (+) or two normal genes (0). These individuals are asymptomatic, but the latter group may become anemic during pregnancy.
- In α-thalassemia major (Hb Barts) there are no functional α-genes and the condition is incompatible with life, with the fetus becoming severely hydropic and often born prematurely.
- Patients with β-thalassemia trait have one defective β-globin gene and are asymptomatic, although they may become anemic in pregnancy.
- Individuals with β-thalassemia major have two defective β-globin genes and therefore become transfusion dependent. Survival of these children has improved, now reaching the second and third decade. Repeated transfusions gradually lead to iron overload and endocrine, hepatic, and cardiac dysfunction—cardiac failure being a common mode of demise. Puberty is often delayed and incomplete, and there have only been anecdotal reports of successful pregnancy in truly transfusion-dependent patients.

α-Thalassemia major is not compatible with life, while patients with β-thalassemia major are not encountered in obstetric practice. Patients with α-thalassemia trait and β-thalassemia trait need to be counseled preferably prior to pregnancy and their partners screened so that, if the partner is also thalassemia trait/minor, then appropriate prenatal diagnosis can be offered to the couple. These patients will need folate supplementation at 4 mg/day and oral iron supplementation if iron deficient, but no parenteral iron. In cases of severe anemia, blood transfusion may be required.

Renal disease

Introduction

In pregnancy, the glomerular filtration rate (GFR) is increased by 50% because renal plasma flow is increased by 40–50% compared with the nonpregnant state. This is due primarily to volume expansion. Thus creatinine clearance increases to about 150–170 mL/min per 1.73 m^2. As a result, creatinine levels of more than 0.8 mg/dL (75 μmol/L) and urea levels of more than 13 mg/dL (4.5 mmol/L) merit further investigation. Glycosuria in pregnancy may reflect altered renal physiology and does not necessarily imply hyperglycemia. Abnormal proteinuria is more than 300 mg per 24 hours.

Underlying renal lesions may result in marked increments in protein excretion during pregnancy. However, this should not be misconstrued as exacerbation of disease. Abnormal blood urate levels are more than 5 mg/dL (300 μmol/L) in singleton pregnancies. There is marked dilatation of the calyces, renal pelvis, and ureters. These changes appear in the first trimester of pregnancy and result more from hormonal changes brought about by progesterone than from back pressure or ureteric obstruction. Vesicoureteric reflux occurs sporadically. The combination of reflux and ureteric dilatation is associated with a high incidence of urinary stasis and an increased tendency to UTI and the development of pyelonephritis, especially in women with asymptomatic bacteriuria.

Urinary tract infection (UTI)

True bacteriuria is defined as more than 100 000 bacteria of the same species per milliliter of urine. The most common infecting organism is *Escherichia coli* and this occurs in 90% of cases. Other organisms frequently responsible include species of *Klebsiella, Proteus,* coagulase-negative *Staphylococcus,* and *Pseudomonas.*

Asymptomatic bacteriuria

This is defined as true bacteriuria without subjective evidence of a UTI. It is found in 2% of sexually active women, and is more common (up to 7%) during pregnancy. Of patients with asymptomatic bacteriuria, 40% will become symptomatic with UTI and acute pyelonephritis. Acute pyelonephritis can cause fetal growth restriction, fetal death, and preterm labor.

This is the argument for screening all women for asymptomatic bacteriuria at booking and again at 28–30 weeks. If present on midstream samples of urine (MSUs), treatment should be given.

- Ampicillin or a cephalosporin are the antibiotics of choice. A single dose of amoxycillin 3 g orally is usually effective. One must test for cure after 1–2 weeks.
- Coagulase-negative infection (*Staphylococcus albus*) should be treated with flucloxacillin 250 mg three times daily.
- Sulfonamides are best avoided because they competitively inhibit the binding of bilirubin to albumin and can increase the risk of neonatal hyperbilirubinemia.

- Nitrofurantoin is best avoided in late pregnancy because of the risk of hemolysis in the newborn because of a possible deficiency of erythrocyte phosphate dehydrogenase.
- Tetracyclines *are absolutely contraindicated* during pregnancy because they predispose to staining and weakening of teeth and long bones and, rarely, may cause acute fatty liver.
- The folic acid antagonist trimethoprim can be an extremely effective antibiotic for UTIs, and may be used on a long-term basis in pregnancy with folic acid supplements. A prophylactic dose of 100 mg nightly with 4 mg folic acid is effective in women with a long-term history of UTI.

Pyelonephritis

The presenting clinical picture may consist of malaise with urinary frequency or a more florid picture with a raised temperature, tachycardia, vomiting, and loin pain. Pyelonephritis occurs in 1–2% of all pregnancies. UTIs should be considered in those with hyperemesis and in women admitted with preterm labor. Treatment is with bed rest and plenty of fluids. Antibiotic sensitivity should be identified within 48 hours and an appropriate antibiotic commenced.

- After blood and urine culture, antibiotics such as cefuroxime 1 g every 8 hours can be given IV, or an alternative antibiotic according to sensitivity results, especially if the patient is vomiting and cannot tolerate oral medication. Treatment should continue for 1–2 weeks and an MSU should be checked every month for the rest of the pregnancy.
- Recurrent infection commonly occurs in up to 30% of women and 15% continue to have positive urinary cultures. These women require long-term low-dose antibiotic suppression with a cephalosporin, ampicillin, or trimethoprim.
- About 20% of women who have pyelonephritis in pregnancy have underlying renal tract abnormalities, and an ultrasound is recommended during pregnancy or an intravenous urogram (IVU) about 12 weeks postpartum.
- Nitrofurantoin suppression, 100 mg every 12–24 hours orally with food, should be given for the rest of pregnancy to prevent recurrences. This drug should be avoided if the GFR is <50 mL/min. Side effects include vomiting, peripheral neuropathy, pulmonary infiltration, and liver damage.

Nephrolithiasis CF { hematuria is seen in ~70% / unilat flank pain ± CVA tenderness
see p. 101
tx { IVF + abx + pain mgt + watch or refer to uro for stent

Hydronephrosis 2/2 stones or physiologic 2/2 uterin pressure
C/F: CVA tenderness, N/V ± Sx of stone (if any)
mgt: renal u/s, formal UA, Cr: BUN

Chronic renal disease

- In women with mild renal deficiency with plasma creatinine <1.4 mg/dL (125 μmol/L) and in those without hypertension and proteinuria of 1 g per day, there is little evidence that pregnancy accelerates renal disorders.
- Women with moderate renal deficiency with plasma creatinine levels of 1.4–2.8 mg/dL (125–250 μmol/L) may progress to serious renal deterioration with uncontrolled hypertension and increase in proteinuria, which may also result in a poor obstetric outcome. Renal function may decline even further in the postpartum period.
- Those with severe renal disease with plasma creatinine levels >2.8 mg/dL (250 μmol/L) and those with marked anemia, hypertension, retinopathy, or heavy proteinuria should avoid pregnancy as further deterioration in renal function may be expected and fetal loss is considerable (up to 60%). These women should be managed in close collaboration with renal physicians during the pregnancy.

Care should include visits at least every 2 weeks until 32 weeks and then weekly.

- Blood pressure monitoring may include domiciliary monitoring and ambulatory monitoring to obtain a profile.
- A 24 hour creatinine clearance and protein excretion should be done fortnightly if there is increased protein excretion on Dipstix testing.
- If blood pressure elevation is noted, especially if there is persistent elevation to ≥140/90 mmHg, every effort should be made to exclude superimposed preeclampsia. This should include a history and physical examination as well as measurements of liver and renal function tests, platelets, and uric acid.

Women on dialysis during pregnancy are prone to complications of fluid overload, hypertension, preeclampsia, and polyhydramnios. A 50% increase in dialysis frequency may be needed and life-threatening complications can occur in up to 50% of women. Outcome is better for women with renal transplant as more than 90% of those who go past the first trimester would have successful pregnancies.

Acute renal failure

This condition should be suspected when the urine volume remains inadequate (<0.5 mL/kg/hour) following adequate fluid replacement. Renal failure could be pre-renal (dehydration) or intra-renal due to acute tubular necrosis or acute cortical necrosis. Causes include septicemia, e.g. from septic abortion or pyelonephritis, hemolysis from sickling crisis or malaria, or hypovolemia, e.g. in preeclampsia, hemorrhage (antepartum, abruptio, or postpartum), DIC, abortion, or adrenal failure (Addisonian crisis) in those on steroids not receiving booster doses to cover labor. Whenever these situations occur, the patient should be catheterized and an hourly urine volume should be measured. Management aims to achieve an output volume of more than 30 mL/hour (>0.5 mL/kg/hour). Monitor renal function with serial measurements of electrolytes, urea, and creatinine in addition to urine output. Dialysis may be needed, especially in cases of anuria.

Urinalysis = microscopic + dipstick (SG, ptn, Glu, Ketones, nitrite, leuk esterase)

- RBC
- WBC, bacteria
- epith cells
- casts, fat bodies, crystals

Adrenal diseases I

The majority of adrenal disorders will have been diagnosed and treated prior to pregnancy. However, atypical presentations of hypertension in pregnancy should prompt consideration of other diagnoses such as pheochromocytoma or Conn's syndrome.

Pheochromocytoma

This is a tumor of the adrenal medulla resulting in excess secretion of catecholamines. The incidence of pheochromocytoma in nonpregnant hypertensive patients is around 1 in 1000, but it is exceedingly rare in pregnancy. Pheochromocytomas are bilateral in 10% of cases, malignant in 10%, and extra-adrenal in 10%. Hypertension in pregnancy is not uncommon, but atypical features such as paroxysms of excessive sweating, palpitations, anxiety, and headaches may indicate patients who need to be screened for the rare possibility of a pheochromocytoma. Diagnosis can be confirmed by measuring 24 hour urinary catecholamines or their metabolites such as vanillylmandelic acid (VMA) or 5-hydroxyindoleacetic acid (5 HIAA). Localization of the tumor is by CT, MRI, or ultrasound. The tumor can also be localized using radiolabeled metaiodobenzylguanidine (MIBG), but MIBG is contraindicated in pregnancy.

The problems associated with pheochromocytoma in pregnancy are the potentially fatal hypertensive crises that may be triggered by the stress of labor or abdominal or vaginal delivery or the pressure exerted by the gravid uterus on the tumor whilst supine. Both maternal and fetal mortality are greatly increased, with maternal mortality of 17% and fetal mortality of 25% in undiagnosed cases. Maternal mortality may be due to arrhythmias, cardiovascular accident (CVA), or pulmonary edema.

- The management in pregnancy involves medical stabilization with α-adrenergic receptor blockade followed by β-blockade to control the tachycardia.
- If the diagnosis is made prior to 24 weeks, surgical management is recommended.
- After 24 weeks, if the patient is medically stabilized, surgery is probably best delayed to achieve further fetal maturity. Definitive surgery may be combined with an elective cesarean delivery. Expert anesthetic involvement is essential, with α-adrenergic receptor blockade for at least 3 days preoperatively.
- Postnatally, the patient needs to be monitored for recurrence.

Cushing's syndrome

This condition represents an excess of glucocorticoids and is rare in pregnancy. It is usually associated with anovulation and therefore subfertility. Glucocorticoid excess presenting in pregnancy requires urgent investigation as there is a 10% chance of malignancy of the adrenal cortex. Diagnosis requires demonstration of raised plasma and urinary cortisol for a given gestational age and low levels of adrenocorticotropic hormone (ACTH). The increased cortisol is not suppressed by dexamethazone, indicating its adrenal origin. Localization of the tumor will require CT or MRI.

Maternal morbidity and mortality are increased, with preeclampsia being a common finding. There is greater postoperative maternal morbidity due to poor tissue healing. There is an increased incidence of fetal loss, prematurity, and perinatal mortality, which is only partly explained by maternal hypertension and diabetes. The neonate is at risk of adrenal insufficiency.

- Drugs used in the management of Cushing' s syndrome include metyrapone, trilostane, and aminoglutethimide, which block various points in the biosynthetic pathway of cortisol, and cyproheptadine, a serotonin antagonist that is used to inhibit corticotrophin-releasing hormone. However, there is very limited experience with the use of these drugs in pregnancy, with only anecdotal reports.
- Surgery is the treatment of choice for both pituitary-dependent and adrenal Cushing's syndrome and has been undertaken successfully in pregnancy.

Conn's syndrome

Primary hyperaldosteronism is caused by an adrenal aldosterone-secreting adenoma or carcinoma or bilateral adrenal hyperplasia. It is a very rare cause of hypertension in pregnancy. Diagnosis is based on a low serum potassium <3 mEq/L (<3 mmol/L) together with raised serum aldosterone and suppressed renin activity. Full investigation may be postponed until after pregnancy, when radiolabeled selenium cholesterol can be used. Management involves control of hypertension (methyldopa, labetalol, or nifedipine) and potassium supplementation to correct the hypokalemia. Spironolactone should be avoided in pregnancy as it is an antiandrogen and may affect a male fetus.

Addison's disease

This presents as adrenocortical failure with deficiency of glucocorticoids and mineralocorticoids. The most common cause in developed countries is autoimmune destruction of both adrenals by adrenal antibodies. Up to 40% of these patients also have other autoimmune conditions such as pernicious anemia, diabetes, or thyroid disease. Worldwide, TB is another significant cause of bilateral adrenal failure. Diagnosis is based on a low cortisol (both free and total cortisol levels rise in pregnancy), a raised ACTH, and no response to synthetic ACTH (Synacthen test).

Pregnancy does not affect the course of Addison's disease other than by possibly delaying the diagnosis as some of the features of the condition are commonly encountered in pregnancy. There may be a requirement for increased doses of steroids to cover certain periods of stress such as intercurrent illness, labor and delivery, or surgery. Provided that the condition is diagnosed and treated appropriately, there is no adverse effect on pregnancy.

- Management of Addison's disease in pregnancy should continue as in the nonpregnant individual, with hydrocortisone (20–30 mg/day) and fludrocortisone (0.05–0.20 mg/day), and appropriate additional hydrocortisone at times of increased stress. Clinical wellbeing and blood pressure provide a good index of adequate steroid replacement.
- Breast-feeding is not contraindicated.

Adrenal diseases II

Congenital adrenal hyperplasia (CAH)

CAH is an autosomal recessive disorder with a gene frequency of 1 in 200–400. The most common abnormality is due to 21-hydroxylase deficiency causing reduced cortisol production and increased androgen synthesis. Pregnancies in women with CAH diagnosed in infancy are uncommon as they are often infertile. Many have anovulation associated with polycystic ovaries, while others often have psychosexual difficulties with anatomical problems following corrective surgery (clitoral surgery, vaginal scarring) performed for virilization of the genitalia.

In the small numbers of pregnancies in women with CAH, there appears to be a higher than average risk of miscarriage, preeclampsia, and IUGR, along with higher rates of cesarean delivery required because of an android pelvis and in an attempt to avoid the risks of vaginal and perineal lacerations in those with previous history of perineal surgery. During pregnancy, increased surveillance is required for preeclampsia and corticosteroid therapy needs to be maintained.

In cases where the fetus is at risk of CAH (i.e. previous child with CAH), a number of options are available.

- Ideally, genetic counseling after the birth of the previous child should have been undertaken along with preconception counseling prior to embarking on the current pregnancy. If this is the case, dexamethazone can be started either preconception or as soon as pregnancy is confirmed prior to differentiation of the external genitalia.
- Prenatal diagnosis by CVS is generally recommended to determine the sex and, if female, the 21-hydroxylase zygosity should be performed.
- If the fetus is male or an unaffected female, treatment *in utero* will not be required and maternal dexamethazone may be discontinued.
- If the fetus is an affected female, the options include continuation with dexamethazone throughout the pregnancy or a termination of pregnancy (TOP).
  - If dexamethazone is continued, maternal estriol levels should be measured every 6–8 weeks to confirm compliance and adrenal suppression, and the mother needs to be monitored for impaired glucose tolerance and hypertension.
- Postnatally, the child needs to be examined carefully for evidence of virilization and the salt-wasting form of the disease, and to receive the appropriate glucocorticoids and mineralocorticoid replacement therapy. Unfortunately, suppression of virilization with this regime is not always successful (especially if the dexamethazone therapy is started after 9 weeks' gestation) and parents must be fully counseled regarding the options available to them.

Hyperprolactinemia

This may be a result of pituitary adenomas, but a variety of other causes include normal pregnancy, hypothalamic or pituitary stalk lesions, empty sella syndrome, hypothyroidism, chronic renal failure, and drugs.

Prolactinomas are divided into microprolactinomas (<1 cm) or macroprolactinomas (>1 cm in size). Women with primary hyperprolactinemia are amenorrheic with anovulation and secondary estrogen deficiency, while others with secondary hyperprolactinemia have ongoing ovarian function. Outside pregnancy, the diagnosis is made on the level of serum prolactin in conjunction with imaging of the pituitary fossa by CT or MRI. In pregnancy, prolactin levels are greatly raised physiologically and, hence, this is unhelpful.

Many patients will require treatment with dopamine receptor agonists (bromocriptine or cabergoline) to restore fertility and achieve conception. In patients with a macroprolactinoma, the general advice is to continue with barrier contraception until imaging confirms shrinkage of the prolactinoma to within the fossa.

- In patients with both micro- and macroprolactinomas, treatment with dopamine receptor agonists should be discontinued upon confirmation of pregnancy.
- Routine visual field testing is not indicated in pregnancy.
- The patient is asked to report symptoms of headache and visual disturbance, which may herald tumor expansion.
  - This can be confirmed by pituitary imaging and treated with bromocriptine.
- The risk of tumor expansion and clinical symptoms is 15% for macroprolactinomas and 1.6% for microprolactinomas, and is highest in the third trimester.
- Hyperprolactinemia has no deleterious effect *per se* on pregnancy, and breast-feeding is not contraindicated.

Hypopituitarism

Anterior pituitary failure may be the result of pituitary surgery, radiotherapy, pituitary or hypothalamic tumors, postpartum pituitary infarction (Sheehan's syndrome), or autoimmune lymphocytic hypophysitis. The diagnosis is based on a combination of signs and symptoms, and confirmed by laboratory investigations. There are reduced levels of thyroxine, TSH, cortisol, ACTH, follicle-stimulating hormone (FSH), luteinizing hormone (LH), and growth hormone (GH). Furthermore, there is a failed response manifest by impaired secretion of ACTH, GH, and prolactin in response to an insulin stress test. Imaging of the pituitary region is required to exclude a space-occupying lesion.

Pregnancy is possible, but gonadotrophin stimulation of ovulation may be required. Once pregnancy is achieved, the fetoplacental unit takes over production of gonadotrophin, estradiol, and progesterone. Provided the condition has been diagnosed and adequately treated, maternal and fetal outcome is normal, but a higher incidence of adverse outcome in terms of maternal morbidity and mortality due to hypotension and hypoglycemia along with increased miscarriage and stillbirth rate is encountered in inadequately treated cases. Management involves replacement therapy with thyroxine and glucocorticoids. Mineralocorticoid replacement is not generally required as mineralocorticoid secretion is independent of the pituitary. Lactation may be impaired because of prolactin deficiency.

Diabetes insipidus and acromegaly

Diabetes insipidus

Posterior pituitary failure results in diabetes insipidus (DI). Deficient production of antidiuretic hormone (ADH) from the posterior pituitary may be caused by an enlarging pituitary adenoma, a craniopharyngioma, skull trauma, or post-neurosurgery. DI may be nephrogenic in origin because of chronic renal disease or it may be related to pregnancy because of increased vasopressinase production by the placenta or reduced vasopressinase breakdown by the liver as with preeclampsia or acute fatty liver of pregnancy (AFLP). Pregnancy may unmask previously subclinical DI. Over half of patients with DI show deterioration in pregnancy, possible mechanisms being increased GFR of pregnancy, vasopressinase production by the placenta, and potential antagonism of vasopressin by prostaglandins. DI has no adverse effects on pregnancy, other than possibly a slight increase in uterine contractility because of the structural similarity of desamino–D-arginyl vasopressin (dDAVP) to oxytocin.

- Treatment of choice for central DI is intranasal dDAVP 10–20 μg two to three times a day.
- For nephrogenic DI in pregnancy, chlorpropamide increases renal responsiveness to ADH, but it is not advisable in pregnancy. Carbamazepine is a safer option in pregnancy.

Acromegaly

This is rarely encountered in pregnancy. Forty percent of patients are infertile because of coexisting hyperprolactinemia. Biochemical diagnosis in pregnancy is unreliable. Growth hormone (GH) secreting adenomas expand during pregnancy and may cause visual symptoms. GH does not cross the placenta. However, there is a greater risk of gestational diabetes and resulting fetal macrosomia. Treatment is by surgery or radiotherapy prior to pregnancy. Medical options include the use of bromocriptine, which may work in 50% of cases, and the somatostatin analogue octreotide, but no data are available on its use in pregnancy.

Recommended further reading

1. Norwitz ER (2003). *Endocrine Disease in Pregnancy*. In Yen SSC, Jaffe RB, Barbieri RL, Strauss J, III eds. *Reproductive Endocrinology: Physiology, Pathophysiology, and Clinical Management* (5th edn). WB Saunders, Philadelphia, PA.

Diagnosis of diabetic pregnancies

Introduction

Pregnancy is a state of insulin resistance, relative glucose intolerance, and maternal hyperinsulinemia. The insulin resistance likely results from placental production of anti-insulin hormones such as human chorionic somatotropin (hCS) (also known as human placental lactogen (hPL)), cortisol, and glucagon. Fasting glucose levels are reduced in pregnancy while postprandial glucose levels are elevated in comparison with the nonpregnant state. Insulin production is increased twofold in normal pregnant women, and the insulin requirements of diabetic women also rise. There is also an increase in glycosuria due to lowering of the renal threshold for glucose.

Diagnosis

The prevalence of pregestational insulin-dependent (type I) diabetes mellitus (IDDM) in women of reproductive age is 0.5%, while the prevalence of non-insulin-dependent (type II) diabetes mellitus (NIDDM) is 2% (10% in Asian women). Gestational diabetes mellitus (GDM) refers to glucose intolerance that is first diagnosed in pregnancy. GDM likely includes a proportion (20–30%) of women with type II pregestational diabetes, although the definitive diagnosis can only be made after delivery.

It is generally recommended that all women are screened for GDM at 24–28 weeks' gestation. Women with risk factors, including GDM in a prior pregnancy, a family history (first-degree relative) with diabetes, prior macrosomic infant, BMI >25, unexplained late intrauterine fetal death (IUFD), persistent glycosuria, polyhydramnios, fetal size greater than expected for gestational age, and/or high risk ethnic groups (Hispanic, African American), should be tested for GDM earlier in pregnancy (at 16–20 weeks of gestation). If this early test is negative, it should be repeated at 24–28 weeks.

Screening for GDM involves a nonfasting glucose load test (GLT), also known as a glucose challenge test (GCT), Women are given a 50 g oral glucose load and serum glucose level is measured 1 hour later, with glucose >140 mg/dL denoting a positive test. A positive GLT screening test should be followed in all cases with a 3 hour glucose tolerance test (GTT). This involves 3 days of glucose loading to 'prime' the pancreas followed by a 100 g oral glucose load. Serum glucose levels are measured fasting and at 1, 2, and 3 hours after the 100 g glucose load. According to the commonly used NDDG criteria, abnormal glucose levels are fasting >105 mg/dL, 1 hour >185 mg/dL, 2 hours >165 mg/dL, and 3 hours >145 mg/dL. Two abnormal values are required for a diagnosis of GDM. Of note, there is no GLT that can make the diagnosis of GDM. However, if the GLT is >200 mg/dL and the fasting level is elevated (>95 mg/dL), the remainder of the GTT can be canceled and a diagnosis of GDM made.

Effect of pregnancy on diabetes

Insulin requirements rise in pregnancy, reaching maximal levels at term when the requirements are at least twice the pre-pregnancy requirements. In patients with diabetic nephropathy, there may be a deterioration of both renal function and proteinuria with a decrease in creatinine clearance in one-third. Any deterioration in renal function during pregnancy is usually reversed after delivery with no long-term detrimental effect. Rapid improvement in glycemic control in early pregnancy may lead to worsening retinopathy through increased retinal blood flow. There is a twofold risk of progression of diabetic retinopathy or the first appearance of retinopathy in pregnancy. Tighter diabetic control also leads to an increased incidence of hypoglycemia, while diabetic ketoacidosis is rare unless associated with hyperemesis, infection, and tocolytic and corticosteroid therapy.

Recommended further reading

1. American College of Obstetricians and Gynecologists (2005). ACOG Practice Bulletin No. 60. Pregestational diabetes mellitus. *Obstet Gynecol* **105**, 675–85.

Effects of diabetes on pregnancy

Preexisting diabetes is associated with an increased risk of congenital abnormalities, and this risk appears to be associated with the degree of glycemic control around the time of conception.

- Specific congenital abnormalities associated with diabetes include sacral agenesis (which is rare but pathognemonic for diabetic embryopathy), congenital heart defects, skeletal abnormalities, and neural tube defects.
- If the hemoglobin A_{1c} (HbA_{1c}) level is < 8%, the risk of congenital abnormalities is around 5% (approximately twice that in non-diabetic women). However, when the HbA_{1c} level is >10%, the risk of congenital abnormalities may be as high as 25%. The risk of spontaneous miscarriage is also related to the degree of glycemic control around the time of conception.
- Perinatal and neonatal mortality figures can be two- to fourfold higher in babies of diabetic mothers. These figures have been decreasing over the last two decades because of improvements in maternal diabetic control and close follow-up of circulating glucose levels in the infant within the first few hours of birth.

Babies of diabetic mothers also appear to be at risk of unexplained intrauterine death towards term, and this appears to be more common in macrosomic babies.

- The fetus can tolerate hypoglycemia relatively well, but maternal hyperglycemia may be detrimental to the fetus and ketoacidosis is associated with a particularly high fetal mortality rate.
- Babies of diabetic mothers tend to be macrosomic (defined as an estimated fetal weight, not birth weight, of greater than or equal to 4500 g). The incidence of macrosomia is greater with poor diabetic control, but not totally eliminated by tight glycemic control.
- Macrosomia carries with it the increased risk of operative vaginal delivery, birth trauma, and shoulder dystocia.
- Fetal polyuria and macrosomia are often associated with polyhydramnios which, in turn, may predispose to prelabor rupture of membranes as well as preterm delivery.
- Prematurity may pose an added problem, since pulmonary surfactant production is slightly delayed in babies of diabetic mothers.
- Antenatal corticosteroids may accelerate pulmonary maturation and should not be withheld despite its deleterious effect on glycemic control for at least 24–48 hours after administration. The issue of glycemic control can be addressed by regular monitoring of blood sugars and adjusting insulin requirements accordingly.
- Postnatally, babies of diabetic mothers are at risk of hypoglycemia and neonatal jaundice. Heel-stick glucose levels in the infant should routinely be checked within 1 hour of birth.
- Diabetic pregnancies, and in particular those with preexisting hypertension, are at increased risk of developing preeclampsia. This risk reaches almost 30% where there is coexisting nephropathy and hypertension.

Management of diabetic pregnancies

Joint obstetric and diabetic management is required to optimize outcome, supported by a multidisciplinary team of specialist dietitians, nurses, and midwives. Preconception counseling is the cornerstone of successful management of diabetic pregnancies. It provides an ideal opportunity to optimize diabetic control prior to pregnancy and thus reduce the risk of congenital abnormalities. It also provides an opportunity to assess the presence and severity of existing diabetic complications and to plan antenatal care. Folate supplementation for at least 3 months prior to conception and throughout the first trimester is advisable to reduce the risk of neural tube defects (NTDs).

The aim of medical management is to achieve maternal normoglycemia as far as possible with fasting glucose <95 mg/dL (<5.0 mmol/L) and 1 hour postprandial levels <140 mg/dL (<7.5 mmol/L). In order to best assess glycemic control, capillary glucose levels should be measured four times daily (fasting and 1 hour after breakfast, lunch, and dinner) to allow for appropriate adjustments to the patient's insulin regimen. Dietary advice on a low-sugar, low-fat, and high-fiber diet will improve glycemic control, but tighter control invariably means more frequent hypoglycemic episodes, and patients and partners/relatives should be educated on how to deal with these. In general, short-acting insulin before meals and intermediate-acting insulin at bedtime will be required to achieve satisfactory control, especially in later pregnancy. In women with pregestational diabetes, the degree of diabetic control needs to be assessed by serial (monthly) HbA_{1c} measurements, and regular ophthalmological examinations should be performed with appropriate treatment if any retinopathy is detected. Where diabetes is complicated by nephropathy, regular monitoring of renal function is required in the form of serum urea, electrolytes, and 24-hour urinary protein excretion and creatinine clearance estimations.

The increased risk of congenital abnormalities associated with diabetes means that detailed ultrasound screening should be offered in the second trimester.

- It is important to bear in mind that biochemical screening for Down syndrome will be affected by diabetes. Hence this should be interpreted using the appropriate normograms.
- Ultrasound scanning for fetal anomalies at 20 weeks should particularly exclude NTDs, sacral agenesis, and cardiac malformations. In women with pregestational diabetes, a further ultrasound scan (fetal echocardiogram) is indicated at 22–24 weeks as the heart is better visualized at this gestation.
- The frequency of antenatal visits needs to be individualized on the basis of a variety of factors such as glycemic control, fetal growth and wellbeing, and the development/worsening of maternal complications such as preeclampsia and deteriorating renal function.

Antenatal fetal surveillance

The increased risks of *in utero* fetal demise in women with pre-gestational diabetes justifies close fetal monitoring, especially in the third trimester, and delivery by 39–40 weeks of gestation.

- Serial ultrasound biometry is recommended to detect polyhydramnios, macrosomia, fetal growth acceleration, or a reduction in growth velocity. Abnormal growth patterns should prompt closer monitoring, as they may be associated with uteroplacental insufficiency.
- Umbilical artery Doppler velocimetry measurements should be used when growth restriction is suspected, but are not of value as a screening test.
- The routine use of biophysical profiles is controversial. In women with vascular disease where there is suggestion of growth restriction or poor glycemic control, closer monitoring by means of cardiotocography as a screening test for fetal acidemia may be useful, while accepting its limitations.

Labor and delivery

Timing and mode of delivery need to be individualized. Where diabetes is well controlled, there is no vascular disease, and the fetus appears appropriately grown, pregnancy can be allowed to go to term awaiting the onset of spontaneous labor.

- Where there are concerns regarding macrosomia or fetal wellbeing, the risks of IUFD need to be weighed against risks of respiratory distress syndrome due to a premature delivery. Cesarean delivery rates of up to 50–60% are reported in women with established diabetes. This is hardly surprising when almost half the babies born to diabetic mothers are over the 90th centile for gestational age.
- Intrapartum care should focus on meticulous diabetic control (maintaining serum glucose levels at 100–120 mg/L in labor by titrating the insulin infusion whilst maintaining a constant rate of 5% dextrose infusion), continuous EFM, and judicious use of oxytocin for poor progression of labor.
- Following delivery of the placenta, the infusion rate of insulin needs to be halved as maternal insulin requirements rapidly return to prepregnancy levels and, with breast-feeding, even less insulin is required.
- In women with GDM, a 75 g GTT is recommended at approximately 6 weeks postpartum.

Recommended further reading

1. Gabbe SG, Gregory RP, Power ML, Williams SB, Schulkin J (2004). Management of diabetes mellitus by obstetrician–gynecologists. *Obstet Gynecol* **103**, 1229–34.
2. American College of Obstetricians and Gynecologists (2005). ACOG Practice Bulletin No. 60. Pregestational diabetes mellitus. *Obstet Gynecol* **105**, 675–85.

Gestational diabetes

This group includes women with carbohydrate intolerance of variable severity diagnosed for the first time during pregnancy. By definition, it will include some women with previously undiagnosed pregestational diabetics. There is a strong variation in prevalence, with the highest incidence of gestational diabetes (GDM) in women from the Indian subcontinent followed by women from Southeast Asia.

Screening for gestational diabetes

There appears to be no consensus as to who, when, how, or even whether to screen for GDM. Universal biochemical screening has been suggested. Other institutions screen on the basis of clinical risk factors (see above). The timing of testing is also controversial, as the later in pregnancy it is performed, the higher the detection rate since glucose tolerance progressively deteriorates. On the other hand, the earlier in pregnancy GDM is diagnosed and hyperglycemia treated, the greater the likelihood of influencing outcome. The current recommendation is routine testing at 24–28 weeks.

Implications of GDM

GDM is associated with increased perinatal mortality and morbidity, but to a far lesser extent than pregestational diabetes. There is no increase in the risk of congenital abnormalities in women with GDM (since it develops after the embryonic period), and macrosomia is the main risk factor for adverse outcome. There is an increased risk of operative delivery as well as maternal risks including a higher incidence of preeclampsia, severe perineal injury (defined as a third or fourth degree perineal laceration), operative vaginal delivery, and cesarean delivery. The long-term implications of GDM provide a further justification for screening. Women identified as having GDM have a significantly increased risk of developing NIDDM in later life. This risk has variously been estimated at around 50% over the following 10–15 years. This awareness of the increased risk of developing NIDDM may enable individuals to alter their diet and lifestyle to prevent or delay the development of diabetes. It may also encourage vigilance by both the patient and her physician such that the diagnosis is made early and therefore before the development of microvascular complications.

Management

A combined diabetic–obstetric approach is essential.

- The initial approach is by dietary modification including calorie reduction in the obese patient.
- The need for insulin is heralded by persistent postprandial hyperglycemia (1 hour >140–150 mg/dL (>7.5–8.0 mmol/L)) or persistent fasting hyperglycemia (>100–105 mg/dL (>5.5–6.0 mmol/L)).
- Regular ultrasound scans to assess fetal growth and wellbeing are recommended, although the risks to the fetus are less than in pre-gestational diabetes and hence early delivery as routine should not be advised unless there are other complicating factors.

- Intrapartum management will depend on whether the patient has been on insulin antenatally and, if so, how much insulin she has been receiving.
  - Patients who are diet controlled or on relatively small doses may not require insulin in labor, while those on larger doses need to be treated as preexisting diabetics and therefore may need a sliding scale or even an insulin drip.
  - Following delivery, any insulin regimen can be discontinued as can postpartum monitoring of glucose levels.
- Patients with GDM should have a GTT at 6 weeks to assess the degree of glucose intolerance outside pregnancy.

Recommended further reading

1. Tuffnell DJ, West J, Walkinshaw SA (2003). Treatments for gestational diabetes and impaired glucose tolerance in pregnancy. *Cochrane Database Syst Rev* **3**, CD003395.

Drug use in pregnancy

Introduction

Approximately 35% of pregnant women take medication (excluding vitamins and iron) at least once in pregnancy, although only 6% do so in the first trimester. This does not include drugs used in labor. The proportion of women taking medication in pregnancy has dropped from around 80% in the 1960s, the reduction being driven by the continued attention in the news media to drug-induced fetal abnormalities. However, the increasing age at which women elect to have children means that more women are already on long-term medication for chronic conditions at the time they embark on pregnancy. Women suffering from certain medical conditions that were considered in the past to be incompatible with pregnancy (SLE, chronic renal disease, certain types of heart disease) now have the opportunity of motherhood because of dramatic improvements in medical care and pregnancy outcome.

Timing of exposure and pregnancy outcome

Medication taken in pregnancy can harm the unborn child through teratogenic effects. Teratogenesis is defined as dysgenesis of fetal organs in terms either of structural integrity or function. Teratogenic effects may take the form of malformations that occur during the period of organogenesis or, subsequently, by causing alterations in the structure or function of organ systems formed during organogenesis. Other manifestations of teratogens include growth restriction, fetal death, and carcinogenesis. In addition, some drugs such as retinoids, which are high-grade teratogens, may exert their effect for up to 2 years after the last dose.

The timing of exposure to a particular drug treatment is a critical factor in assessing the nature and extent of any potential adverse effects. Three important phases are recognized in human development:

1 *Pre-embryonic phase*. This extends from conception to 17 days post-conception (or 3 days after the first missed period). During this period of implantation and blastocyst formation, any adverse effect is an 'all or nothing phenomenon' and the result of an insult will be either death and abortion/resorption or intact survival through multiplication of the totipotent stem cells.

2 *Embryonic phase*. This period extends from post-conception day 18 to day 55 and is the most crucial period of organogenesis. It is the period of greatest theoretical sensitivity and risk of congenital malformation with rapidly differentiating tissues, so that any damage becomes irreparable. The earlier in this period the insult occurs, the more marked is the likely effect. The following lesions have been identified with time of exposure (approximate days postconception): anencephaly, day 24; limb reduction defects, days 12–40; transposition of the great vessels, day 34; cleft lip, day 36; ventricular septal defects, day 42; syndactyly, day 42; hypospadius, day 84.

3 *Fetal phase*. This phase runs from post-conception age 8 weeks through to term. The impact of drugs that can cross the placenta affects fetal growth and development rather than causing gross structural malformations.

Prescribing principles

When prescribing in pregnancy it is important to consider the following principles:

- Drugs should be prescribed only for clear indications and where the benefits (usually for the mother) outweigh the potential risks (usually to the fetus). Question the need for any drug in pregnancy.
- If possible, it is better to try and avoid all drugs (including nonprescription medications) in the first trimester.
- Medication should be used in the smallest effective dose for the shortest period of time.
- It is preferable to prescribe medications that have been widely used in pregnancy and have a good safety track record, rather than newer agents that may have theoretical though as yet unproved advantages.
- All women of reproductive age are at risk of pregnancy.
- Most drugs with a molecular weight of less than 1500 Da are capable of crossing the placenta and therefore of potentially affecting the fetus, but very few drugs have been conclusively shown to be teratogenic.
- Encourage preconception counseling in all patients with chronic medical disorders and, in particular, those on long-term drug therapy. If this has not been possible, review all drug regimens as early in pregnancy as possible, avoiding polypharmacy as far as possible.

Breast-feeding

The vast majority of drugs cross into breast milk. In general terms, the doses of drugs reaching the baby are clinically insignificant when one considers dilution of the drug in the mother and the small volumes of milk the neonate feeds on.

Drugs can be considered in three broad categories with respect to breast-feeding:

- Drugs that cannot be detected in the baby. Examples include the anticoagulant warfarin and the group of antibiotics known as aminoglycosides, which are not absorbed from the gastrointestinal tract of normal infants.
- Drugs that are detectable in the baby in clinically insignificant amounts, such as non-narcotic analgesics, NSAIDs, penicillins, cephalosporins, antihypertensive drugs, bronchodilators, and most anticonvulsants except barbiturates.
- Drugs that reach the neonate in sufficient amounts to cause side effects. Examples in this group include benzodiazepines reported to cause lethargy, barbiturates causing drowsiness, amiodarone with a theoretical risk of hypothyroidism, tetracyclines because of the potential risk of discoloration of teeth, combined oral contraceptive pills (OCPs) because of the risk of diminishing milk supply, ephedrine which is associated with irritability, cytotoxic drugs because of immune suppression/neutropenia, and aspirin with its risk of Reye's syndrome.

Management of pregnancy and potential teratogenesis

The risk of teratogenesis is present in two broad groups of patients. The first group comprises patients on long-term medication for a chronic condition. Ideally, they should be counseled prior to pregnancy and made aware of the risks of fetal malformation and how these risks could be reduced. Often, however, this has not been the case. The second group comprises those patients taking a single course of treatment and unaware of early pregnancy.

The management of exposure to potential teratogens in pregnancy relies on accurate determination of the history of exposure including the gestational age at exposure, as well as up-to-date information on the teratogenic potential of the agent in question at the particular gestation of exposure. Accurate dating of pregnancy is essential, and this can be performed by a combination of early dating scan and menstrual and conception history. Fetal malformations associated with exposure to a teratogen may affect the CNS, cardiovascular system, arms and legs, and orofacial region (clefting). Multiple organ systems may also be involved. The majority of major malformations are detectable on detailed ultrasound scanning at 18–20 weeks. Where cardiac abnormality is suspected, a repeat scan and fetal echocardiogram at around 22 weeks may be helpful. In cases where open NTDs are one of the manifestations of exposure to a particular teratogen, maternal serum α-fetoprotein (MSAFP) estimation at 15–20 weeks may also be of value. Further management will depend on the established risks from exposure to the given teratogen at a particular gestation time along with the wishes of the couple after comprehensive counseling, preferably by experts in the field.

Table 5.1 summarizes the teratogenic and fetal effects of common medications.

Recommended further reading

1. Rubin PC, Craig GS, Gavin K, Sumner D. (1986). Prospective survey of use of therapeutic drugs, alcohol and cigarettes during pregnancy. *Br Med J*, **292**, 81–3.
2. Moore KL (1988). *The Developing Human: Clinically Oriented Embryology*, (4th edn), p. 131. WB Saunders, Philadelphia, PA.
3. Rubin PC (1995). General principles. In: Rubin PC, ed. *Prescribing in pregnancy* (2nd edn) pp. 1–8. BMJ Publications, London.
4. Little BB (1999). Medication during pregnancy. In: James DK, Steer PJ, Weiner CP, Gonik B, eds. *High Risk Pregnancy—Management Options* (2nd edn), pp. 617–38. WB Saunders, London.
5. De Swiet M (2000). Anticoagulants. In: Rubin PC, ed. *Prescribing in Pregnancy* (3rd edn) pp. 47–64. BMJ Books, London.
6. Koren G, Pastuszak A, Ito S (1998). Drug therapy. Drugs in pregnancy. *N Eng J Med* **338** 1128–37.
7. Briggs GG, Freeman RK, Yaffe SJ (2002) *Drugs in Pregnancy and Lactation* (6th edn). Lippincott–Williams & Wilkins, Philadelphia PA.
8. Weiner CP, Buhimschi CS (2004) *Drugs for Pregnant and Lactating Women*. Churchill Livingstone, Philadelphia, PA.

Table 5.1 Drugs with proven teratogenic and fetal effects in humans

Category	Drug	Teratogenic effect
Antibiotics	Aminoglycosides Tetracycline Quinolones Sulfonamides	Deafness, vestibular damage Anomalies of teeth and bone Animal studies only—irreversible arthropathy Hyperbilirubinemia, kernicterus
Anticholinergics		Neonatal meconium ileus
Anticoagulants	Warfarin	Skeletal and CNS defects, Dandy–Walker syndrome
Anticonvulsants	Carbamazepine Phenytoin Valproic acid Paramethadione	NTDs Growth restriction, CNS defects NTDs CNS and facial abnormalities
Antidepressants	Lithium carbonate	Ebstein's anomaly, hypotonia, reduced suckling, hyporeflexia
Antihypertensives	ACE inhibitors	Prolonged renal failure in neonates, decreased skull ossification, renal tubular dysgenesis
	β-Blockers	Growth restriction, neonatal bradycardia, hypoglycemia
Antithyroid drugs	Propylthiouracil	Fetal and neonatal goiter and hypothyroidism
	Methimazole	Aplasia cutis, fetal and neonatal goiter, hypothyroidism
Cytotoxic drugs	Aminopterin, methotrexate	CNS and limb malformations
	Cyclophosphamide	CNS malformations, secondary cancer
Diuretics	Furosemide	Decreased uterine blood flow, hyperbilirubinemia
	Thiazides	Neonatal thrombocytopenia
Hypoglycemics		Neonatal hypoglycemia
NSAIDS	Indomethacin	Premature closure of ductus arteriosus, necrotizing enterocolitis, neonatal pulmonary hypertension
Prostaglandin analogs	Misoprostol	Moebius sequence, abortion, induction of labor
Recreational drugs	Ethanol	Fetal alcohol syndrome (pre- and postnatal growth restriction, CNS anomalies, characteristic facial features)
	Cocaine	Growth restriction, placental abruption, uterine rupture
Systemic retinoids	Isotretinoin, etretinate	CNS, craniofacial, cardiovascular, and other defects
Sex hormones	Danazol and other androgenic drugs	Masculinization of female fetuses
	Diethylstilbestrol	Vaginal carcinoma, genitourinary defects in male and female offspring
	Diethylstilbestrol	Masculinization of female fetuses
Sedatives	Thalidomide	Limb shortening and internal organ defects
Psychoactive drugs	Barbiturates, opioids, benzodiazepines	Neonatal withdrawal syndromes when drugs taken in late pregnancy
Phenothiazines		Neonatal effects of impaired thermoregulation, extrapyramidal effects

Chapter 6

Labor and delivery

Term premature rupture of membranes

Introduction

Premature rupture of the membranes (PROM) refers to the spontaneous rupture of membranes prior to the onset of labor and can occur at any gestational age. PROM complicates 8% of term pregnancies. The majority of women with term PROM (also known as prelabor rupture of membranes) will go into active labor spontaneously within the following 48 hours. Term PROM presents a number of potential complications and management dilemmas.

Diagnosis

Most patients with term PROM will present with a history of fluid loss vaginally. This may constitute a sudden gush of fluid or a continuous trickle remote from micturition. Although amniotic fluid may be seen on the patient's underwear or sanitary towel, urinary incontinence may confound the diagnosis. Hence a speculum examination should be performed to confirm the diagnosis of ruptured membranes, at which time amniotic fluid should be seen pooling in the upper vagina or trickling from the cervical os. Transiently raising intraabdominal pressure by asking the woman to cough or performing a Valsalva maneuver may help to demonstrate this if amniotic fluid is not immediately obvious.

The presence of other vaginal discharge may confuse the detection of amniotic fluid, and detection aids, such as nitrazine sticks (color changes from yellow to dark blue because of the alkaline pH of amniotic fluid as opposed to acidic vaginal secretions) and 'ferning' (crystallization of amniotic fluid on drying), have been advocated to clarify diagnosis, but may lead to overdiagnosis (e.g. contamination with blood, semen, etc.). Newer diagnostic tests based on the identification of amniotic fluid/fetal-specific proteins (such as fetal fibronectin [fFN] and placental α-microglobulin-1 (PAMG-1)) in cervicovaginal secretions are currently under investigation.

Management

Evaluation

Following speculum examination to confirm the diagnosis and exclude cord prolapse, any evidence of fetal or maternal compromise must be ruled out. A fetal cardiotocograph (CTG) should be commenced. Evidence of possible fetal hypoxia, such as meconium staining of the liquor or a suspicious or pathological CTG, should lead to expedition of delivery by induction of labor or cesarean delivery as deemed appropriate. Any clinical signs of chorioamnionitis indicated by fetal tachycardia, maternal tachycardia, maternal pyrexia, and/or uterine tenderness or irritability with or without a rising leukocyte count must be sought. Unstable lie of the fetus should be identified as it is associated with the risk of cord prolapse whilst the onset of contractions is awaited.

Conservative management

If none of the previous problems are identified, conservative management to allow the possibility of spontaneous onset of labor is a reasonable approach.

- A high vaginal swab can be taken at speculum examination and sent for culture. Prolonged rupture of membranes (defined as >18 hours) may be followed by pyrexia in labor or neonatal infection, and early identification of pathogens facilitates optimization of antibiotic therapy.
- If labor does not occur spontaneously, the timing of induction remains a matter for debate. The majority of institutions recommend induction of labor 24–36 hours after term PROM to allow time for the spontaneous onset of contractions and to reduce the risk of chorioamnionitis. Earlier induction of labor may be appropriate if the patient is known to be colonized with GBS.

Labor and delivery

The mode of induction of labor also varies, with either prostaglandins (vaginally, rectally, or orally) or synthetic oxytocin (pitocin). In the presence of ruptured membranes, there is no difference in the mean induction to delivery interval whether prostaglandin or pitocin is used. However, the protocols of most units differentiate between an unfavorable cervix, where the use of prostaglandins is favored, and a favorable cervix, when use of intravenous pitocin infusion is preferred.

Fetuses who have marked oligohydramnios secondary to PROM may demonstrate cord compression with corresponding CTG changes (variable decelerations) with uterine contractions. Amnioinfusion has been used in some centers to alleviate the effects of cord compression with variable success. The majority of studies suggest that amnioinfusion in this setting does not change the cesarean delivery rate or perinatal outcome.

Recommended further reading

1. Royal I, Parry S, Strauss JF (1998). Premature rupture of the fetal membranes. *N Eng J Med* **338**, 663–70.
2. Duff P (1998). Premature rupture of the membranes in term patients: induction of labour versus expectant management. *Clin Obstet Gynecol* **41**, 883–91.
3. Mozurkewich E (1999). Management of premature rupture of membranes at term: an evidence-based approach. *Clin Obstet Gynecol* **42**, 749–56.
4. Hannah ME, Hodnett ED, Willan A, Foster GA, Di Cecco R, Helewa M (2000). Prelabor rupture of the membranes at term: expectant management at home or in hospital? The Term PROM Study Group. *Obstet Gynecol*, **96**, 533–8.
5. Seaward PG, Hannah ME, Myhr TL, *et al.* (1998). International multicenter term PROM study: evaluation of predictors of neonatal infection in infants born to patients with premature rupture of membranes at term. Premature Rupture of the Membranes. *Am J Obstet Gynecol*, **179**, 635–9.
6. Dare M, Middleton P, Crowther C, Flenady V, Varatharaju B (2006). Planned early birth versus expectant management (waiting) for prelabour rupture of membranes at term (37 weeks or more). *Cochrane Database Syst Rev*, **1**, CD005302.

Prolonged pregnancy

Introduction

Prolonged pregnancy is a matter of concern to women and obstetricians because of its association with fetal morbidity and mortality. It remains the most common cause of induction of labor.

Prolonged pregnancy, also known as post-term pregnancy, refers to a pregnancy that has gone beyond 42 weeks 0 days (294 days) from the first day of the last menstrual period (LMP) in a woman with regular 28 day cycles (EDD + 2 weeks). The terms 'post-dates pregnancy' or 'postdatism' are poorly defined and therefore are best avoided.

Incidence

The incidence of prolonged pregnancy varies from 3% to 10% depending on population mix (low-risk versus high-risk pregnancies) and local practice patterns (such as the rate of routine induction of labor and management of women with a prior cesarean delivery). It will also vary depending on whether gestational age dating is based on history and clinical examination alone or whether an ultrasound scan was used to calculate the gestation in the first half of the pregnancy. Naegele's rule has traditionally been used to determine the EDD.

Dates cannot be relied upon in the following circumstances:

- About 10–30% of women give a doubtful date of their LMP.
- Irregular periods.
- Recent use of contraception, including combined oral contraceptive pills and injectable contraceptives.
- Conception during lactational amenorrhea.

Perinatal mortality is increased in those with unknown dates and every effort should be made to establish the EDD in early pregnancy. Ultrasound has changed our practice. Routine early pregnancy ultrasound reduces the incidence of post-term pregnancy by approximately 50%.

Fetal risks

Perinatal mortality and morbidity

It has long been recognized that prolonged pregnancy is associated with increased risks of perinatal mortality and morbidity. After exclusion of congenital malformations, intrapartum deaths were four times more common and early neonatal deaths were three times more common in infants born after 42 weeks of gestation. In addition, meconium staining of amniotic fluid and non-reassuring fetal testing (previously known as 'fetal distress') during labor were much more common in prolonged pregnancies. Meconium aspiration syndrome is caused by chronic *in utero* aspiration of meconium-stained amniotic fluid leading to a chemical pneumonitis, which may require assisted ventilation to treat the infant at birth. It is not believed to be caused by acute aspiration of meconium-stained amniotic fluid at birth, which explains why suctioning of the nasopharynx at delivery has not been shown to prevent this disorder. Meconium aspiration syndrome is almost exclusively a disease of post-term infants.

With the development and application of modern techniques of fetal monitoring, the perinatal risk in prolonged pregnancy has been reduced but is still significantly elevated over women delivering spontaneously at term.

Ultrasound is now used routinely for dating pregnancy in many units, and the prevalence of prolonged pregnancy in a well-dated population is small.

Fetal postmaturity syndrome

Postmaturity syndrome is the term used to describe post-term infants exhibiting physical signs of intrauterine malnutrition. They constitute only a small proportion of babies born after 42 weeks. It is now known that a baby born with such features can present at an earlier gestational period. Therefore the term 'prolonged pregnancy' should be reserved for post-maturity for pregnancies beyond 42 weeks.

The following features characterize this syndrome:

- Absence of vernix caseosa.
- Absence of lanugo hair.
- Abundant scalp hair.
- Long fingernails.
- Dry cracked desquamated skin.
- Body length increased in relation to body weight.
- Alert and apprehensive facies.
- Meconium staining of skin and mucous membranes.

Other risks

The incidence of birth injury is higher in post-term pregnancies and is related to the higher incidence of macrosomia (defined as an antepartum estimated fetal weight, not birthweight, ≥4500 g) compared with that in term infants. Macrosomic infants are susceptible to birth injuries such as skull and long-bone fractures, cephalohematomas, and neurologic injuries (including facial nerve and brachial plexus palsies).

Other neonatal complications such as hypothermia, hypoglycemia, and polycythemia are mainly due to the presence of associated growth restriction. Birth after 42 weeks is also an independent risk factor for cerebral palsy and sudden infant death syndrome (SIDS).

Maternal risks

- Maternal anxiety increases once the estimated delivery date is passed.
- Maternal risks in prolonged pregnancy include increased cesarean delivery, operative vaginal delivery, severe perineal injury (defined as third- or fourth-degree perineal lacerations), postpartum hemorrhage, puerperal infection, and psychological morbidity.

Management of prolonged pregnancy

The first step in the management of prolonged pregnancy is to confirm the dates and to assess the presence of any risk factors. Debate exists between the active approach of routine elective induction of labor at 41 weeks and the conservative approach of awaiting spontaneous onset of labor with appropriate fetal surveillance. The available evidence is reviewed here.

Confirmation of dates

Evidence should be sought from the antenatal records to confirm gestational age dating. Clinical methods are not always accurate. Ultrasound examination in the first or early second trimester is likely to give an accurate estimation of the dates within an error margin of 1 and 2 weeks, respectively. Ultrasound dating of pregnancy in the late second or third trimester of pregnancy is less reliable, with an error of approximately 3 weeks.

Assessment of risk factors

There is a small but significant risk of increased perinatal mortality when pregnancy is prolonged beyond 42 weeks. Therefore it is important to assess any risk factors complicating the pregnancy. Pregnancies with risk factors for adverse pregnancy outcome (such as pregestational diabetes, preeclampsia, recurrent antepartum hemorrhage, and IUGR) should probably be delivered at 39–40 weeks' gestation and should not be allowed to progress post-term.

Counseling for induction of labor or conservative approach

Women's preference is often given as reason for conservative management. Many women will see elective induction of labor as interference with a natural process. Therefore appropriate facilities should exist for fetal surveillance if the conservative approach of waiting for spontaneous onset of labor is decided. In reality, few women choose to wait beyond 42 weeks.

Elective induction versus conservative approach

In a low-risk uncomplicated pregnancy, controversy still exists between induction of labor by 42 weeks and conservative approach of waiting for spontaneous onset of labor.

- Present evidence favors a policy of routine induction of labor by 41–42 weeks because of reduced perinatal mortality, decreased meconium staining of amniotic fluid, and a small decrease in cesarean delivery rates compared with conservative management.
- Proponents of a conservative approach argue that a conservative policy of waiting until spontaneous onset of labor is safe provided that appropriate fetal surveillance is performed. However, what constitutes an appropriate method of fetal surveillance beyond 42 weeks is not clearly established. Moreover, routine fetal surveillance beyond 40 weeks has not been shown to definitely improve perinatal outcome. The next section details the tests used for fetal surveillance in pregnancies that go beyond 42 weeks.

Recommended further reading

1. American College of Obstetricians and Gynecologists (2004). Management of postterm pregnancy. ACOG Practice Bulletin No. 55. *Obstet Gynecol* **104**, 639–46.
2. Rand L, Robinson JN, Economy KE, Norwitz ER (2000). Post-term induction of labor revisited. *Obstet Gynecol* **96**, 779–83.
3. Smith GC (2001). Life-table analysis of the risk of perinatal death at term and post term in singleton pregnancies. *Am J Obstet Gynecol* **184**, 489–96.
4. Alexander JM, McIntire DD, Leveno KJ (2000). Forty weeks and beyond: pregnancy outcomes by week of gestation. *Obstet Gynecol* **96**, 291–4.
5. Treger M, Hallak M, Silberstein T, Friger M, Katz M, Mazor M (2002). Post-term pregnancy: should induction of labor be considered before 42 weeks? *J Matern Fetal Neonatal Med* **11**, 50–3.
6. Hannah ME, Hannah WJ, Hellmann J, Hewson S, Milner R, Willan A (1992). Induction of labor as compared with serial antenatal monitoring in post-term pregnancy. A randomized controlled trial. The Canadian Multicenter Post-Term Pregnancy Trial Group. *N Engl J Med* **326**, 1587–92.
7. Crowley P (2000). Interventions for preventing or improving the outcome of delivery at or beyond term. *Cochrane Database Syst Rev* **2**, CD000170.
8. Anonymous (1994). A clinical trial of induction of labor versus expectant management in post-term pregnancy. The National Institute of Child Health and Human Development Network of Maternal–Fetal Medicine Units. *Am J Obstet Gynecol* **170**, 716–23.
9. Shime J, Librach CL, Gare DJ, Cook CJ (1986). The influence of prolonged pregnancy on infant development at one and two years of age: a prospective controlled study. *Am J Obstet Gynecol* **154**, 341–5.

Fetal surveillance

Fetal movement chart

Fetal activity in the form of fetal movements has been found to be a useful indicator of fetal health. Although inexpensive, its value in monitoring prolonged pregnancy has not been validated. Based on current data, the fetal movement chart alone cannot be relied upon for monitoring fetal health in prolonged pregnancy.

Cardiotocography (nonstress test)

A recording of the fetal heart rate (FHR) for a period of 20–40 minutes, called the nonstress test, has become one of the most popular methods of antenatal fetal surveillance. Definitions of normal, suspicious and abnormal FHR patterns have been described by the International Federation of Gynecologists and Obstetricians (FIGO) and ACOG. The fetal acoustic stimulation (FAS) test where a vibroacoustic stimulus is used to elicit accelerations of FHR during a nonstress test is a useful way of reducing the number of nonreactive traces and shortening the testing time. Compromise to the fetus in prolonged pregnancy is generally due to oligohydramnios (reduced amniotic fluid volume). If the trace is not reactive despite stimulating the fetus or if it shows significant decelerations, it indicates possible compromise and should be an indication for delivery.

Assessment of amniotic fluid volume

Fetal urine contributes significantly to the volume of amniotic fluid. With diminished placental function, selective perfusion of the brain and heart and reduced perfusion of other systems, including the kidneys, take place. This leads to reduction of fetal urine formation and thus the sequelae of oligohydramnios in severe IUGR. Thus, in prolonged pregnancy, assessing the amniotic fluid volume can help to monitor fetal compromise that is due to gradual decline in placental function. Evaluation by palpation may be deceptive, and impression of the adequacy on ultrasonographic examination is more reliable. Amniotic fluid index (AFI) is used for the assessment of amniotic fluid volume in these pregnancies. In prolonged pregnancy, an AFI of 5 cm or less is suggestive of reduced placental function. An alternative and equally accepted definition is a maximal vertical pocket (MVP) of amniotic fluid of less than 2 cm.

Other methods

More complex fetal monitoring incorporating a formal biophysical profile (BPP) has been suggested for monitoring prolonged pregnancy. This test involves sonographic evaluation of amniotic fluid volume, fetal movement, fetal tone, and fetal breathing movements. Indeed, the BPP was first developed to evaluate fetal wellbeing in the setting of post-term pregnancy, although it has since been validated for use in term and preterm pregnancies. The role of Doppler ultrasound has been evaluated in high-risk pregnancy, e.g. IUGR or severe preeclampsia, but its role in prolonged pregnancy has not been properly evaluated.

Conclusions

Prolonged pregnancy remains a matter of concern for obstetric care providers and women. The absolute risk of fetal demise is small (approximately 1 in 650 post-term pregnancies). With the use of routine ultrasound examination, the incidence of prolonged pregnancy has decreased. Current evidence supports elective induction of labor by 42 weeks of gestation because of reduced perinatal mortality, decreased meconium staining of amniotic fluid, and a small but significant decrease in the cesarean delivery rate compared with conservative management. Nevertheless, some women may see induction as an unnecessary intervention in a natural process of childbirth and may opt for conservative management. Fetal surveillance is necessary when a conservative approach is adopted beyond 42 weeks. Surveillance should probably include twice-weekly assessment of fetal wellbeing (nonstress test) with assessment of amniotic fluid volume at least once weekly.

Recommended further reading

1. American College of Obstetricians and Gynecologists (2004). Management of postterm pregnancy. ACOG Practice Bulletin No. 55. *Obstet Gynecol* **104**, 639–46.
2. Smith GC (2001). Life-table analysis of the risk of perinatal death at term and post term in singleton pregnancies. *Am J Obstet Gynecol* **184**, 489–96.
3. Shime J, Librach CL, Gare DJ, Cook CJ (1986). The influence of prolonged pregnancy on infant development at one and two years of age: a prospective controlled study. *Am J Obstet Gynecol* **154**, 341–5.

Induction of labor

Induction of labor is the artificial initiation of uterine contractions prior to their spontaneous onset in an attempt to achieve progressive effacement and dilatation of the cervix and delivery of the baby. The term is usually restricted to pregnancies at gestations greater than the limit of fetal viability (currently regarded as 24 weeks).

The aim of successful induction is to achieve vaginal delivery when continuation of pregnancy presents a threat to the life or wellbeing of the mother or her unborn child. The infant should be delivered in good condition within an acceptable time-frame and with a minimum of maternal discomfort or side effects. In current obstetric practice, induction is usually performed for obstetrical or medical indications. Social induction comprises a small proportion of the total inductions, and is not generally recommended.

Indications for induction of labor

The most common indication is prolonged pregnancy. There is good evidence that induction of labor should be offered routinely to all women whose pregnancies continue beyond 42 weeks' gestation. Induction during this period is associated with beneficial outcome in terms of reduced cesarean delivery rate, reduced operative vaginal delivery rate, reduced chance of nonreassuring fetal testing ('fetal distress'), meconium staining of the amniotic fluid, and macrosomia (defined as an estimated fetal weight ≥4500 g), and reduced risk of fetal and neonatal death.

While in a few circumstances the advantages of elective delivery by induction are clear, e.g. to prevent maternal morbidity in fulminating preeclampsia, the advantages are less clear when it is done for fetal macrosomia. Indeed, routine induction of labor for macrosomia has not been shown to reduce cesarean delivery rate or improve perinatal outcome. Maternal indications for induction are few, as the pregnant mother is directly accessible for examination and investigation. The majority of inductions are done for fetal indications and are mainly based on epidemiological evidence. The tests available for fetal wellbeing also influence the induction rates.

Attention should be paid to women's views on induction, especially when the indications for induction are not strong. Many women believe that induced labor, not being natural, is more painful than spontaneous labor and that in induced labor they are not in control of what is happening to them during childbirth. Such negative attitudes may partly reflect inadequate provision of information regarding induction. Some of the common indications for induction are:

- gestational or insulin-dependent diabetes
- preeclampsia
- chronic hypertension
- renal disease.

Recommended further reading

1. Bishop EH (1964). Pelvic scoring for elective induction. *Obstet Gynecol* **24**, 266–8.
2. Keirse MJNC, Chalmers I (1989). Methods for inducing labour. In: Chalmers I, Enkin M, Keirse MJNC, eds. *Effective Care in Pregnancy and Childbirth*. Oxford: Oxford University Press.
3. Kelly AJ, Kavanagh J, Thomas J (2003). Vaginal prostaglandin (PGE2 and PGF2a) for induction of labour at term. *Cochrane Database Syst Rev* **4**, CD003101.
4. Hofmeyr GJ, Gulmezoglu AM (2003). Vaginal misoprostol for cervical ripening and induction of labour. *Cochrane Database Syst Rev* **1**, CD000941.

Factors influencing the outcome of induced labor

- Favorability or 'ripeness' of the cervix.
- Parity.
- The method chosen for induction.

Failed induction is diagnosed when, in the absence of nonreassuring fetal testing ('fetal distress'), acute events such as abruption or cord prolapse, or failure to progress due to cephalopelvic disproportion or malposition, a woman who was induced did not deliver vaginally because she did not enter the active phase of labor despite adequate uterine contractions for at least 12 hours.

The success of induction depends largely on the state of the cervix at the beginning of induction. The parity and the method of induction, the process of cervical softening, and eventually dilatation (cervical ripening) is part of a continuum that culminates in labor. Bishop's score, or a modified version of it, is used to assess the favorability of the cervix. The characteristics of the cervix and the station of the head are considered. The modified scoring system used most commonly is given in Table 6.1.

Table 6.1 A scoring system used to assess the favorability of the cervix and the station of the head for labor

	Score		
	0	**1**	**2**
Position of cervix	Posterior	Axial	Anterior
Length of cervix	2 cm	1 cm	<0.5 cm
Dilatation of cervix	0 cm	1 cm	>2 cm
Consistency of cervix	Firm	Soft	Soft and stretchable
Station of presenting part	–2	–1	0

Recommended further reading

1. Bishop EH (1964). Pelvic scoring for elective induction. *Obstet and Gynecol* **24**, 266–8.

Methods of cervical priming

The process of functional transformation of the cervix from a sphincteric organ acting to preserve and contain the growing fetus within the uterus to a canal that softens, shortens, and dilates to facilitate the passage of the fetus starts well before the actual labor itself. During this transformation process, a method used for cervical priming might act as a method to induce labor.

Pharmacological methods

- *Prostaglandins.* If induction is necessary, 'ripening' of the cervix with prostaglandins is useful. There are advantages to the use of prostaglandins (PGs) for ripening the cervix and induction of labor compared with oxytocin alone, including decreased need for analgesia in labor, fewer cases undelivered within 12–24 hours of painful contractions, and decreased operative delivery. This is at the expense of increased gastrointestinal side effects and uterine hypertonus, which occurs in up to 7% of cases. Intravaginal PGE_2 (either gel or tablets) may be marginally superior to intracervical PGE_2 gel with higher successful induction rates and decreased need for oxytocin.
- *Misoprostol* (a PGE_1 analogue) is much cheaper and more easily stored than other prostaglandins. Recent studies have shown it to be as safe and effective as other PGs, and it is now commonly used throughout the world. A dosage regimen of 25 μg administered vaginally, rectally, or orally every 4–6 hours appears to be almost as effective as 50 μg every 4–6 hours with reduced side effects (especially fewer cases of uterine hyperstimulation).
- *Oxytocin.* Regular uterine contractions achieved with IV infusions of oxytocin would result in cervical ripening in most cases. Control studies have shown it to be a less satisfactory method than local prostaglandin application.
- *Other topical pharmacological agents* that have been tried but are not in regular use are *estradiol* (150–300 mg) in tylose gel, *purified porcine ovarian relaxin* (1–4 mg) in a gel applied vaginally or intracervically, and *mifepristone* (an antiprogestin) in a dose of 200 mg orally for 48 hours before the formal induction.

Mechanical methods of cervical ripening

- *Hygroscopic tents,* such as natural laminaria tents (seaweed) or synthetic sponges impregnated with magnesium sulfate (Lamicel), need to be inserted into the cervical os 4–12 hours before labor.
- *Foley's catheter* in the cervix with the balloon inflated with 30 mL of saline. This approach can be used with oxytocin infusion.

Since it appears that mechanical agents bring about cervical ripening through a local release of tissue prostaglandins in the cervix or the lower uterine segment, there seems little rationale for their use where topical prostaglandins are available.

Conclusion

In summary, intravaginal PGs (either PGE_2 or PGE_1) are currently the best agents to use for cervical ripening prior to induction of labor.

Recommended further reading

1. Hofmeyr GJ, Gulmezoglu AM (2003). Vaginal misoprostol for cervical ripening and induction of labour. *Cochrane Database Syst Rev* **1**, CD000941.

Methods of induction of labor

A wide variety of mechanical and chemical methods have been used for labor induction namely:

- amniotomy.
- uterotonic agents (oxytocin or one of the prostaglandins).
- sweeping or stripping of the membranes (rarely used as a formal method of induction).

Amniotomy

Amniotomy or artificial rupture of the membranes is one of the most irrevocable interventions in pregnancy and, more than any other procedure, calls for a firm commitment to delivery. A combination of mechanical induction by amniotomy followed by oxytocin, if necessary, is often used. If oxytocin infusion is commenced at the time of amniotomy rather than delayed, there are advantages of a significantly shorter induction–delivery interval, reduced operative delivery rates, and a reduction in postpartum hemorrhage. Conversely, up to 88% of women with a favorable cervix will go into labor within 24 hours after amniotomy alone.

Oxytocin

Since the introduction of oxytocin as an IV infusion in the 1940s, it has come to be the most widely used method of labor induction. The oxytocin infusion should be given via an infusion pump, and fluid load minimized. Most infusion regimens commence at low rates (1–4 mU/min) and increased by 1–2 mU/min titrated against contractions, arithmetically or logarithmically, at intervals of 20–30 minutes up to a maximum of approximately 20–30 mU/min. Most studies suggest that low-dose 30-minute titration protocols are as effective as high-dose 20-minute titration protocols with reduced uterine hypertonus, decreased maximum and total dose of oxytocin, and decreased rate of cesarean deliveries for FHR abnormalities. Moreover, there appears to be no adverse effect on induction–delivery intervals.

Prostaglandins for induction of labor

Both $PGF_{2\alpha}$ and PGE (PGE_2 and PGE_1) have been used for cervical priming as well as for labor induction depending on the cervical score and the dosage. The most widely adopted mode of administration of prostaglandins has become the vaginal route. When the cervical score is good, a single vaginal application of prostaglandin can induce labor and avoid the necessity for formal oxytocin–amniotomy induction in nulliparas and multiparas with a concomitant reduction in cesarean delivery rates. For women with a good cervical score, amniotomy and oxytocin infusion could be the preferred method as it is less expensive and allows better control of uterine contractions than vaginal prostaglandins. For nulliparous women with a poor cervical score, vaginal prostaglandins are preferable. This could be followed by amniotomy when the cervix is favorable and oxytocin infusion if uterine contractions are inadequate or if there is poor progress of labor.

Intrauterine fetal death

Prostaglandins PGE_2 and $PGF_{2\alpha}$ and their various analogs have been used via different routes for induction of labor in the presence of intrauterine death. Intraamniotic instillation is best avoided because of the risk of sepsis and erratic absorption through devitalized membranes.

Previous cesarean delivery, breech presentation, and multiple pregnancy

Although the above conditions are considered as relative contraindications to induction of labor, labor can be induced in such cases under compelling circumstances and only after careful selection and counseling.

- For women with a previous lower segment cesarean scar, induction of labor with rupture of the membranes and oxytocin infusion can be carried out when the cervix is favorable and the pelvis appears clinically adequate. Use of PG has been associated with greater incidence of uterine rupture (25 in 1000) compared with those in spontaneous labor (5 in 1000) or those receiving oxytocin infusion (8 in 1000). Therefore cervical ripening is not recommended in such women.
- In twin pregnancy when the first twin is in cephalic presentation and cervical score is favorable, induction of labor by amniotomy and oxytocin infusion is usually effective. A PG pessary or gel can be used for cervical priming in the presence of an unfavorable cervix. Fortunately, with twin pregnancies, an unfavorable cervical score is rare at term.
- Current evidence favors elective cesarean delivery for breech presentation. If the woman insists on vaginal breech delivery, where chances of achieving vaginal delivery are reasonable, labor may be induced by amniotomy and oxytocin infusion, especially in cases of extended breech with the presenting part well settled in the pelvis. Because of the significant risk of cord prolapse with membrane rupture in those with incomplete breech presentations, it is best to opt for a cesarean delivery in this setting. Such a management plan should only be undertaken by an experienced provider and after careful counseling about the risks of vaginal breech delivery, including head entrapment, long-term neurologic injury, and fetal or neonatal death.

In these special circumstances (previous cesarean delivery, twins, breech presentation), the rate of progress of labor, especially in the active phase, should be monitored closely and early recourse to cesarean delivery should be taken when the progress is slow.

Stabilizing induction

In patients with a transverse or oblique lie with no apparent cause, especially in multipara, stabilizing the fetal lie and induction of labor at 39–40 weeks may be a valid option of management. External cephalic version should allow the head to be in the lower segment. Artificial rupture of membranes, after excluding cord presentation, and use of oxytocin to initiate uterine contractions should stabilize the presentation. The accoucheur should hold the head in position till no shift is felt in between a few uterine contractions. Abdominal binders to stabilize the fetal lie are rarely effective and may adversely effect uteroplacental perfusion by compressing the uterus against the inferior vena cava. Therefore they are not usually recommended.

Induction of labor in special circumstances

Risks and complications of induction of labor

Induction of labor is a potentially hazardous obstetric intervention. There are three broad groups of risks associated with induction of labor:

1. Risks associated with termination of pregnancy artificially before the spontaneous onset of labor.
2. Risks associated with artificial stimulation of uterine contraction.
3. Risks attributable to the specific method of labor induction.

Risks can be summarized as follows:

- Failed induction leading to cesarean delivery.
- Inadvertent preterm delivery is a risk with any induction.
- Uterine hyperstimulation could lead to fetal hypoxia, neurologic injury, and death.
- In grandmultipara and patients with a previous cesarean delivery, uterine hyperstimulation could lead to uterine rupture.
- Postpartum hemorrhage due to uterine atony occurs more commonly following induced labor than with spontaneous labor and may be related to the length of labor, which is usually longer with induction. It occurs less commonly following prostaglandin induction than following oxytocin induction.
- Low amniotomy may cause prolapse of the cord, especially with a high and poorly applied presenting part, and possible introduction of pathogenic organisms.
- Use of oxytocin, if excessive, may result in neonatal jaundice.
- Prolonged infusion of relatively high doses of oxytocin in dilute solutions can lead to maternal water intoxication, hyponatremia, coma, and even death. Similar disturbances in neonatal biochemistry, leading to seizures, could also occur in severe cases.
- Prostaglandins may produce gastrointestinal tract side effects. This is greater with $PGE_{2\alpha}$ and occurs less commonly with endocervical and extraamniotic administration than with oral, intravenous, or vaginal use.
- PGE_2 and PGE_1 may cause pyrexia because of their direct effect on thermoregulatory centers in the brain.

The spontaneous onset of labor is a robust and effective mechanism and should be given the chance to operate. We should only induce labor when we are sure that we can do better.

Recommended further reading

1. Bishop EH (1964). Pelvic scoring for elective induction. *Obstet Gynecol* **24**, 266–8.
2. Keirse MJNC, Chalmers I (1989). Methods for inducing labour. In: Chalmers I, Enkin M, Keirse MJNC, eds. *Effective Care in Pregnancy and Childbirth*. Oxford University Press, Oxford.
3. Kelly AJ, Kavanagh J, Thomas J (2003). Vaginal prostaglandin (PGE_2 and $PGF_{2\alpha}$) for induction of labour at term. *Cochrane Database Syst Rev* **4**, CD003101.
4. Hofmeyr GJ, Gulmezoglu AM (2003). Vaginal misoprostol for cervical ripening and induction of labour. *Cochrane Database Syst Rev* **1**, CD000941.
5. Boulvain M, Kelly A, Lohse C, Stan C, Irion O (2001). Mechanical methods for induction of labour. *Cochrane Database Syst Rev* **4**, CD001233.

Labor

Introduction

Labor is the process whereby the products of conception are delivered from the uterus after the 20th week of gestation. Although it is difficult to time the onset of labor, it can be defined as that point at which uterine contractions become regular and cervical effacement and dilatation begin. For scientific studies, the observed lengths of the various stages of labor following admission to hospital are considered. Labor is characterized by:

- The spontaneous onset of uterine contractions which increase in frequency, duration, and strength with the progress of time.
- The time taken for cervical effacement (shortening of the cervix) and dilatation which is slow until 3–4 cm (latent phase) followed by a rate of cervical dilatation of 1 cm/hour (active phase) until full dilatation of the cervix (10 cm) is the *first stage of labor.*
- The process of labor is usually accompanied by rupture of membranes with leakage of amniotic fluid, which should normally be clear.
- Once the cervix is fully dilated, the *second stage* is diagnosed. Descent of the presenting part through the birth canal is more during this stage. If the woman has an epidural *in situ,* then it is often common practice to wait for a further hour (passive second stage) to allow descent of the head before commencing pushing in time with contraction.
- Birth of the baby is expected after approximately 1 hour of bearing-down efforts in a primigravid woman, while a considerably shorter second stage is anticipated in a multiparous woman.
- The *third stage* is from delivery of the baby to delivery of the placenta and membranes, and is usually about 10 minutes.
- The normal blood loss associated with placental separation is less than 500 mL. Blood loss more than this amount is termed a postpartum hemorrhage (PPH).

The mechanism of labor

The head usually engages in the transverse position and the passage of the head and trunk follows a well-defined pattern through the pelvis (Fig. 6.1). Not all the diameters of the fetal head can pass through a normal pelvis. Therefore the process of labor involves the adaptation of the fetal head to the various segments of the pelvis.

The normal process of movement of the head in labor for a normal vertex presentation involves the following sequence (also know as the cardinal movements of labor):

1. *Descent* with increased flexion as the head enters the cavity. The sagittal suture lies in the transverse diameter of the pelvic inlet (brim).
2. *Internal rotation* occurs at the level of the ischial spines because of the grooved gutter of the levator ani muscles. Flexion produces a small diameter of presentation, changing to the suboccipito-bragmatic diameter from the occipito-frontal diameter.
3. Distension of the perineum with crowning is followed by extension of the head as it comes out of the vulva.
4. *Restitution.* The head rotates back for the occiput to be in line with the spine.

5. *External rotation.* The shoulders rotate when they reach the levators until the bisacromial diameter is anteroposterior. Accordingly, the head externally rotates by the same amount.
6. Delivery of the posterior shoulder occurs by lateral flexion of the trunk anteriorly.
7. Delivery of the anterior shoulder occurs by lateral flexion of the trunk posteriorly.
8. Delivery of the buttocks and legs follows the delivery of body.

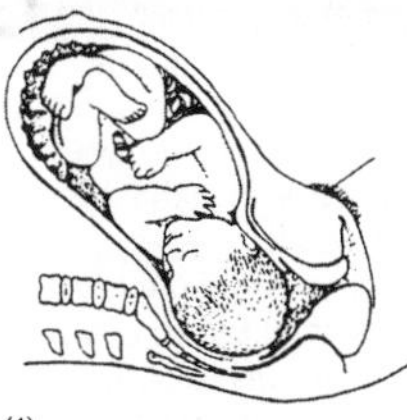

(1)
1st stage of labor. The cervix dilates. After full dilatation the head flexes further and descends further into the pelvis.

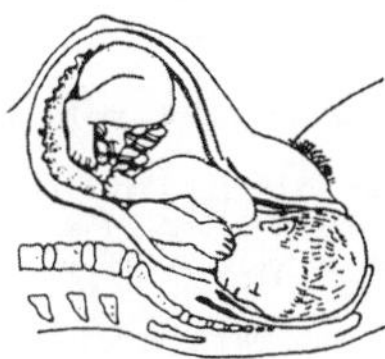

(2)
During the early second stage the head rotates at the level of the ischial spine so the occiput lies in the anterior part of pelvis.
In late second stage the head broaches the vulval ring (crowning) and the perineum stretches over the head.

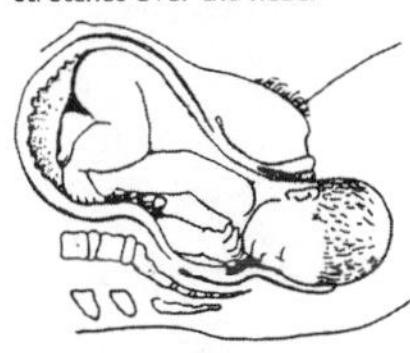

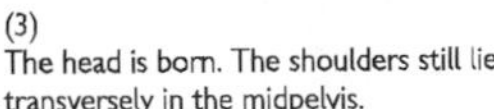

(3)
The head is born. The shoulders still lie transversely in the midpelvis.

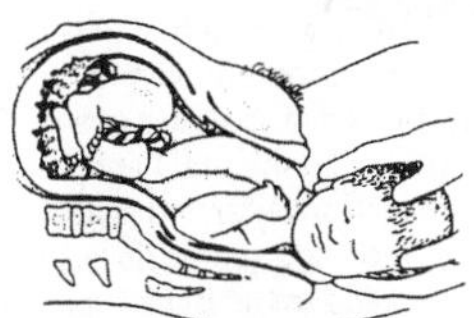

(4)
Birth of the anterior shoulder. The shoulders rotate to lie in the anteroposterior diameter of the pelvic outlet. The head rotates externally, restitute, to its direction at onset of labor. Downward and backward traction of the head by the birth attendant aids delivery of the anterior shoulder.

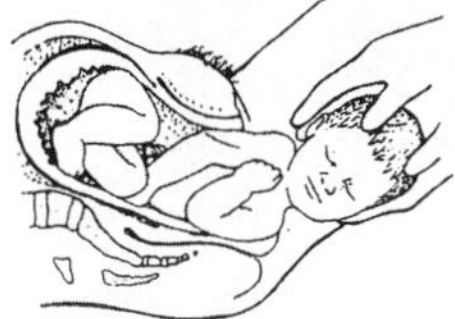

(5)
Birth of the posterior shoulder is aided by lifting the head upwards whilst maintaining traction.

Fig. 6.1 Mechanism of labor and delivery. (Reproduced from Collier J, Longmore M, Brown TD (eds). *Oxford Handbook of Clinical Specialties* (5th edn), p. 83, © 1999, by permission of the publisher Oxford University Press.)

The first stage of labor

Braxton–Hicks contractions are non-painful contractions (15 mmHg pressure) of the uterus which occur from 30 weeks' gestation and are more common after 36 weeks. Contractions in labor are painful, and contraction pressure, as well as the frequency and duration, gradually increases.

The minimum acceptable rate for cervical dilatation is 1 cm/hour. The active first stage usually takes up to 8–12 hours in a primipara and 6–8 hours in a multipara.

- During the first stage maternal pulse, blood pressure (BP), and temperature are checked every 30 minutes.
- The contractions are assessed every 30 minutes to record the frequency (every 10 minutes) and duration in seconds.
- Vaginal examination is carried out every 4 hours to assess the rate of cervical dilatation and the position and station of the head (measured in centimeters above the ischial spines). Note is also made of the degree of the caput and molding and the state of the amniotic fluid.
- The fetal heart rate (FHR) is monitored by auscultation every 30 minutes in nullipara (15 minutes in multipara) if it is not being continuously monitored electronically. The FHR before, during, and immediately after a contraction is noted.

Recommended further reading

1. American College of Obstetricians and Gynecologists (2005). ACOG Practice Bulletin No. 62. Intrapartum fetal heart rate monitoring. *Obstet Gynecol* **105**, 1161–9.
2. Norwitz ER, Robinson JN, Challis JRG (1999). The control of labor. *N Engl J Med* **341**, 660–6.
3. Norwitz ER, Robinson JN, Repke JT (2001). Labor and delivery. In: Gabbe SG, Niebyl JR, Simpson JL, eds. *Obstetrics: Normal and Problem Pregnancies*, (4th edn), pp. 353–94. WB Saunders, New York.
4. Thacker SB, Stroup D, Chang M (2001). Continuous electronic heart rate monitoring for fetal assessment during labor. *Cochrane Database Syst Rev* **2**, CD000063.
5. East CE, Chan FY, Colditz PB (2004). Fetal pulse oximetry for fetal assessment in labour. *Cochrane Database Syst Rev* **4**, CD004075.
6. Neilson JP (2003). Fetal electrocardiogram (ECG) for fetal monitoring during labour. *Cochrane Database Syst Rev* **2**, CD000116.

Failure to progress in the first stage

Delay in the first stage of labor is identified when progress in the 'active phase' falls to the right of the action line drawn parallel and 1–2 hours to the right of the alert line drawn at a rate of 1 cm/hour from the admission cervical dilatation (Fig. 6.2). If the labor is slow from the early active phase, it is termed primary dysfunctional labor. If the rate of progress is slow after initial adequate progress, it is termed secondary arrest of labor. In some cases, the labor may be prolonged in the latent phase. The causes of poor progress in the first stage are inefficient uterine activity (power), malposition or malpresentation, cephalopelvic disproportion (passenger), inadequate pelvis (passage), or a combination of the three. Rare causes include pelvic tumors or a contacted pelvis.

Management relies on careful assessment and appropriate corrective action.

- Assessment begins with a review of the history and patient records, abdominal palpation for lie, presentation, and engagement (as fifths of head palpable above the brim), estimated fetal size, and frequency and duration of contractions.
- The fetal condition needs to be assessed by reviewing the FHR recording or cardiotocograph (CTG) and the color and quantity of amniotic fluid if membranes are ruptured. Maternal hydration and analgesia should be reviewed.
- A vaginal assessment should identify the presentation and, if vertex, the amount of caput and molding and the position. The station of the leading bony skull and the degree of flexion should be noted along with the assessment of the bony pelvic adequacy.

In grandmultiparous women (parity of 5 or more) and in women with a uterine scar, an experienced obstetrician should review the case prior to commencement of oxytocin.

- The management options are cesarean delivery if there is obvious cephalopelvic disproportion (CPD) or non-reassuring fetal testing ('fetal distress').
- If uterine activity is inadequate with no contraindications for augmentation, oxytocin infusion can be administered and titrated to achieve optimal contractions (four in 10 minutes, each lasting >40 seconds). Follow-up assessment should be performed in 2 hours to confirm that adequate progress is being made after the contractions were augmented.

Recommended further reading

1. Norwitz ER, Robinson JN, Repke JT. Labor and delivery. In: Gabbe SG, Niebyl JR, Simpson JL, eds. *Obstetrics: Normal and Problem Pregnancies* (4th edn), pp. 353–94. WB Saunders, New York.

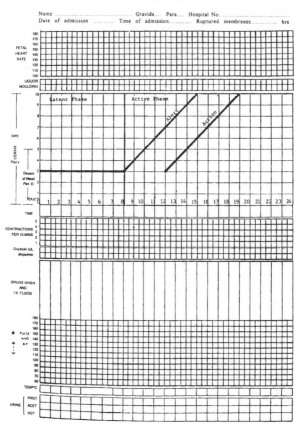

PARTOGRAPH

Name .... Gravida.... Para.... Hospital No. ....
Date of admission .... Time of admission............ Ruptured membranes.............. hrs

FETAL HEART RATE: 180, 170, 160, 150, 140, 130, 120, 110, 100

LIQUOR
MOULDING

CERVIX (cm) Plot x: 10, 9, 8, 7, 6, 5, 4, 3, 2, 1, 0

Desent of Mead Plot O

Latent Phase

Active Phase

Alert

Action

Hours: 0, 1, 2, 3, 4, 5, 6, 7, 8, 9, 10, 11, 12, 13, 14, 15, 16, 17, 18, 19, 20, 21, 22, 23, 24

TIME

CONTRACTIONS PER 10 MINS: 5, 4, 3, 2, 1

Oxytocin U/L drops/min

DRUGS GIVEN AND I.V. FLUIDS

PULSE AND BP: 180, 170, 160, 150, 140, 130, 120, 110, 100, 90, 80, 70, 60

TEMP°C

URINE: PROT, ACET, VOT

Fig. 6.2 Partogram.

The second and third stages of labor

The second stage

The second stage is the time from complete cervical dilatation until the baby is born. During this time, the mother has a desire to bear down when the cervix is fully dilated. She uses her abdominal muscles with the Valsalva maneuver to deliver the baby.

- With the attendant scrubbed, gowned, and gloved, the mother is placed in either the supine (with the head of the bed tilted upwards), left lateral, or lithotomy position. Some women prefer to deliver in the squatting position.
- As the head is pushed down with each contraction, it distends the perineum and the anus. The anus is covered with a pad and the descent of the occiput controlled with the left hand, the head being kept well flexed until crowned when it is allowed to extend. In this way, perineal distension is minimized and a precipitous delivery is prevented.
- Once the head is delivered, the eyes and nasal pharynx are cleaned.
- If the perineum appears to be tearing extensively, an episiotomy can be performed. Adequate analgesia is required, either epidural analgesia or by infiltrating the perineum with a local anesthetic.
- With the next contraction, the head is gently pulled towards the perineum until the anterior shoulder is delivered under the subpubic arch.
- Gentle traction downwards and anteriorly helps to deliver the posterior shoulder and the remainder of the trunk.

The normal time for second stage is 60 minutes in a nullipara and 30 minutes in a multipara.

In the management of the second stage of labor, if the woman has an epidural *in situ* and the FHR pattern is normal, 1 hour may be allowed for the presenting part to descend with uterine contractions before starting to push. During this hour, it is important to ensure that good contractions are present and, if there are any concerns regarding the FHR, delivery could be expedited.

- In a nulliparous woman if, after 2 hours of effective expulsive efforts, delivery is not imminent and there has been no significant progress, the situation needs to be reassessed with a view to an assisted instrumental (operative) vaginal delivery.
- In a multiparous woman, delivery is generally expected within 60 minutes of effective expulsive efforts, and failure to achieve this should raise suspicions of malposition, malpresentation, or disproportion.

Cutting the cord between clamps after pulsations stop allows m... blood to the baby. Holding the baby below the introitus and delaying clamping for 30 seconds results in higher hematocrit levels, but this is of unclear clinical benefit. The condition of the baby is assessed at 1 and 5 minutes using the Apgar scoring system, and the baby is handed to the mother.

The third stage

The third stage is the duration from delivery of the baby to delivery of the placenta and fetal membranes.

- The mother is turned on to her back if she is not already in the supine position. A dish is placed under the cord and at the introitus to collect any blood loss. The left hand is placed on the abdomen over the uterine fundus.
- Routine use of oxytocin (5–10 IU IM) or Syntometrine (ergometrine maleate 0.5 mg IM + oxytocin 5 IU IM) after delivery of the anterior shoulder of the baby in some institutions has decreased third-stage time (to about 5 minutes), and has also decreased the incidence of PPH. One should be sure to exclude multiple pregnancy with such practice.
- As the uterus contracts to a 20 week size after the baby is born, the placenta separates from the uterus through the spongy layer of the decidua basalis.
- At this point, the uterus will be felt to become firmer and more globular, the cord will appear to lengthen, and there will be a trickle of fresh blood. These are the three signs of placental separation.
- Controlled cord traction is applied with the right hand whilst supporting the fundus with the left hand to prevent uterine inversion (Brandt–Andrew's technique).

Assisted delivery of the placenta is usually completed within 5 minutes of delivery. The placenta and membranes are checked for missing cotyledons and to see if the membranes are complete. The estimated blood loss is recorded.

Most complications of the third stage, such as PPH, uterine inversion, or vulval or perineal hematoma, occur in the first 2 hours after delivery. Usually the women are kept in the delivery unit for these 2 hours to observe their pulse, BP, temperature, uterine size and contractions, fresh vaginal bleeding, or painful swelling of the vulva or perineum. Effort is also taken to support the mother in breast-feeding the baby, to clean and weigh the baby, and to clean the mother and offer her some refreshments. If there were no complications during the 2 hours, she can be transferred to the postnatal ward. Relaxation of the uterus may lead to postpartum hemorrhage. In situations where the uterus is overstretched (as in multiple pregnancy, big babies, or polyhydramnios) or in prolonged labor or placenta previa, an oxytocin infusion, e.g. 20–40 units in 500 mL of saline, can be set up as an IV infusion over 3–4 hours to manage this complication.

Fetal surveillance in labor

Introduction

Labor has been defined as the most dangerous journey made by anyone, and, therefore the fetus needs all the help it can get to complete this journey successfully. Each fetus enters labor with different resources and reserves and hence a different capacity to withstand the stresses of labor. It is estimated that only 10% of cerebral palsy (CP) is due to intrapartum ischemic hypoxic events, the rest being attributed to antenatal events. However, given the relatively short duration of labor compared with the antenatal period, the 'risk per unit time' is greatest in labor. The blood supply to the placental pool is restricted with each contraction and this is further aggravated by voluntary bearing-down efforts in the second stage. Therefore a fetus that was coping well in the antenatal period but has little extra reserve capacity may decompensate in labor. Thus intrapartum surveillance should begin with a review of antenatal risk factors which affect the reserves and hence the capacity with which each fetus enters labor.

Electronic fetal monitoring (EFM)

When EFM was introduced, it was expected to reduce perinatal morbidity and CP dramatically. However, it has resulted in increased intervention and operative delivery rates without a significant reduction in the rate of CP. The reason for this is that CTG is very sensitive but not specific in detecting fetal hypoxia. Additional tests such as fetal scalp blood sampling in labor are required to improve the specificity. Interest is also growing in the use of fetal electrocardiographic ST waveform analysis and pulse oximetry as adjuncts to improve the positive predictive value of CTG, although both these techniques should be regarded as investigational at this time.

The options for intrapartum surveillance are intermittent auscultation or continuous EFM. It is recommended that, on admission in labor, an admission assessment is made to identify fetal or maternal risk factors which will help determine which is the better option for fetal monitoring for that pregnancy.

- *Maternal risk factors* include previous cesarean delivery, preeclampsia, post-term pregnancy, prolonged rupture of membranes, induced labor, diabetes, antepartum hemorrhage, and other maternal medical conditions.
- *Fetal risk factors* include IUGR, prematurity, oligohydramnios, abnormal Doppler velocimetry, multiple pregnancy, meconium-stained amniotic fluid, and breech presentation.
- Although low risk on admission, *intrapartum risk factors* may develop, such as the need for oxytocin augmentation, epidural analgesia, intrapartum vaginal bleeding, fever, and fresh meconium staining of the amniotic fluid or abnormal FHR on intermittent auscultation. If none of the above apply, the woman may be suitable for intermittent auscultation. This should be performed for a full minute before, during, and after a contraction at least every 15 minutes in the first stage (30 minutes in a nullipara) and every 5 minutes or after every other contraction in the second stage.

Recommended further reading

1. American College of Obstetricians and Gynecologists (2005). ACOG Practice Bulletin No. 62. Intrapartum fetal heart rate monitoring. *Obstet Gynecol* **105**, 1161–9.
2. Norwitz ER, Robinson JN, Repke JT (2004). Labor and delivery. In: Gabbe SG, Niebyl JR, Simpson JL, editors. *Obstetrics: Normal and Problem Pregnancies* (4th edn), pp. 353–94. WB Saunders, New York.
3. Thacker SB, Stroup D, Chang M (2001). Continuous electronic heart rate monitoring for fetal assessment during labor. *Cochrane Database Syst Rev* **2**, CD000063.
4. East CE, Chan FY, Colditz PB (2004). Fetal pulse oximetry for fetal assessment in labour. *Cochrane Database Syst Rev* **4**, CD004075.
5. Neilson JP (2003). Fetal electrocardiogram (ECG) for fetal monitoring during labour. *Cochrane Database Syst Rev* **2**, CD000116.

Definitions of terms used in EFM

- *Baseline rate* is the mean level of the FHR when accelerations and decelerations have been excluded. Normal baseline, FHR is 110–160 beats/min.
- A *bradycardia* is a baseline FHR of less than 110 beats/min (100–110 beats/min is termed moderate baseline bradycardia and, provided that other parameters are normal, may be normal). A baseline below 100 beats/min should raise the possibility of hypoxia or other pathology (beware of the maternal heart rate being recorded as the FHR).
- A *tachycardia* is a baseline FHR of more than 160 beats/min. A baseline of 160–180 beats/min is termed moderate baseline tachycardia and, provided that other features are normal, is not regarded as indicative of hypoxia.
- An *acceleration* is a transient rise in FHR by at least 15 beats over the baseline lasting for a total of 15 seconds or more (Fig. 6.3). A prolonged acceleration lasts more than 2 minutes but less than 10 minutes. An acceleration lasting longer than 10 minutes is a change in baseline.
- A *deceleration* refers to any transient reduction in the baseline FHR. A prolonged deceleration is one lasting longer than 2 minutes but less than 10 minutes. A deceleration lasting longer than 10 minutes is a change in baseline.
    - Decelerations can be uniform in appearance and timing, not drop below 30 beats/min below the baseline, synchronous with contractions, and form a 'mirror-image' of the contraction. These are known as *early decelerations* and are associated with head compression (Fig. 6.4).
    - Decelerations can be uniform in appearance, not drop below 30 beats/min below the baseline, but start after the contraction has started, nadir after the peak of the contraction, and resolve after the contractions has dissipated. These are known as *late decelerations* and are likely associated with uteroplacental insufficiency (Fig. 6.5). They are late in timing because they result from a fetal chemoreceptor rather than baroreceptor response, although both are mediated through the parasympathetic nervous system (vagus nerve).
    - However, the majority of decelerations are variable in their appearance and timing. They generally have a rapid (steep) deceleration phase lasting less than 30 seconds and a rapid recovery phase lasting less than 30 seconds. These are known as *variable decelerations*, and are typically associated with cord compression (Fig. 6.6). Features of concern include variable decelerations lasting longer than 60 seconds with a loss of more than 60 beats from the baseline, slow recovery to baseline, a combined variable and a late deceleration component, and a rising baseline rate.
    - Repetitive decelerations refers to decelerations occurring with more than 50% of contractions.

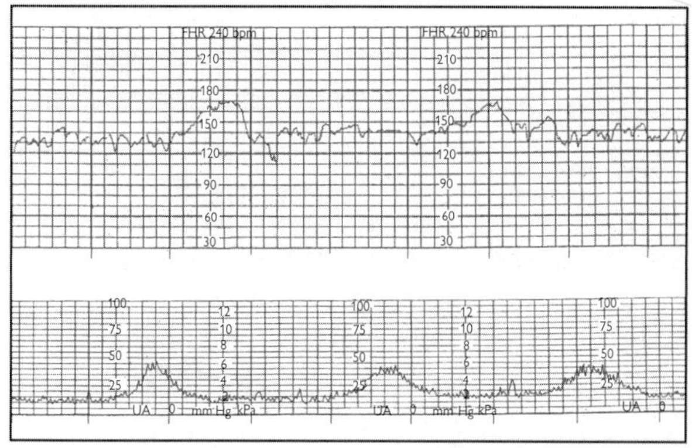

Fig. 6.3 A CTG trace showing normal baseline rate accelerations and moderate baseline variability.

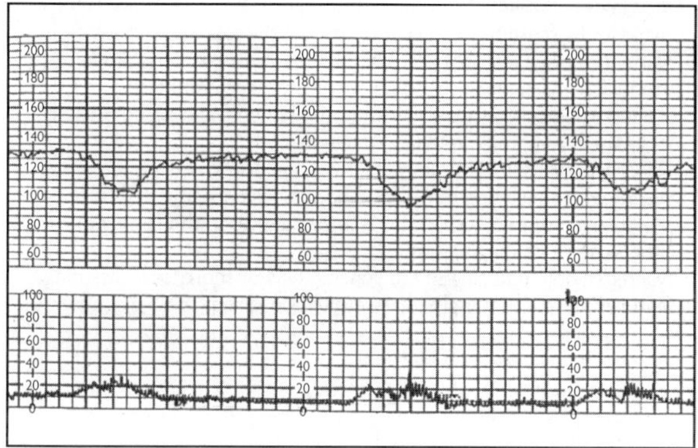

Fig. 6.4 CTG with early decelerations.

- *Baseline variability* is the degree to which the baseline varies, i.e. the bandwidth of the baseline after exclusion of accelerations and decelerations. A variability of 0 beats/min is defined as 'absent', 0–5 beats/min as 'minimal', 6–25 beats/min as 'moderate', and >25 beats/min as 'marked'.

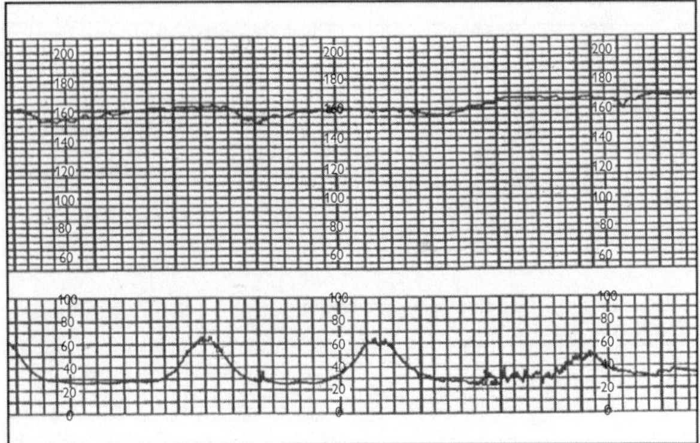

Fig. 6.5 CTG with late decelerations.

The CTG is classified as reactive (normal), nonreactive (suspicious), or nonreassuring (pathological) on the basis of the following criteria:

- *Normal* All four features are reassuring: normal baseline, moderate variability, accelerations, and no significant decelerations. For a CTG tracing to be called 'reactive,' all these elements should be present including two accelerations in 20 minutes.
- *Nonreactive (suspicious)* No more than one nonreassuring feature is resent when analysing the CTG. This term is typically used to denote the absence of two accelerations in 20 minutes in the setting of an otherwise reassuring tracing.
- *Nonreassuring (pathological)* In general, two or more nonreassuring features are present. Immediate evaluation is required.

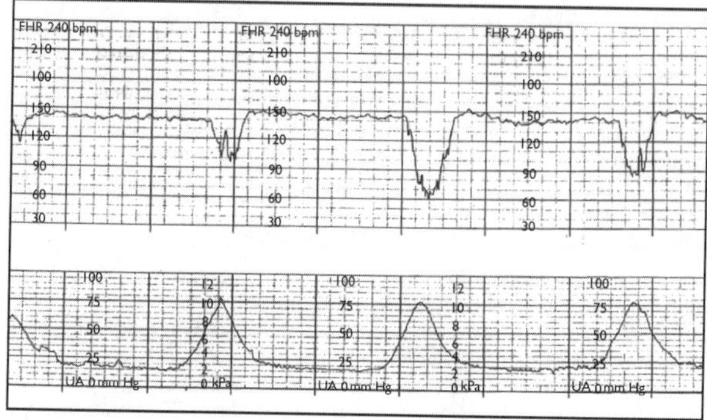

Fig. 6.6 CTG with variable decelerations.

Reassuring, nonreassuring, and abnormal features include the following:

- *Reassuring features* Baseline rate of 110–160 beats/min, baseline variability >5 beats/min, no decelerations, and two accelerations per 20 minutes. (The absence of accelerations in an otherwise normal CTG is of uncertain significance.)
- *Nonreassuring features* Baseline 100–109 or 161–180 beats/min, variability <5 beats/min, or uncomplicated variable deceleration.
- *Abnormal features* Baseline rate of <100 beats/min or >180 beats/min, sinusoidal pattern for more than 10 minutes (suggestive of fetal anemia), baseline variability of <5 beats/min for more than 30 minutes, repetitive atypical variable or late decelerations, and a prolonged deceleration.

Recommended further reading

1. American College of Obstetricians and Gynecologists (2005). ACOG Practice Bulletin No. 62. Intrapartum fetal heart rate monitoring. *Obstet Gynecol* **105**, 1161–9.
2. Thacker SB, Stroup D, Chang M (2001). Continuous electronic heart rate monitoring for fetal assessment during labor. *Cochrane Database Syst Rev* **2**, CD000063.
3. East CE, Chan FY, Colditz PB (2004). Fetal pulse oximetry for fetal assessment in labour. *Cochrane Database Syst Rev* **4**, CD004075.
4. Neilson JP (2003). Fetal electrocardiogram (ECG) for fetal monitoring during labour. *Cochrane Database Syst Rev* **2**, CD000116.

Action with nonreassuring CTGs

Where abnormal or nonreassuring features are encountered on the CTG, it is important to search for and correct any causes such as uterine hyperstimulation, hypotension, maternal dehydration/fever, infection, and the need for pain relief. Routine action should include turning the patient onto her side, discontinuing any oxytocin infusion, immediate oxygen supplementation 10 L/min by face mask, and administering IV fluids, if indicated.

If no remediable cause is found, it is important to gain reassurance about fetal wellbeing before proceeding with the labor. Biophysical profile (BPP) has no proven benefit in labor. An acceleration on CTG with fetal scalp stimulation is predictive of a cord pH >7.20 and is reassuring. In some situations a fetal scalp blood sample may be appropriate to determine fetal acid–base status. A scalp blood pH <7.20 should prompt immediate delivery, usually by cesarean; a pH of 7.20–7.25 gives short-term reassurance, but should lead to a repeat of fetal blood sampling in 20–30 minutes to determine the trend in relation to progress of labor; a pH >7.25 is reassuring and should only be repeated with persistent CTG abnormality.

The assessment of CTGs should always be done in the context of the clinical picture. A normal baseline rate does not exclude hypoxia, and the change in baseline may indicate gradually developing hypoxia. Good baseline variability is an indicator of adequate oxygenation of the autonomic system and, in conjunction with a reactive CTG, is an indicator of good fetal health. A CTG trace with no accelerations, baseline variability <5 beats/min, and shallow deceleration (even <15 beats/min) may indicate the possibility of longstanding hypoxia. With repetitive prolonged decelerations lasting >2 minutes and reaching <80 beats/min, the fetus may become hypoxic within a short period of time (<60 min). Hypoxia may develop rapidly when the FHR remains <80 beats/min for >10 min (prolonged bradycardia). A rising baseline with loss of variability and/or slow recovery of prolonged decelerations indicates the need for scalp blood pH or delivery and, in the active second stage, may be an indication for operative vaginal delivery if spontaneous delivery is not imminent. If the CTG is abnormal without decelerations in labor, the possibility of infection, drugs, cerebral hemorrhage, and congenital/chromosomal malformation should be considered.

It is important to remember always that the true monitors of fetal wellbeing are the attending obstetricians and midwives, and that the EFM equipment is merely a recording device.

Recommended further reading

1. American College of Obstetricians and Gynecologists (2005). ACOG Practice Bulletin No. 62. Intrapartum fetal heart rate monitoring. *Obstet Gynecol* **105**,1161–9.
2. Thacker SB, Stroup D, Chang M (2001). Continuous electronic heart rate monitoring for fetal assessment during labor. *Cochrane Database Syst Rev* **2**, CD000063.
3. East CE, Chan FY, Colditz PB (2004). Fetal pulse oximetry for fetal assessment in labour. *Cochrane Database Syst Rev* **4**, CD004075.
4. Neilson JP (2003). Fetal electrocardiogram (ECG) for fetal monitoring during labour. *Cochrane Database Syst Rev* **2**, CD000116.

Meconium-stained amniotic fluid

There are two principal reasons why meconium is passed. One is a function of fetal maturity, but it may also indicate possible fetal compromise. The incidence of meconium staining of the amniotic fluid increases from 36 to 42 weeks, reaching around 20% at 42 weeks. Thus it can be a marker of maturation of the CNS and the gastrointestinal system. However, passage of meconium in the preterm fetus is rare and should raise the possibility of intrauterine infection.

Traditionally, three grades of meconium are described.

- Grade 1 meconium (light) is diluted by a large volume of amniotic fluid that is lightly stained by meconium.
- Grade 2 (moderate) meconium is a reasonable amount of amniotic fluid with a heavy suspension of meconium.
- Grade 3 (thick) meconium suggests the presence of meconium in small amounts of amniotic fluid and the meconium may be particulate.
  - If no amniotic fluid is obtained at artificial rupture of membranes, one should consider this as being in the same risk category as thick meconium and the fetal condition should be observed closely.

The significance of meconium varies with presentation. Thus, where there is a breech presentation in the late first or second stage, the passage of meconium is likely to be due to mechanical causes and therefore less sinister than in a cephalic presentation.

The presence of scanty fluid with thick meconium is suggestive of oligohydramnios and, if there are added CTG abnormalities in early labor, delivery by cesarean may be preferable. Some studies have suggested that amnioinfusion of warm sterile saline into the uterus may dilute the meconium, relieve the spasm of the umbilical vessels, and improve the FHR tracing resulting in fewer cesarean deliveries and an improvement in perinatal outcome; however, more recent large clinical trails have shown no benefit to amnioinfusion.

Meconium aspiration syndrome (MAS) has an incidence of 1 in 1000 live births. It is seen most commonly in infants born post-term. Meconium can be aspirated *in utero* or after birth. Although fetuses do not normally draw amniotic fluid into the airway, they gasp when asphyxiated. Therefore the coexistence of asphyxia and acidosis may precipitate meconium aspiration. Asphyxia also causes added damage to the lungs and may further complicate the management of MAS. Meconium creates a ball valve effect in the airways because of its chemical irritant properties. Aggressive tracheal toilet at delivery has been proposed to protect against MAS, but large clinical trials have shown no benefit. This is likely because the weight of evidence in the literature suggests that MAS is the result of chronic *in utero* aspiration and not aspiration at delivery. Interventions that may be effective in decreasing the incidence of MAS would include avoidance of intrauterine hypoxia/acidosis (which may make the fetus pass meconium and gasp) and delivery at an earlier gestational age.

Recommended further reading

1. Hofmeyr GJ (2002). Amnioinfusion for meconium-stained liquor in labour. *Cochrane Database Syst Rev* **1**, CD000014.

Pain relief in labor

Undoubtedly labor is a painful process and adequate provision of analgesia is important. The request for analgesia in childbirth varies in different cultures and is also influenced by the previous obstetric experience of the woman, the course of labor, and its anticipated duration. Professionals are expected to provide expert advice about analgesia, but the final decision rests with the woman. Most importantly, there is no medical reason to withhold analgesia in labor. Maternal request is sufficient reason to administer pain relief.

Nonpharmacological means

Relaxation techniques including lying in warm water and breathing exercises do not relieve pain as such, but may help the woman cope with or manage her pain better. Homeopathy, acupuncture, and hypnosis, although used occasionally, have not been demonstrated conclusively to alter objective assessments of pain or the need for conventional analgesia.

Transcutaneous electrical nerve stimulation (TENS) works on the principle of blocking pain fibers in the posterior ganglia by stimulation of the small afferent fibers. Low-intensity continuous stimulation is applied to the dermatomes associated with pain. It is a safe form of analgesia and is often found useful in the very early stages of labor. It may postpone the need for stronger analgesia, but will not often be adequate throughout the course of labor.

Pharmacological means

Nitrous oxide (Entonox)

This is self-administered premixed inhaled nitrous oxide and oxygen in a 1:1 ratio. It has a quick onset of action and is short-lasting. The main side effects are transient lightheadedness and nausea. Appropriate use of Entonox can be highly effective and is safe for mother and baby.

Narcotic agents

- Pethidine is a synthetic analgesic and antispasmodic and is very useful in labor. It can cause nausea in 20% of women and therefore it is best co-administered with an antiemetic. It is used in doses of 50–150 mg IM or 50–100 mg IV. If given within 2 hours of delivery it is important to be aware of the possibility of neonatal respiratory depression.
- Morphine is an alkaloid of opium and is a stronger analgesic without antispasmodic properties. It is used in IM doses of 10 mg and is also associated with side effects of nausea and vomiting. Hence it is co-administered with an antiemetic. There is a risk of neonatal respiratory depression with a delivery within 2 hours of the previous dose.
- Diamorphine is a very powerful opiate and particularly useful for the anxious mother with a prolonged labor. It is used in doses of 5–10 mg IM and may cause neonatal respiratory depression for 3–4 hours after the last dose.

The main advantages of IM narcotic analgesia are the ease of administration and reasonably rapid action with a relatively low incidence of side effects. The main disadvantages, in addition to nausea and vomiting, are that they may be inadequate in terms of analgesia for up to 40% of women, and may cause confusion and inability to cooperate and delay in gastric emptying.

Pudendal nerve block/local anesthesia

A pudendal nerve block involves blocking the pudendal nerve with 10 mL xylocaine 0.5–1% as it exits Alcock's canal about 1–2 cm medial and below the ischial spine. It is usually performed transvaginally but can be performed through the perineum. This form of anesthesia is sufficient for outlet forceps and vacuum deliveries, and for repair of episiotomies and vaginal lacerations. Local infiltration of the vulva, vagina, labia, and perineum are useful for cutting episiotomies and prior to repair of perineal lacerations and episiotomies.

Regional anesthesia

This is a form of analgesia that relies on blocking nerve roots at their point of outflow to prevent reception and transmission of painful impulses.

- *Epidural block.* An epidural cannula is inserted into the peridural fat at the L2–3, L3–4, or L4–5 interspace and, after confirming that no blood or cerebrospinal fluid (CSF) can be aspirated, bupivicaine 1% or marcain 0.25–0.5% is administered after an initial test dose.
  - Epidural anesthesia can be administered as intermittent top-up boluses every 2–3 hours as required or as a continuous infusion, and it aims to block the nerve root T11–S4.
  - Contraindications to the use of epidural analgesia are the lack of experienced personnel to site and monitor the epidural, infection at the injection site or systemic sepsis, coagulation defects or bleeding diathesis, anticoagulation, shock and hypovolemia, bony abnormalities of the spinal column, and idiosyncratic reactions to local anesthetics.
  - In addition to pain relief in labor, operative deliveries can be performed under epidural anesthesia.
- *Spinal block.* A fine-gauge spinal needle is inserted into the subarachnoid space and a small volume of 'heavy' local anesthetic ± opiate is administered at the level of L3–4 after which the spinal needle is withdrawn. The main use of spinal anesthesia in obstetrics is for operative deliveries and repairs of extensive genital tract trauma (i.e. third- or fourth-degree tears or extensive vaginal lacerations). It can also be used for cesarean delivery, but only gives 1–2 hours of surgical anesthesia.
- *Caudal block.* This is a form of localized epidural through the sacral hiatus and gives good anesthesia for operative deliveries, but is effective in only 80% of cases.

The complications of regional anesthesia are discussed on 📖 *p.330.*

Recommended further reading

1. Norwitz ER, Robinson JN, Challis JRG (1999). The control of labor. *N Engl J Med* **341**, 60–6.
2. Norwitz ER, Robinson JN, Repke JT (2001). Labor and delivery. In: Gabbe SG, Niebyl JR, Simpson JL, eds. *Obstetrics: Normal and Problem Pregnancies* (4th edn), pp. 353–394. WB Saunders, New York.
3. American College of Obstetricians and Gynecologists. Committee Opinion No. 279. (2002). Prevention of early-onset group B streptococcal disease in newborns. *Obstet Gynecol* **100**, 1405–12.

Episiotomy and tears

An episiotomy is a surgical incision of the perineum to increase the diameter of the vulval outlet during childbirth. Episiotomy is cut at the judgment/discretion of the attending professional, and should only be done with the woman's consent. The popularity of episiotomy has waned over the years from a high of 90% in primigravidas in the 1970s to the WHO's recommendation for an episiotomy rate of only 10% in normal deliveries.

Indications for an episiotomy

- Where perineal tearing appears inevitable.
- In association with forceps delivery, at the discretion of the obstetric care provider.
- To expedite a spontaneous delivery where there are concerns about fetal wellbeing in the second stage of labor.
- Failure to progress late in the second stage due to perineal rigidity.
- During a breech delivery.
- Previous perineal reconstructive surgery.
- Previous pelvic floor surgery.
- To avoid severe perineal laceration in women with inflammatory bowel disease, especially Crohn's disease.

Types of episiotomy

- *Midline episiotomy* is a vertical cut from the fourchette towards the anus. It is used more commonly in the USA. The principal problem associated with midline episiotomies is the high incidence of associated third- and fourth-degree tears—hence its unpopularity in the UK. Midline episiotomies are associated with less bleeding, better healing, and possibly less pain in the puerperium and are easier to repair, but this must be set against the higher incidence of third- and fourth-degree perineal lacerations.
- *Mediolateral episiotomy* starts in the midline in the fourchette and is directed laterally to avoid the anal sphincter. It is used more commonly in the UK.

An episiotomy should be performed at the correct time. Too early an incision increases blood loss. Adequate analgesia should be used—regional block topped up or local infiltration. Sharp straight scissors should be used to make a single cut rather than repeated small extensions that would invariably result in a zigzag incision. Repair should be performed as soon as possible after delivery.

Side effects of episiotomies/perineal lacerations

- *Pain.* This can be reduced by prompt, careful, and expert repair.
- *Bleeding.* This can be kept to a minimum by timely episiotomy and early repair. If a large vessel is bleeding, this can be tied off or artery forceps applied to it while waiting to commence repair.
- *Breakdown* is often a consequence of infection, bad technique, or inappropriate suture material. Management depends on the merits of the case.
- *Dyspareunia.*

Perineal lacerations

- First-degree tears involve the skin only.
- Second-degree tears involve perineal muscles (most episiotomies fall into this group).
- A third-degree tear is a perineal tear leading to partial or complete disruption of the anal sphincter.
- The fourth-degree tear is the same as the third-degree tear with involvement of the anal epithelium.

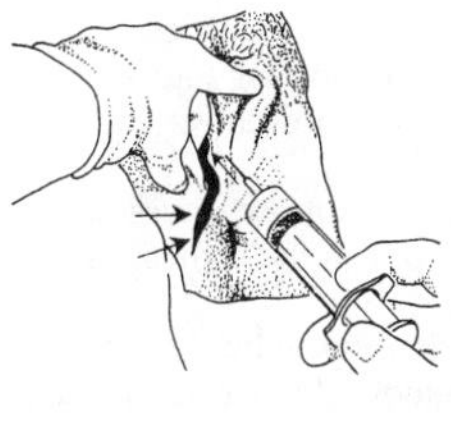

(1)
Swab the vulva towards the perineum. Infiltrate with 1% lignocaine → (*arrows*).

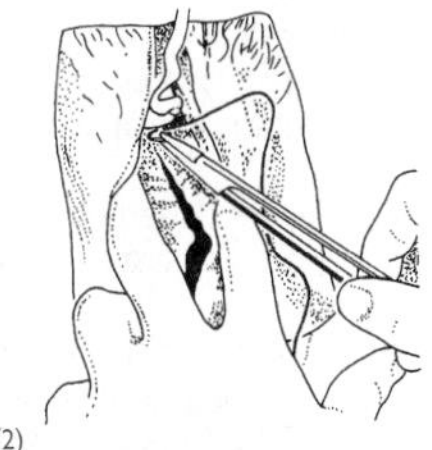

(2)
Place tampon with attached tape in upper vagina. Insert 1st suture above apex of vaginal cut (not too deep as underlying rectal mucosa nearby).

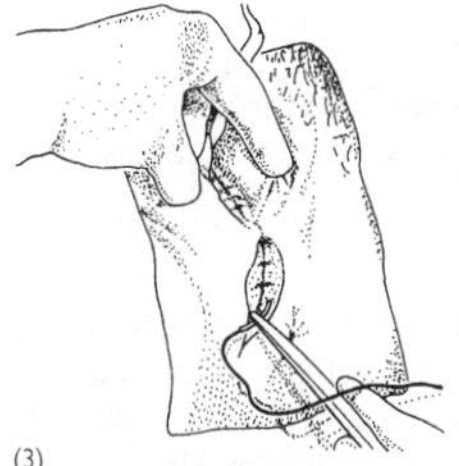

(3)
Bring together vaginal edges with continuous stitches placed 1 cm apart. Knot at introitus under the skin. Appose divided levator animuscles with 2 or 3 interrupted sutures.

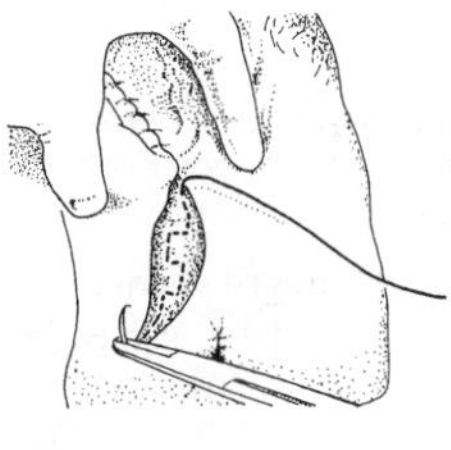

(4)
Close perineal skin (subcuticular continuous stitch is shown here).

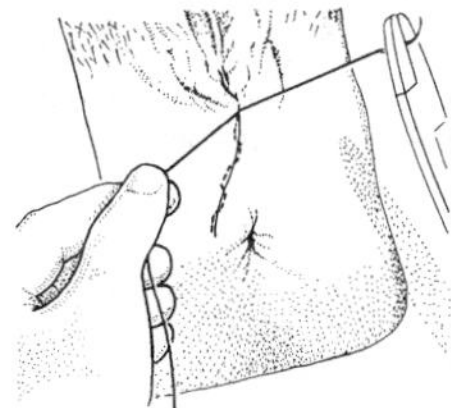

(5)
When stitching is finished, remove tampon and examine vagina (to check for retained swabs). Do a rectal examination to check that apical sutures have not penetrated the rectum.

Fig. 6.7 Steps in repairing an episiotomy. (Reproduced from Collier J, Longmore M, Brown TD (eds) *Oxford Handbook of Clinical Specialties* (5th edn), p. 147, © 1999, by permission of the publisher Oxford University Press.)

Principles of perineal repair (Fig 6.7)

- Adequate exposure and lighting.
- Adequate analgesia.
- Identification and securing the apex. Failure to do so at onset of repair will result in continuous bleeding or the development of a paravaginal hematoma.
- Absorbable synthetic suture material.
- Good anatomical approximation.
- Deep perineal tissues can be sutured with interrupted stitches.
- The vaginal wall is approximated with continuous locking sutures to achieve better hemostasis and approximation and prevent vaginal shortening.
- The perineal skin may be closed by interrupted mattress sutures but subcuticular sutures are associated with less pain in the immediate postpartum period.
- On completion of repair, a vaginal examination should be done to confirm hemostasis, check alignment, and remove the tampon and any accumulated blood clots. A rectal examination also needs to be performed to exclude accidental suture involvement of the rectum.
- Instruments, swabs, and needle numbers should be checked, detailed documentation with estimated blood loss should be recorded, and analgesia and stool softeners should be prescribed.

Complications

- Immediate: bleeding, distorted anatomy, pain, suture through rectum.
- Delayed: hematoma, infection, scarring, dyspareunia, fistula formation, scar endometriosis.

Third- and fourth-degree tears

The important feature here is recognition and reconstitution of the disrupted muscle and/or epithelium. The two surgical techniques of repair are the end-to-end or the overlapping method, and both appear to be equally effective. This procedure needs to be done with adequate lighting, assistance, and appropriate instruments and suture material. All patients need to receive laxative and stool softeners routinely. Routine administration of antibiotics has not been shown to improve short- or long-term results. Because of the significant risk of short-term incontinence of feces and flatus, these women should be seen for follow-up in 1–2 weeks to check on symptoms.

Postpartum hemorrhage management I

- *Early PPH* is traditionally defined as the loss of more than 500 mL of blood from the genital tract in the first 24 hours after delivery or any loss less than 500 mL if associated with hemodynamic changes in the mother. Since clinicians routinely underestimate blood loss at delivery, more recent definitions of PPH include a 10% drop in hematocrit or women requiring blood transfusion.
- If the loss occurs between 24 hours and 6 weeks post-delivery, it is defined as *late PPH*.
- PPH occurs in 2–11% of deliveries, but in most situations when blood loss is estimated visually, it is underestimated.
- Quantitative measurements of blood loss increase the PPH rate to 20%, but life-threatening hemorrhage occurs in approximately 1 in 1000 deliveries.
- Early PPH is one of the major causes of maternal deaths, with the majority of deaths occurring after cesarean delivery.
- Worldwide, over 125 000 women die of PPH each year.

The main causes of early PPH are uterine atony, retained placenta or placental fragments, and lower genital tract trauma together with coagulopathy, which compounds the problem. Uterine inversion and uterine rupture are less common causes. Ninety percent of all cases of early PPH are due to uterine atony.

Management of early PPH

The two main aspects of management of PPH that should be performed simultaneously are resuscitation of the patient and identification of the specific cause of PPH in order to institute immediate appropriate management.

Resuscitation

Resuscitation involves fluid replacement, investigations, and monitoring. All appropriate staff should be alerted and made available. Essential staff include an experienced obstetrician, anesthesiologist, midwives, operating room personnel, blood bank/hematologist, as well as staff to ferry samples and blood products to and from the labs.

- At a minimum, two large-bore IV cannulae (size 14 gauge) should be inserted with colloid (Haemaccel, Gelofusine) running through one line and with crystalloid (Hartmann's, 0.9% saline, etc.) through the other until blood becomes available. When transfusing under such conditions, blood is preferred, and a compression cuff and blood warmer should be used. It is preferable not to transfuse more than 2000 mL of crystalloids, 1500 mL of colloid, and two units of uncrossmatched group-specific blood while awaiting cross-matched blood.
- The aim of fluid replacement should be to replace all previous loss in the first hour, followed by maintenance fluids to replace continuing loss, and maintain normal vital parameters of pulse, blood pressure, and respiration.
- If coagulopathy develops, liaison with a medical hematologist is imperative to obtain fresh frozen plasma (FFP), cryoprecipitate, and platelets.

Monitoring of the patient's condition is vital. This should include:

- continuous pulse oximetry.
- pulse and blood pressure measurement every 15 minutes.
- indwelling urinary catheter and hourly urine output measurements.
- central hemodynamic monitoring with a central venous pressure (CVP), if indicated.
- an arterial line if indicated to facilitate BP monitoring or blood draws.

The information should be recorded as it would be in an intensive care unit (ICU) to allow easy assessment of any change in the patient's condition.

The primary cycle of investigations should include CBC, cross-match 4–6 units of blood, coagulation screen, and estimation of fibrinogen and fibrin degradation products. Other investigations may be required such as chest X-ray if a CVP line is inserted and arterial gases if oxygen saturation falls on oximetry. Electrolytes, urea, and creatinine should be measured every 4–6 hours to monitor serum levels, which may be deranged with IV fluids, blood transfusion, and diminished renal function secondary to acute hypotension. The primary cycle of investigations should be repeated as deemed necessary until the patient's condition is stabilized.

Subsequent care in a high-dependency unit (HDU) or ICU setting should be considered if massive transfusion (>12 units), respiratory problems, persistent oliguria, or persistent coagulopathy are encountered.

Postpartum hemorrhage management II

Establishing a cause

Establishing a cause should be done in parallel to stabilization. Assessment should be in the operating room, if required, to identify and remove retained placental tissue or repair lower genital tract soft tissue trauma.

- If uterine atony appears to be the underlying problem, the bladder needs to be emptied and uterine contractions induced manually using fundal massage, whilst pharmacological agents (uterotonics) are employed to contract the uterus.
- Whilst an infusion of oxytocin (40 IU oxytocin in 0.9% saline) is being prepared, a bolus of 250 μg of ergometrine can be administered IV.
- If the bleeding persists, an IV bolus dose of oxytocin (10 IU) should be administered and bimanual compression applied.
- If the hemorrhage continues, 15-methylprostaglandin $F_{2\alpha}$ (Hemobate) 250 μg IM can be administered either into the thigh/gluteal muscle or directly into the myometrium, and can be repeated up to three more times at 15 minute intervals.
- For PPH unresponsive to oxytocin and/or ergometrine or when ergometrine is contraindicated, misoprostol administered rectally may have a role. Sustained uterine contractions can be produced within a few minutes of a rectal dose of 800–1000 μg (4–5 tablets) of misoprostol.
- If bleeding still remains refractory and other potential causes (retained products, soft tissue trauma, coagulation disorder) have been excluded, a number of surgical options are described for dealing with intractable hemorrhage and a senior obstetrician/consultant should be available by this stage to expedite them.

Surgical management of primary PPH

Surgical management of PPH has traditionally relied on ligation of internal iliac (hypogastric) arteries and puerperal hysterectomy as a last resort. Over the last few years, a number of new and simpler techniques (which also preserve fertility) have come to be used before resorting to complex and risky major surgical procedures.

- Undersuturing the placental bed. Where PPH follows a placenta previa or low-lying placenta, the large sinuses that are responsible for the bleeding must be undersewn.
- The 'tamponade test.' Where coagulopathy has been excluded or corrected but intractable hemorrhage remains a problem despite all pharmacological means, the 'tamponade test' provides a means of selecting those patients who require further surgery.
  - A Sengstaken–Blakemore tube or Rusch balloon catheter can be inserted into the uterine cavity and the balloon filled with 100–500 mL warm saline. The warm saline speeds up the rate of the clotting cascade. If minimal bleeding is observed, the test is considered successful and a laparotomy could be avoided.

- Uterine 'compression sutures.' B-Lynch suture and modifications. The B-Lynch suturing technique involves a pair of vertical brace sutures around the uterus essentially to appose the anterior and posterior walls and to apply continuing compression. The brace sutures probably work by direct application of pressure on the placental bed bleeding and also by reducing blood flow to the uterus.
- Uterine artery ligation. The uterus receives 90% of its blood supply from the uterine arteries, and therefore bilateral uterine artery ligation has a role in the management of PPH. This is not useful if a bilateral hypogastric artery ligation has already been performed.
- Utero-ovarian artery anastomosis ligation. The utero-ovarian anastomosis can be ligated after identifying an avascular area in the meso-ovarium.
- Internal iliac (hypogastric) artery ligation. Internal iliac artery ligation may help control uterine and vaginal bleeding as the vagina is supplied by the vaginal branch of the internal iliac artery. Bilateral internal iliac artery ligation results in 85% reduction in pulse pressure in the arteries distal to the ligation and 50% reduction in blood flow in the distal vessel, turning an arterial pressure system into one with pressures approaching those in the venous system and more amenable to hemostasis via clot formation. The success rate of the procedure in achieving its target is reported to be around 40%.
- Arterial embolization. This procedure is usually available in a small number of tertiary centers with appropriately trained interventional radiologists. Access is usually gained via the femoral artery. The catheter is advanced above the bifurcation of the aorta and the bleeding point is identified by contrast injection. The feeder artery is catheterized and embolized with Gelfoam or absorbable gelatine sponge, which is usually resorbed in about 10 days.
- Puerperal hysterectomy. Hysterectomy is the last resort in the management of PPH due to uterine causes. In most instances, a subtotal or supracervical hysterectomy, which is quicker, simpler, safer, and associated with less blood loss, is adequate. Total hysterectomy is needed in cases where bleeding is in the lower segment such as in cases with placenta previa/accreta or a laceration in the lower segment. Hysterectomy is only considered when all other avenues available have been exhausted, where bleeding continues, in a severely shocked patient or where further delay may compromise the patient, and in cases of coagulopathy where no replacement blood products are available.

Other causes of postpartum hemorrhage

Injuries to the genital tract

Bleeding from soft tissue injuries in the genital tract (cervical and vaginal lacerations) can be torrential, leading to cardiovascular compromise if appropriate resuscitative measures are not carried out while the bleeding is being brought under control. Optimal repair of genital tract lacerations requires correct positioning of the patient, satisfactory analgesia/anesthesia, adequate lighting and exposure, together with appropriate assistance and instruments such as retractors and long needle holders. These prerequisites often mean that the patient needs to be moved to the operating room. While this is being organized, blood loss can be reduced by vaginal packing or, if a bleeding source is identifiable, this can be clamped with artery forceps.

Disseminated intravascular coagulopathy (DIC)

DIC may compound all the above causes of obstetric hemorrhage. In such cases, it is not until the deranged coagulation is corrected that PPH can be effectively controlled whatever other measures are required and employed. DIC may be a result of abruptio placentae, sepsis, massive blood loss or transfusion, severe preeclampsia, or amniotic fluid embolism. Dealing with the underlying pathology (emptying the uterus in sepsis or abruption) may prevent the onset or progression of DIC.

Uncontrolled bleeding without clot formation may result from consumption of platelets, fibrinogen, and coagulation factors (in the DIC process or during bleeding) or from elevated levels of fibrinogen degradation products (FDPs). Unless FDP levels are very high, the presence of minimum levels of clotting factors will usually serve to arrest bleeding. The D-dimer component is the most commonly used parameter to assess FDP levels as it is specific for fibrin breakdown. Levels are normally <200 ng/mL, but often exceed 2000 ng/mL in cases of DIC.

In situations of massive obstetric hemorrhage, it is essential to involve a senior medical hematologist who will advise about the appropriate investigations and provide the appropriate blood products to correct coagulation disturbances.

Blood products used in the correction of deranged coagulation include:

- Cryoprecipitate. Each unit is approximately 200 mL in volume and contains the equivalent of 0.2 g of fibrinogen and 80 units of factor VIII. Contains no platelets. The usual requirement is 10–15 units.
- Fresh frozen plasma (FFP). Each unit is approximately 200 mL in volume and contains 0.4 g of fibrinogen and all clotting factors. The usual requirement is 5 units.
- Platelet concentrate. Each unit is approximately 60 mL in volume and contains a minimum of 5.5×10^{10}/L platelets. The usual requirement is 5–6 units. These are usually pooled from multiple donors.

Retained placenta

The average length of the third stage of labor is 10 minutes. Failure to expel the placenta and fetal membranes within 30 minutes of delivery of the baby is defined as a prolonged third stage. Where there is no significant bleeding, 1 hour is commonly allowed before manual removal is performed. Varying degrees of success have been reported when 10 IU of oxytocin is milked up the umbilical vein to enhance expulsion of the placenta. An infusion of oxytocin (40 IU oxytocin in 500 mL 0.9% saline at a rate of 125 mL/hour) is set up to maintain uterine contraction while preparing for a manual removal of the placenta. The procedure requires an effective regional block (functioning epidural or spinal) or general anesthesia.

Blood needs to be sent for hemoglobin estimation, group and screen, or cross-match.

- At the onset of the procedure, broad-spectrum antibiotics should be administered intravenously.
- During the procedure, the external hand should steady the uterus to facilitate removal of the placenta and reduce the risk of perforating the uterus by pressing firmly on the fundus.
- Once an adequate level of analgesia has been achieved, the internal hand should be placed through the vagina and into the uterus. Using the fingers in a side to side shearing motion, the plane between the placenta and uterine wall should be identified and developed so as to separate and remove the placenta.
- Once the placenta has been removed, the placenta and membranes should be carefully inspected, the uterine cavity checked and confirmed as empty, and the oxytocin infusion continued to maintain uterine contractions.

Morbidly adherent placenta

Abnormal attachment of the placental villi to the myometrium because of absence of the decidua basalis or imperfect development of the fibrinoid layer is known as placenta accreta, while invasion of the myometrium and penetration through to the peritoneum are known as placenta increta and percreta, respectively.

The risk of morbid adherence of the placenta is increased in women with a history of repeated surgical terminations of pregnancy, cesarean deliveries, and full-thickness myomectomies.

- In most instances of morbidly adherent placenta, especially with heavy bleeding, the treatment is immediate blood replacement and recourse to hysterectomy.
- If bleeding is minimal and not of concern, a conservative approach of leaving the placenta *in situ* with no further treatment may be adopted. This is an option only if adequate facilities for monitoring and management of the patient are available and in the absence of infection.
- An alternative course of action involves no attempt at placental separation and the administration of cytotoxic agents such as methotrexate in addition to antibiotics and follow-up with serial serum β-hCG measurements and ultrasound scans.

Uterine inversion

Complete inversion of the uterus is due most commonly to mismanagement of the third stage either by excessive cord traction on a fundally implanted placenta that has not yet separated or secondary to fundal pressure erroneously thought to aid placental expulsion. However, uterine inversion may also occur spontaneously with an atonic uterus and sudden increase in intraabdominal pressure (coughing/sneezing). Although often associated with massive hemorrhage, the shock is typically disproportionate to the blood loss and probably partly neurogenic due to traction on the uterine supports.

If diagnosed within a short time following inversion, the best course of action is immediate replacement by pushing up on the fundus with the palm of the hand and fingers in the direction of the long axis of the vagina. If this is not successful or diagnosis is delayed, assistance should be summoned and resuscitation commenced with IV fluids and blood products, as appropriate. If the placenta is still attached, it should be left *in situ* (unless there is partial separation and bleeding) until you are prepared to reduce the uterus. When the patient is hemodynamically stable, correction of the uterine inversion is performed followed by removal of placenta (unless removal of the placenta first facilitates reduction). The rationale for this course of action is to minimize further hemorrhage.

Before attempting replacement of the uterine fundus, a tocolytic such as terbutaline 0.25 mg or glyceryl trinitrate 100–200 μg may be administered IV for uterine relaxation. The replacement is attempted manually as described above or by the hydrostatic method. The latter (known as the O'Sullivan method) involves replacing the inverted uterus in the vagina and rapid infusion of ≥2 liters of warm saline into the vagina with one hand sealing the labia. This leads to ballooning of the vaginal fornices and exerts an even hydrostatic pressure that gradually forces open the constricting cervix and pushes the rim of inverted uterine wall upwards, thereby reducing the inverted uterus. If the placenta is intact, this can be removed and an oxytocin infusion commenced after the uterus has been restored to its normal configuration. Removal of the placenta just prior to reduction may make the procedure easy.

In the rare circumstance where manual and hydrostatic methods of restoring the uterus are not successful, possibly because of a dense constriction ring, laparotomy may be required. At laparotomy, traction is placed on the round ligaments with Allis forceps while an assistant pushes from below. The process may be aided by placement of a suture in the fundus to use for traction. Occasionally, where the constriction ring still prohibits repositioning, the Haultain technique of making a vertical incision in the posterior cervico-isthmic portion of the constriction ring to expose and restore the fundus to its normal configuration can be used. Operative procedures should be the last resort as, in most cases, persistent pressure from below to reduce the uterus under anesthesia yields good results.

Forceps delivery

Forceps consist of a pair of fenestrated blades with a handle connected to the blades by a shank. They are designed with a cephalic curve that fits around the fetal head and a pelvic curve that fits the pelvis. They are mainly used for traction. Kielland's forceps have a reduced pelvic curve and sliding lock, making them suitable for rotation of the fetal head in cases of malpresentation (only in experienced hands).

Conditions for use

On abdominal examination, the fetus should not be too large, suggestive of possible disproportion, and the head should be one-fifth or less palpable above the pelvic brim (engaged in the pelvis). There should be good uterine contractions. The bladder should be empty. On vaginal examination, the cervix must be fully dilated with ruptured membranes and a vertex presentation with no excess caput (scalp edema) or molding. The position of the vertex should be known (e.g. left occipitoanterior (LOA), left occipitotransverse (LOT), etc.), the station should be below +2 out of +5 (centimeters below ischial spines), and there should be descent of the head with contraction and bearing-down effort.

Adequate analgesia must be achieved before application of forceps using one of the following.

- Local analgesia: pudendal block and perineal infiltration (not suitable for Kielland's forceps).
- An existing epidural block, usually with a top-up.
- Spinal anesthesia.

Verbal consent should be obtained from the mother, explaining the indication for the instrumental delivery, the steps in the procedure, and the advantages and disadvantages. Options should be reviewed, including ventouse and cesarean delivery.

Indications for use

- Forceps may be used when there is delay in the second stage as a result of poor maternal expulsive efforts or due to malposition. Often it may be related to the absence of the urge to bear down with epidural anesthesia and inadequate uterine activity. Prolonged second stage is defined as >2 hours in nullipara without regional anesthesia (>3 hours with regional anesthesia) and >1 hour in multipara without regional anesthesia (>2 hours with regional anesthesia).
- Forceps may also be used when there is nonreassuring fetal testing ('fetal distress').
- Forceps are also used to prevent undue maternal expulsive efforts in women with certain cardiac and respiratory diseases.
- They can also be applied to the after-coming head in a breech presentation and to extract the fetal head at cesarean delivery.

Recommended further reading

1. American College of Obstetricians and Gynecologists (1994). ACOG Technical Bulletin No. 196. Operative vaginal delivery. *Int J Gynecol Obstet* **47**, 179–85.

Techniques for forceps delivery

- The mother is placed in the lithotomy position with her buttocks just over the edge of the delivery bed.
- The vulva and perineum are cleansed. The bladder should be emptied.
- The position of the fetal head is identified. Molding may make this difficult. The inverted Y shape described by the occipital bone on the parietal bone identifies the posterior fontanelle. The overriding of the parietal bones on the frontal bones identifies the anterior fontanelle. There are four sutures that delineate the anterior fontanelle. Alternatively, one can feel for the fetal ear and check in which direction the ear flicks to identify the direction of the occiput.
- Adequate analgesia is required. If the mother has no epidural, a pudendal block can be performed to block the pudendal nerve as it exits Alcock's canal adjacent to the ischial spines. This should be performed bilaterally with infiltration of up to 20 mL of 1% lidocaine hydrochloride (plain).
- For occipitoanterior positions, Simpson's or Tucker-McLane forceps can be used.

The blades are assembled to check that they fit, and positioned assembled in front of the perineum with the pelvic curve pointing upwards (the so-called 'phantom application') to allow the practitioner to orientate themselves. The handle that lies on the left hand is the left blade and is inserted first (to the mother's left side), negotiating the pelvic and cephalic curve with a curved movement of the blade between the fetal head and the accoucheur's hand kept along the left vaginal wall. The right blade is inserted in a similar manner. If the blades are applied correctly, the handles should lock easily. Traction should be applied in the direction of the pelvic curve and must not be excessive. Traction is synchronized with contractions and maternal bearing-down efforts, guiding the head downward initially. An episiotomy may be performed when the head is at the vulva, but is not required. The direction of traction is changed to up and out as the head passes out of the vulva.

Kielland's forceps

Before Kielland's forceps are used, it is essential to identify abdominally the side of the baby's back. The forceps are applied with the 'knobs' facing toward the baby's occiput to orientate the accoucheur. The anterior or posterior blade may be applied first directly depending on the preference of the obstetrician. The anterior blade is usually positioned by the 'wandering method' (first placed over the face and then moved to lie on the side of the fetal head) and the posterior blade directly. The blades are locked and asynclitism corrected by sliding the blades on each other into position. If the asynclitism is corrected, the sagittal suture of the fetus will lie equidistant from the two blades of the forceps. If the blades cannot be locked easily, the application of the forceps should be checked and reapplied if necessary.

An abnormal position (e.g. occipitotransverse) is corrected by rotating the handles of the forceps blades in the long axis of the mother (remembering that these forceps do not have a pelvic curvature) and directing the fetal occiput to the anterior position to emerge underneath the symphysis pubis. The head can be flexed at the same time. An excessive twisting force should not be used. Rotational forceps deliveries are best done by an experienced person. Once the rotation has been successfully achieved, the rotational forceps are typically replaced with Simpson's or Tucker–McLane forceps (or vacuum) to facilitate traction and to complete the delivery.

Complications of forceps

- *Maternal trauma.* Labial, vaginal, and perineal tears (including third- and fourth-degree perineal lacerations involving the anal sphincter).
- *Fetal trauma.* Fetal facial bruising, seventh nerve paralysis (usually resolves completely), and skin abrasions are seen relatively commonly. Cephalhematomas, fracture of the skull, and other neurologic injuries (such as brachial plexus injuries) are seen less commonly.

Recommended further reading

1. American College of Obstetricians and Gynecologists (1994). ACOG Technical Bulletin No. 196. Operative vaginal delivery. *Int J Gynecol Obstet* **47**, 179–85.

Ventouse delivery

An alternative to forceps delivery is the application of a suction cup to the fetal scalp and extraction by traction. The ventouse or vacuum extractor is associated with less maternal trauma but more fetal trauma than forceps. It may be used in preference to rotational forceps because, as traction is applied with the cup over the fetal occiput, spontaneous rotation to the occipitoanterior position often occurs during delivery. Ventouse should be avoided in preterm (<34 weeks) babies, face presentations, and those with bleeding disorders.

A silicon or metal cup should be applied on the 'median flexion point' (defined as symmetrically astride the sagittal suture and 3–4 cm anterior to the posterior fontanelle). A suction force of up to 0.2 kg/cm^2 is created initially. The rim of the cup is checked to make sure that there is no maternal tissue caught inadvertently under the suction cup. The pressure is then increased to 0.8 kg/cm^2 and traction exerted with uterine contractions and maternal bearing-down effort. The baby's scalp is often sucked up to form a 'chignon' (artificial caput), which resolves in 2–3 days. A posterior cup (metal or rigid cup) should be the choice for occipitotransverse or posterior positions to facilitate traction.

The use of the vacuum extractor rather than forceps for assisted vaginal delivery appears to reduce maternal morbidity and perineal injury. However, cephalhematoma, retinal hemorrhage, and jaundice are more common with vacuum, although no long-term ill effects are attributed to these complications. Follow-up studies show no consistent trend to physical or cognitive impairment from low outlet instrumental deliveries.

Combined forceps and ventouse delivery

As a rule, combined forceps and ventouse deliveries are associated with increased risk of adverse outcome to both mother and fetus. Therefore they are not generally recommended.

Trial of instrumental delivery

At times it is difficult to assess whether instrumental vaginal delivery could be carried out safely or whether to opt for a cesarean delivery. If nonreassuring fetal testing ('fetal distress') is present, delivery should be affected in the quickest and safest manner. This relies, in part, on the experience and judgment of the care provider. If time permits, a trial of instrumental delivery can be offered. Such procedures should be done in the operating room under adequate epidural or spinal anesthesia and with the surgical team, anesthesiologist, and pediatrician present. The intent is to abandon instrumental vaginal delivery should there be any difficulties and to proceed immediately to cesarean delivery. This should be explicitly explained to the mother and her partner prior to the trial of instrumental delivery, and appropriate written consent obtained prior to cesarean delivery.

Recommended further reading

1. American College of Obstetricians and Gynecologists (1999). ACOG Committee Opinion No. 208. Delivery by vacuum extraction. *Int J Gynecol Obstet* **64**, 96.
2. American College of Obstetricians and Gynecologists (1994). ACOG Technical Bulletin No. 196. Operative vaginal delivery. *Int J Gynecol Obstet* **47**, 179–85.

Malpresentations in labor

Malpresentation is said to occur when the fetus is not presenting by the vertex. The vertex is a diamond-shaped area defined by the parietal eminences, the anterior fontanelle, and the posterior fontanelle. Breech, brow, face, and shoulder presentations fall into this category.

Breech presentation is the most common malpresentation (3–4% at term). The appropriate clinical management of breech presentation antenatally and in labor is discussed on 📖 *p.84*.

Brow presentation

The incidence is 1 in 1500 deliveries. It may be associated with a contracted pelvis or a very large baby. The engaging diameter is the mentovertical (13 cm). In a normal-sized baby, if the presentation does not correct itself in labor, cesarean delivery is indicated. Occasionally a brow may extend to become a face and delivers spontaneously if it is mentoanterior. To ensure that this happens, the mother should have a vaginal examination every 2 hours to identify satisfactory progress. Failure to progress is an indication of disproportion due to the presenting diameter and oxytocin augmentation should not be used.

- *Diagnosis and management.* The head remains high and does not engage.Therefore it is easily palpable on abdominal examination. On vaginal examination, the forehead is palpable and, with additional vigilance, the brow is palpable between the bridge of the nose and the supraorbital ridges. The mentovertical diameter that is presented is 13.5 cm. The safest delivery is by cesarean.

Face presentation

This occurs in approximately 1 in 500 deliveries. Fifteen percent of these are due to congenital abnormalities such as anencephaly, a tumor in the neck or a thyroid goiter, or shortened fetal neck muscles. Most occur by chance as the head extends rather than flexes as it emerges. The diameters of the face are the biparietal diameter (9.5 cm) and submentobragmatic (9.5 cm).

- *Diagnosis and management.* Abdominally, the fetal spine feels S-shaped, the uterus is ovoid without fullness in the flanks, and there is a deep groove between the occiput and the back. On early vaginal examination, the nose and eyes may be felt. Later in labor, however, the nose and eyes may not be easily felt because of edema. Most engage in the transverse (submentobragmatic diameter, 9.5 cm). Ninety percent rotate so that the chin lies behind the symphysis pubis (mentoanterior) and the head can be born by flexion. If the chin rotates posteriorly (mentoposterior), there is a large area of skull comprising the vertex and occiput that cannot follow the face under the mother's symphysis pubis. Cesarean delivery is then indicated.

Shoulder presentation

This occurs in 1 in 400 deliveries and usually in multiparous women. If labor starts when the lie is transverse, it is clear that vaginal delivery cannot occur unless the fetus is very small or macerated. Placenta previa, fibroids, ovarian cysts, fetal malformations, multiple pregnancy, and abnormal uterus should be excluded. The transverse lie may evolve into a shoulder presentation and, as the cervix dilates, the arm may prolapse.

- *Diagnosis and management.* If the shoulder is presenting, no attempt should be made to replace or apply traction to the arm. Unless the lie can be corrected before the situation occurs, the only appropriate method of delivery is by cesarean. Uterine relaxants such as 0.25 mg terbutaline in 5 mL saline may be given IV to relax the uterus to accomplish the delivery through a lower-segment transverse incision. At the time of the cesarean, a classical hysterotomy (vertical incision in the upper segment) may be required if the membranes have ruptured and the uterus has been contracting as there will be considerable difficulty delivering the baby through a lower segment incision.

Cesarean delivery

Cesarean delivery is the process whereby the child is removed from the uterus by direct incision through the abdominal wall and the uterus. The incidence of cesarean delivery varies widely throughout the world, and appears to be rising. In the US, the cesarean delivery rate is 25–30%, in the UK, it is 10–20%, and in parts of South America (such as Brazil), it is of the order of 80–85%. It has an associated maternal mortality of 0.33 per 1000 deliveries.

Types of cesarean deliveries

Two main uterine incisions (hysterotomies) are commonly used for cesarean delivery.

Lower uterine segment incision

This is the most commonly performed procedure. The bladder is reflected from the lower segment, and a transverse uterine incision is made. The presenting part is then delivered through the lower segment. The lower-segment hysterotomy is closed in two layers. Compared with the classical (high vertical) incision, the surgery is much easier, is associated with less blood loss, and heals better, and the chance of uterine and intraabdominal infection is low. Uterine rupture in subsequent spontaneous labor is about 5 in 1000 deliveries; with the use of oxytocin it is 8 in 1000, and with prostaglandins for induction of labor it is 25 in 1000.

Classical (high vertical) cesarean incision

In this procedure, a vertical incision is made in the upper segment of the uterus and the child is delivered through this incision. This is not widely used because it has a much higher morbidity postoperatively and a much higher incidence of subsequent rupture of the scar (4–8% with half of these uterine ruptures occurring before the onset of labor). The indications for this type of incision include the following:

- Transverse lie of the fetus with ruptured membranes and oligohydramnios.
- Structural fetal abnormality making lower-segment approach difficult.
- Constriction ring (Bandle's ring) present because of neglected labor.
- Fibroids in the lower uterine segment.
- Anterior placenta previa with abnormally vascular lower segment.
- Perimortum cesarean delivery requiring rapid delivery.
- Very premature fetus (especially breech presentation) where the lower segment is poorly formed.

Puerperal hysterectomy

Cesarean delivery and hysterectomy are sometimes performed at the same time, e.g. where there is uterine rupture, placenta accreta, uncontrollable postpartum hemorrhage, and in cases of cervical malignant disease.

Indications for cesarean delivery

Cesarean delivery can be performed either as an emergency or as an elective procedure. Indications for elective cesarean delivery before the onset of labor include absolute cephalopelvic disproportion (CPD), complete placenta previa, some malpresentations (e.g. breech or brow presentation), history of a prior suburethral repair or vesicovaginal fistula repair, prior full-thickness myomectomy, prior uterine rupture, certain fetal conditions (e.g. monochorionic monoamniotic twin pregnancy), and maternal infections (e.g. active genital herpes, HIV with an elevated viral load). Approximately one-third of all elective cesarean deliveries are elective repeat procedures. In the case of a repeat section, it is important to localize the placenta on ultrasound to exclude placenta previa as this is more common in women with a uterine scar and more likely to be complicated by placenta accreta—hence the risk of massive intrapartum and postpartum hemorrhage and the possibility of needing a hysterectomy.

Emergency cesarean delivery may be needed because of antenatal complications, e.g. severe preeclampsia, IUGR, abruptio placentae (baby still alive). The need for emergency cesarean may become apparent during labor if there is nonreassuring fetal testing ('fetal distress') in the first stage of labor, failure to progress in the first stage of labor, prolapsed cord (if fetus is alive), obstructed labor, CPD becoming evident during labor, and after failed induction of labor.

- *Fetal indications.* On occasion, cesarean delivery is carried out almost entirely in the interest of the fetus, e.g. severe IUGR, preterm fetus needing delivery that is in the breech presentation, although the evidence for the latter practice is not strong. Perimortem cesarean delivery occasionally may be performed to save the life of the baby if it is still alive and to facilitate resuscitation of the mother. In this case, a classical type of operation may be indicated to extract a child with the utmost speed.
- *Maternal indications.* Cesarean delivery may be performed because of previous surgery, e.g. a previous hysterotomy or myomectomy. Previous myomectomy does not constitute an absolute indication for cesarean delivery if the prior surgery did not enter the uterine cavity. If a vaginal delivery is allowed in these circumstances, great care must be taken during labor to look out for signs of imminent rupture of the uterus.

Recommended further reading

1. McDonagh MS, Osterweil P, Guise JM (2005). The benefits and risks of inducing labour in patients with prior caesarean delivery: a systematic review. *Br J Obstet Gynecol* **112**, 1007–15.
2. American College of Obstetricians and Gynecologists (1999). Vaginal birth after previous cesarean delivery. ACOG Practice Bulletin No. 2. *Int J Gynecol Obstet* **64**, 201–8.

Elective and emergency cesarean deliveries

Timing of elective cesarean delivery

When a cesarean delivery is carried out in the maternal interests (such as severe preeclampsia), there is usually little choice in the timing of the procedure. When the fetal interest is paramount, timing of the operation is influenced by two main factors: fetal maturity (gestational age) and fetal condition. Elective cesarean deliveries are usually performed after 39 weeks' gestation, although in special cases they can be done before that time after confirmation of fetal lung maturity. Clinical knowledge and experience are important in making the decision about when the infant is at less risk in the nursery than in the uterus.

Before an emergency cesarean delivery

- Explain to the mother and her partner/family about the need for an emergency cesarean delivery and obtain written consent.
- Activate the anesthesiologist, operating room staff, and neonatologist.
- Have the mother breathe 100% oxygen if there is nonreassuring fetal testing.
- Neutralize gastric contents with 20 mL of 0.3 sodium citrate. Gastric emptying can be promoted with metoclopramide 10 mg IV (ranitidine 150 mg, an H_2 agonist, can be given for elective cesarean deliveries 2 hours before surgery).
- Consider preoperative emptying of the stomach (e.g. if prolonged labor or if the patient had a meal recently or if an opiate was given). These measures will minimize the risk of postoperative aspiration (Mendelson's syndrome).
- Transfer to the operating room. Set up an IV infusion with a 14 cannula and take blood for CBC and coagulation profile (if indicated), and consider cross-matching blood, e.g. two units (four units if anterior placenta previa or placental abruption).
- Catheterize the bladder.
- Tilt the mother to left lateral position by 15° on operating table using a wedge.
- Consider pneumatic compression boots on the lower extremities to reduce the incidence of deep vein thrombosis (DVT).
- Use pulse oximetry both peri- and postoperatively.
- Use prophylactic antibiotics routinely after clamping the umbilical cord to reduce the incidence of infection.
- Inform the pediatrician if the mother has had opiates in the last 4 hours.

Halothane is not used for obstetric procedures because uterine muscle relaxation increases bleeding. Other anesthetic problems include vomiting on induction and light anesthesia, resulting in awareness although the woman is paralysed. Most cesarean deliveries are now performed under spinal/epidural anesthesia. It is important to have an experienced anesthesiologist in order to reduce maternal morbidity.

Recommended further reading

1. McDonagh MS, Osterweil P, Guise JM (2005). The benefits and risks of inducing labour in patients with prior caesarean delivery: a systematic review. *Br J Obstet Gynecol* **112**, 1007–15.
2. American College of Obstetricians and Gynecologists (1999). Vaginal birth after previous cesarean delivery. ACOG Practice Bulletin No. 2. *Int J Gynecol Obstet* **64**, 201–8.

Complications of cesarean delivery

The immediate complications are those of hemorrhage (primary or secondary) which may lead to shock and the complications of anesthesia. There may be inadvertent damage to the bladder, ureters, or colon, a vesicouterine fistula, or retained placental tissue and bleeding (this should be rare as the uterine cavity should be inspected and cleaned during the cesarean delivery). Injury to the fetus (such as a facial laceration) can also occur at the time of cesarean.

After a cesarean delivery, all excess blood should be removed from the peritoneal cavity, the peritoneal cavity irrigated, and the ovaries and tubes visually inspected. Rh(D)-negative mothers with an Rh(D)-positive baby should be given anti-D immunoglobulin 300 µg IM within 72 hours of delivery. A Kleihauer–Betke test should be sent to determine if further doses of anti-D immunoglobulin are required. The mother should be mobilized early.

Prophylaxis against venous thromboembolism

Low risk

Women with no risk factors undergoing elective cesarean delivery in an uncomplicated pregnancy require only early mobilization and good hydration.

Moderate risk

- Age over 35 years
- Obesity over 80 kg
- Para 4+
- Preeclampsia
- Emergency cesarean in labor
- Gross varicose veins
- Current infection
- More than 4 days of prior immobility
- Major concurrent illness (heart disease, nephritic syndrome, cancer).

These women require heparin prophylaxis (e.g. unfractionated heparin 7500 IU SC twice daily, enoxaparin 40 mg SC once daily, dalteparin 5000 IU SC once daily) and/or mechanical methods (physiotherapy before and after surgery, pneumatic boots during surgery, graded elastic stockings postoperatively, early mobilization).

High risk

These women should all receive heparin until 5 days postoperatively or until fully mobilized. The use of leg stockings confers additional benefit. Those at high risk include the following:

- Any women with three risk factors under the 'Moderate risk' heading.
- Extended surgery, e.g. puerperal hysterectomy.
- Past history of thromboembolism or known inherited thrombophilia.
- Strong family history of thromboembolism.
- Paralysed lower limbs.
- Women with antiphospholipid antibody syndrome.

Women at high risk of a venous thromboembolic event (including DVT or pulmonary embolus), such as women who have had a thromboembolic event in the index pregnancy, should receive thromboprophylaxis as mentioned above for a minimum of 6 weeks postpartum.

Recommended further reading

1. McDonagh MS, Osterweil P, Guise JM (2005). The benefits and risks of inducing labour in patients with prior caesarean delivery: a systematic review. *Br J Obtet Gynecol* **112**, 1007–15.
2. American College of Obstetricians and Gynecologists (1999). Vaginal birth after previous cesarean delivery. ACOG Practice Bulletin No. 2. *Int J Gynecol Obstet* **64**, 201–8.
3. Smail F, Hofmeyr GJ (2002). Antibiotic prophylaxis for cesarean section. *Cochrane Database Syst Rev*, **3**, CD000933.

Obstetric analgesia

The role of the anesthesiologist in an obstetric unit is to administer safe analgesia and anesthesia and to be part of the multidisciplinary team concerned in the management of the sick parturient.

Adequate pain relief in labor is not available to the majority of women in the world. Anesthetists are usually not involved in pain management unless an epidural is requested/required. Epidural anesthesia for pain relief is discussed earlier on 📖 *p.304*. More details related to epidural anesthesia are discussed here.

Advantages of epidurals

- Epidurals are the most effective method of providing pain relief in labor.
- A good working epidural can be topped up for an instrumental delivery, if required.
- Epidurals can be converted to provide anesthesia for an operative delivery or for the removal of a retained placenta.
- Epidurals can be used as an adjuvant in the control of blood pressure in preeclamptic women.
- Epidural opiates (diamorphine or morphine) provide good postoperative pain relief for many hours.
- Epidural analgesia allows a woman to be clear-headed and thus to be in control of her labor.

Disadvantages of epidurals

- Epidurals are invasive procedures with side effects and complications.
- Women with epidurals *in situ* require close monitoring, ideally with a one-to-one care provider.

Side effects and complications of epidurals

- The blood pressure may drop (from blockade of sympathetic nerves).
- The block may be unilateral or patchy.
- Motor nerves as well as sensory nerves may be blocked (with loss of mobility).
- There is a less than 1% possibility of a dural tap by the needle or catheter. Approximately 60% of women who have had a dural tap develop a severe headache, which may require an epidermal blood patch as treatment.
- Loss of sensation of a full bladder can lead to retention, breakthrough pain, and the need for catheterization for a period of time.
- Neuropathy: the majority of postpartum neuropathies occur in women who have not had any anesthetic intervention. However, there is an incidence of nerve damage to both the cord and the peripheral nerves because of incorrect drug administration, direct trauma from the needle tip, or from infarction during a hypotensive episode.
- Meningitis (both bacterial and chemical).
- Epidural abscess.
- Epidural hematoma.
- Short-term backache (it is now established that women who have had epidurals for labor are no more likely to suffer long-term backache than those women who did not have epidurals for labor).

Consent issues

It is often difficult for the anesthesiologist to ensure that the woman has adequate understanding to give valid consent if she is in the throes of labor. Ideally, anesthesiologists should be involved antenatally or early in the course of labor to review the options for pain management.

Performing an epidural

- Consent must be obtained.
- Blood should be taken for a baseline CBC and coagulation studies, if indicated.
- A large-bore IV cannula for administration of fluids should be established (to counteract any fall in blood pressure).
- For epidural placement, the woman may be lying on her side or sitting, but her back should be curved to open up the intervertebral spaces.
- Using an aseptic technique, the anesthesiologist infiltrates local anesthetic into the skin over L2–3 or L3–4 (if a combined spinal epidural technique is being used then the space should be L3–4 to avoid the possibility of the spinal needle damaging the spinal cord which usually ends at L1 level). The average epidural space is approximately 4–5 cm deep. The Tuohy needle is marked at 1 cm intervals to allow depth to be gauged.
- The epidural space is identified using a loss of resistance technique to saline or air.
- The epidural catheter is threaded through the needle and the needle withdrawn.
- Local anesthetic, usually bupivacaine, is often given initially in a test dose to ensure that the epidural catheter has not inadvertently entered the subarachnoid space giving a consequent drop in blood pressure.
- A bolus dose is then given and the epidural is run either on bolus top-up doses every 1–2 hours as required or, more effectively, as a continuous infusion. Some anesthesiologists offer women a patient-controlled epidural with or without a continuous infusion. Mobility can be encouraged.
- Blood pressure readings must be taken at 5 minute intervals for 20 minutes after each top-up and at 30 minute intervals once established.
- The level of block height must be monitored by testing the dermatome level to which the block has spread using cold or touch sensation. Motor power is tested by the ability to lift the leg and bend the knee.
- Blood pressure, block height, and motor block must be documented.

With low-dose epidural infusions, good analgesia can be established particularly when small doses of opiate (usually fentanyl) are added. The incidence of instrumental delivery (ventouse or forceps) was greater in women who had large volumes of high-concentration bupivacaine, which caused increased motor block. With low-dose weak concentration, there is no higher risk of instrumental delivery except when the epidural has been running for a long time and there is some motor block combined with maternal fatigue.

Recommended further reading

1 American College of Obstetricians and Gynecologists (2004). ACOG Committee Opinion No. 295. Pain relief during labor. *Obstet Gynecol* **104**, 213.

Obstetric anesthesia: emergency

Epidurals

Conversion of a working epidural from analgesia to anesthesia is the anesthetic of choice for a laboring woman who requires instrumental vaginal or operative delivery. The indication for cesarean delivery (e.g. a cord prolapse or sudden massive obstetric hemorrhage) may mean that there is no time to top up the epidural adequately (which typically takes 10–20 minutes) and a general anesthetic will be required.

When epidurals are in place:

- ephedrine should be available at all times to counteract any fall in blood pressure
- continuous fetal heart rate monitoring is recommended.

Facilities and drugs should always be ready for rapid conversion to general anesthesia:

- if the block progresses too high
- if the woman experiences pain and requests a general anesthetic
- if the surgery is complicated and may proceed to cesarean hysterectomy.

NB. To put a woman to sleep against her wishes constitutes assault. Prior discussion about the possibility should obviate potential complaint. Consent is required. In an emergent situation, verbal consent may be adequate.

Spinals

When there is no epidural *in situ* and a woman requires an emergency cesarean delivery, there may be time for the anesthesiologist to administer a spinal anesthetic.

Recommended further reading

1. Datta S, edr. (2004). *Anesthetic and Obstetric Management of High-Risk Pregnancy*, pp. 381–402. Springer-Verlag, New York.
2. Anim-Somuah M, Smyth R, Howell C, Anim-Somuah M (2005). Epidural versus non-epidural or no analgesia in labour. *Cochrane Database Syst Rev*, **4**, CD000331.
3. American College of Obstetricians and Gynecologists (2002). ACOG Practice Bulletin No. 36. Obstetric analgesia and anesthesia. *Int J Gynecol Obstet* **78**, 321–35.

Obstetric anesthesia: elective

An elective cesarean delivery can be performed under either general or regional anesthesia. Regional anesthesia can be epidural, spinal, or combined spinal epidural (CSE).

Regional anesthesia is generally preferred because it is:

- safer for mother
- safer for baby
- allows immediate bonding
- allows birth partner to be present
- allows better management of postoperative pain especially when opiates are used.

Epidurals

Disadvantages of epidural over spinal anesthesia:

- Can take up to three-quarters of an hour to establish an adequate block *de novo*.
- Block may be unilateral.
- Fewer operative cases can be performed on a given operative list.
- On occasion, conversion level to general anesthetic may be required.
- Higher chance of CSF leak with subsequent spinal headache.

Advantages of epidural over spinal anesthesia:

- Can be topped up during surgery if the operation is taking a long time.
- Catheter may be left in for postoperative pain management.

Spinals

Disadvantages of spinals:

- may wear off if surgery is prolonged.
- less control over a fall of blood pressure.
- may cause more nausea and vomiting.
- more likely to cause nerve damage.

Advantages of spinals:

- technically easier to perform.
- definite endpoint to confirm correct placement (i.e. evidence of CSF in the spinal needle).
- block less likely to be unilateral.
- gives a good dense block within a few minutes.

Combined spinal epidurals

These are usually performed by the 'needle-though-needle' technique, i.e. the spinal needle is passed through the Tuohy needle into the CSF, but can be performed as two separate injections.

Disadvantages:

- Technically more difficult.
- Higher risk of chemical and bacterial meningitis.
- Spinal may be unilateral if performed in the lateral position and there is difficulty threading the epidural catheter.

Advantages:

- Have the advantages of both epidurals and spinals.

The majority of elective cesarean deliveries in developed countries are performed under spinal anesthesia.

General anesthesia

General anesthesia is indicated when:

- The mother requests to be put to sleep.
- Regional anesthesia is contraindicated:
  - In the presence of documented coagulopathies.
  - In a patient who is anticoagulated.
  - Where there is local infection at the injection site.
  - When there is systemic bacteremia or septicemia.
  - In certain cases of back injury or previous back surgery.
  - In certain cardiac diseases.
  - Where there is allergy to local anesthetic agents.

There are some relative contraindications to regional procedures, e.g. certain neurologic diseases. In such cases, it is best to arrange for an antepartum anesthetic consultation to address the issue.

Dangers of general anesthesia:

- Risk of difficult intubation (especially in preeclampsia).
- Risk of inhalation of gastric content (Mendelson's syndrome).
- General anesthetics cross the placenta and can depress the baby.
- There may be delayed bonding of mother and baby.

There is a decrease in lower esophageal tone, which increases the risk of passive reflux. All pregnant women having a general anesthetic for whatever reason from 20 weeks onward should have a rapid-sequence induction (preoxygenation and cricoid pressure) to minimize the risk of gastric reflux and aspiration.

In all obstetric units, there should be good communication between midwives, obstetricians, and anesthesiologists as it is important for the successful management of women with known pre-existing medical problems. There should be a plan as to the management and mode of delivery of these women which should be documented in the antenatal notes.

Recommended further reading

1. Datta S, edr. (2004). *Anesthetic and Obstetric Management of High-Risk Pregnancy.* pp. 381-402. Springer-Verag, New York.
2. Anim-Somuah M, Smyth R, Howell C, Anim-Somuah M (2005). Epidural versus non-epidural or no analgesia in labour. *Cochrane Database Syst Rev* **4**, CD000331.
3. American College of Obstetricians and Gynecologists (2002). ACOG Practice Bulletin No. 36. Obstetric analgesia and anesthesia. *Int J Gynecol Obstet* **78**, 321–35.

Physiological changes of pregnancy affecting anesthesia

The obstetric patient presents the anesthesiologist with particular challenges. The physiological changes that occur in a woman during pregnancy add to the potential risk of anesthesia.

- *Changes in blood volume.*
  - There is an increase in plasma volume (40–50%).
  - There is an increase in red cell volume (15–20%).
  - There is consequently 'physiological anemia of pregnancy'.
  - Clotting factors increase for maternal cardiovascular protection at the time of delivery such that the woman is in a hypercoaguable state.
- *Cardiovascular changes.*
  - There is an increase in cardiac output (30–40%).
  - There is an increase in heart rate (15–20 beats/min).
  - There is downregulation of α and β receptors.
  - There is a profound effect on venous return when the large gravid uterus compresses the inferior vena cava and also the aorta (which can lead to aortacaval compression or supine hypotension syndrome if the women lies supine).
  - A pregnant woman must never lie flat on her back. Care must be taken especially when she is being transferred on to a trolley or operating table. Her hips should be tilted to one side by at least 15° using a wedge or pillow. Alternatively, the operating table can be in left lateral tilt.
- *Respiratory effects.*
  - An increase in minute ventilation (40%).
  - An increase in respiratory rate (15%).
  - A decrease in functional residual capacity.
  - A decrease in expiratory reserve volume.
  - A decrease in residual volume.
  - Increased oxygen consumption and decreased functional residual capacity mean that women develop hypoxemia very rapidly. Anesthesiologists must preoxygenate for a longer time before induction of general anesthesia.
  - There is a decrease in minimum alveolar concentration (MAC) which increases susceptibility to inhalation anesthetic agents.
- *Gastrointestinal effects*: In order that the fetus can grow, maternal nutrition must provide the placenta with adequate nutrients.
  - To maximize absorption, particularly of iron, gastrointestinal motility is decreased.
  - There is an increased secretion of gastric acid stimulated by the hormone gastrin towards term.
  - Gastric pH is low and there is delayed gastric emptying.
  - The lower esophageal tone is lowered and hence reflux of acid gastric content can occur.
  - Inhalation of gastric contents in pregnancy was first described by Mendelson (Mendelson's syndrome or acid aspiration syndrome).

- *Antacid prophylaxis.* H_2 receptor antagonists (ranitidine), which make gastric secretion less acidic, and sodium citrate, which neutralizes acid already in the stomach, should be prescribed. Women should be given ranitidine every 6 hours during labor.
- *Weight gain.*
  - The average parturient gains approximately 25 kg (55 lb) in weight.
  - This weight gain can cause difficulty when lifting patients.
  - Difficulty with venous access.
  - Potential intubation difficulties (every pregnant woman is given a rapid-sequence induction for general anesthesia).
- *Large patient.*
  - Large pendulous breasts hinder laryngoscope movements.
  - Edema, especially in preeclamptic patients when there is often laryngeal edema.
  - High oxygen demand leading to rapid desaturation.
  - Potential of inhalation of gastric contents increased.

Resuscitation

Cardiac arrest during pregnancy is rare.

- *Causes:*
  - Cardiac disease, especially after delivery when there is an increase in blood volume by autotransfusion from involution of the uterus.
  - Cocaine abuse, now the most common cause of cardiac arrest at term in the USA.
  - Hemorrhage.
  - Iatrogenic: anaphylaxis, general anesthesia (e.g. failed intubation), and regional anesthesia (inadvertent IV injection of local anesthetic, inadvertent total spinal from subarachnoid injection of local anesthetic).
- *Management:*
  - ABC (airway, breathing, and circulation) as for all cardiac arrests.
  - Left lateral tilt (it is impossible to resuscitate a woman when the venous return to the heart is blocked).
  - Cricoid pressure (if enough personnel available).
  - Immediate delivery of the baby (the chances of successful resuscitation of the mother are small but are increased by the delivery of the baby). A perimortem cesarean delivery may be required if the mother cannot be effectively resuscitated within 5 minutes.

Recommended further reading

1. Datta S, edr. (2004) *Anesthetic and Obstetric Management of High-Risk Pregnancy*, pp. 381–402. Springer-Verlag, New York.
2. Anim-Somuah M, Smyth R, Howell C, Anim-Somuah M (2005). Epidural versus non-epidural or no analgesia in labour. *Cochrane Database Syst Rev* **4**, CD000331.
3. American College of Obstetricians and Gynecologists (2002). ACOG Practice Bulletin No. 36. Obstetric analgesia and anesthesia. *Int J Gynecol Obstet* **78**, 321–35.
4. American College of Obstetricians and Gynecologists (2004). ACOG Committee Opinion No. 295. Pain relief during labor. *Obstet Gynecol* **104**, 213.

Neonatal resuscitation

Anticipating problems is the key to effective resuscitation. Call the pediatrician in good time for deliveries where problems may occur.

- Preterm deliveries <35 weeks of gestation.
- All emergency cesarean deliveries.
- Breech birth.
- Nonreassuring fetal test ('fetal distress').
- Thick meconium.
- Expected major fetal abnormality.
- Concern for other reasons, e.g. maternal drug addiction.

Term infants requiring resuscitation often respond to simple measures: dry and warm; clear the airway; mild stimulation. An inverted pyramid (Fig. 6.8) illustrates the relative frequencies and priorities of neonatal resuscitation.

Practical aspects of resuscitation

Before delivery

Check resuscitation cart and equipment.

- Heater on.
- Oxygen supply connected.
- Pressure valves set at 25–30 cmH_2O.
- Laryngoscope illuminating effectively.
- Suction device functioning and suction catheters available.
- Endotracheal tubes (ETTs) available.
- Emergency resuscitation box available.

At delivery

This section assumes that there is no meconium-stained amniotic fluid. Resuscitation of the infant with meconium-stained amniotic fluid is discussed later (in the eponymous section).

- Start clock.
- Transfer baby to resuscitation table.
- Dry baby and wrap in warm towel/gauze.
- Assess condition:
    - *Breathing*. Assess rate and quality.
    - *Heart rate*. Listen to the apex beat with a stethoscope. Palpate the brachial or femoral pulse or palpate the base of the umbilical cord.
    - *Color*. Look at the trunk, lips, and tongue. Note if the baby is centrally pink, cyanosed, or pale. Peripheral cyanosis is common and, by itself, does not indicate hypoxemia.

Condition of the newborn infant at birth

After assessment of breathing, heart rate, and color, the baby can usually be placed in one of four broad categories.

1 Healthy. Pink; crying lustily; heart rate >100 beats/minute.
    - *Action*. Dry and give to mother.

2 Primary apnea. Cyanosed; heart rate >100 beats/minute; some respiratory effort, tone, and response to stimulation.
 - *Action.* Gentle stimulation and facial oxygen. This baby is likely to begin to breathe spontaneously—a short wait of not more than 1 minute is acceptable. Stimulate by rubbing with a dry towel, gentle oral or nasal suction oxygen to the face. If no response by 1 minute, use bag and mask ventilation.

3 Terminal apnea. Pale; heart rate < 60 beats/minute; floppy and apneic.
 - *Action.* Bag and mask ventilation immediately. This baby will not breathe without help. If not improving quickly, intubation and cardiac compressions may be required.

4 Fresh stillbirth. Apneic; pale; floppy; no heart rate.
 - *Action.* Full cardiopulmonary resuscitation immediately (follow ABC set out in the next section).
 - Assist breathing: positive pressure ventilation via ETT (or with bag and mask until skilled help for intubation available).
 - Give cardiac compressions (this will be of no benefit unless effective ventilation is established).

Assess (support): temperature (warm and dry)

Airway (position and suctioning)

Breathing (stimulate to cry)

Circulation (heart rate and colour)

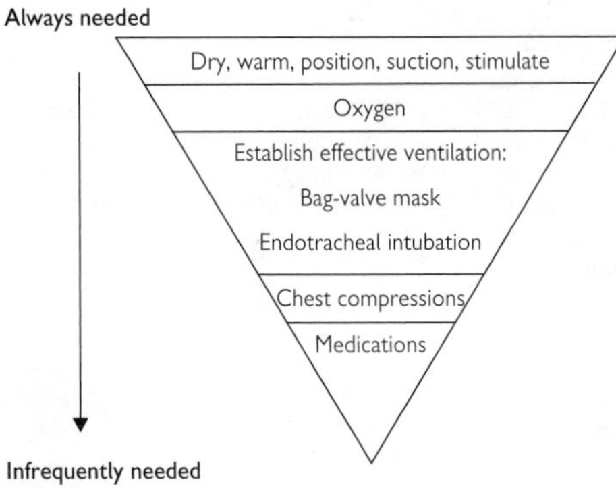

Fig. 6.8 An inverted pyramid illustrating the relative frequencies and priorities of neonatal resuscitation.

ABC of resuscitation

'ABC' stands for attention to airway, breathing, and circulation. To these should be added temperature control.

Temperature control

Keep the baby dry and warm. This reduces the risk of hypoglycemia and acidosis and minimizes oxygen consumption.

Airway

- Position baby face upward with head in the neutral position.
- Use soft suction catheters and a negative pressure of 5–10 kPa to gently clear airway. Avoid deep pharyngeal suction as vagal stimulation can cause bradycardia or laryngospasm.

Breathing

Bag and mask ventilation

Indications for use:

- Shallow irregular respiration with heart rate < 100 beats/minute and falling.
- Apnea.

Choose a mask large enough to cover the face from the bridge of the nose to below the mouth. Connect the bag to an indirect O_2 supply. Without a reservoir bag, you will only be able to deliver about 40–50% O_2. The bag usually has a blow-off valve that operates at 30–40 cmH_2O. If a greater inflation pressure is necessary, put your finger on top of the valve to override it. Squeeze bag to achieve adequate chest expansion and establish a rate of 30–40 breaths/minute.

On some resuscitation carts, it is also possible to give effective ventilation via a T-piece system connected to the O_2 outlet. Ensure blow-off valve is set at the correct pressure. The hole on the connector is occluded with your finger to allow the pressure to build up, and ventilation is delivered by releasing and re-occluding the hole on the connector at the desired rate (Fig. 6.9).

Endotracheal intubation

- Indications for use:
  - Primary apnea that does not respond promptly to bag and mask ventilation.
  - Terminal apnea or asystole.
- For small babies, use size 2.5 mm ETT.
- For term babies, use 3.0–3.5 mm ETT.

Hold the first inflation for 2 or 3 seconds to allow proper expansion of the lungs and establish a functional residual capacity. After the first few breaths, establish a rate of 30–40 breaths/minute with inspiratory times of approximately 0.5–1 second. If there is poor chest movement, the pressure can be increased sequentially up to 40 cm of water.

Following intubation check for:

- Bilateral chest movement.
- Breath sounds bilateral and equal on auscultation.
- Absence of breath sounds over the stomach.

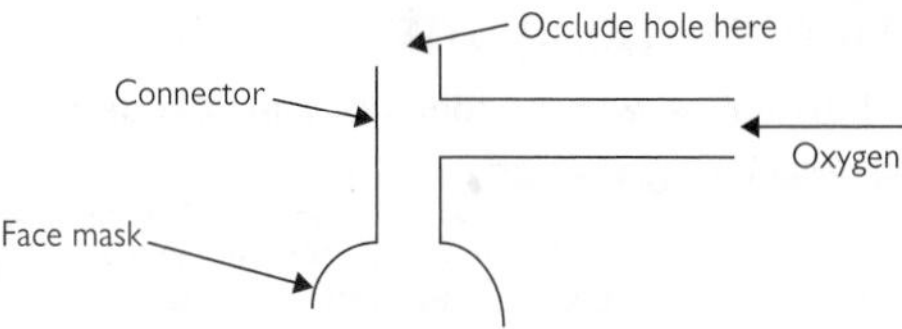

Fig. 6.9 Diagram showing procedure for giving effective ventilation via a T-piece system connected to the O_2 outlet.

Circulation

Cardiac compression

- Indication for use: heart rate <60 beats/minute despite effective ventilation.

Cardiac compression may be performed in one of two ways.

1. Encircle chest with both hands so that fingers lie behind the baby and thumbs are opposed over the mid-sternum.
2. Place two fingers over sternum 1 cm below the internipple line.

Depress sternum at a rate of 120 compressions/minute to a depth of 1–2 cm. Give three chest compressions for every inhalation.

Drugs

The use of drugs is indicated if adequate ventilation with 100% oxygen and effective chest compressions have failed to increase the heart rate above 60 beats/minute.

- Epinephrine is the most important drug. It can be given either intravenously (via umbilical venous catheter) or down the ETT.
  - *Doses.* 10 μg/kg (0.1 mL/kg, 1: 10 000) IV or 20 μg/kg via ETT. Epinephrine 10–30 μg/kg every 3–5 minutes if there is no response.
- Sodium bicarbonate is indicated if the heart rate remains <60 beats/minute despite good ventilation, chest compressions, and IV epinephrine.
  - *Dose.* 1 mmol/kg intravenously (use 2 mL/kg of 4.2% solution (= 0.5 mmol/mL)).
- Volume expanders are indicated if there is no response to resuscitation, especially if any evidence of hypovolemia. Use 0.9% saline or 4.5% human albumin solution.
  - *Dose.* 10–20 mL/kg over 5–10 minutes. O Rh(D)-negative blood is given when significant acute blood loss is suspected.
- Dextrose 10% is given intravenously at 2–3 mL/kg.
- Naloxone is only indicated for persisting apnea related to maternal opiate analgesia in an otherwise well baby. It does not improve cardiac performance and should not be given to an asphyxiated baby or a baby whose heart rate is <60 beats/minute or if mother is opiate dependent.
  - *Dose.* 100 μg/kg IM.

Resuscitation of the infant

Resuscitation of the infant with meconium-stained liquor

When thick meconium is present at delivery:

- Aspirate the mouth and nostrils with a wide-bore suction catheter when the head is delivered. Although commonly used, this approach has not been shown to improve the outcome in such infants.
- Following delivery, move the baby quickly to the resuscitation table.

For a pink and vigorous baby:

- Continue suction of oropharynx if meconium is still present.
- Intubation is not usually required.

If the baby shows depression of respiratory effort:

- Suck out pharynx before the baby is either encouraged to breathe or given artificial respiratory support.
- If there is meconium in the mouth, visualize larynx and the vocal cords with laryngoscope.
- If there is meconium at the level of or below the vocal cords, intubate and apply suction. Remove ETT slowly, reintubate with a clean tube, and repeat the procedure. This can be continued for up to 2 minutes in an infant with a good heart rate. Where the heart rate is <60 beats/minute, full resuscitation should be commenced at 1 minute even if all the meconium has not been removed.

Actions in the event of poor initial response to resuscitation

1. Check for technical fault.
    - Is oxygen connected?
    - Is ETT in the trachea? If in doubt remove ETT and replace.
    - Is ETT down one bronchus? If in doubt remove ETT and replace.
    - Is ETT blocked? If in doubt remove ETT and replace.
    - Check that blow-off valve is set at 30 cmH_2O
    - Check flow rate of oxygen at 5–8 L/min.
2. Does the baby have lung pathology, e.g.
    - Pneumothorax (transillumination of the thorax will make the diagnosis quickly).
    - Congenital diaphragmatic hernia.
    - Hypoplastic lungs.
    - Hydrops.
3. If the baby has good chest movement has there been:
    - Fetal hemorrhage? Consider plasma or O Rh-negative blood 20–30 mL/kg via umbilical vein.
    - Severe asphyxia?

Resuscitation of the preterm infant

Preterm babies are likely to be deficient in surfactant and may require relative higher inflation pressures than term babies. Start resuscitation with a pressure of 20–25 cmH_2O but increase if this does not produce satisfactory chest wall movement. Consider administering artificial surfactant down the ETT.

When should resuscitation be stopped

If signs of life were present shortly before delivery, it is justifiable to carry out full cardiopulmonary resuscitation on a fresh stillbirth. However published data suggest that if there are still no signs of life by 15 minutes then very few babies will survive. If there is no response to full resuscitation, the decision to discontinue should be made by the most senior pediatrician available. The parent's wishes should be taken into account as much as possible; however, the ultimate decision of whether or not to continue with aggressive resuscitative efforts lies with the senior neonatologist or pediatrician.

Recommended further reading

1. Advanced Life Support Group (2000). *Advanced Paediatric Life Support* (3rd edn). BMJ Books, London.
2. Chameides L, Hazinski MF, eds (1997). *Pediatric Advanced Life Support*. American Heart Association, Washington, DC.
3. Hamilton P (1999). Care of the newborn in the delivery room. *BMJ* **318**, 1403–6.

Home birth

Introduction

Current evidence suggests that, for low-risk women and their babies, outcomes attributed to birth at home may be as good as those for birth in hospital. Positive outcomes are both clinical and psychological. However, in some instances, the lack of access to emergency cesarean delivery may be detrimental. There will need to be a discussion on a case-by-case basis. Anyone considering a home birth should be strongly advised to discuss this request with her primary obstetric care provider as soon as possible.

Providing information

Information should be tailored to the particular woman and her baby. Factors to be discussed include the following:

- The woman's clinical history.
- The progress of her current pregnancy.
- Her plans and expectations for labor and birth, and those of her partner.
- Available obstetric/midwifery expertise in the community.
- Availability to the family of transport.
- Time needed to travel to the nearest acute obstetric unit at all times of day and night.
- Access to a telephone.
- Available family and community support.

Information should be given in an unbiased, non-threatening, and sensitive manner. It should take into account medical, obstetric, and psychiatric history and social factors.

Explanations need to be specific, concise, realistic, and tailored to the individual situation. Statements based on absolute risk may be more useful than those based on relative risk. For example, the statement: 'the risk of perinatal death when the pregnancy is continued beyond 41 weeks' gestation is 7 per 3000 compared with 1 per 3000 when labor is induced' may be more helpful than stating that 'the risk is seven times greater'.

Establishing risks and benefits

The theoretical risk of a problem in pregnancy does not automatically rule out the option of a home birth. In the event of the risk materializing during the course of the pregnancy, the plan can be changed. Conversely, if a risk factor is identified early in pregnancy but subsequently resolves (e.g. screening for fetal abnormality), a home birth can again be considered.

In discussing risk, a distinction should be made between the following:

- Any actual condition with a high imminent risk to mother or baby (e.g. pregestational diabetes, placenta previa, preeclampsia, or prior cesarean delivery).

- Any actual condition or history of a condition with a low risk of acute adverse event in labor or with a nonimminent risk of recurrence (e.g. nulliparity, maternal age over 35, or previous forceps for failure to progress).
- History of a risk that is minimized before labor (e.g. previous history of congenital fetal abnormality when no screening tests in this pregnancy signify risk).

In some unusual cases, such as a baby with a lethal congenital abnormality or a known intrauterine death, where there are no anticipated maternal complications, a woman and her family may seek a home birth. They should be informed of the likely maternal risks in their particular case.

Legal issues

- Until delivered, the fetus has very limited legal rights. Therefore decisions about safety cannot be made for the fetus against the wishes of a mentally competent mother.
- Even where mental incompetence is suspected, intervention cannot take place against her expressed wishes without the ratification of a court order.
- The legal position on the right of access to a home birth in most countries is currently unclear.

General points

- Only the woman and her family can make the final assessment of the relative risks and benefits to them and their baby. Although you may not actually support the mother's decision, you should make every effort to respect her considered choice.
- All discussions about a patient's desire for home birth and her final decision should be recorded in detail in the medical record.
- Failure or the inability to support a home birth does not preclude the capacity to administer care in an emergency situation should a patient present to an Emergency Room or Labor & Birth unit with a labor-related complication.

Recommended further reading

1. Hodnett ED, Downe S, Edwards N, Walsh D (2005). Home-like versus conventional institutional settings for birth. *Cochrane Database Syst Rev* **1**, CD000012.
2. Chamberlain G, Wraight A, Crowley P, eds (1997). *Home Births*. Parthenon, Carnforth.

Chapter 7

Postnatal care

Care in the puerperium

Introduction

The puerperium is the time when the mother's body is returning to its prepregnant state. Most of the physical changes are complete by 6 weeks. The puerperium is also a time for psychological adjustment—the mother's joy at the arrival of the new baby may be tempered by anxiety about her child's welfare and her ability to cope, and these anxieties may be compounded if she is tired after labor or if there were medical complications during labor. Although the puerperium is a time of great importance for mother and baby, it is an aspect of maternity care that has received little attention.

Physiological changes to the uterus and lower genitourinary tract in the puerperium

Involution of the uterus and renal system

The postpartum uterus, which weighs about 1 kg, returns to its pre-pregnancy weight of around 80 g. Post-delivery, the uterine fundus lies just below the umbilicus but, by 2 weeks, it can no longer be felt above the symphysis. This process of involution involves autolysis of muscle cells, with absorption of the protein into the circulation and excretion with the urine.

- The most common causes of delayed involution include full bladder, loaded rectum, uterine infection, retained placental fragments or membranes, fibroids, or possible broad ligament hematoma.
- By the end of the second week, the cervical internal os is closed and unable to admit a finger, while the stretched, smooth, and edematous vaginal walls regain their ruggae by the third week postnatally.
- If lactation is suppressed, the uterine cavity is covered by new endometrium by 3 weeks and the first menstruation occurs by 6 weeks. In breast-feeding mothers, ovarian activity is suppressed and resumption of menstruation may be delayed for many months.
- During the first few days, the bladder and the urethra may show evidence of minor trauma sustained at delivery, but this resolves rapidly. Within 2–3 weeks the calyceal dilatation and hydorureter become less evident, although complete return to normality takes 6–8 weeks.

Lochia

This blood-stained uterine discharge consists of blood and necrotic superficial decidua. During the first few days the lochia is red, then it gradually changes to pink, and by the end of the second week it becomes serous.

- Persistent red lochia may be associated with infection or retained products of conception.
- Uterine tenderness with pyrexia and offensive lochia is highly suggestive of intrauterine infection (postpartum endometritis) and justifies immediate treatment with broad-spectrum antibiotics and, if there are retained products, surgical evacuation of the uterus with antibiotic cover.

Problems in the puerperium I

Thrombosis and thromboembolism

Venous thromboembolic events account for the largest proportion of maternal deaths in the puerperium. Over half of all cases of pregnancy-related maternal death occur in the puerperium, and the majority follow cesarean delivery. Therefore it is essential to adhere to thromboprophylaxis guidelines and to have a high index of suspicion in women who have recently given birth when they present with signs or symptoms that raise the possibility of thromboembolic disease and to investigate them appropriately.

Perineal pain/discomfort

Perineal discomfort is the most common problem encountered postnatally, occurring in 42% of women immediately after spontaneous vaginal delivery and persisting for more than 2 months in 8–10%. These figures following operative vaginal delivery are 84% and 30%, respectively. Perineal pain is worse following instrumental delivery, episiotomy, or spontaneous vaginal tears. Treatments such as local cooling and topical applications of local anesthetic provide short-term relief (24 hours), with longer relief being provided by NSAIDs. It is important to exclude infection as a result of bacterial contamination. If there are signs of infection, this needs to be aggressively treated with antibiotics and drainage of any collection of pus. Where an episiotomy or tear repair breaks down, resuturing is contraindicated in the presence of infection and healing by secondary intention should be allowed.

Bladder dysfunction

- Voiding difficulties and urinary retention may occur after delivery, especially if regional anesthesia has been used. Loss of bladder sensation with epidural or spinal anesthetic may lead to overstretching of the detrusor muscle, dampening bladder sensation with subsequent voiding difficulties.
- Difficult instrumental delivery and multiple or extended perineal lacerations may cause pain and periurethral edema which may impede voiding.
- Other sources of pain, such as prolapsed hemorrhoids, abdominal wound pain, or even fecal impaction, may all contribute to voiding difficulties.
- In general, after a cesarean delivery under regional anesthesia, an indwelling catheter is left for 12–24 hours to avoid bladder overdistention, and it may also be advisable to use this approach where a difficult instrumental delivery with extensive perineal repair has been performed.
- If there is any difficulty voiding, it is always good practice to send a specimen of urine for culture and sensitivity to exclude underlying infection.
- Incontinence early in puerperium should be investigated to exclude the rare possibility of a vesicovaginal fistula.

- Urinary tract infection (UTI) is not uncommon in the puerperium with 3–5% reporting a UTI in the first year after delivery and a further 5% reporting urinary frequency for the first time after delivery. The increased incidence of UTIs may be due to bladder stasis, voiding difficulties, and catheterization in labor. Management involves the appropriate use of antibiotics.

Bowel function

Constipation is common in pregnancy and remains so in the puerperium. The problem of constipation may be further exacerbated by fear of defecation due to pain of prolapsed hemorrhoids (affecting 18% of women), anal fissure, or the sutured perineum. The importance of avoiding straining at defecation is greatest where there has been a third- or fourth-degree tear repair. Narcotic analgesics can exacerbate the problem. Hence, such women should have stool softeners prescribed routinely.

It is now becoming clear that the trauma to the anal sphincter is greater than previously thought, with 35% of primiparas having occult anal sphincter trauma on anal endosonography, but only 13% admitting to bowel symptoms by 6 weeks postpartum. Both direct trauma and nerve damage following spontaneous or operative vaginal delivery contribute to this. Incontinence of flatus or feces is reported in 4% of women after delivery. Furthermore, 20–50% of women who had primary third- and fourth-degree repairs may suffer some degree of fecal or flatus incontinence. Thus follow-up in the hospital setting should be arranged as a routine after third- or fourth-degree tear repairs. It is essential that such women are encouraged to come forward for proper investigation and treatment.

Problems in the puerperium II

Postnatal depression and tiredness

10–15% of women experience postnatal depression within the first year after delivery. Tiredness is the most commonly reported problem post-delivery, affecting 42% of women while in hospital and rising to 54% at 2 months. Extreme exhaustion lasting at least 6 weeks is reported in 12%, but may well represent underlying postpartum depression.

Breast problems

Two-thirds of women who start breast-feeding report problems. These problems (nipple pain, engorgement, cracks, and bleeding) are preventable or surmountable with advice regarding positioning of the baby's mouth coupled with sympathetic supportive counseling. In cases of mastitis, feeding should continue to overcome the blocked duct, while a breast abscess will need incision and drainage. Both conditions may need a course of antibiotics.

Late postpartum hemorrhage

The most common presentation is at 7–14 days after delivery, and is generally due to retained placental tissues. The differential diagnosis includes endometritis, hormonal contraception, bleeding disorders, and choriocarcinoma. Management is according to the underlying cause but, if bleeding is heavy, resuscitation of the patient is the first priority followed by careful examination in the operating room and curettage of the uterus under antibiotic cover, if indicated.

Traumatic neuritis

This may present with footdrop, paresthesia, hypoesthesia, sciatic pain, and muscle wasting in one or both lower limbs following delivery. The mechanism is as yet not fully elucidated, but may be associated with herniation of the lumbosacral discs at L4–5 due to exaggerated lithotomy and instrumental delivery. The management entails bed rest, physiotherapy, and spinal/orthopedic opinion with appropriate imaging.

Perineal neuritis may result from compression of the perineal nerve between the head of the fibula and the lithotomy pole, and presents as footdrop. Treatment is supportive with physiotherapy. Resolution is almost always complete.

Diastasis of the symphysis pubis

The incidence is around 0.1% after spontaneous vaginal delivery. It may be associated with a forceps delivery, a rapid second stage, or exaggerated flexion and abduction of maternal thighs such as in McRobert's maneuver. The symptoms are of pain over the symphysis, which is exaggerated by weight-bearing. The clinical signs are a waddling gait, tenderness over the joint, and, occasionally, a palpable interpubic gap. Management is supportive with bed rest, physiotherapy, analgesia and anti-inflammatory drugs, and a pelvic support brace.

Puerperal pyrexia

Puerperal pyrexia is defined as a maternal temperature >38°C (100.4°F) on more than one occasion in the first 14 days after delivery.

Etiology

- 90% of infections are genital or urinary tract in origin. Genital tract infections are commonly due to *E.coli, Streptococcus A* or *B*, or *Clostridium*. Urinary tract infections are predominantly due to *E.coli, Proteus*, or *Klebsiella*.
- Other causes are mastitis (usually staphylococcal), infected perineal or cesarean delivery wounds, chest infections, and infected pelvic hematomas.
- Venous thrombosis may be associated with pyrexia, as may breast engorgement without infection.
- Uterine infections are more likely following prolonged rupture of the membranes (>18 hours) and after instrumental delivery.

Diagnosis

History

- Check for prolonged rupture of membranes, intrapartum pyrexia, prolonged labor, operative delivery, and any difficulty with the delivery of the placenta.
- Ask about associated symptoms of offensive or unusually heavy lochia and abdominal, breast, or wound pain.
- Ask about any previous treatment and allergies.
- Perineal infections usually present around the second day after delivery.

Examination

- Check the patient's general condition, pulse, and blood pressure.
- Check the breasts for any areas of tenderness and erythema and listen to the chest.
- Inspect abdominal wound for swelling or associated cellulitis.
- Check the fundal height and tenderness of the uterus.
- Perform a gentle pelvic examination and check the appearance of the perineum.
- Assess for tenderness of the uterus on bimanual examination and look for evidence of swelling in the adnexae. Endometritis is associated with lower abdominal pain, offensive liquor, and a tender uterus on bimanual vaginal examination.
- Check legs for signs of superficial thrombophlebitis or deep vein thrombosis.

Investigations

- Send a midstream urine sample for culture.
- Take swabs for bacterial culture and for *Chlamydia* from the cervix and lochia.
- Take sample of sputum or any discharge from wounds or nipples for culture.
- Take blood for CBC and cultures.

Management

Initial therapy depends on diagnosis, allergies, and whether the patient is breast-feeding (e.g. avoid tetracyclines if breast-feeding). For suspected pelvic infections, start with Amoxil 500 mg three times a day (erythromycin if allergic to penicillin) and metronidazole 400 mg three times a day or Augmentin 675 mg three time a day. Substitute flucloxacillin 250 mg three times a day for Amoxil for wound or breast infections. Encourage the patient to continue milk expression to prevent blockage of the milk ducts and breast engorgement. Trimethoprim 200 mg twice a day is a suitable alternative for UTIs.

- *Intravenous therapy* should be used if the patient is vomiting, systemically unwell, has diabetes mellitus, or you suspect pyelonephritis or necrotizing fasciitis.
- *If the patient fails to respond* to initial therapy, review the results of the initial cultures, assess her clinically, and arrange a pelvic ultrasound scan to exclude pelvic collection. If there is a wound or a pelvic or breast abscess, it may need draining. Otherwise, change antibiotics according to sensitivities or, if these are not available, consider adding gentamicin or a third-generation cephalosporin.

Early involvement of microbiologists is invaluable in severely ill patients and those who fail to respond to treatment. If group B β-hemolytic *Streptococcus*, *Chlamydia*, or *Neisseria gonorrhea* are cultured, inform the pediatricians if the patient is still in hospital or the patient's primary care provider if she has been discharged home so that the baby can be tested for infection. Early surgical referral is essential if there is any evidence of rapidly evolving cellulitis with necrosis of the overlying skin and breast infection not responding to treatment with antibiotics. A diagnosis of necrotizing fasciitis should be entertained, especially if the patient is diabetic and delivered by cesarean.

Breast-feeding

Breast-feeding is the healthiest way to feed a baby and has important health benefits for both mother and baby. The WHO/UNICEF Baby Friendly Hospital Initiative summarizes the practices necessary to support breast-feeding in the hospital and community.

In order to make an informed decision about how to feed a baby, it is vital that information is available to women before they give birth.

Benefits

- Protects baby against:
  - gastroenteritis
  - urinary tract infections
  - ear infections
  - chest infections.
- Reduces the risk of accidental scalding/burns.
- Reduces risk of allergies and juvenile-onset diabetes.
- Babies have better mental, tooth, and jaw development.
- Protects mother against:
  - premenopausal breast cancer
  - ovarian cancer
  - osteoporosis.
- Contraceptive effect, if exclusively breast-feeding (but should not be relied upon).
- Reduces risk of postpartum hemorrhage and aids uterine involution.

Disadvantages of formula

Formula-fed infants are disadvantaged because of constituents of the formula, production problems that lead to excesses or deficiencies in substances, and accidental contamination. Immunologically, formula cannot compete with breast milk.

Steps to success

- *Skin-to-skin contact after delivery*. Encourage contact within 30 minutes of birth. This helps to keep the baby warm and to stabilize the baby's heart rate and breathing. It calms the baby, promotes bonding, and can help to start off breast-feeding.
- *Initiating the first breast-feed*. Encourage babies to breast-feed soon after they are born. Babies can be weighed and have a neonatal check before initiating skin-to-skin contact and feeding.
- *Rooming in*. Baby stays with mother all the time. This builds the mother's confidence in caring for the baby and helps her to learn feeding signals, and how to comfort the baby.
- *Demand feeding*. Healthy term babies can feed whenever they want, for as long as they want. This helps in establishing and maintaining a good milk supply.
- *Help and support*. Midwives, infant-feeding advisors, health visitors, and breast-feeding/lactation counselors are available for support. Peer support groups can also be vital in increasing the number of women who continue to breast-feed. It is important not to give conflicting advice. Positively supporting the mother's efforts is vital even when advising change.

- Importance of good positioning and attachment.
  - In the mother this prevents sore nipples, breast engorgement, poor milk supply, blocked ducts, and mastitis.
  - In the baby, this prevents a hungry baby, an unsettled baby, low weight gain, and prolonged feeding.
- *Pacifiers and teats whilst breast-feeding.* Avoid using until breast-feeding is established. This helps to prevent a poor supply of breast milk and nipple–teat confusion.

Recommended further reading

1. Sikorski J, Renfrew MJ (2000). Support for breastfeeding mothers. *Cochrane Database Syst Rev* **2**, CD001141.
2. Dyson L, McCormick F, Renfrew MJ (2005). Interventions for promoting the initiation of breastfeeding. *Cochrane Database Syst Rev* **2**, CD001688.

Initiating breast-feeding and expressing breast milk

Initiating breast-feeding

Remember, breast-feeding is natural but it is not always instinctive. Some babies need to learn how and some learn faster than others. Before feeding, women should make themselves comfortable—a chair may be more practical than sitting on a bed. A pillow to help support baby may be required. Initially, it may be better to undress the baby down to its nappy to prevent overheating.

Holding the baby

The mother can hold the baby in a number of positions for feeding. One way is to hold the baby horizontally, head opposite the nipple, turned completely on its side with legs under the arm. The baby's bottom is brought close with the elbow and the baby's neck and shoulder are supported between spread-out fingers and thumb. The baby's head should fall back gently between the V-shape that the finger and thumb create, which helps raise the baby's chin off its chest so that its mouth can be opened wide.

Attaching baby to the breast

- Cup breast underneath with the hand, the little finger touching the ribs and the thumb resting on edge of areola in a C-shape.
- Fingers are then kept away from areola and nipple. The nipple should be lined up with baby's nose and not be aimed centrally into the mouth. The baby will smell the milk and open its mouth wide.
- The baby should be brought to the breast and the bottom lip should make contact with the areola, well away from the base of the nipple. The mother's thumb quickly slides or rolls forward the nipple under the palate.
- Once a good feeding rhythm is established, the hand should be slowly released from the breast and brought to rest under the baby. The baby should be held firm and close as if gently 'squashing' him or her.
- A drawing sensation is felt on initial attachment; thereafter no pain should be felt. The baby initially suckles quickly to facilitate the let-down reflex, and then nutritive feeding is established with a rhythmical slow suck–swallow pattern.

Early days

Healthy term babies may not feed very much in the first 48 hours. Colostrum (first milk) is high density and low volume; the neonate's immature kidneys cannot cope with large volumes of fluid without metabolic stress. Despite the small quantity, colostrum provides sufficient fluid and nutrients for healthy term babies. A busy feeding period usually follows and soon passes. Frequent feeds according to the baby's demands will reduce the risk of engorgement and maintain milk supply. Breast milk changes to meet the needs of the baby as he or she grows and matures.

Expressing breast milk

This is an essential skill that enables a mother to know where her milk reservoirs are. Expressed milk on the nipple can tease the baby to open his or her mouth and can help relieve engorgement or blocked ducts.

Gently massage the breast and stimulate the nipple to encourage the let-down reflex.

1. Position the thumb and the first two fingers about 2.5–3.5 cm behind the nipple. Place the thumb above the nipple and the fingers below in a C-shape. The fingers are positioned so that the milk reservoirs lie beneath them.
2. Push straight into the chest wall—avoid spreading the fingers apart. For large breasts, first lift and then push into the chest wall.
3. Roll thumb and fingers forward as if making thumb and finger prints at the same time. The rolling motion of the thumb and fingers compresses and empties the milk reservoirs without hurting sensitive breast tissue.
4. Repeat rhythmically to drain the reservoirs, i.e. position, push, roll, release; position, push, roll, release.
5. Rotate the thumb and finger position to milk the other reservoirs. Use both hands on each breast for more effective expressing.

Recommended further reading

1. Sikorski J, Renfrew MJ (2000). Support for breastfeeding mothers. *Cochrane Database Syst Rev* **2**, CD001141.
2. Dyson L, McCormick F, Renfrew MJ (2005). Interventions for promoting the initiation of breastfeeding. *Cochrane Database Syst Rev* **2**, CD001688.

Problems associated with breast-feeding

Women who experience problems with breast-feeding should have access to trained staff and voluntary breast-feeding counselors.

- *Sore and cracked nipples* should not occur if the baby is correctly attached at the breast. Expressed breast milk can be helpful during the healing phase.
- *Nipple sensitivity* is usually transient. It is due to enhanced lactational hormones, prolactin, and oxytocin. On examination, there is usually no obvious nipple damage, only occasional redness, and the mother needs reassurance that this will resolve.
- *Breast fullness (engorgement)*. Breasts can become full when the milk comes in. This should not occur if the baby is demand feeding and attached correctly to the breast. If breasts become red and painful, it is resolved by correctly attaching the baby to the breast and should quickly improve. Simple analgesia may be helpful; ice packs or hot flannels should be used with caution.
- *Mastitis (noninfective)* is characterized by a pink-red flushing over the breast, which may or may not be associated with lumpy areas and influenza-like symptoms. It is caused by a build-up of breast milk which has not been effectively removed from the breast. Antibiotics are not usually required; correct positioning and attachment is essential. Hand expressing to improve quality of attachment before feeding or after feeding may be beneficial. Symptoms should subside quickly and usually resolve within 24 hours. If noninfective mastitis is incorrectly managed, it may lead to infective mastitis.
- *Mastitis (infective)* is characterized by a red lumpy area of breast, usually wedge-shaped, pyrexia, pain, and influenza-like symptoms. It may be caused by a blocked duct, infection, or poor attachment. It is important to find the cause of mastitis as it can lead to abscess formation if left untreated. Breast-feeding should continue. Breast-feeding from the infected breast first is recommended to facilitate effective milk removal, but if breast-feeding at the affected breast is too painful, milk should be expressed to facilitate milk removal and maintain the milk supply. If symptoms do not improve, treatment with antibiotics may be necessary and breast-feeding should be continued.
- *Breast abscess* is a possible complication of infective mastitis which is poorly managed, and is most likely to occur when breast-feeding is stopped abruptly. Breast-feeding from the infected breast can continue, but if this is too painful, milk should be expressed to facilitate milk removal and maintain the milk supply. Symptoms include elevated temperature, red swollen area, and possible discharge from the affected area. It is important that medical opinion is sought and that antibiotics are administered. Abscesses require surgical incision and drainage, and breast-feeding may cease if symptoms do not resolve.
- There are, on rare occasions, a number of situations where infants cannot breast-feed or should not be breast-fed, e.g. when mother is on certain medications or has certain infections (such as HIV or hepatitis C). If in doubt, consult a specialist in neonatology or maternal–fetal medicine.

Inborn errors of metabolism with implications for breast-feeding

Some congenital and hereditary disorders are characterized by specific enzyme deficiencies and severely limit the use of certain milk components. Some of these disorders present as failure to thrive while breast-feeding and a sudden worsening of symptoms when weaned while others are alleviated by breast-feeding.

- *Galactosemia*. There are two main forms of this disease. One is characterized by a deficiency of galactokinase in which infants who are fed breast milk or given any lactose-containing preparation can develop cataracts. The other form, which is even more serious, is due to a deficiency of galactose-1 phosphate uridyl transferase. The resulting metabolite accumulates in the blood, causing considerable damage. Symptoms include diarrhea, vomiting, hepatomegaly, jaundice, and splenomegaly. Cataracts, hepatic cirrhosis, and mental retardation will result unless lactose is excluded from the diet.
- *Phenylketonuria* is characterized by defective metabolism in the amino acid phenylalanine hydroxylase. This can result in moderate to severe mental retardation. Routine genetic screening can confirm the diagnosis, and the clinical condition can be almost entirely avoided by providing a low-phenylalanine diet. Fortunately, breast milk contains a low concentration of this amino acid (far lower than that in cow's milk). Thus babies suffering from phenylketonuria may be breastfed while their phenylalanine levels are monitored. Breast milk can then be replaced by low-phenylalanine milk formula.
  - Incidence: 1–20 per 100 000 population.
- *Maple syrup urine disease*. This rare disease is due to a defect in the metabolism of the branch-chain amino acids valine, leucine, and isoleucine. It is characterized by the typical maple-syrup color of the urine, refusal of food, vomiting, metabolic acidosis, and progressive neurological and mental retardation. Special synthetic formulas have been developed for feeding such infants, although outcomes are usually poor.
  - Incidence: 0.5 per 100 000 population.

Recommended further reading

1. Sikorski J, Renfrew MJ (2000). Support for breastfeeding mothers. *Cochrane Database Syst Rev* **2**, CD001141.
2. Dyson L, McCormick F, Renfrew MJ (2005). Interventions for promoting the initiation of breastfeeding. *Cochrane Database Syst Rev* **2**, CD001688.

Chapter 8

Obstetric emergencies

Maternal collapse

The causes of maternal collapse are numerous. They may be related to pregnancy or may be incidental causes which may have been aggravated by pregnancy. The management needs to concentrate on resuscitation of the patient whilst simultaneously working out the diagnosis to institute appropriate treatment.

Obstetric causes

- Postpartum hemorrhage (PPH) is by far the most common cause and is discussed separately
- Eclampsia
- Amniotic fluid embolism
- Uterine inversion
- Uterine rupture
- Intraabdominal bleeding such as broad ligament hematoma
- Unrecognized genital tract hematoma (especially if not associated with external trauma)

Incidental causes

- Massive thromboembolic event (including pulmonary embolism)
- Ruptured hepatic, splenic, or aortic aneurysm
- Ruptured liver or spleen
- Myocardial infarction
- Cardiac cause, e.g. arrhythmia or cardiac failure
- Cerebrovascular accident
- Subarachnoid hemorrhage
- Anaphylactic shock
- Septic shock
- Metabolic/endocrine cause
- Abuse of medication/substance abuse

Management

Maternal resuscitation is the first priority. This involves securing an airway (A), ensuring ventilation if necessary by bag and mask or intubation and administration of 100% oxygen (B), and maintaining the circulation if necessary by extenal cardiac massage (C). Assistance from an experienced obstetrician and anesthesiologist should be summoned. Operating room staff should be forewarned that there may be a need for urgent laparotomy. The direction of initial investigations will be dictated by symptoms and signs and events leading up to the collapse from the primary provider or from the patient if she is alert/conscious.

A full clinical examination including a neurological assessment should be made. In general, adequate IV access by two large-bore cannulas is always useful for administration of fluids to support the circulation as well as to administer drugs required in the resuscitation process.

- Baseline blood tests (CBC, cross-match specimen, coagulation screen, electrolytes, blood glucose, and liver function) should be performed.

- Monitoring of pulse, blood pressure, oxygen saturation, and urine output needs to be instituted, and the need for invasive monitoring addressed.
- If a cardiorespiratory cause is suspected, a chest x-ray, arterial blood gases, electrocardiography (EKG), and possibly echocardiogram may be required.
- Alteration in consciousness in the absence of cardiorespiratory signs raises the possibility of a neurologic lesion (cerebrovascular accident, subarachnoid hemorrhage (SAH), or previously undiagnosed space-occupying lesion (SOL)) but may also suggest a metabolic or endocrine problem.
- Where a neurologic cause is suspected, imaging of the brain and consultation with a neurologist are the investigations of choice.

Where there is no excessive external bleeding or any other cause to account for the maternal collapse, the possibility of massive internal hemorrhage should be considered. This may be a consequence of a ruptured uterus due to a previous scar, ruptured viscus such as liver or spleen, or a ruptured splenic, hepatic, or aortic aneurysm. Intraperitoneal bleeding will cause peritonism and circulatory changes out of proportion to external signs. Abdominal girth may be noted to be increasing and abdominal ultrasound may reveal free fluid in the peritoneal cavity. If the maternal collapse is due to massive internal bleeding, an emergency laparotomy will be required to bring it under control, possibly with the involvement of other disciplines such as general surgery, with postoperative care in an intensive care setting.

The possibility of occult genital tract hematoma should also be remembered as, in certain situations (such as operative vaginal delivery), there may be a large supralevator hematoma presenting with shock and maternal collapse without external evidence of hemorrhage or trauma. Bimanual examination may reveal a mass in either iliac fossa or a mass in the vaginal fornix displacing the uterus.

The management of specific obstetric causes such as eclampsia, massive PPH, uterine inversion, and amniotic fluid embolism are discussed in other chapters.

The general principles of management are to resuscitate and stabilize maternal condition, organize initial investigations on the basis of the working diagnoses, involve senior members of the clinical team, and obtain assistance from other relevant disciplines whilst ensuring adequate documentation of events and management. If the fetus is viable (>24 weeks), continuous fetal heart rate monitoring is recommended and delivery considered if there is evidence of continued nonreassuring fetal testing ('fetal distress').

Recommended further reading

1. American College of Obstetricians and Gynecologists (1995). ACOG Technical Bulletin No. 199. Blood component therapy. *Int J Gynaecol Obstet* **48**, 233–8.

Shoulder dystocia

Introduction

Shoulder dystocia refers to a difficulty in delivery of the shoulders after delivery of the head. This is due to the anterior shoulder being impacted under the symphysis pubis or, very rarely, the posterior shoulder being impacted against the sacral promontory.

This occurs in approximately 1 in 200 deliveries. When it occurs, shoulder dystocia is an acute obstetric emergency which necessitates prompt and skilful intervention in order to prevent serious fetal trauma or death. Anticipation and stepwise management are the keys to a successful outcome.

Associations

Fetal macrosomia (defined as an estimated fetal weight ≥4500 g) and diabetes are the most important factors associated with shoulder dystocia. It occurs in 9% of babies with a birth weight >4000 g, 15% if >4500 g, and 40% if >5000 g. However, even in the presence of risk factors (below), it is difficult to predict the occurrence of shoulder dystocia accurately. The majority of shoulder dystocia cases occur in nondiabetic women delivering babies weighing <4000 g.

Anticipation—antenatal associations

Several risk factors for shoulder dystocia have been identified:

- Multiparity.
- Prepregnancy obesity.
- Previous large baby.
- History of a previous shoulder dystocia (recurrence rate is about 10%).
- Excessive weight gain in pregnancy.
- Diabetes—both pregestational and gestational.
- A clinically large baby with a symphyseal–fundal height larger than expected for gestational age.
- Post-term pregnancies.
- Ultrasound estimation of fetal weight >90th percentile for gestational age or >5000 g in nondiabetic women (>4500 g in diabetic women).

Anticipation—intrapartum associations

- Prolonged labor, especially protracted late first stage with loosely applied cervix.
- Prolonged second stage of labor. However, shoulder dystocia is also associated with a precipitous second stage (<30 minutes).
- Midpelvic instrumental vaginal delivery.

In couples at risk of shoulder dystocia, a detailed discussion about the optimum mode of delivery should be held before the onset of labor. On occasion (such as women who have had a prior shoulder dystocia and have a recurrence risk of 10%), it may be appropriate to proceed with elective cesarean delivery.

Recommended further reading

1. American College of Obstetricians and Gynecologists (2003). ACOG Practice Bulletin No. 40. Shoulder dystocia. *Int J Gynaecol Obstet* **80**, 87–92.

Diagnosis of shoulder dystocia

Shoulder dystocia is diagnosed when the fetal head delivers and the shoulder does not emerge with the next bearing-down effort. Evidence of 'rosy fat cheeks' may suggest a large baby, especially if the mother is diabetic. On occasion, the fetal head will retract or recoil against the maternal perineum (the so-called 'turtle' sign), which is often a sign of a severe shoulder dystocia. Immediate assistance should be sought as soon as the diagnosis is suspected or made.

Management

- Call for help.
- Note the time.
- ***Primary maneuver*** Place the mother in McRobert's position so that her legs are slightly abducted and hyperflexed at 45° to the maternal abdomen. This position flattens the sacral promontory and increases the pelvic outlet. This maneuver is usually performed along with firm suprapubic (not fundal) pressure applied at an angle in an attempt to reduce the bisacromial diameter and dislodge the impacted anterior shoulder.
- Consider performing a generous episiotomy to help with manipulations.
- Avoid excessive downward traction on the fetal head as this can lead to a traction injury to the brachial plexus or even to the cervical spine and spinal cord.
- ***Secondary maneuvers*** McRobert's maneuver will resolve upwards of 85% of all cases of shoulder dystocia. If not successful, a secondary maneuver is indicated. Which maneuver to use depends on the clinical situation and the experience of the obstetric care provider. The maneuvers include the following:
  - Performing a copro-episiotomy.
  - Placing the patient in the knee–chest position to disimpact the anterior shoulder from behind the pubic symphysis.
  - Woods' screw maneuver in which operator places two fingers in front of the posterior shoulder and increases and splints the bisacromial diameter with a view to 'screwing' the baby out of the pelvis. In this way, the posterior shoulder moves anteriorly and the bisacromial diameter enters the larger oblique inlet diameter of the pelvis.
  - Rubin modification of Woods' maneuver in which the operator attempts to decrease the bisacromial diameter so that the fetus can squeeze through the pelvis.
  - Delivery of the posterior arm and shoulder by inserting the fingers into the restricted space available in the back of the baby's chest in order to flex the posterior arm at the elbow and then bring it down. Once the posterior arm has been brought down, there is more space in the pelvis and the anterior shoulder can be slipped behind the symphysis pubis, effecting the delivery. The major risk of this maneuver is fracture of the humerus.

- If these secondary maneuvers are also unsuccessful, it may be reasonable to attempt a ***salvage maneuver***. These include the following.
  - Cutting or fracture of the clavicle of the anterior shoulder (cleidotomy).
  - A symphysiotomy.
  - Replacement of the fetal head back into the uterus followed by cesarean delivery (Zavanelli maneuver).
- If the baby dies prior to delivery, cutting through both clavicles (cleidotomy) with strong scissors may assist delivery.
- A neonatologist or pediatrician and anesthesiologist should be on standby for assistance with both the mother and baby. The baby should be checked for possible damage, e.g. brachial plexus injury (Erb's palsy) or fractured clavicle or humerus.
- After the delivery, the procedure and the outcome should be explained to the parents and documented in the medical record.
- Should there be evidence of birth injury (orthopedic, peripheral nerve damage, or asphyxia), a postnatal visit should be arranged to counsel the parents about delivery options for future pregnancies.

Recommended further reading

1. American College of Obstetricians and Gynecologists (2003). ACOG Practice Bulletin No. 40. Shoulder dystocia. *Int J Gynaecol Obstet* **80**, 87–92.

Cord prolapse

The umbilical cord is said to be presenting (known as a funic presentation) when it lies over the cervix below the presenting part and the membranes are intact. If the membranes rupture, the cord may prolapse into the vagina. Cord prolapse is an obstetric emergency because of the risk of mechanical cord compression and/or occlusion of the umbilical arteries because of vasospasm causing fetal asphyxia. Delivery must be effected as quickly as possible. There is an increased incidence of cord prolapse with fetal malpresentations (such as breech or shoulder presentation), a high unengaged head, a premature or small fetus, an unduly long cord, or polyhydramnios. Artificial rupture of the membranes when the presenting part is poorly applied to the cervix is also a risk factor for cord prolapse. It is less likely to occur with spontaneous rupture of the membranes in labor as the presenting part is likely to be pushed down into the pelvis by uterine contractions.

Diagnosis

The diagnosis is made when a loop of cord is felt in the vagina or, rarely, may be seen at the vulva. In a woman at risk for this complication, it is good practice to perform an immediate vaginal examination after rupture of the membranes, whether or not she is having contractions, in order to exclude the diagnosis. A nonreassuring fetal heart rate pattern on CTG may suggest the diagnosis. The loop of cord should be felt to see if pulsations are present and the fetal heart should be auscultated at the same time (pulsations may be absent and the fetus may still be alive). If in doubt, perform an immediate ultrasound examination. The degree of cervical dilatation should be noted.

Management

The first goal of management is to replace the umbilical cord into the uterine cavity and prevent the presenting part from mechanically compressing and occluding the cord. This can be effected by putting a hand in the vagina and pushing the presenting part up to avoid pressure on the cord, especially during contractions. In addition, the woman may be placed either in a knee–elbow position (kneeling so her rump is higher than her head) or by backfilling the bladder with 500 mL of warm saline through a size 16 catheter. The cord should be kept in the vagina to keep it warm and moist to prevent the arteries going into spasm.

Delivery needs to be expedited. Attempts to replace the cord back into the uterine cavity above the presenting part and continue with attempted vaginal delivery are usually unsuccessful, and may also produce spasm of the cord vessels. If the cervix is fully dilated and the presenting part is sufficiently low in the pelvis, an immediate operative vaginal delivery may be performed. However, in the vast majority of cases, emergent cesarean delivery is indicated if the fetus is alive. If it is certain that the fetus is dead, labor can be continued with a view to achieving a vaginal delivery.

Massive obstetric hemorrhage

Massive obstetric hemorrhage is defined as blood loss >1500 mL or >25% of the circulating blood volume. Hemorrhage is the third most common cause of direct maternal mortality, accounting for 6.5% of all maternal deaths. Of all cases of massive obstetric hemorrhage, 50% are due to PPH, 25% to placenta previa, and 25% to placental abruption.

Normal response to blood loss

Normal blood flow to the uterus at term is 500 mL/minute. After delivery of the placenta, blood flow from the placental bed is controlled mainly by myometrial contraction, prostaglandin-mediated spasm of the spiral arterioles, and the formation of a fibrin clot over the placental bed. The higher plasma volume and red cell mass of the pregnant woman compensate for the blood loss associated with parturition.

The response to *excess blood loss* (10–15% of circulating volume) is to maintain blood flow to critical organs by a combination of increasing cardiac output and reducing the effective vascular volume. These changes are mediated through a combination of neural and hormonal mechanisms. Increased cardiac output occurs mainly as a result of an increase in heart rate with some increase in stroke volume. Endovascular volume is reduced by peripheral vasoconstriction. Blood flow to skin, skeletal muscle, gut, and kidney is reduced, while cerebral and myocardial perfusion are preserved.

Pathological response to blood loss

Fear, anxiety, and pain may lead to a counterproductive increase in blood pressure, whilst the release of endorphins counters the beneficial effects of increased sympathetic tone. Table 8.1 gives the clinical signs and symptoms associated with blood loss.

- *Cellular/microvascular level changes*. As tissue perfusion is reduced, anaerobic respiration leads to the release of lactic acid. When cellular adenosine triphosphate (ATP) production is insufficient to maintain membrane integrity, there is an influx of sodium, calcium, and water into the cells, release of potassium into the circulation, and cell death. Lysosomal contents from autolysis are then released into the circulation and locally acting vasodilators such as 5-HT overcome centrally mediated vasoconstriction and trigger DIC.
- *Tissue level changes*. Endothelial breakdown allows bacteria and toxins to enter the circulation. Impaired hepatic function cannot clear these, and this stimulates the development of defects in the clotting mechanism, allowing further blood loss.

Table 8.1 Clinical signs and symptoms

% Blood loss	Heart rate	Systolic blood pressure	Signs of tissue perfusion
10–15	Increased	Normal	Postural hypotension
15–30	Increased +	Normal	Peripheral vasoconstriction
30–40	Increased ++	70–80	Pallor, restlessness, oliguria
40+	Increased ++	50	Collapse, anuria, air hunger

Management of massive obstetric hemorrhage

The aim is to control blood loss and restore oxygen-carrying volume to the tissues. For the treatment of specific causes of blood loss see Chapter 2 📖 *p.90* on antepartum hemorrhage and the section of Chapter 6 📖 *p.310* covering postpartum hemorrhage.

Immediate treatment

1. Summon help. This should include the obstetrician attending if not already present, maternal–fetal medicine specialist, anesthesiologist, additional nursing and operating room staff, and possibly the hematologist on call.
2. Set up two large-bore IV lines (16 gauge or larger).
3. Take 30 mL of blood for cross-matching (minimum six units), CBC, and clotting studies.
4. Replace circulating volume with crystalloid (lactated Ringer's, dextrose saline, or 0.9% sodium chloride solution) or a plasma expander (such as albumin). Crystalloids lack oncotic pressure and fluid will tend to move into the extravascular space over time, and so they should not be over-used. However, an initial fluid challenge of up to 2 L in a young woman is unlikely to cause pulmonary edema unless there are other causes of endothelial damage such as preeclampsia.
5. Commence oxygen by face mask at 8–10 L/minute.
6. Catheterize to follow urinary output.
7. Give blood as soon as possible. Restoration of normovolemia is the first priority. If the bleeding is controlled and the blood pressure stable after IV fluids, transfusion can be delayed until cross-matched blood is available. If a more urgent transfusion is required, ABO and Rh (D) compatible blood should be given. The use of non-cross-matched O-negative blood is usually only indicated where the estimated blood loss exceeds 40% of circulating volume and the patient is severely compromised. Blood should be given using a suitable compression cuff and a blood warmer once more than two units have been given. Blood filters are generally unnecessary and serve only to slow transfusion in an emergency situation.
8. Stop active bleeding. Attempts at aggressive resuscitation will not be successful if there is ongoing blood loss. Bleeding may be evident clinically (such as ongoing vaginal bleeding) or may be concealed (such as intraabdominal bleeding in the setting of uterine rupture or broad ligament hematoma). If the patient is stable, imaging studies (such as CT or MRI) may identify the source of the bleeding. Selective arterial embolization by interventional radiology can help to stem ongoing bleeding, but only if time permits. Emergent explorative laparotomy may be required.

If more than 40% (six units) of blood volume have been lost

- Give additional colloid (and possibly human serum albumin) with further packed cells.
- In consultation with the on-call hematologist, replace clotting factors, fresh frozen plasma, cryoprecipitate, and platelets as indicated. Repeat platelet count and coagulation studies.
- Give additional calcium if indicated by serum biochemistry, using 10% calcium chloride.
- Replete other electrolytes, including potassium and magnesium.
- Site central venous and arterial lines.
- Continue to monitor for ongoing bleeding.

Once the bleeding is controlled

- Monitor pulse, blood pressure, central venous pressure, blood gases, electrolytes, and urinary output.
- Repeat the coagulation profile as indicated.
- Consider transfer to an intensive ICU in consultation with the consultant obstetrician, anesthesiologist, and internist.

Early involvement of senior staff is essential, especially where there is ongoing bleeding or evidence of deranged clotting.

Recommended further reading

1. Mousa HA, Alfirevic Z (2003). Treatment for primary postpartum haemorrhage. *Cochrane Database Syst Rev* **1**, CD003249.
2. Neilson JP (2003). Interventions for treating placental abruption. *Cochrane Database Syst Rev* **1**, CD003247.
3. American College of Obstetricians and Gynecologists (1995). ACOG Technical Bulletin No. 199. Blood component therapy. *Int J Gynaecol Obstet* **48**, 233–8.

Amniotic fluid embolism

Amniotic fluid embolism (AFE) is a rare event estimated to occur in 1 in 20 000–80 000 deliveries. It remains a major cause of maternal death. In those who develop AFE, maternal mortality is around 60–70%. Maternal morbidity is significant and the fetus fares little better. The onset is rapid and death ensues quickly in many cases. The etiology remains obscure and management of the condition is mainly supportive care.

Pathophysiology

The similarities between the clinical presentations of AFE and anaphylactic and septic shock suggest a similar pathophysiology. Therefore the name 'anaphylactoid syndrome of pregnancy' has been suggested. AFE may involve an anaphylactoid response involving the nonimmunological release of endogenous mediators such as arachidonic acid metabolites. Another view of the development of AFE is that it is an immunoglobulin-mediated anaphylactic reaction. There is not enough evidence to support or refute either mechanism.

- Hypotension is an essential feature of AFE and is due to poor ventricular function.
- The other classic feature of this condition, namely profound hypoxia, leads to the neurological sequelae often seen in survivors of AFE.
- Even if the patient survives the initial insult, she may die from massive hemorrhage as a result of profound coagulopathy.

Clinical presentation

AFE may occur in the antenatal period, in a woman in labor, or in a woman who has just undergone vaginal delivery, cesarean delivery, or termination of pregnancy. It has even occurred up to 48 hours postpartum. It has also been known to complicate amniocentesis. The onset is sudden with cardiovascular collapse, hypoxia, cyanosis, and hypotension followed by cardiopulmonary arrest. It may be heralded by seizures.

If undelivered, there may be tetanic uterine contraction with subsequent fetal compromise. It was initially thought that the tetanic contractions precipitated the embolism of amniotic fluid into the uterine veins and maternal circulation. However, it now appears that the tetanic contractions are the result of AFE and are caused by a direct effect of high circulating levels of norepinephrine on the uterine musculature. The previously held belief that AFE was precipitated by oxytocin-induced labor and uterine hyperstimulation has not been borne out by recent studies.

Any one of the major features of AFE may dominate the clinical picture or not occur at all, which can confuse the initial picture. Death will result in 61–86% of cases, although this may be an overestimate as there may be milder presentations that currently remain undiagnosed. Because of the initial profound hypoxia—only 15% of the survivors remain neurologically intact.

The fetus fares badly as well. If it is *in utero* at the time of AFE, 80% survive but half have neurological sequelae secondary to profound hypoxia. Not surprisingly, survival is related to the timing of delivery. If delivered within 15 minutes, intact survival occurs in 67%. Thereafter, death or neurological sequelae are the most likely outcome.

The diagnosis of AFE can be problematic. Histological findings of fetal squames or mucin in the pulmonary vessels or aspirates from pulmonary artery catheter lines are neither sensitive nor specific, and the diagnosis of AFE remains clinical.

Management

Management is mainly supportive care aimed at maintaining blood pressure >90 mmHg systolic, urine output >25 mL/hour, and arterial oxygen tension >8 kPa, and correcting any clotting abnormality. Help should be summoned immediately and appropriate consultations made, e.g. with a hematologist, anesthesiologist, and respiratory physician. Standard cardiopulmonary resuscitation (CPR) should be instituted immediately if indicated because of either cardiac arrest or dysrhythmia.

- High-concentration oxygen should be administered and the woman intubated, if indicated.
- Left ventricular failure leading to hypotension is common, but may be treated with volume expansion to increase preload, followed by pressor support (dopamine) if hypotension persists.
- Invasive hemodynamic monitoring with pulmonary artery catheterization aids fluid replacement, which may be complicated.
- After the initial volume expansion, fluid should be restricted to prevent pulmonary edema and respiratory distress which may rapidly ensue.
- Clotting anomalies should be treated aggressively with fresh frozen plasma or fresh whole blood, if available.
- High-dose steroids may be given, although there is no consistent evidence supporting their use.
- In the event of cardiopulmonary arrest, maternal survival is very low. The resuscitation is more difficult in the presence of a gravid uterus, especially if >20 weeks in size. Therefore, if maternal resuscitation is not successful within 5 minutes, an immediate perimortem cesarean delivery should be undertaken for the sake of the fetus and to facilitate resuscitation of the mother.

Recommended further reading

1. Clark SL, Hankins GD, Dudley DA, Dildy GA, Porter TF (1995). Amniotic fluid embolism: analysis of the national registry. *Am J Obstet Gynecol* **172**, 1158–67.
2. Hankins GD, Snyder R, Dinh T, Van Hook J, Clark S, Vandelan A (2002). Documentation of amniotic fluid embolism via lung histopathology. Fact or fiction? *J Reprod Med* **47**, 1021–4.
3. Tuffnell DJ (2005). United Kingdom amniotic fluid embolism register. *Br J Obstet Gynecol* **112**, 1625–9.

Venous thromboembolism in pregnancy

Thromboembolic disease remains the leading cause of maternal death (approximately 2.1 in 10 000 pregnancies in developed countries). VTE risk rises sixfold in pregnancy (0.3–1.6% of all pregnancies; 20–50% occur antenatally, in any trimester, but they become more common as pregnancy advances).

There is an increased risk with the following:

- Immobility.
- Increased body mass index (BMI).
- Increasing maternal age.
- Increasing parity.
- Smoking.
- Air travel.
- Surgery (including cesarean delivery).
- Family history of deep vein thrombosis (DVT)/VTE (50% of those with VTE have thrombophilia syndrome).
- Caucasian race.
- Sickle cell disease.
- Women with antiphospholipid antibody syndrome with risk of arterial and venous thrombosis, which may occur in atypical sites such as in the arm on in the portal circulation.

Investigate any unexplained calf or chest symptoms on the same day. Often symptoms/signs are not obvious.

Previous or family history

In patients with a recurrent history of VTE or a family history strongly suggestive of VTE, a screen for inherited and acquired thrombophilias should be performed.

- *Factor V Leiden mutation.* Factor V is degraded by protein C. A genetic mutation in the factor V molecule (known as the Leiden mutation) affords resistance to activated protein C resulting in persistent activation of factor V leading to thrombosis. Many laboratories will only proceed with definitive DNA analysis if there is evidence of activated protein C resistance. The Leiden mutation is the most common abnormality seen in approximately 5% of Caucasian women. Heterozygotes for this mutation have a 10-fold increased risk of DVT. Homozygotes are rarely seen, but have a 100-fold increased risk of DVT.
- *Prothrombin (factor II) gene mutation.* This is the second most common inherited thrombophilia and is present in 2% of Caucasian women.
- *Antithrombin III deficiency.* This is very rare, but is the most thrombogenic of all inherited thrombophilias. As with the other disorders, it is autosomal dominant. A heterozygote has a 50–70% risk of having a significant venous thromboembolic event in pregnancy.
- *Protein C deficiency.*
- *Protein S deficiency.* This is a difficult diagnosis to make, because circulating protein S levels normally decrease in pregnancy.

- *Homocysteinemia*. The methylene tetrahydrofolate reductase gene 'mutation' is seen in 40–50% of Caucasian women. Therefore screening for this mutation is not recommended. A fasting serum homocysteine level should be measured in high-risk women. Treatment involves folic acid supplementation.
- *Antiphospholipid antibody syndrome*. This diagnosis requires two elements: the correct clinical setting (recurrent miscarriage, unexplained thromboembolic event, or autoimmune thrombocytopenia) and one or more confirmatory serologic tests, including positive lupus anticoagulant (LAC) and high-positive IgG anticardiolipin antibodies (ACA) or other identifiable antiphospholipid antibodies (such as anti-phosphatidylcholine, antiphosphatidylethanolamine). A false-positive serologic test for syphilis is not sufficient to make the diagnosis.

Liaise with hematologists if there is any doubt about the risk of DVT/pulmonary embolism (PE).

Recommended further reading

1. Lockwood CJ (2002). Inherited thrombophilias in pregnant patients: detection and treatment paradigm. *Obstet Gynecol* **99**, 333–41.
2. American College of Obstetricians and Gynecologists (2001). ACOG Practice Bulletin. Thromboembolism in pregnancy. *Int J Gynaecol Obstet* **75**, 203–12.

Deep vein thrombosis and pulmonary embolism

Deep vein thrombosis (DVT)

- *Incidence in pregnancy* 0.5–1.4%.
- *Presentation* Acutely painful swollen leg in the absence of trauma.
- *Signs*
  - Dorsiflexion of the calf may elicit pain (Homan's sign—poor clinical discriminator with a sensitivity of only 50%).
  - Calf and thigh commonly affected—turgid and tender.
  - Thirty percent of such patients do not have a DVT when assessed by venography.
- *Risks* PE and postphlebitic syndrome (skin swelling, ulceration).
- *Investigations*
  - Ultrasound imaging with Doppler flow studies (clot imaging, lack of vein compressibility, lack of vein dilatation during Valsalva maneuver) are good techniques for diagnosing proximal vein thromboses (iliac etc.) but not distal vein thromboses (e.g. in calf veins). Of note, calf vein thromboses seldom embolize.
  - Radionucleotide venography is the gold standard for the diagnosis, but the use of radioisotopes is not recommended in pregnancy.
  - Limited venography with shielding of the maternal abdomen in second or third trimesters may be undertaken if clinically indicated.
  - Consider MRI for investigation of suspected pelvic vein thromboses.

Pulmonary embolism (PE)

- *Incidence in pregnancy*. 0.3–1.2%. Small emboli may cause unexplained pyrexia, syncope, cough, chest pain, and breathlessness.
- Pleurisy should be considered to be caused by PE unless there is high fever or purulent sputum (which suggests pneumonia).
- Large emboli may present as collapse with chest pain, breathlessness, and cyanosis.
- *Signs* include raised jugular venous pressure (JVP), third heart sound, and parasternal heave.
- *Risks*. Untreated PE carries a maternal mortality of 13%.
- *Investigations:*
  - Chest X-ray.
  - EKG may be normal. Maternal tachycardia is the most sensitive sign of PE, but is not specific. The classic EKG pattern suggestive of PE is S1, Q3, T3.
  - Blood gases may show decreased p_aO_2 (partial arterial pressure of oxygen) and decreased or normal p_aCO_2 (due to hyperventilation as a consequence of chest pain and hypoxia). Arterial blood gas measurements are not particularly useful for the diagnosis of PE.
  - Ventilation–perfusion scans are safe in pregnancy. If the clinical suspicion of PE is high, consider instigating treatment whilst awaiting the test.
  - Consider spiral CT scan or MRI to confirm the diagnosis.

Recommended further reading

1. American College of Obstetricians and Gynecologists (2001). ACOG Practice Bulletin. Thromboembolism in pregnancy. *Int J Gynaecol Obstet* **75**, 203–12.

Counseling and prophylaxis

During prepregnancy counseling, initiate a thrombophilia screen when indicated and explain the risks to the mother and fetus from VTE and its treatment.

Prophylaxis

- *Low-risk group*, e.g. single episode of thromboembolism prior to pregnancy with no additional risk factors including no documented thrombophilia. Antenatal prophylaxis should be considered, but is not mandated. Postpartum prophylaxis should be employed.
  - Start unfractionated heparin (UFH) 7500 IU SC twice daily or low-molecular weight heparin (LMWH) (also known as fractionated heparin) once daily after delivery. Start oral warfarin (coumadin) on postpartum day 1 and overlap with heparin for 5–7 days. Then continue warfarin for at least 6 weeks.
- *High-risk group*, e.g. multiple thromboembolic episodes or single episode with a risk factor (such as a positive thrombophilia screen).
  - Start prophylactic UFH 10 000 IU SC twice daily or LMWH (enoxaparin 40 mg once daily or fragmin 5000 IU SC once daily) once pregnancy is confirmed. Prophylactic UFH does not change the activated partial thromboplastin time (aPTT). Prophylactic LMWH should be titrated to give an anti-factor Xa activity level measured 4 hours after SC injection of 0.1–0.3 U/mL.
  - Counsel regarding risk of thrombocytopenia and bone demineralization. Encourage calcium supplementation. CBC should be checked on days 3 and 7 after initiation of UFH and then every 4–6 weeks throughout gestation.
  - If on LMWH, switch to UFH at 35–36 weeks in preparation for labor. This is because UFH has a shorter half-life than LMWH (1 hour vs 8 hours), and it can be rapidly reversed using protamine sulfate, if necessary.
  - If on UFH, discontinue the night before a timed delivery at 39 weeks. Check immediate coagulation studies on the morning of induction.
  - Early consultation with anesthesiology regarding the use of regional anesthesia.
  - After delivery, restart UFH or LMWH in 6–8 hours. Start oral warfarin (coumadin) on postpartum day 1 and overlap with heparin for 5–7 days. Then continue warfarin for at least 6 weeks.
- *Thrombophilia screen positive patients*, e.g. those women who are 'screen positive' but have not had a VTE event themselves.
  - It is unclear whether such women need antenatal or postpartum prophylaxis. In general, only women with very high risk thrombophilias should be considered candidates for anticoagulation, e.g. women with antithrombin III deficiency or homozygous/compound heterozygous for prothrombin gene mutation or factor V Leiden mutation.

   - Women who are 'screen positive' for the other thrombophilias but without a history of VTE should only be considered for postpartum anticoagulation if they are obese, are immobilized, or were delivered by cesarean.
- *Patients with prosthetic heart valves.*
   - For such women, therapeutic anticoagulation with UFH is essential throughout pregnancy with aPTT levels at 2- to 2.5-fold control. LMWH is generally regarded as contraindicated in women with mechanical heart values because of a high failure rate.
   - Ideally, such patients should be switched from warfarin to UFH prior to conception, because of the risk of warfarin embryopathy in the first trimester.
   - Such women should have an anesthesia consultation in the third trimester and a timed delivery at 39 weeks, and should be off their anticoagulation for as short a time as possible. An elective cesarean and restarting anticoagulation with UFH within 4–6 hours of delivery may be appropriate in such women.
   - Warfarin can then be restarted on the first postoperative day and, once a therapeutic INR has been reached, UFH can be discontinued within 5–7 days. Women on warfarin can breast-feed.
   - Liaise with hematologists throughout the pregnancy.

Recommended further reading

1. Gates S, Brocklehurst P, Davis LJ (2002). Prophylaxis for venous thromboembolic disease in pregnancy and the early postnatal period. *Cochrane Database Syst Rev* **2**, CD001689.
2. American College of Obstetricians and Gynecologists (2001). ACOG Practice Bulletin. Thromboembolism in pregnancy. *Int J Gynaecol Obstet* **75**, 203–12.

Treatment of venous thromboembolism

Acute phase

An acute PE may present with massive cardiac collapse that is usually fatal. Treatment consists of cardiac resuscitation with consideration of pulmonary embolectomy. Although generally regarded as contraindicated in pregnancy, streptokinase or tissue plasminogen activator treatment in life-threatening emergencies may be considered if surgery is not immediately available.

Give bolus IV injection of up to 10 000 IU UFH and then commence an infusion aiming to achieve an aPTT value that is 2- to 2.5-fold that of control. This can usually be achieved with infusion rates of 1000–2000 IU/hour, but may require individual dose regimens.

Chronic phase

Antenatal treatment

Treat for 1 week on IV UFH, and then consider long-term therapeutic SC heparin (10 000–15 000 IU twice daily) or LMWH equivalent (enoxaparin 40 mg once daily with final dose dependent on patient's weight and titrated to give an anti-factor Xa activity level measured 4 hours after SC injection of 0.6–1.0 U/mL). Warfarin can be substituted if postpartum.

- Heparin use (primarily UFH) is associated with osteopenia (occurs in 1 in 100 patients and is reversible) and thrombocytopenia (rare and unpredictable, but is reversible). May be mild and symptomless or may be due to the development of heparin-dependent antibodies.
- In the event of osteopenia or thrombocytopenia, stop UFH. Consider switching to LMWH or warfarin, if appropriate.
- Alopecia (very rare and unpredictable, but reversible) with long-term use.
- No known fetal risks from heparin, as it does not cross the placenta.
- Heparin should be continued throughout gestation and discontinued for the shortest possible time for a timed delivery at 39 weeks. Warfarin can be given postpartum.
- Epidural anesthesia is contraindicated if the patient received heparin within the previous 8–12 hours (for UFH) or 24–48 hours (for LMWH).
- There is no evidence of increased risk of PPH. If there is significant bleeding at delivery, consider protamine sulfate administration (reverses effect of heparin—dose calculated by neutralization test).

Warfarin

Fetal risks of warfarin prevent its use. It is teratogenic, with warfarin embryopathy seen most commonly following exposure at 6–8 weeks of gestation. However, warfarin can cause fetal injury at any stage of pregnancy (chondrodysplasia punctata, asplenia, diaphragmatic hernia, optic neuritis). It may be associated with bleeding problems in the fetus, resulting in optic atrophy, microcephaly, and other CNS defects.

Postnatal treatment

Heparin (either UFH or LMWH) can be started within 6–8 hours of a vaginal delivery and 8–12 hours of a cesarean delivery, depending on the indication. Warfarin can be started as early as postpartum day 1, although it generally takes 48 hours before the INR increases. Once a therapeutic INR has been reached, heparin can be discontinued after 5–7 days. The reason for overlap is because of the transient hypercoagulable state which occurs after starting warfarin therapy (because of a decrease in protein C which precedes the decrease in the vitamin K-dependent clotting factors, i.e. II, VII, IX, and X). Treatment should be continued for a minimum of 6 weeks postpartum or post-thrombosis if the embolism occurs postnatally. Breast-feeding is safe with warfarin. Liaise with the hematology department for better control.

Treatment failure despite adequate anticoagulation

- *DVT*. In the setting of recurrent DVT despite anticoagulation, consider delivery as symptoms are exacerbated by obstruction to venous flow by the gravid uterus.
- *PE*. If PE recurs, consider placement of an inferior vena cava filter above the aortic bifurcation but below renal vessels. Use a local anesthetic procedure via percutaneous puncture of an unaffected femoral vein.
- *Septic PE (rare)*. The DVT source is often the pelvic veins (septic pelvic thrombophlebitis). It is characterized by recurrent PEs with high fever and secondary bronchopneumonia. Treatment is with antibiotics in addition to anticoagulants.

Prophylaxis against VTE at cesarean delivery

Delivery by lower-segment cesarean increases the risk of VTE by two- to tenfold. A risk assessment of all patients undergoing cesarean delivery should be performed and prophylaxis instituted as appropriate. This is discussed further in Chapter 6 📖 *p.328*.

Recommended further reading

1. Walker MC, Ferguson SE, Allen VM (2003). Heparin for pregnant women with acquired or inherited thrombophilias. *Cochrane Database Syst Rev* **2**, CD003580.
2. American College of Obstetricians and Gynecologists (2001). ACOG Practice Bulletin. Thromboembolism in pregnancy. *Int J Gynaecol Obstet* **75**, 203–12.

Chapter 9

Miscellaneous obstetrics

Fibroids in pregnancy

Fibroids (myomas) are benign smooth muscle tumors of the myometrium and may be present in as many as one in five women over the age of 35. They are more common in Black than in Caucasian women.

Effects of fibroids on pregnancy

Fibroids tend to be responsive to estrogen and therefore generally enlarge in size during pregnancy because of increased vascularity, edema, hypertrophy, and hyperplasia of fibromuscular tissues.

- Occasionally fibroids may be mistaken for fetal parts.
- Fibroids may also undergo softening and flattening during pregnancy, and this may make them indistinguishable from the normal uterus.
- The presence of fibroids often results in the uterus measuring large for dates.
- Implantation over a submucous fibroid may be associated with a risk of miscarriage.
- In early pregnancy, impaction of the fibroid may lead to urinary retention and the initial management is that of a retroverted gravid uterus. This is a rare complication.
- Later in pregnancy, fibroids in the lower segment or cervical fibroids may prevent engagement of the head and result in persistent abnormalities of fetal lie or presentation.
- Fibroids *per se* do not appear to interfere with uterine action during labor, but they may predispose to PPH as fibroids in the lower segment may interfere with contraction and retraction of the uterus. Therefore it may be worthwhile having IV access *in situ* with cross-matched blood if there are large or multiple fibroids, especially if they are localized to the lower uterine segment.
- If cesarean delivery is required, it is best to avoid the fibroids altogether. The only reason to remove a fibroid at the time of cesarean is if it is impossible to close the uterine incision with it *in situ*. Even removal of a pedunculated subserosal fibroid may lead to uncontrollable bleeding and a need for puerperal hysterectomy.
- In the puerperium, uterine involution may appear to be slower than expected.
- Other potential problems in the puerperium may be infection in the fibroid and secondary PPH.

Two of the complications that fibroids may undergo are more common in pregnancy: infarction (red degeneration) and torsion.

Red degeneration

Red degeneration (infarction) is thought to be a result of the fibroid outgrowing its blood supply. It presents with acute abdominal pain requiring opiate analgesia and localized tenderness over the fibroid. Clinical signs may include localized peritonism and guarding. There may be associated constitutional symptoms, such as vomiting and pyrexia, and a leukocytosis. Management involves supportive care with bed rest, analgesia, and reassurance. It is common for signs or symptoms to persist for 7–10 days. The differential diagnosis includes placental abruption, appendicitis, or UTI/pyelonephritis. The pattern of illness together with results of bacteriological investigations and observation of the clinical course will lead to the correct diagnosis.

Torsion

Torsion of a pedunculated fibroid may occur during pregnancy or soon after delivery in the puerperium where uterine involution and laxity of the previously tense abdomen predispose to increased mobility of the abdominal contents.

- Presentation may be as an acute abdomen, the diagnosis being suspected in the presence of a known history of one or more pedunculated fibroids.
- The differential diagnosis includes ovarian cyst rupture or hemorrhage, appendicitis, spontaneous rectus sheath hematoma, small bowel obstruction, or renal colic/pyelonephritis.
- Management is surgical removal of the fibroid.

Recommended further reading

1. Benecke C, Kruger TF, Siebert TI, Van der Merwe JP, Steyn DW (2005). Effect of fibroids on fertility in patients undergoing assisted reproduction. A structured literature review. *Gynecol Obstet Invest* **59**, 225–30.
2. American College of Obstetricians and Gynecologists (1994). Uterine leiomyomata. ACOG Technical Bulletin No. 192. *Int J Gynaecol Obstet* **46**, 73–82.
3. American College of Obstetricians and Gynecologists (2001). ACOG Practice Bulletin No. 16. Surgical alternatives to hysterectomy in the management of leiomyomas. *Int J Gynaecol Obstet* **73**, 285–93.
4. American College of Obstetricians and Gynecologists (2004). ACOG Committee Opinion. Uterine artery embolization. *Obstet Gynecol* **103**, 403–4.
5. Gupta J, Sinha A, Lumsden M, Hickey M (2006). Uterine artery embolization for symptomatic uterine fibroids. *Cochrane Database Syst Rev* **1**, CD005073.

Ovarian cysts in pregnancy

Ovarian cysts of varying sizes may occur. The majority are small (3–4 cm) and represent persistent follicular cysts. The other main groups of benign ovarian tumors in pregnancy are the cystadenomas and dermoid cysts. The latter are twice as common in pregnancy than in the nonpregnant state. Malignant disease of the ovary in pregnancy is rare.

Effects of ovarian cysts on pregnancy

Impaction of a large ovarian cyst may lead to urinary retention. The sheer size of the ovarian cyst may be responsible for discomfort. Later in pregnancy, a large ovarian cyst may predispose to failure of engagement of the fetal head and malpresentation and there may be a risk of obstructed labor.

Ovarian cysts in pregnancy may undergo the same complications as in the nonpregnant state. Torsion of an ovarian pedicle is most likely to occur in early pregnancy, in particular at the end of the first trimester, or in the puerperium. Hemorrhage into the cyst may occur as a result of increased vascularity and this, in turn, may lead to rupture of the cyst. Cyst rupture may also occur in labor. However, in the majority of cases the cyst remains asymptomatic.

Management

Management of ovarian cysts in pregnancy depends on the size, ultrasound appearance, symptoms, and complications. In general, with cystadenomas and dermoids that are asymptomatic, treatment is deferred until after the delivery. If acute complications such as torsion arise, these need to be dealt with at any gestation. If elective surgery in pregnancy is contemplated, this is best done at around 16 weeks where the risk of miscarriage and preterm labor are less and access to the adnexae is relatively easy. Provided that engagement of the head has occurred and labor is progressing satisfactorily, no special action needs to be taken. If a cesarean delivery is needed for obstetric indications, the cyst should be dealt with at the same time. Written consent for cesarean delivery should include permission for peritoneal washings, ovarian cystectomy, and possible unilateral salpingo-oophorectomy. Alternatively, further evaluation can be arranged for the postnatal period.

Recommended further reading

1. American College of Obstetricians and Gynecologists (1994). Uterine leiomyomata. ACOG Technical Bulletin No. 192. *Int J Gynaecol Obstet* **46**, 73–82.
2. American College of Obstetricians and Gynecologists (2004). ACOG Committee Opinion. Uterine artery embolization. *Obstet Gynecol* **103**, 403–4.
3. Gupta J, Sinha A, Lumsden M, Hickey M (2006). Uterine artery embolization for symptomatic uterine fibroids. *Cochrane Database Syst Rev* **1**, CD005073.

Malignancy and premalignancy: cervix

Cervical cancer complicates 0.02–0.4% of pregnancies. Up to 7% of cervical carcinomas are diagnosed at the time of pregnancy. Cervical carcinoma is the most common genital tract malignancy to present in pregnancy.

Presentation

Between one- and two-thirds of women with invasive lesions are asymptomatic. Roughly 50% of these are detected by cervical cytology. The most common presenting symptom is vaginal bleeding. Any woman with a history of recurrent painless bleeding in pregnancy not due to placenta previa should be referred for colposcopy to exclude cervical neoplasia.

Management

- *Early invasive disease.* Diagnosis is usually made by a colposcopically directed biopsy or wedge biopsy of the cervix. Treatment is by cone biopsy. There is an increased risk of hemorrhage. Despite the increased risk of miscarriage following cone biopsy in pregnancy, 80% of pregnancies will deliver at term and the overall fetal survival rate is 90%. Further treatment can then be deferred until 6 weeks postpartum.
- *Stage 1B.* If the disease is diagnosed after 24 weeks, the pregnancy can be allowed to continue until viability. Treatment is then by radical hysterectomy and lymphadenectomy or radiotherapy. If delivery is by cesarean section, this can be combined with radical hysterectomy. The prognosis is the same whichever method of treatment is used.
  If disease is diagnosed before 24 weeks, a delay in treatment is not recommended. Termination of pregnancy can be combined with surgical treatment. If radiotherapy is used this will usually induce miscarriage, although, after 16 weeks, termination of pregnancy may be required before proceeding to intracavity radiotherapy.
- *Advanced disease.* Stage 2b or more advanced disease should be treated by radiotherapy. If the pregnancy has reached viability, this can be carried out after delivery of the fetus by cesarean section.

Prognosis

Five-year survival depends mainly on the stage of disease at the time of diagnosis. It ranges from 74% for patients with stage 1B lesions to 16% for stage 3/4 disease. The prognosis for stage 1 disease is the same as that for nonpregnant women, although the prognosis for advanced disease is poorer. The overall prognosis tends to be worse for women diagnosed in the later stages of pregnancy because a higher proportion of women have stage 2 or more disease. When analyzed by stage there is no significant difference in survival between patients diagnosed in the first and third trimesters. Delaying treatment of early-stage disease by up to 16 weeks to allow the fetus to reach viability does not appear to affect long-term prognosis.

Preinvasive disease

Interpretation of cervical cytology can be difficult during pregnancy. Women with evidence of dysplasia on cervical cytology should be referred for colposcopy to differentiate premalignant from invasive disease. The increased vascularity of the cervix accentuates the color difference between normal and (aceto-white) neoplastic epithelium. If an area of atypical epithelium is identified, this should be biopsied if clinically suspicious of high-grade cervical intraepithelial neoplasia (CIN) or invasive disease. There is some increased risk of bleeding following biopsy during pregnancy, but the risk of miscarriage is low. Colposcopic assessment without biopsy may be acceptable if there is no suggestion of invasive disease on cytology and colposcopy and the assessment is carried out by an experienced colposcopist. If biopsy confirms CIN, a conservative approach to treatment is usually adopted. Repeat colposcopy is carried out between 24 and 34 weeks and again at 8–12 weeks postpartum. If this confirms the continued presence of CIN, treatment should be delayed until the third or fourth month postpartum because of the increased risk of bleeding prior to this. Pregnancy does not appear to affect the rate of progression from low- to high-grade CIN nor from CIN to invasive disease.

Recommended further reading

1. Singer, A. (1989). Malignancy and premalignancy of the genital tract in pregnancy. In: Chamberian G, ed. *Turnbull's Obstetrics*, Chapter 43, p. 657. Churchill Livingstone, Edinburgh.

Ovarian carcinoma

One in 80–300 pregnancies are complicated by the presence of ovarian cysts. The majority of these will be benign, the most common being functional ovarian cysts (follicular cysts, corpus luteum). The most common solid benign ovarian cysts found in pregnancy are mature cystic teratomas (dermoid cysts). Mucinous cystadenomas are the most common epithelial neoplasm. Between 2% and 5% of ovarian cysts in pregnancy will be malignant, with an overall incidence of 1 in 8000–20 000 pregnancies. Twenty-five percent of all malignant tumors in pregnancy will be dysgerminomas.

Diagnosis

Most lesions are asymptomatic and diagnosed following palpation of an abdominal or pelvic mass or on routine ultrasound scanning for fetal viability or abnormality. Symptoms usually arise as a result of complications such as torsion or rupture of the cyst, causing abdominal pain, nausea, vomiting, and local tenderness. Torsion (but not hemorrhage and rupture) is more common in pregnancy and in the puerperium than at other times (complicates 10–15% of tumors). Torsion occurs most commonly between 10 and 16 weeks. Ultrasound examination should be arranged to distinguish ovarian cysts from other types of pelvic mass. Definitive diagnosis can only be made by removal of the cyst at laparotomy.

Management

Asymptomatic cysts <5 cm can be left and monitored by ultrasound. They will usually resolve without treatment after delivery. Cysts of size 5–10 cm with no abnormal features on ultrasound can be either managed conservatively or aspirated under ultrasound guidance and the fluid examined cytologically. Laparotomy is indicated for cysts that are persistently >10 cm in diameter, are enlarging, or contain abnormal features on ultrasound scan (complex multilocular or solid areas). Unless indicated earlier because of an acute surgical complication of the cyst such as torsion, laparotomy is usually performed during the mid-trimester at 16 weeks (by which time the pregnancy is not dependent on the corpus luteum and miscarriage is less likely).

- Benign lesions are treated by unilateral cystectomy or salpingo-oophorectomy.
- Stage 1 ovarian carcinoma can be treated by unilateral salpingo-oophorectomy provided that there is no obvious invasion of the capsule or involvement of the contralateral ovary and no ascites.
- Patients with more advanced disease should ideally be treated by total abdominal hysterectomy and bilateral salpingo-oophorectomy.
- Where the diagnosis is made in the second trimester, a decision will need to be made on a case-by-case basis as to whether to delay treatment to allow the pregnancy to reach viability.

- Where possible, patients with suspected ovarian cancer should be managed in a specialist cancer unit. This is especially important for patients with malignant germ cell tumors where it may be possible to preserve reproductive function and even the pregnancy in which the tumor is diagnosed by appropriate chemotherapy.
- Although chemotherapeutic agents are teratogenic in the first trimester, malformation rates do not appear to be increased in women treated in the second or third trimesters.

Recommended further reading

1. Singer, A. (1989). Malignancy and premalignancy of the genital tract in pregnancy. In: Chamberian G, ed. *Turnbull's Obstetrics*, Chapter 43, p. 657. Churchill Livingstone, Edinburgh.

Vulval malignancy

Vulval carcinoma is rare in pregnancy, since the peak incidence of the disease is in the 60–70 year age group. However, vulval intraepithelial neoplasia (VIN) is seen in younger women.

Diagnosis

Premalignant disease is commonly asymptomatic. The most common presenting symptom is pruritus. Signs such as fissuring, ulceration, or raised areas indicate the possibility of invasive disease. Colposcopic assessment may be helpful in identifying the extent of disease, but the diagnosis should be confirmed by biopsy.

Treatment

- *Premalignant disease.* Treatment of VIN can be deferred until after the pregnancy is completed.
- *Malignant lesions.* Management is essentially the same as for the nonpregnant woman. Early invasive disease confirmed pathologically where the depth of penetration is no more than 1 mm can be treated by wide local excision. Where more invasive disease is diagnosed after 36 weeks, treatment is usually deferred until after delivery. At earlier gestations, vulvectomy and node dissection can be performed without having to terminate the pregnancy. If the vulval wound has healed, there is no contraindication to vaginal delivery.

Recommended further reading

1. Singer, A. (1989). Malignancy and premalignancy of the genital tract in pregnancy. In: Chamberlain G, ed. *Turnbull's Obstetrics*, Chapter 43, p. 657. Churchill Livingstone, Edinburgh.

Perinatal mortality

Introduction

In the USA, the *perinatal mortality rate* is defined as the total number of stillbirths (fetuses born dead at or after 20 weeks' gestation) and early neonatal deaths (live born babies who die within the first week of life regardless of gestational age at birth) per 1000 total births. In the UK, a stillbirth refers to delivery of a non-viable fetus at or after 24 weeks' gestation. A late neonatal death is one that occurs from 7 days to 28 days of life, whereas a postneonatal death includes deaths from 28 days onward but under 1 year. *Infant mortality rate* refers to the number of live born babies who die within the first year of life regardless of gestational age at birth expressed per 1000 total births.

The perinatal mortality rate in developed countries is around 8–9 per 1000 births. Direct comparison between developed countries may be somewhat misleading because of slight variations in definitions (see above). Perinatal mortality rates are up to 10-fold higher in the developing world. Possible causes for this vast discrepancy are malnutrition and susceptibility to infection.

There has been a steady improvement in perinatal mortality over the last 60 years. Not surprisingly, the major contribution to the improvement has been through public health measures leading to a healthier population through better nutrition and health education. However, the role of the medical profession must not be underestimated.

Classification of perinatal deaths

The Wigglesworth classification of perinatal deaths uses a pathophysiological approach where causes of death are arranged in a hierarchical mutually exclusive order. This classification has been extended for use in the CESDI reports as follows:

- Congenital malformations (lethal or severe)
- Antepartum fetal deaths
- Deaths due to intrapartum asphyxia, anoxia, or trauma
- Neonatal deaths due to immaturity
- Infection
- Other specific causes
- Accident or non-intrapartum trauma
- Sudden infant death (cause unknown)
- Unclassifiable

Causes of perinatal mortality

The four most common causes of perinatal mortality in developed countries are prematurity, congenital malformations, antepartum fetal death, and intrapartum asphyxia.

Prematurity

Although prematurity accounts for only 1 in 10 births, this group is overrepresented among the neonatal deaths with approximately one in two neonatal deaths having been premature babies. There have been dramatic improvements in the survival of very premature infants through improvements in neonatal care and antenatal corticosteroid administration. The most common causes of morbidity and mortality in premature babies are respiratory distress syndrome, overwhelming sepsis, and neurologic and gastrointestinal problems.

Congenital malformations

Malformations account for one in six perinatal deaths. There has been a change in the pattern of congenital abnormalities over the last two decades with a reduction in open neural tube defects (NTDs). This has been brought about by improved prenatal diagnosis with maternal serum α-fetoprotein (MS-AFP) screening and routine ultrasound scanning in pregnancy. Detection of the abnormality offers the woman the possibility of termination of the affected pregnancy. It is hoped that the recent advice regarding periconceptual folic acid will further reduce the incidence of NTDs. With the reduction in open NTDs, the predominant group of lethal abnormalities is those of the cardiovascular system, where prenatal ultrasound is not as sensitive as that for NTD screening.

Antepartum deaths

Antepartum fetal death includes not only fetal loss due to a variety of causes (such as placental abruption), but also a significant proportion of unexplained fetal losses. Despite intensive efforts, almost one-third of cases of antepartum fetal death remain unexplained, although IUFGR can be seen in up to a quarter of cases. The incidence of placental abruption and abnormal glucose tolerance in this group is around 10%.

Intrapartum asphyxia

The risk of a baby dying in labor is less than 1 in 1000 births. Some of these deaths are clearly related to inadequate intrapartum management, including inadequate recognition of antenatal risk factors, poor interpretation of and failure to act on CTG abnormalities, and poor resuscitation of the newborn. Every effort is currently being made to minimize these events through critical appraisal of the training, supervision, and practice of both obstetricians and midwives, and through the development of guidelines and educational programs to achieve and maintain the competence required for intrapartum care and fetal monitoring.

Conclusion

The perinatal mortality rate appears to have plateaued since the late 1980s. If further improvements are to be made, it is important to reduce the avoidable causes of perinatal loss, particularly suboptimal intrapartum care. There is also a need to direct research efforts towards antepartum fetal loss and how this can be predicted and prevented.

Maternal mortality

Introduction

There are in excess of half a million maternal deaths worldwide each year and there is a huge worldwide variation in maternal mortality rates. Based on the WHO figures for 1988, developed countries accounted for just 1.6% of that year's total number of maternal deaths worldwide. The high maternal mortality in the developing world can be attributed to the high fertility rate with poor access to contraception, unsafe abortion practices, absence of a primary healthcare system, and often lack of access to any form of healthcare professional or institution.

Steps taken in the past

Maternal mortality has decreased dramatically in developed countries over the past 50 years for the following reasons:

- General improvement in public health.
- Better training of obstetric care providers, including midwives and obstetricians.
- The use of antibiotics such as penicillin and sulfonamides has dramatically cut down the deaths due to puerperal sepsis.
- Prevention and treatment of PPH.
- Development of safe blood transfusion practice.
- The introduction of effective and simple family planning options such as the combined oral contraceptive pill has helped reduce parity and average family size.
- The legalization of abortion has led to the elimination of illegal abortion and associated complications.

Classification of maternal deaths

In order to understand better the causes of maternal death, it is useful to ensure that appropriate definitions are being used.

- *Maternal death.* Death of a woman while pregnant or within 42 days of termination of pregnancy from any cause related to or aggravated by pregnancy or its management, but excluding accidental or incidental causes.
- *Direct death.* Death resulting from obstetric complications of the pregnant state; from interventions, omissions, or incorrect treatment; or a chain of events resulting from the above.
- *Indirect deaths.* Deaths resulting from previous existing disease or disease which developed during pregnancy and was not due to obstetric causes, but was aggravated by the physiologic effects of pregnancy.
- *Late deaths.* Deaths occurring between 42 days and 1 year after abortion, miscarriage, or delivery because of direct or indirect maternal causes.
- *Fortuitous deaths.* Deaths from unrelated causes which happen to occur in pregnancy or the puerperium.

Causes of maternal mortality

Direct causes

Thrombosis and thromboembolism

The maternal mortality rate from complications of venous thromboembolism accounts for 16.5 deaths per million maternities. Deaths from thromboembolism are predominantly after PE and can occur at any stage of pregnancy (including the first trimester) and the puerperium (slightly more common compared with the antenatal period). Close attention is needed with symptoms such as chest and leg pains to exclude PE or DVT by means of the appropriate investigations. Thrombosis and thromboembolism have always been among the leading causes of maternal mortality. Guidelines have been drawn up to identify patients at high risk for such events and to prevent their development using appropriate thromboprophylaxis. The last triennium has seen a decline in maternal deaths due to this cause.

Hypertensive disorders

These conditions account for 7.1 maternal deaths per million maternities. In this group, cerebral and hepatic complications in the setting of preeclampsia are the main causes of maternal mortality. Protocols for the management of preeclampsia have been developed, including the use of magnesium sulfate seizure prophylaxis to prevent eclampsia (seizures or coma) and the appropriate use of antihypertensive agents to prevent CVA (stroke). Antenatal education of all women to recognize the symptoms associated with preeclampsia and seek professional help urgently is also recommended.

Amniotic fluid embolism

To date, AFE remains a clinical diagnosis without the absolute requirement of postmortem histopathological confirmation. The diagnostic criteria are cardiac arrest or acute hypotension, acute hypoxia (cyanosis, dyspnea, or respiratory arrest), coagulopathy, or any combination of the above during labor, at cesarean delivery, or within 30 minutes of delivery with no other clinical condition or potential explanation. There appear to be no consistent common factors to identify women at risk.

Early pregnancy deaths

Such maternal deaths may follow ectopic pregnancy, spontaneous miscarriage, or termination of pregnancy (TOP). The major cause of deaths in the setting of ectopic pregnancy is delay in diagnosis and inappropriate management. An empty uterus on transvaginal ultrasound in a woman with a positive pregnancy test (especially if the serum β-hCG is >2000 IU/mL) should be regarded as an ectopic pregnancy until proven otherwise.

Sepsis

Routine use of prophylactic antibiotics at cesarean delivery has significantly decreased maternal deaths from sepsis. Women with prolonged rupture of membranes (>18 hours) who develop fever should be carefully assessed to exclude sepsis. Where patients are systemically ill, antibiotic treatment should be instituted immediately while awaiting bacteriological cultures.

Hemorrhage

Anterior placenta previa with a previous uterine scar may be associated with severe uncontrollable hemorrhage at the time of cesarean delivery, necessitating puerperal hysterectomy. Hence an experienced surgeon should be involved in such cases from the onset. Regular 'practice drills' and agreed protocols for the management of emergencies such as obstetric hemorrhage can save lives.

Genital tract trauma

This includes uterine ruptures and uterine and/or vaginal lacerations following instrumental delivery. Recent guidelines for the intrapartum management of women attempting vaginal birth after cesarean (VBAC), e.g. reluctance to induce labor in such women, will likely minimize such complications and resultant maternal deaths.

Anesthesia

The safety of obstetric anesthesia is such that the risk of maternal death is only one per million maternities. This has been achieved through greater use of epidural and regional anesthesia in place of general anesthesia, and ready access to intensive care facilities when required.

Indirect causes of maternal mortality

Cardiac deaths

Preexisting maternal heart disease is the most common cause of maternal death. Indeed, women who have pulmonary vascular disease (such as pulmonary hypertension) have a 30% risk of mortality. Women with severe or complex heart disease should be managed by a multidisciplinary team of obstetricians and cardiologists. Excessive use of oxytocin or iatrogenic fluid overload may compromise a woman with severe cardiac disease. An obscure febrile illness may suggest the possibility of endocarditis. Aortic dissection in pregnancy should be kept in mind in women with severe chest pain in pregnancy. Chest X-rays should not be withheld. Echocardiography is the investigation of choice for diagnosis of aortic root dissection.

Psychiatric deaths

Suicide is a major cause of maternal mortality in pregnancy. Screening for psychiatric disorders and substance abuse at booking as well as the availability of a psychiatrist with an interest in perinatal mental health is important. Women who have serious mental illness should be counseled about possible recurrence following the pregnancy.

Other indirect deaths

This group includes women with diseases of the CNS, including subarachnoid hemorrhage and seizure disorder. Again, optimal management of such women in the acute setting requires a multidisciplinary approach. As regards women with a preexisting seizure disorder, mortality can be decreased by educating relatives about positioning patients in the 'recovery position' following a seizure and educating the pregnant women herself to avoid having a bath when alone and to use a shower instead to avoid the possibility of drowning following a seizure.

Chapter 10

Psychiatric disorders and substance abuse

Substance abuse in pregnancy

Substances of abuse (psychoactive drugs) are those that lead to relatively rapid effects on the CNS, including changes in the level of consciousness or the state of mind. These include those available for general use (e.g. alcohol) and illegal substances (e.g. cocaine and heroin). Substance abuse in pregnancy has effects on the mother and the developing fetus. Abuse in early pregnancy carries the potential risk of fetal abnormality, while in late pregnancy fetal dependence and neonatal withdrawal are potential complications.

Most users abuse more than one substance. The quality and potency of street drugs vary from time to time and place to place. This is a growing problem as most pregnancies are in young women, and young people are the group most likely to be exposed to drugs on either a regular or occasional/experimental basis. However, reliable statistics are difficult to obtain as most drug abuse goes undetected and a history of drug abuse may not be given even when specific inquiry is made. It is estimated that 1–2% of the adult population routinely use illicit drugs.

Definitions

- *Harmful use.* Pattern of use that causes physical damage (e.g. hepatitis from needle-sharing) or mental damage (e.g. depression following drug use).
- *Tolerance.* Diminishing CNS effects from repeated drug use, such that increasing doses are needed to achieve the same effects.
- *Dependence.* Condition in which the use of a drug takes higher priority for the individual than behaviors which previously had a higher value. Dependence may be physical, psychological, or combined.
- *Withdrawal state.* Physical or psychological symptoms occurring on partial or complete withdrawal of a drug after prolonged use or high dose. It may be complicated by delirium and convulsions.

Maternal problems

Drug abuse has a chronic relapsing course and a mortality risk (usually from accidental overdose) of 10–15% over 10 years. The risk of such overdose is highest after enforced abstinence leading to loss of tolerance. Other maternal problems include the following:

- *Suboptimal use of healthcare facilities.* Drug abusers are likely to avoid medical and social services facilities. Late booking in pregnancy and poor attendance at antenatal clinic are common problems.
- *Crime.* Drug abuse often results in disinhibition of behavior and impairment of judgment, leading to violence and criminal activity, including theft and prostitution, to finance the drug habit. Many of the crimes committed by users are petty in terms of scale, but they are vast in terms of numbers.
- *Nutrition.* This is likely to be poor as funds are diverted to buy drugs. Deficiencies of iron, vitamins, and folic acid may occur.

- *Vascular and skin complications*. Superficial and deep vein thromboses may result from venous injection of drugs. Subcutaneous extravasation or accidental subcutaneous injection may result in tissue necrosis and abscesses.
- *Infections*. Systemic infection may occur from IV injection, including septicemia, bacterial endocarditis, hepatitis B and C, and HIV. Multiple sexual partners or prostitution predispose to sexually transmitted diseases, including heterosexually transmitted HIV.
- *Overdose*. Inconsistent drug quality can produce accidental overdose or withdrawal symptoms, especially with IV drug abuse.

Fetal/neonatal problems

The effects of substance abuse on the fetus are not necessarily due to the drugs alone, but rather are a combination of poor nutrition, smoking, poor personal care, and social deprivation associated with drug abuse. Effects observed in childhood may also be partly due to the continuing adverse family and social environment rather than purely a lasting effect of the intrauterine exposure.

Problems include the following:

- Teratogenicity risk with some substances.
- Dating problems resulting from late booking. Screening tests for fetal abnormality are of limited or no value with late booking and poor attendance.
- Prematurity.
- IUGR.
- Stillbirth.
- Withdrawal symptoms in neonatal period.
- Vertical transmission of infection.
- Neglect of the baby.

Drugs I

Morphine and diamorphine (heroin)

These are natural opiates and are the most widely abused opiates in developed countries. They can be administered by most routes, although abuse is usually by inhalation or IV injection. Clinical effects of opiate use include euphoria, analgesia, respiratory depression, pupillary constriction, constipation, reduced appetite, and reduced libido. Tolerance develops rapidly, leading to the need for increasingly higher doses. However, tolerance also diminishes rapidly such that after a period of abstinence, e.g. hospitalization for detoxification, fatal respiratory depression may result from using a previously tolerated quantity of opiate.

Symptoms of maternal withdrawal include intense craving for the drug, nausea and vomiting, body aches, joint pains, runny nose and eyes, dilated pupils, sweating, pyrexia, insomnia, tachycardia, abdominal pains, and diarrhea. Withdrawal symptoms usually start about 6 hours after the last dose and reach a peak after 36–48 hours. A person in good health is not likely to suffer fatality from withdrawal symptoms, but the great distress caused drives her to seek further supplies. It should be borne in mind that a drug abuser presenting with nonspecific abdominal pain may be exaggerating the symptoms to obtain further opiates, e.g. morphine or pethidine.

Opiates do not carry a teratogenic effect, but opiate addiction is associated with IUGR and prematurity. A fetus born to a heroin-dependent mother is likely to develop withdrawal symptoms within 48 hours of birth. Severity is related to the amount and duration of drug used by the mother. Symptoms include irritability, jitteriness, tremors, poor feeding, respiratory distress, sneezing, and a high-pitched cry. The onset of withdrawal symptoms may be delayed by days or weeks when the mother has been on methadone as it is stored in fetal tissues and has a long half-life. The likelihood of neonatal withdrawal symptoms depends on the amount of drugs used in the antenatal period, but most babies have minor symptoms, if any. Management is mainly supportive and symptoms usually resolve within a few days. There are no substantiated long-term neurological defects in the baby.

Methadone

This is a synthetic opiate similar to heroin. It is available on controlled prescription from methadone maintenance treatment programs. Methadone is available in liquid or tablet form, but is usually dispensed in liquid form. However, patients on methadone may still resort to illicit narcotics to 'top-up', thereby subjecting themselves and their fetuses to the risks that the treatment programs aim to minimize. Methadone is nearly as potent as morphine and causes similar withdrawal symptoms. Because of its long half-life, methadone withdrawal manifests after 36 hours and peaks after 3–5 days.

Cocaine

Derived mainly from the leaves of the coca plant, cocaine is a potent vasoconstrictor and local anesthetic. It can be ingested from chewing coca leaves, smoking coca paste, inhaling or injecting cocaine hydrochloride powder, or smoking crack cocaine, an alkaloid form of cocaine. Because it is a potent vasoconstrictor, nasal inhalation (snorting) leads to delayed absorption. However, smoking and IV injection produce a rapid and intense effect. Features of cocaine intoxication include tachycardia, elevated blood pressure, sweating, nausea, and vomiting. Behavioral changes include impairment of judgment, euphoria, agitation, grandiosity, and visual or tactile hallucinations, especially the feeling of insects crawling under the skin (formication, 'cocaine bug').

The euphoria produced by cocaine use is followed by a 'crash' characterized by mood disturbance, anxiety, fatigue, and a craving for more cocaine. Some users will use heroin to alleviate the intensity of the 'crash' following cocaine use. Sudden withdrawal can lead to delirium within 24 hours, and withdrawal following chronic use can lead to paranoid and suicidal thoughts.

Although placental vasoconstriction reduces the quantity of cocaine reaching the fetus, the transfer of oxygen and nutrients is similarly impaired. Such placental vasoconstriction may cause spontaneous miscarriage, stillbirth, and placental abruption. Less severe fetal effects include IUGR and subtle neurologic signs, persisting for months after birth. The effects appear to be proportionate to maternal drug use in the second and third trimesters.

Amphetamines

Amphetamines are CNS stimulants with similar effects to those of cocaine. Fenfluramine and dexfenfluramine are related substances which are sometimes used as appetite suppressants, but can cause psychological dependence. Amphetamine abuse is usually oral, but can also be IV or nasal inhalation, e.g. metamphetamine ('speed'). Amphetamines produce euphoria, excitement, a feeling of wellbeing, increased confidence, increased drive and energy, and a feeling of alertness and less need for sleep. Physical effects include tachycardia, pupillary dilatation, and raised blood pressure. Effects of chronic use and cessation of chronic use may be similar to those due to opiates. Chronic use of large doses may produce a state similar to schizophrenia.

Amphetamine causes vasoconstriction and hypertension, leading to chronic fetal hypoxia. There may be an association with cleft palate. Like cocaine, it increases the risks of placental abruption, IUGR, preterm delivery, and perinatal mortality. Neonatal effects include hyperactivity, tremors, poor feeding, and disordered sleep.

Recommended further reading

1. Puri BK, Laking PJ, Treasaden IH (1996). Psychoactive substance use disorders. In: *Textbook of Psychiatry*, pp. 119–37. Churchill Livingstone, Edinburgh.

Drugs II

Hallucinogens

These include lysergic acid diethylamine (LSD), dimethyltryptamine (DMT), mescaline, phencyclidine (PCP), and 3,4-methylenedioxy-methamphetamine (MDMA, ecstasy). These are usually taken orally in tablet or capsule form. Physical effects include sweating, pupillary dilatation, blurring of vision, tachycardia, palpitations, tremors, and loss of coordination. Psychological effects may depend on the personality of the user and include anxiety, depression, impairment of judgment, paranoid thoughts, and life-threatening delusions. Hallucinogens have been responsible for people jumping off tall buildings under the delusion that they could fly. MDMA produces feelings of euphoria, sociability, and intimacy. MDMA deaths have been attributed to hyperthermia, cardiac arrhythmias, intracerebral hemorrhage, and toxic hepatitis. Tolerance to MDMA develops quickly, but no clear withdrawal syndrome has yet been described.

Solvent abuse (glue sniffing)

Solvents, petrol, adhesives, butane gas, and paint thinners give off psychoactive vapors that can be inhaled either directly or from plastic bags. The latter route carries the additional risk of loss of consciousness or suffocation. Toxicity from these substances can cause death. Physical effects include dizziness, blurring of vision, poor coordination, poor concentration, slurring of speech, ataxia, muscle weakness, and tremors. Psychological effects include apathy, psychomotor retardation, and impairment of judgment and social functioning. Some solvents may cross the placenta, leading to growth restriction, microcephaly, prematurity, perinatal mortality, and developmental delay.

Cannabinoids

The major active substance in this group is tetrahydrocannabinol. The main source is the cannabis plant, the leaves of which may be smoked or chewed. Cannabinoids can lead to marked psychological dependence but not physical dependence. Cannabinoids can cause euphoria, anxiety, suspiciousness (sometimes leading to delusions of persecution), impairment of judgment, and social withdrawal. There are no substantiated adverse fetal effects. However, cannabis use may be a gateway to the abuse of harder drugs with more established negative maternal and fetal effects.

Benzodiazepines

Benzodiazepines are commonly prescribed to patients of all ages, and initial exposure often occurs in the form of medically indicated prescription. Subsequent abuse of benzodiazepines is usually from illicit procurement. The quality and purity are variable and high doses are common. Neonatal withdrawal effects include hypotonia, feeding difficulties, and respiratory depression.

Alcohol

Total abstinence or minimal consumption of alcohol is recommended in pregnancy. Excessive consumption can lead to permanent fetal damage. Alcohol intake of over 140 g (14 units) per week may lead to fetal alcohol syndrome (FAS). Features of FAS include IUGR, microcephaly, typical facies, mild to moderate mental restriction, and increased perinatal mortality.

Tobacco

Tobacco is the substance most commonly abused in pregnancy. Complications include increased risk of placental abruption, low birth-weight, neonatal death, and sudden infant death syndrome. The risk is related to the number of cigarettes smoked per day.

Recommended further reading

1. Puri BK, Laking PJ, Treasaden IH (1996). Psychoactive substance use disorders. In: *Textbook of Psychiatry*, pp. 119–37. Churchill Livingstone, Edinburgh.
2. Gelder M, Gath D, Mayou R, Cowen P (1996). The abuse of alcohol and drugs. In: *Oxford Textbook of Psychiatry*, pp. 438–81. Oxford University Press, Oxford.

Management of opiate addiction

Management of opiate addiction is more formalized than for other substances of abuse but the principles are similar. Management in pregnancy is based on a multidisciplinary approach involving obstetricians, midwives, neonatologists, addiction counselors, social workers, and health visitors. All efforts should be made to keep the pregnant woman within the service, reducing the risk to herself and the fetus, and improving her long-term prospects of being weaned off her addiction.

- It is important to avoid a judgmental approach as this may drive the woman away from the care needed.
- The risks to the mother and fetus should be carefully outlined.
- The woman should be reassured of confidentiality. It is useful to have a record of friends and family who know of her addiction, as their support may be valuable.
- Recommending cessation of drug abuse is often counterproductive, but this is the only way forward for some substances (e.g. cocaine, hallucinogens, amphetamines, and solvents) as there are no substitutes to use as replacement.
- Screen for hepatitis B and C, sexually transmitted diseases, and HIV after appropriate counseling.
- Screen for fetal abnormality and IUGR by ultrasound in the second and third trimesters, respectively.
- Providers on labor and delivery should be informed and the neonatal unit alerted to the delivery of a baby who may have withdrawal symptoms.

Many mothers will use their opiate before coming into hospital for labor and delivery. This complicates fetal monitoring and analgesia in labor and potentiates neonatal withdrawal. Epidural analgesia is preferable to using more opiates in large doses.

When necessary, drug use can be confirmed from analysis of urine sample, although hair analysis is more informative in investigating long-term abuse.

Planned withdrawal

Eventual drug withdrawal is the ultimate aim of a treatment program, but will not succeed on its own without psychological treatment and social support. Treatment usually takes place in psychiatric units or special treatment clinics. Return to drug abuse after such hospitalization carries a high risk of accidental overdose due to loss of tolerance.

Drug maintenance

This approach is adopted for patients unwilling or unable to give up drug abuse. A less addictive drug with a slower action/longer half-life is prescribed. This form of management is of particular use in opiate addiction, with methadone used as the alternative. There are no suitable substitutes for many abused substances, e.g. cocaine, amphetamines.

Maintenance therapy removes the need to obtain illicit supplies and the associated criminal tendencies. It needs to be combined with social and psychological support to enable eventual withdrawal. However, it should be borne in mind that some subjects on maintenance programs continue to use illicit drugs and supplement these with the supplies from the maintenance program. They may also obtain large amounts by registering in more than one center. Regular urine or hair testing can be used to monitor compliance. Many pregnant women return to illicit opiates, especially after delivery. Relapse is usually related to the circumstances that made the woman an addict in the first place.

Harm reduction

This is a more controversial approach which aims to reduce the risk of serious infections, e.g. HIV, for drug abusers not willing or able to change by offering education/counseling and practical help. The practical help includes the supply of sterile syringes and needles or advice to adopt noninjection modes of drug use.

Recommended further reading

1. Walker JJ (1999). Drug addiction. In: James DK, Steer PJ, Weiner CP, Gonik B, eds. *High Risk Pregnancy—Management Options* (2nd edn), pp. 599–616. WB Saunders, London.

Psychiatric disorders in pregnancy

Introduction

Pregnancy evokes joy in the majority of women with planned pregnancies, but still constitutes a very stressful event. Psychiatric illness in pregnancy may be an onset of a new disorder or an exacerbation of an old problem.

Up to two-thirds of pregnant women have some psychological symptoms in pregnancy. These include anxiety, labile mood, irritability, and depression. However, serious psychiatric disorders are probably less common in pregnant than in nonpregnant women.

- 1–2% of pregnant women have a psychiatric disorder, although not all will seek or need treatment.
- The incidence of psychiatric disorder in pregnancy is higher in the first and third trimesters than in the second trimester.
- An unplanned pregnancy may be associated with anxiety and depression in the first trimester.
- General discomfort, poor sleep, and fears about the impending labor and delivery and normality of the baby may cause anxiety and depression in the third trimester.
- The stress of childbirth and the lifestyle changes that come with a newborn baby may precipitate psychiatric illness after delivery. This is more likely in the presence of domestic/marital problems, unplanned/ unwanted pregnancy, or a personal/family history of mental illness.

The booking history should include history of mental illness and abuse of alcohol and psychoactive substances. The classification of psychiatric disorders is outlined in the American Psychiatric Association's *Diagnostic and Statistical Manual*, 4th edition (DSM-IV) of 1993.

Antenatal disorders

Major mood disorders include depression (unipolar affective disorder) and manic–depressive illness (bipolar affective disorder).

- Features of depression include fatigue, feelings of worthlessness, poor concentration, poor appetite, and suicidal thoughts.
- Severe depression in pregnancy is usually a preexisting illness and the treatment needs to be continued.
- Schizophrenia has higher psychiatric morbidity than any other psychiatric disorder. Its main clinical features include delusions, hallucinations, incoherence, and inappropriate affect. It also has a significant genetic component—the offspring carries a 5–10% schizophrenia risk when one parent is affected. Women have a later age of onset compared with men, such that the illness may not manifest until well into the childbearing age.

Effects of medication on pregnancy

- *Risks to the pregnant woman.* A severe preexisting psychiatric illness, if untreated, is a major threat to the life and wellbeing of a pregnant woman. It is necessary for her to continue with medication until medical advice can be sought regarding alteration or discontinuation. Cessation of medication carries the risks of relapse and self-harm, which may far outweigh possible risks to the fetus.

- *Substance abuse.* Psychiatric disorders may be associated with substance abuse, e.g. alcohol, tobacco, and narcotic drugs, with the associated risks to mother and baby (see earlier).
- *Teratogenicity.* Before prescribing medication, the physician should ask a psychiatric patient if she is intending to become pregnant as it may be possible to avoid medication with established teratogenicity. Associations between psychotropic drugs and fetal malformation include the following.
  - Lithium carries a teratogenic effect on the fetal heart, associated with 1% risk of Ebstein's anomaly. There is also a risk of lithium toxicity in the newborn.
  - Phenytoin is associated with cleft lip and palate, cardiac malformations, microcephaly, and growth restriction.
  - Benzodiazepines have an unconfirmed link with cleft lip and palate, but neonatal hypotonia and respiratory depression are established risks.
  - Antidepressants include tricyclic antidepressants, monoamine oxidase inhibitors (MAOIs), and selective serotonin-uptake inhibitors (SSRIs). Although SSRIs are newer than the other two groups, antidepressants generally have not been shown to have a teratogenic effect. Recent studies suggest that congenital cardiac anomalies may be increased twofold in women on paroxetine (Paxil).
  - Phenothiazines make up the largest group of antipsychotic medications. They are not associated with an increased risk of teratogenicity. Most patients on antipsychotics have a high risk of relapse if their medication is withheld.
- *Neonatal withdrawal symptoms.* As psychotropic drugs cross the placenta, a neonate may manifest signs of exposure to the drugs, e.g. floppiness, poor feeding, and respiratory depression from benzodiazepine therapy or neonatal goiter from lithium.
- *Breast-feeding.* Most psychotropic drugs are secreted into breast milk. Maternal therapeutic doses of benzodiazepines and lithium may result in breast milk levels sufficient to affect a neonate. Breast-feeding may have to be avoided in mothers on these medications, especially if the neonates show signs of toxicity (excessive lethargy, poor feeding, failure to thrive). The amounts of antidepressant and anticonvulsant medication secreted into breast milk do not have a significant effect on babies.

Recommended further reading

1. Gelder M, Gath D, Mayou R, Cowen P (1996). Psychiatric aspects of obstetrics and gynaecology. In: *Oxford Textbook of Psychiatry* pp. 394–9. Oxford University Press, Oxford.
2. Puri BK, Laking PJ, Treasaden IH (1996). Psychiatry of menstruation and pregnancy. In: *Textbook of Psychiatry* pp. 231–44. Churchill Livingstone, Edinburgh.

Postpartum disorders

Mental illness predating a pregnancy has a high risk of recurrence in the puerperium.

Postpartum 'blues'

About 70% of postpartum women experience brief episodes of mood lability, tearfulness, poor sleep, and irritability, starting around the third postpartum day and reaching a peak lasting 1–2 days. This is most common in primiparous women and is not related to delivery complications. There is often a background of anxiety and depressive symptoms in the third trimester of pregnancy. The condition usually resolves spontaneously without treatment in a few days. Reassurance and support are the mainstays of management.

Postnatal depression

This is a nonpsychotic depressive illness in the postnatal period affecting about 10% of women in the postnatal period. Clinical features include poor sleep, poor concentration, irritability, poor appetite, and decreased libido. The recurrence rate in subsequent pregnancies may be up to 70%. Mild cases either need no treatment or can be treated by their family practitioner and rarely see a psychiatrist. Most cases resolve within 6 months of delivery. However, many mild cases are missed and may continue to suffer from depression, and up to 75% of sufferers may be inadequately treated. Lack of social and domestic support may precipitate or compound postnatal depression, with the extra pressures of caring for a child being an unbearable additional burden. Postnatal depression may lead to a disturbed mother–infant relationship which progresses into a vicious cycle of worsening of the mother's condition and further poor relationship with the child.

Management should involve reassurance and support from the partner and other family members. Input from a social worker and attendance at support groups of women with similar problems may be of value. Severe cases should be referred to a psychiatrist, and treatment options include anxiolytics, antidepressants, and electroconvulsive therapy (ECT). Antidepressant medication is indicated if the depression lasts for longer than a month.

Puerperal psychosis

Puerperal psychosis has an incidence of up to 1 in 200, resulting in 1 in 600 postpartum women being admitted into a psychiatric unit. Peak incidence is at about 2 weeks' postpartum. Primiparous women are more susceptible, and up to 20% of these patients have a previous history of bipolar mood disorder. The recurrence risk in a future pregnancy is up to 25%. The condition may be depressive, manic, or schizophrenic. Onset is usually within 2 weeks of delivery. There is an associated suicide rate of up to 5% and an infanticide rate of up to 4%. The patient needs to be hospitalized for treatment as well as for the protection of the baby from neglect, mishandling, or infanticide. Despite the risk to the baby, it is inappropriate except in cases of severe psychotic disturbance to separate the baby from the mother. Admission into a 'mother and baby unit' is ideal. Mothers who keep their babies with them, bond, recover better, and stay in hospital for shorter periods than those separated from their babies. The underlying psychosis is treated with appropriate antidepressant or antipsychotic medication or ECT.

Seventy percent of cases of puerperal psychosis make a full recovery, but the risk of further psychosis is up to 50% overall and 20% in a future puerperium.

Recommended further reading

1. Cunningham FG, MacDonald PC, Gant NF, *et al.* (1997). Neurological and psychiatric disorders. In *William's obstetrics* pp. 1255–72. Appleton and Lange, Stamford, CT.
2. Gelder M, Gath D, Mayou R, Cowen P (1996). Psychiatric aspects of obstetrics and gynaecology. In *Oxford Textbook of Psychiatry* pp. 394–9. Oxford University Press, Oxford.
3. Puri BK, Laking PJ, Treasaden IH (1996). Psychiatry of menstruation and pregnancy. In *Textbook of Psychiatry* pp. 231–44. Churchill Livingstone, Edinburgh.

Chapter 11

Gynecological history, examination, anatomy, and development

History of the gynecological patient

It is best to have an outline on which the gynecological history can be taken and presented. This avoids inadvertent omission of important details (both positive and negative) and allows for a systematic and concise presentation of the facts. Please be polite. Introduce yourself (your name and designation) to the patient and explain the purpose of your discussion. A suggested outline is as follows:

Current history

- Name, age, and parity
- Detailed history of present complaint. One should be able to establish the presenting complaints. A brief history relevant to the presenting complaints must be taken. There must be some organizational logic in history taking.
    - *Abnormal menstrual loss* Distinguish between a regular or irregular pattern of bleeding. Attempt to quantify amount of loss by indicating the number of sanitary pads used in a day, presence of blood clots, and the need to use two pads at one time ('flooding'). The social impact of the heavy periods such as absence from work during menses because of associated pain, weakness, or 'flooding' is important.
    - *Pelvic pain* Establish the duration, site, and nature of pain and possible relationship with the time in the menstrual cycle. Determine aggravating and relieving factors. Ask about radiation of the pain and associated symptoms, e.g. vomiting, fever, dysuria.
    - *Vaginal discharge* Describe the odor, color, consistency, amount, and presence of blood. Relationship to the period and associated itching or irritation is relevant.

Past medical, family, and social history

This is an inquiry into the reproductive history that includes past obstetric, gynecological, menstrual, contraceptive, and cervical smear histories. This should be followed by past medical and surgical history. Family and social history should not be forgotten.

- *Menstrual history*
    - Menarche (age when periods began)
    - Cycle (interval between the first days of two consecutive periods)
    - Duration of period
    - State first day of the last menstrual period (LMP)
- *Past obstetric history* Describe outcomes and details of previous pregnancies. If there were many pregnancies, it is appropriate to summarize, e.g. five previous full-term spontaneous vaginal deliveries. Operative deliveries and any important issue such as miscarriage and fetal loss should be noted.
- *Past gynecological history* Details of gynecological history other than the presenting complaint should include previous cervical smears, previous gynecological problems, and any surgery (e.g. pelvic inflammatory disease or endometriosis).

- *Contraceptive history* The methods used, duration of use, acceptance, current method, side effects, and plan for the future.
- *Past medical and surgical history* Past medical and surgical history may have some bearing on the current problem or its management.
- *Drug allergies* This is vital information and should be prominently displayed in the notes. Failure to do so may cause severe illness or death of the patient.
- *Social history* This should include the impact of the present problem on the patient's life. Smoking, drinking, drug abuse, and living conditions may be relevant to the current problem or to the management planned.

Physical examination

This should always start with a general examination of the patient followed by cardiovascular and respiratory systems.

The gynecological examination encompasses both an abdominal and a vaginal pelvic examination which includes bimanual palpation. A bimanual examination should be preceded by inspection of the vulva, vagina, and cervix using a speculum. In specific circumstances, a rectal examination may be indicated.

Abdominal examination

The fundamental steps in an abdominal examination should be followed, i.e. inspection, palpation, and percussion. Auscultation may be relevant, especially in cases of acute abdomen and postoperative examinations.

Inspection

Abdominal distension, if any, should be noted and, if present, look for visible evidence of masses. If surgical scars are present, they should be correlated with the past history.

Palpation

Guarding, tenderness, and rebound tenderness are important signs to elicit in any one presenting with an acute abdomen. After performing a routine light palpation of the whole abdomen with the right hand, it is important to switch to the left hand and feel for pelvic masses. This is an important difference between gynecological and surgical examination which allows the clinician to detect any masses that may rise out of the pelvis.

Percussion/auscultation

Percussion is useful to distinguish between a solid mass (dull) and distended bowel (tympanic). In the presence of a vague mass on palpation in an obese individual or when one is tensing the abdominal wall, percussion is useful to identify the possibility of the mass and to define the borders. It is useful to demonstrate ascites or collection of blood. Shifting dullness and fluid thrill need to be demonstrated appropriately to the situation.

The pelvic examination

The pelvic or vaginal examination is the most challenging part of the gynecological physical examination. It is a potential source of embarrassment to the woman and should be conducted in a sensitive manner in privacy accompanied by a suitable chaperon. Exposure should be in a manner needed to carry out the examination. The abdomen should be covered up to and just below the knees. The examination should be performed gently, otherwise it can be uncomfortable. A well-performed pelvic examination gives good information about the genital tract and pelvic organs. Thus it is an indispensable part of the gynecological assessment.

Position

The pelvic examination can be performed in the dorsal, lithotomy, or Sim's position. Sim's position is a modification of the left lateral position and is ideal for examination of a woman with uterovaginal prolapse or vesicovaginal fistulae. The lithotomy position, in which both thighs are abducted and the feet suspended from lithotomy poles, is usually adopted when performing vaginal surgery. The dorsal position is most commonly used for routine outpatient gynecological examinations such as when obtaining a cervical smear.

Technique

The steps in performing a pelvic examination are as follows:

- Inspection of the external genitalia
- Speculum examination of the vagina and cervix
- Bimanual examination of the uterus and adnexae.

Inspection

Inspect the vulva and external genitalia. It is useful to imagine a series of circles surrounding the vaginal introitus and then to describe your findings from the outermost to the innermost circle. For example, one could begin with describing the mons pubis and pubic hair distribution, the labia majora and minora, the clitoris, urethral meatus and vaginal introitus.

Speculum examination

Two vaginal speculae are commonly used: Sim's (duck-billed) speculum and Cusco's (bivalve) speculum. Sim's speculum is used in the Sim's position and is most useful for the examination of uterovaginal prolapse. Cusco's speculum is most frequently used and is described below.

The labia minora are parted with the index and middle fingers of the left hand to obtain a good view of the introitus. A well-lubricated and warm bivalve speculum is held in the right hand with the main body of the speculum in the palm and the closed blades projecting between the index and middle fingers. This grasp is intended to keep the blades opposed and prevent inadvertent opening of the speculum while it is being inserted. In the lithotomy position, the speculum is usually inserted with the handle inferior while in the dorsal position, the handle should be superior. The speculum is advanced gently along with gentle pressure on the posterior wall of the vagina to open the potential space. Take note that the axis of the vagina is directed slightly towards the rectum. Open the speculum only when it cannot be advanced further. The cervix may be visualized. If it cannot be seen, the speculum is either above or below the cervix as the blades are in the anterior or posterior fornix of the vagina. It will then be necessary to close the speculum, withdraw it slightly, change its direction, and advance it before opening it again. The vaginal skin is rugose and that over the cervix is smooth. Usually there is mucus close to the cervical os, and there will be a convex anterior vaginal fornix or a concave posterior fornix. One or more of these features may come into view and may help to change the direction of the speculum.

Removal of the speculum requires as much care as insertion. It is essential that the blades are held open as the speculum is withdrawn until the ends of the blades are distal to the cervix. Otherwise, closing the blades on the cervix will cause pain. The speculum must be completely closed as the ends of the blades come out through the introitus.

Digital examination

The digital bimanual examination helps to identify the pelvic organs. The bladder should be emptied prior to this examination. The index and middle fingers of the right hand are inserted into the vagina with the palmar aspect facing upwards. Feel the consistency of the cervix. The left hand is placed on the abdomen and bimanual palpation commenced. The purpose of bimanual palpation is to bring the abdominal wall close to the pelvic organs by pressing on the appropriate place on the abdominal wall and also by shifting the pelvic organs or masses towards that hand. One should feel these organs or masses between the vaginal and abdominal hands. First, the uterus is felt with the vaginal fingers placed on the cervix and the hand on the lower midline above the uterine fundus. Then the adnexae can be palpated between the vaginal fingers placed in the lateral fornices and the abdominal hand over the respective iliac fossa. An anteverted uterus is easily palpated bimanually, but a retroverted one may not be. Retroverted uteri can be assessed by feeling the body of the uterus with the vaginal fingers via the vaginal wall of the posterior fornix.

If a pelvic mass is discovered, its size, consistency, and mobility are determined. Uterine masses may be felt to move with the cervix when the uterus is shifted upwards, while adnexal masses will not. If adnexal masses are suspected there should be a line of separation between the uterus and the mass, and the mass should be felt distinctly from the uterus. However, pedunculated masses from the uterus may give the impression of an adnexal mass and an adnexal mass adherent to the uterus may give the impression of a uterine mass. The consistency of the mass may be of help in distinguishing the origin in some cases. An ultrasound examination may be necessary to define it better.

Summary of the clinical problem

At the end of history taking and examination, the clinical problem should be summarized in a manner that will provide the important differential diagnosis and some guidelines toward the investigations needed to derive at the diagnosis. The summary should include salient points from the past medical, surgical, obstetric, and gynecological history which may influence the treatment.

This summary should be explained to the patient and the information provided should be understood by her in order for her to decide whether to proceed with the investigations and/or to accept the treatment. This summary should also be made available to her primary care provider if she so desires.

The pelvic walls and cavity

The anatomy of the female genital tract comprises the pelvic wall, the pelvic cavity and its contents, and the perineum.

The pelvic walls

These consist of the bony pelvis and pelvic floor muscles.

- *Anterior wall* Pubic bone and its rami, symphysis pubis, and urogenital membrane.
- *Posterior wall* Sacrum, coccyx, piriformis muscle, and sacrotuberous and sacrospinous ligaments.
- *Lateral wall* Part of the pubic bone below the pelvic inlet, obturator membrane, sacrotuberous and sacrospinous ligaments, and obturator internus muscle with its covering fascia.
- *Inferior wall (pelvic floor)* Levator ani and coccygeus muscles and their covering fascia. It is incomplete anteriorly to allow the passage of the urethra and vagina.

The pelvic cavity

This contains the rectum, sigmoid colon, terminal coils of the ileum, ureters, bladder, female genital organs, visceral pelvic fascia, and peritoneum.

Ovaries

Each ovary is oval, measuring 4 × 2 cm, and is attached to the broad ligament by the mesovarium. The ovarian ligament supports the ovary and connects it to the lateral margin of the uterus. Before puberty, the ovaries are smooth, but they become progressively scarred with age. Postmenopausal ovaries are shrunken and have a surface pitted with scars.

Tubes (fallopian tubes)

Each tube is about 10 cm long, lies in the upper border of broad ligament, and runs laterally from the uterine cornu to the ovary. The fallopian tube is divided functionally into four parts: the funnel-shaped infundibulum and its fimbriae, the wide ampulla, the narrow isthmus, and the intramural part which pierces the uterine wall.

The fallopian tubes, ovaries, and associated connective tissue (parametria) are collectively called the *adnexae*. They are palpated bimanually in the lateral fornices and, if normal, cannot be felt except in a very relaxed and slim woman.

- On pelvic examination, feel for masses and tenderness.

Uterus

This is a hollow pear-shaped organ with thick muscular walls that measures about 8 cm (length) × 5 cm (breadth) × 2.5 cm (anteroposterior) in a young nulliparous adult. It is divided into the fundus, body, and cervix. The mucin-secreting glands on the surface of the cervix lubricate the vagina. The opening (os) of the cervical canal is circular in nulliparous women and slit-like in parous women. The peritoneum is draped over the uterus, forming an anterior uterovesical fold, a posterior recto-uterine fold, and, laterally, the broad ligament.

Relations of the uterus

- Anterior: uterovesical pouch, superior surface of the bladder, anterior fornix of the vagina.
- Posterior: recto-uterine pouch (of Douglas), coils of ileum or sigmoid colon.
- Lateral: contents of the broad ligament (fallopian tubes, round ligament, ovarian ligament, uterine and ovarian vessels, vestigial mesonephric remnants), ureter, lateral vaginal fornix.

Positions

In most women, the uterus lies in an anteverted and somewhat anteflexed position.

- *Anteverted* The long axis of the uterus is bent forward on the long axis of the vagina, almost at right angles.
- *Anteflexion* The long axis of the body of the uterus is bent forward at the level of the internal os with the long axis of the cervix.
- *Retroversion* The fundus and body are bent backward and therefore lie in the pouch of Douglas.
- *Retroflexed* The body of the uterus is bent backward on the cervix.

Ten to twenty percent of normal women have a retroverted uterus. A full bladder will push the uterus backward and mimic retroversion.

Supports

The supports of the uterus are the levator ani and perineal body, the transverse cervical ligaments (also called cardinal ligament or Mackenrodt ligament), the uterosacral ligaments, and the pubocervical ligament.

- *Look for:* uterine position, size, mobility, and tenderness; cervical ectopy; cervicitis; discharge; polyps and pain on moving the cervix (cervical excitation tenderness).

Vagina

The vagina is an empty distensible muscular tube, extending upward and backward from the vulva to the uterus. It is about 8 cm long, with its upper half above the pelvic floor and its lower half within the perineum. It is attached circumferentially at its upper end to the cervix, which divides the vaginal lumen into an anterior, a posterior, and two lateral fornices.

- Relations
  - Anteriorly: bladder and urethra.
  - Posteriorly: pouch of Douglas, ampulla of the rectum, and perineal body.
  - Laterally: ureter, levator ani, urogenital diaphragm, and bulb of the vestibule.
- *Look for:* inflammation, discharge, prolapse.

Perineum

This is the part of the pelvic inlet which lies inferior to the pelvic diaphragm. When seen from below with the thighs abducted, it is diamond-shaped and bounded anteriorly by the symphysis pubis, posteriorly by the tip of the coccyx, and laterally by the ischial tuberosity. The perineum is artificially divided into an anterior urogenital and a posterior anal triangle.

- *Contents of urogenital triangle* Vulva and urethral and vaginal orifices.
- *Contents of anal triangle* Anus and ischiorectal fossa with the pudendal canal of Alcock in its extreme lateral position.

Vulva

This is the name applied to the external female genitalia (Fig. 11.1). It consists of the mons pubis, labia minora, labia majora, the vestibule (with the clitoris, ducts of paraurethral glands, ducts of Bartholin's glands, hymen, and vaginal and urethral orifices), and the perineum. When broken (by tampons or intercourse), the hymen leaves tags at the entrance to the vagina.

- *Look for:* rashes, atrophy, ulcers, lumps, and deficient perineum.

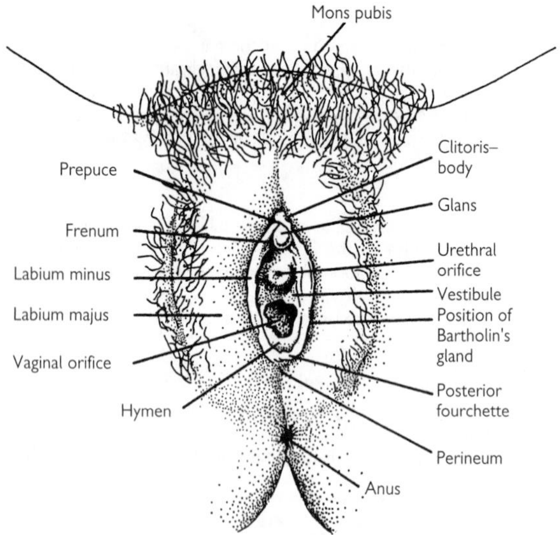

Fig. 11.1 External genitalia. (Reproduced from Collier J, Longmore M, Scally P, eds. *Oxford Handbook of Clinical Specialties*, 6th edn, p. 9, © 2003 by permission of the publisher Oxford University Press.)

Malformations of the female genital tract

Malformations of the female genital tract

The incidence is difficult to ascertain but it is estimated that 1% of phenotypic females have some abnormality of the genital tract. Of these, 40–50% are associated with renal tract abnormalities and 15% with an absent kidney. Vulval and gonadal anomalies are dealt with later in this chapter 📖 *p.436*.

Malformations of the uterus

The incidence is difficult to define. Malformations include absent uterus (Müllerian agenesis or hypoplasia), fusion anomalies of the uterus, and cervical atresia.

Absence of the uterus

The uterus may be absent or so rudimentary as to be incapable of functioning. This is usually associated with absence of vagina and primary amenorrhea (no menses). It may be associated with a blindly ending lower vagina, suggesting androgen insensitivity (XY with testes) or XX chromosome complement with ovaries.

Treatment

There is no corrective treatment available. Give psychological support. If there is androgen insensitivity, remove any testicular tissue to avoid risk of malignancy and provide estrogen replacement therapy.

Fusion anomalies

These are more common and result in a variety of well-recognized uterine shapes such as bicornuate uterus and subseptate uterus.

- Diethylstilbestrol (DES) exposure is associated with a T-shaped uterus.
- Unilateral atresia of one mesonephric duct results in a unicornuate uterus with a single fallopian tube, usually associated with unilateral absence of a kidney.
- Unilateral partial atresia of the mesonephric duct results in the presence of a rudimentary horn, which may communicate with the well-developed side.
- In a didelphic uterus, there are two completely separate uterine cavities, two cervices (which often unite externally), the vagina may be septate, and there may be associated ipsilateral absence of the kidney. It could be asymptomatic or present with cryptomenorrhea and hematoma. Cervical smears for cervical cancer screening (Pap smears) should be taken from both cervices.

Presentation

Fusion anomalies may be asymptomatic and only diagnosed on investigation of recurrent pregnancy loss, primary infertility, urological abnormalities, or menstrual disorders. In pregnancy, they may be associated with miscarriage, poor intrauterine fetal growth, malpresentation, and abnormal placentation.

Investigations

Hysterosalpingogram (HSG): if a double cervix, contrast should be injected into both cervical canals. Cervical atresia is a rare but serious malformation, which is due to the failure of the cervical portion of the fused Müllerian ducts to develop. The uterus may be normal or didelphic. If attempts to create a cervical opening are not effective, tubo-ovarian masses and peritonitis could develop, requiring hysterectomy. Sonohysterography (transabdominal ultrasound with instillation of sterile saline through the cervical os to facilitate visualization) has replaced HSG at many institutions.

Ultrasound or MRI may be needed to distinguish a separate uterus from uterus didelphys.

Malformations of the vagina

These occur in 1 in 4000–10 000 female births. They are the second most common cause of primary amenorrhea. Fifty percent are associated with renal anomalies and 12% with anomalies of the bony skeleton.

Absence

- If there is a rudimentary or no uterus due to congenital absence of the Müllerian duct (Mayer–Rokitansky–Kuster–Hauser syndrome), it presents at about age 16 years with primary amenorrhea. Sexual characteristics are normal because the ovaries are normal.
- If secondary sexual characteristics are not well developed, consider androgen insensitivity syndrome (XY female).
- Fifteen percent have major renal defects.
- If the uterus is present and the majority of the vagina is absent, the presentation is with amenorrhea, cyclical abdominal pain, and hematometra with a palpable mass. Sexual characteristics are normal.

Disorders of vertical fusion

There could be a high (46%), middle (35%), or low (19%) transverse vaginal septum or intact hymen. The usual presentation is as a teenager with cryptomenorrhea, cyclical abdominal pain, and hematocolpos. She may also have pressure symptoms of urinary frequency or retention.

Lateral fusion defects

There may be a complete or partial septum lying in the midline in the sagittal plane. These defects may be associated with a double uterus and cervix or with a single uterus. They are usually an incidental finding or they may present with dyspareunia (pain with intercourse). When associated with unilateral vaginal obstruction, they present with abdominal pain, hematometra, and hematocolpos. Careful examination is needed. Otherwise, it will be missed, as it is associated with menstrual flow from the other side.

Diagnosis

- There should be a careful examination of the vulval appearance and sexual characteristics, and evidence of retained blood in the vagina or upper or lower part of the genital tract should be sought.
- There should be an ultrasound scan of the pelvis investigating the uterus, ovaries, hematometra, hematocolpos, and the level of defect.
- Intravenous urogram (IVU).
- Chromosomal analysis is needed if the vagina is absent. May require gonadectomy if XY.

Management

- *Absence.*
    - Psychological counseling.
    - If nonfunctioning uterus: vaginal dilators or vaginoplasty.
    - If coexisting functional uterus: release of retained menstrual blood; creation of a neovagina.

- *Vertical fusion defect.*
  - Obstructed hymen: cruciate incision through hymen.
  - Low/middle septum: transvaginal removal of septum and reanastomosis of vaginal segments.
  - High septum: abdominoperineal surgery.
- *Lateral fusion defect.* Resection of septum.

Wolffian duct anomalies

Remnants of the lower part may present as vaginal cysts and those of the upper part as paraovarian cysts (epoophoron and paroophoron). Small vaginal cysts do not necessarily need removal. If causing symptoms (usually dyspareunia), it should be removed surgically. Large or painful paraovarian cysts require surgical exploration.

Basic concepts in sex differentiation

Understanding intersex requires an insight into factors that are required for sexual development. The gonads, genital ducts, and external genitalia (Table 11.1) are normally interlinked in their development, but they can develop independently in aberrant conditions.

- *The gonads.* All gonads are genetically programmed to develop into ovaries unless 'rescued' by products of the SRY (sex-related Y) gene to become testes. The SRY gene is located on the Y chromosome. We do not know whether SRY is an activator of genes involved in testis determination, a suppressor of genes involved in ovarian differentiation, or both. Genes other than SRY may also be important in gonadal differentiation.
- *The genital ducts.* During early embryonic development, males and females have both Wolffian (male) and Müllerian (female) genital ducts. The neutral state is the female genital ducts. Its suppression and regression requires the production of Müllerian inhibitory factor (MIF) released from the testes.
- *External genitalia.* These develop under hormonal influence. The genital tubercle forms the phallus or the clitoris. The urethral fold forms the shaft of the penis or the labia minora. The genital swelling forms the scrotum or labia majora.

Basic principles in management

- The fundamental step at the birth of an intersex neonate is to rule out a life-threatening process.
  - Immediate threat to life: congenital adrenal hyperplasia (CAH).
  - Late threat to life: gonadal tumor formation particularly in neonates with 45,X/46,XY or neonates with 46,XY and gonadal dysgenesis. Tumor formation in women with androgen insensitivity syndrome (previously known as testicular feminization syndrome) increases after the age of 15.
- Decision-making on the gender. Expert advice may be required to determine the sex of rearing with the aim of providing close to natural secondary sexual organs and preserving fertility. The suitability of external genitalia for sexual life should be an important determinant in one or the other gender role. The determination of the sex of rearing and any simple corrective feminizing surgery may be performed before discharge. The decision on sex of rearing should be reinforced by continued support and counseling to parents, relatives, and the child as he or she continues to develop.
- Preservation of fertility. CAH patients can be fertile if treated early, and true hermaphrodites are potentially fertile if an ipsilateral ovary is present.

Some conditions of intersex are described in Table 11.2.

Table 11.1 Basic concepts in sex differentiation

	Differentiation of ducts		
	Wolffian duct	**Müllerian duct**	**Mesonephros**
In the male	Epididymis, ductus deferens, seminal vesicles	Remnant forms appendix testes	Regress, may form ductuli efferentes joining rete testis
In the female	Remnant may form Gartner's cyst at side of uterus or vagina	Tubes, uterus, upper four-fifths of vagina	Regress, may form epoophoron or paroophoron in the broad ligament

Table 11.2 Conditions of intersex

Congenital adrenal hyperplasia (CAH)

Autosomal recessive, enzymatic defect in cortisol synthesis (most common is 21-hydroxylase). Lack of negative feedback leads to excess ACTH which over stimulates the mineralocorticoid and the androgen pathways. Severity depends on degree of enzyme defect:

- Severe neonatal CAH: virilization of female fetus and salt losing; vomiting, diarrhea, weight loss, dehydration. Diagnosis may be delayed in males as no physical finding at birth.
- Non-salt-losing CAH: mild virilization; may present in childhood with genital overgrowth and increase in weight.
- Late-onset CAH: presents at puberty; early and excess sexual hair; clitoromegaly; delayed menarche; lack of puberty progression.
- Diagnosis: family history; clinical findings; excess metabolites proximal to 21-hydroxylase particularly 17-hydroxyprogesterone. Electrolyte levels will indicate the mineralocorticoid status; genetic studies confirm the diagnosis.
- Treatment. Cortisol replacement; salt supplementation to neonates; correction surgery of female genitalia if necessary; psychological support to parents and child.

The XY female

Failure of androgen production due to anatomical testicular failure (pure gonadal dysgenesis or mosaicism). There is a uterus and an upper vagina.

Failure of androgen production due to enzymatic testicular failure. There is no uterus or upper vagina.

End-organ insensitivity: 5-α reductase deficiency resulting in no conversion of testosterone to DHT. There is no uterus or upper vagina. Inactive androgen receptors (absent gene on X)

The XX male

Normal external genitalia, but underdeveloped with hypospadias. Positive H-Y antigen. Unlikely to present to gynecologist.

True hermaphrodites

Both ovary and testis are present. Male or female may dominate. Most are 46, XX, but also can be 46,XX/XY, 46,XY, 46,XY/47,XXY.

Androgens from luteoma, polycystic ovary, Krukenberg tumor.
Gestogens derived from testosterone

Variable masculinization but no metabolic defect.

Management of intersex

Even mild deviations from normal anatomy at birth or in childhood may represent potential intersex disorders. This should encourage specific questioning about drug use during pregnancy, the family history of women without periods, and queries about family members who had ambiguous external genitalia. A full examination for other endocrine and other physical anomalies should be undertaken.

Examination

It is imperative that an experienced clinician performs the examination. This should include evaluating the size of the genital tubercle (clitoris/ phallus), palpating the labioscrotal pouches and inguinal canals for any masses, identifying the urethra, and identifying the vagina and cervix if necessary by using a pediatric cystoscope. Rectal examination may at times be helpful in palpating the uterus. Table 11.3 lists anomalies that may be found and their possible causes.

Conditions confused with intersex

- Labial adhesion (confused with vaginal agenesis) is rare at birth. It can be acquired as early as 6 weeks of age and occurs more frequently before 12 months. The etiology remains unclear and infection does not necessarily result in fusion. However, *Candida* and Herpes simplex infection can cause labial adhesions.
- The presence of notches and bumps on the hymen's rim are common findings at birth. The decrease in estrogen levels after birth and aging to prepuberty results in a decrease in the number of these findings.
- Hymenal septa, hymenal clefts, and imperforated hymen are abnormal findings but are not intersex.
- In prepubertal girls, a vaginal opening more than 4 mm is distinctly rare in the absence of a history of sexual abuse.

Virilizing adrenal tumors may produce sufficient masculinization of the external genitalia to simulate sexual ambiguity. Evaluate for the presence of Y DNA. 17-Hydroxyprogesterone, electrolytes, and renin will indicate the mineralocorticoid status and are diagnostic for CAH.

Investigation

- Ultrasonography with Doppler may be useful for hydrocele or inguinal masses.
- Cord blood (risk of contamination) and peripheral blood samples should be sent for karyotyping, testosterone, and 17-hydroxyprogesterone.
- Fluorescent *in situ* hybridization (FISH) and polymerase chain reaction (PCR) are particularly valuable to document the presence of Y DNA.
- The HLA complex in families can be studied as necessary to determine whether they are normal, heterozygotes, or affected.

Table 11.3 Differential diagnosis of intersex

Anomaly	Possible causes
Clitoral enlargement	CAH, asymmetrical gonadal dysgenesis; hermaphroditism
Cryptorchidism	Undescended testes, but also 46XX, 45,X/47,XYY.
Inguinal or labioscrotal masses	Androgen insensitivity syndrome; Rokitansky syndrome
Large testicles with hypospadias	Fragile-X syndrome
Sex ambiguity	CAH, XY female, XX male, true hermaphrodite, excess androgens

Recommended further reading

1. McCann J *et al.* (1990). Genital findings in prepubertal girls selected for non-abuse: a descriptive study. *Pediatrics* **86**, 428–39.
2. Berenson AB (1993). Appearance of the hymen at birth and one year of age: a longitudinal study. *Pediatrics* **91**, 820–5.
3. Goff CW *et al.* (1989). Vaginal opening measurement. *Ame Jo Disea Child* **143**, 166–8.
4. Haqq CM, King CY, Ukiyama E, *et al.* (1994). Molecular basis of mammalian sexual determination: activation of Mullerian inhibiting substance gene expression by SRY. *Science* **266**, 1494–500.
5. McElreavey K, Vilain E, Abbas N, Herkowitz I, Fellous M (1993). A regulatory cascade hypothesis for mammalian sex determination: SRY represses a negative regulator of male development. *Proc Natl Acad Sci USA* **90**, 3368–72.
6. Birk OS *et al.* (2000). The LIM homeobox gene Lhx9 is essential for mouse gonad formation. *Nature* **403**, 900–13.

Treatment of intersex

Physiological replacement of cortisol in CAH patients, plus mineralocorticoid if needed, will suppress ACTH secretion and remove the stimulation of excessive androgen synthesis. Increased dosages are needed during periods of stress, but excessive therapy may suppress growth. A subsequent pregnancy in couples with a CAH child has a 1 in 4 chance of being affected. Steroids can be given. However, to be effective this should begin shortly after conception before the diagnosis can be made by chorionic villus sampling (CVS). This will involve treating seven or eight pregnancies (males or unaffected females) for each affected female diagnosed. The safety of long-term steroid treatment is yet unknown.

The decision on the sex of rearing should be made on the basis of the suitability of external genitalia for sexual life in one or other gender role. The female role is often chosen in the XY female. Inappropriate gonads for the chosen gender role should be removed and hormone replacement therapy (HRT) is given at puberty.

In true hermaphrodites, menstruation and/or breast development may occur and, if brought up as male, then total abdominal hysterectomy (TAH) and bilateral salpingo-oophorectomy (BSO) should be performed. Bilateral mastectomy may also be required. Traditionally, surgical construction of female genitalia has been done. Further studies are needed to assess a possible psychosocial impact of CNS exposure to high androgens in the female and the presence of ambiguous genitalia.

Follow-up during childhood is essential to monitor for tumor formation, Remove contradictory pelvic gonads, perform reconstruction surgery, and measure levels of follicle-stimulating hormone (FSH), luteinizing hormone (LH), and testosterone. Support groups and continued counseling of the child and parents are essential as the child continues to develop. New possible therapies are anti-androgens and aromatase inhibitors.

Recommended further reading

1. Merke DP, Cutler GB, Jr (1997). New approaches to the treatment of congenital adrenal hyperplasia. *JAMA* **277**, 1073–6.
2. Schober JM (2004). Feminizing genitoplasty: a synopsis of issues relating to genital surgery in intersex individuals. *J Pediatr Endocrinol Metab* **17**, 697–703.

Common childhood conditions

Vaginal discharge

Neonates

Circulating maternal estrogens exert a physiological effect on the female fetus and it is normal to see a clear odorless vaginal discharge in the early neonatal period. In around 10% of cases, it will be bloodstained as a result of endometrial stimulation by the maternal estrogens. The discharge settles as the levels of maternal hormone in the newborn decline after birth.

Older children (ages 2–7 years most commonly)

Vulvovaginitis (infection of the vaginal introitus) often presents with recurrent green-yellow discharge, pruritis, or inflammation. Swabs should be taken from the introitus below the hymen. The infection is almost exclusively bacterial in origin (*Haemophilus influenzae, Staphylococcus, Streptococcus,* coliform bacteria) and is rarely due to *Candida* in this age group. Growth of *Gonococcus, Trichomonas, or Gardnerella* suggests sexual abuse. Treatment consists of appropriate antibiotics, hygiene and clothing advice, and avoidance of constipation.

Pruritis vulvae

This is a collective term for vulval irritation due to a variety of causes in the absence of discharge.

- Threadworms (*Enterobius vermicularis*). Common, diagnose using the perianal tape test.
- Nonspecific vulvitis. This may be due to a number of dermatological conditions, e.g. eczema, psoriasis, contact dermatitis. They are rarely confined to the vulva.
- Lichen sclerosus. Usually a self-limiting condition in childhood without malignant predisposition. Relapses are not uncommon.
- Warts. Usually due to autoinoculation from hand lesions or transmitted from the hands of carers. Usually self-limiting, but may require more definitive treatment.

Labial adhesions

These are the most commonly seen condition in toddlers. They develop secondary to chronic inflammation and are usually asymptomatic, but may obscure the urethral opening and give rise to urinary symptoms. Treatment consists of reassurance and topical estrogen cream in two weekly cycles until the adhesions separate. Surgery is rarely needed.

Bleeding from the vagina/bloodstained discharge

This should always be investigated. Around 90% will be due to the presence of a foreign body causing an offensive bloody discharge. This typically requires an examination under anesthesia (EUA) to remove the foreign body.

- Trauma (e.g. straddle injuries) is a common cause of genital bleeding. Tears involving the posterior fourchette or hymen are *not* typically caused by this mechanism and are suspicious of sexual abuse.
- If no obvious cause is found, rarer causes must be considered, e.g. vaginal tumors, Munchausen's syndrome by proxy.

Recommended further reading

1. Emans SJ, Laufer MR, Goldstein DP (2004). *Pediatric and Adolescent Gynecology* (5th edn). Lippincott–Williams & Wilkins, Philadelphia, PA.

Puberty

Puberty is a recognized continuum of changes that begins around the age of 9 years in girls. Marshall and Tanner[1] described and staged the changes occurring in puberty in terms of breast development or thelarche (stages 1–5), pubic hair development or adrenarche (stages 1–5), and an end growth spurt, with the onset of menstruation or menarche occurring on the downward slope of the growth velocity curve (current average age of menarche is 12.8 years).

Precocious puberty

Pubertal changes before the age of 8 years are considered to be precocious and are divided into two categories.

- True or central precocious puberty: premature activation of the hypothalamic–pituitary–ovarian axis (HPO axis)
  - *Causes.* Largely idiopathic. Can be secondary to brain abnormalities, e.g. hamartomas, hydrocephalus.
  - *Treatment* depends on the cause. Gonadotropin-releasing hormone (GnRH) analogs are used to postpone puberty until a more appropriate age and to optimize adult height potential.
- Pseudo-precocious puberty. A process independent of the HPO axis. It is much rarer than true precocious puberty.
  - *Causes.* In girls it is often due to an estrogen-secreting tumor, McCune–Albright syndrome.

When hirsutism/virilization occurs with precocious puberty, late-onset adrenal hyperplasia and adrenal tumors must be excluded.

Delayed puberty

This presents with primary amenorrhea (no menses) with or without the presence of secondary sexual characteristics.

Girls with absence of both menses and secondary sexual characteristics by age 14

Possible causes are as follows:

- *Constitutional delay* is by far the most common cause, often with a positive family history.
  - Treatment consists of ruling out other causes and reassurance. The induction of puberty can be considered if there are psychological problems.
- *Chronic systemic disease*, e.g. endocrine disorders, cystic fibrosis, chronic renal failure, celiac disease, emotional or physical neglect.
  - Treating the underlying cause usually triggers puberty.
- *Absence of ovarian function*, e.g. due to premature ovarian failure or abnormal gonadal development or gonadal dysgenesis. The majority will have Turner's syndrome (46, X).
  - Treatment relies on good psychological support, especially regarding fertility issues, induction of puberty, and long-term maintenance of estrogen levels. Gonadectomy may be necessary if any Y chromosome is present because of increased malignant potential.

- *Hypothalamic-pituitary dysfunction* due to tumors, genetic conditions, or idiopathic.
  - The underlying cause should be treated if possible and, if due to a nonreversible cause, puberty should be induced.

Girls with normal secondary sexual characteristics but absent menses by age 16

Possible causes are the following.

- *Constitutional delay* is again the most common cause, usually with a family history.
- Absent uterus/endometrium because of:
  - *Complete androgen insensitivity syndrome* (46,XY female). Treatment is with estrogen replacement and gonadectomy because of malignant potential. Vaginal reconstruction surgery may be needed and psychological support is vital.
  - *Rokitansky–Kutser–Hauser syndrome* (46,XX, absent uterus and upper vagina, associated renal and vertebral anomalies). Treatment might involve vaginal reconstructive surgery. Psychological support is essential, especially regarding fertility issues (assisted conception).
- *Absent vagina/imperforate hymen* presents with cyclical abdominal pain, pelvic mass, and absent menses. Treatment is to incise hymen, excise septum, or fashion lower vaginal opening to allow menstrual flow to pass.

Induction of puberty

This aims to mimic the gradual increase in ovarian function at puberty. Treatment is with an increasing ethinyl estradiol regime in six-monthly increments. When breakthrough bleeding occurs or when the 20–30 mg dose is reached, progesterone is added for endometrial protection. This is usually the combined oral contraceptive but HRT preparations are also used.

Recommended further reading

1. Marshall WA, Tanner JM (1969). Variations in the pattern of pubertal changes in girls. *Archi Dis Child* **44**, 944–54.
2. Emans SJ, Laufer MR, Goldstein DP (2004). *Pediatric and Adolescent Gynecology* (5th edn). Lippincott–Williams & Wilkins, Philadelphia, PA.

Chapter 12

Normal menstruation and its disorders

Physiology of normal menstruation

Menstruation is the shedding of the functional layer (upper two-thirds) of the endometrium after sex steroid withdrawal. The role of the functional layer is to prepare the uterus for implantation. The basal endometrial layer (lower one-third) provides tissue for regeneration during the following cycle. This shedding process, which consists of three phases (menstrual, proliferative, and secretory), is repeated approximately 300–400 times during a woman's reproductive life. It also occurs in primates and bats. Menstruation indicates that conception has not occurred.

Phases of the endometrial cycle (Fig. 12.1)

The proliferative phase

This phase is associated with increasing ovarian follicular growth and therefore increasing levels of ovarian estrogen, which leads to repair and growth of the glandular, stromal, and vascular components of the endometrium. Toward the end of the proliferative or follicular phase endometrial glands are short, straight, and narrow, measuring up to 5 mm in height.

The secretory phase

After ovulation, progesterone becomes the dominant steroid, and its early effect is to inhibit and stop epithelial proliferation, which occurs 2–3 days after ovulation. During this secretory or luteal phase, initial glandular and vessel growth within a progesterone-dominated endometrium leads to increasing tortuosity of glands and coiling of spiral vessels. The *lumina* of the endometrial glands gradually fill with glycogen-rich secretion. This phase lasts around 14 days, and is ended by the demise of the corpus luteum and therefore progesterone production, unless implantation occurs.

Implantation, on days 21–22 of a 28-day menstrual cycle, is followed by further dramatic morphological changes. In the absence of implantation, the gradual fall of progestogen and estrogen from the mid-secretory phase onward causes other changes (below) which finally lead to menstruation.

The menstrual phase

Gradual withdrawal of ovarian sex steroids causes slight shrinking of the endometrium, and therefore the blood flow of spiral vessels is reduced. This, together with spiral arteriolar spasms, leads to distal endometrial ischemia and stasis. Extravasation of blood and endometrial tissue breakdown leads to the onset of menstruation.

Fifty percent of the menstrual blood loss is thought to occur during the first 24 hours, and the rest thereafter. An estimated volume of approximately 80 mL is expelled. A loss of over 80 mL is considered to be heavy (menorrhagia), although the volume lost is poorly related to patient perception of loss. Various mechanisms are thought to have an important role to play in the control of menstrual loss.

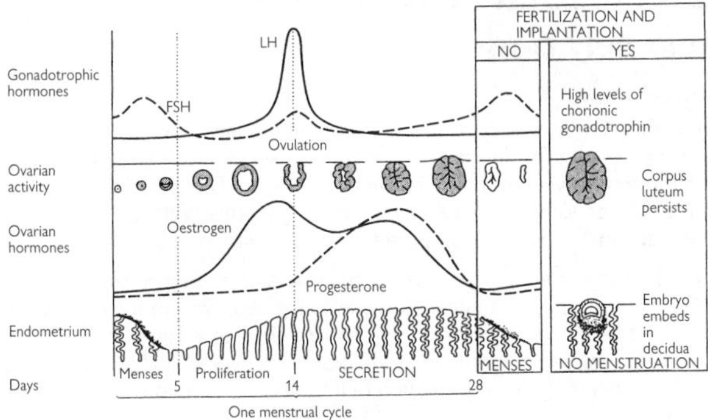

Fig. 12.1 Pituitary, ovarian, and endometrial cycles. (Reproduced form Collier J, Longmore M, Scally P, eds. *The Oxford Handbook of Clinical Specialities* (6th edn), p. 9, © 2003 by permission of the publisher Oxford University Press.)

Recommended further reading

1. Hallberg L, Hogdahl AM, Nilsson L, *et al.* (1966). Menstrual blood loss—a population study. *Acta Obstet Gynecol Scand* **45**, 320–51.
2. Chimbira TH, Anderson AB, Turnbull A (1980). Relation between measured blood loss and patient's subjective assessment of loss, duration of bleeding, number of sanitary towels used, uterine weight and endometrial surface area. *Br J Obstet and Gynecol* **87**, 603–9.
3. Baird DT, *et al.* (1996). Prostaglandins and menstruation. *Euro J Obstet and Gynecol Reproduct Bio* **70**, 15–17.
4. Campbell S, Cameron IT, (1998). The origins and physiology of menstruation. In: Cameron IT, Fraser IS Smith SK, eds. *Clinical Disorders of the Endometrium and Menstrual Cycle*, pp. 13–30. Oxford University Press, Oxford.

Endometrial hemostasis and regeneration

Introduction

In parallel with the endometrial ischemic changes already described, progesterone also destabilizes lysosome membranes, leading to the release of active enzymes and prostaglandins. These active enzymes cause further local tissue necrosis, including vascular damage. Therefore the functional endometrium is shed in tandem with local bleeding.

On shedding the functional endometrium and ending a sequence of changes designed to nourish an implanting embryo, various complex mechanisms come into play to control and limit bleeding balanced with active fibrinolysis to avoid clot formation. Absence of fibrinolysis would subsequently lead to the formation of intrauterine adhesions and reduced fertility.

Prostaglandins

Endometrial prostaglandin (PG) concentrations are now known to be low during the proliferative phase of the menstrual cycle, and increase during the latter part of the secretory phase. The two main endometrial PGs have antagonistic effects on the spiral arteriolar system. PGE_2 is a vasodilator and $PGF_{2\alpha}$ is a vasoconstrictor. Women with menorrhagia are thought to have a higher local concentration of the vasodilator PGE_2, which can respond to therapeutic doses of prostaglandin synthetase inhibitors.

- Prostacyclin (or PGI_2), predominantly from the myometrium, is also a vasodilator and reduces platelet aggregation.
- Prostaglandins are known to play a key role in the onset of human parturition and myometrial contractility and also promote endometrial hemostasis by inducing uterine contractions.

Other agents

Platelet activation factors likely to make a direct contribution to endometrial hemostasis have also been shown to stimulate the release of vasoconstricting PGE_2 but not $PGF_{2\alpha}$. Other potent vasoconstrictors of small vessels in the human uterus include a group of peptides termed *endothelins*.

Endometrial regeneration

At the end of menstruation, the basal endometrium (glandular, stromal, and vascular) grows and develops to form the subsequent functional endometrial component. This process begins soon after the onset of menstruation. The aim of certain surgical approaches for women with menorrhagia is the complete or near-complete destruction of the basal endometrium leading to amenorrhea.

The cellular and molecular processes of endometrial repair are poorly understood, but several agents are thought to play a role in endometrial regeneration. These include:

- interleukins
- interferons
- epidermal growth factors
- insulin-like growth factors.

The proliferative effect of estradiol on the endometrium is probably mediated by basal endometrial tissue release of the above factors and many others not yet clearly implicated.

Recommended further reading

1. Hallberg L, Hogdahl AM, Nilsson L, *et al.* (1966). Menstrual blood loss—a population study. *Acta Obstet Gynecol Scand* **45**, 320–51.
2. Chimbira TH, Anderson AB, Turnbull A (1980). Relation between measured blood loss and patient's subjective assessment of loss, duration of bleeding, number of sanitary towels used, uterine weight and endometrial surface area. *Br J Obstet Gynecol* **87**, 603–9.
3. Baird DT, *et al.* (1996). Prostaglandins and menstruation. *Europ J Obstet Gynecol and Reprod Bio* **70**, 15–17.
4. Campbell S, Cameron IT (1998). The origins and physiology of menstruation. In: Cameron IT, Fraser IS, Smith SK, eds. *Clinical Disorders of the Endometrium and Menstrual Cycle*, pp. 13–30. Oxford University Press, Oxford.

The ovarian and pituitary cycle

The ovarian cycle

The uterus is a target organ and menstruation is an active response to changes in the ovarian steroid signals. Therefore no account of normal menstruation would be complete without a brief review of the ovarian cycle and its physiology.

Follicular growth

Each ovary contains approximately 250 follicles at birth. In every menstrual cycle, a small cohort of follicles develops and some become sensitive to the pituitary gonadotropin FSH. What induces initial follicular growth and renders a few follicles responsive to FSH remains speculative, but increased FSH sensitivity is paramount to antral follicular development. Follicular estrogen synthesis is essential for uterine priming, but is also part of the positive feedback that induces a surge in release of the pituitary LH which triggers ovulation. The growth of the follicle and oocyte over such a short period of time is dramatic. A preovular human follicle can grow up to 25 mm, and an oocyte enlarge from 15 μm to >100 μm. Inhibin is also thought to be produced by the dominant preovulatory follicle. Its role is probably to suppress FSH levels, therefore causing other follicles to become atretic.

Corpus luteum

Progesterone production by the corpus luteum is regulated initially by LH and subsequently, if a pregnancy occurs, by human chorionic gonadotropin (hCG). The continuation or cessation of secretion of progesterone by the corpus luteum then controls the onset of menstruation. If pregnancy fails to occur, luteal regression leads to reduced responsiveness to LH and subsequent luteolysis. With implantation of a blastocyst and hCG secretion, the endometrium is sustained and menstruation delayed.

Implantation is a process which includes an embryo reaching the inner uterine wall and penetrating the epithelium and the underlying circulation of the receptive endometrium. This process starts 2–3 days after the fertilized egg enters the uterus. Soon after trophoblastic invasion of the myometrium, hCG produced by the conceptus can be detected in the maternal circulation and urine. This luteal support with sustained progesterone production is crucial during the first weeks of pregnancy to avert endometrial regression.

The pituitary cycle

Follicular development and ovarian steroidogenesis are regulated by the gonadotropins, FSH and LH, released from the anterior pituitary. Pulsatile release of gonadotropin-releasing hormone (GnRH) from the hypothalmus at the start of the cycle stimulates the release of FSH and follicular development in the ovary. Fourteen days before menstruation in a 28 day cycle, the rising level of estrogen leads to a surge of LH and ovulation.

Recommended further reading

1. Campbell S, Cameron IT (1998). The origins and physiology of menstruation. In: Cameron IT, Fraser IS, Smith SK, eds. *Clinical Disorders of the Endometrium and Menstrual Cycle*, pp. 13–30. Oxford University Press, Oxford.

Menstrual problems

Secondary amenorrhea is defined as complete cessation of menstrual cycles for a minimum of 6 months. Failure to start menstruating by the age of 16 (14 if associated with absent breast development) is described as *primary amenorrhea*. The etiology and management of these symptoms are often similar, apart from a few specific causes of primary amenorrhea. The causes of amenorrhea and their frequencies are given in Table 12.1.

Oligomenorrhea is defined as menstrual bleeding at intervals of between 35 days and 6 months. This occurs frequently in practice but only needs investigating if it is persistent or associated with other problems.

The aims of investigations for these conditions should include the following:

- To reach a diagnosis and to address patients' concerns.
- To detect serious causes requiring specific treatment.
  - Anorexia nervosa.
  - Tumors: hypothalamic, pituitary, ovarian.
- To detect incidental or secondary conditions that affect general health and require further unrelated treatment.
  - Estrogen deficiency.
  - Unopposed estrogen.
- To manage ongoing subfertility: assess the need for ovulation induction and inform woman of prognosis.
- To give sound contraceptive advice on the basis of formal diagnosis.

Genital tract causes

- *Congenital Müllerian duct disorders* cause primary amenorrhea with abnormalities of varying severity. With functioning ovaries, cyclical symptoms are often present and so is secondary sex hair growth—not so in testicular feminization. Similarly, a hematocolpos, most commonly caused by an imperforate hymen, leads to cyclical abdominal pain.
- *Asherman's syndrome* (also known as endometrial fibrosis) is now often induced surgically to achieve amenorrhea or light periods in women with menorrhagia. It is now rarely seen following surgical trauma or pelvic tuberculosis infection.
- *Cervical stenosis* is also very rare and in most cases caused by surgical trauma after repeat surgery for cervical intraepithelial neoplasm (CIN). Laser endocervicectomy is the treatment of choice.

Hypothalamic disorders

The arcuate nucleus of the hypothalamus secretes pulses of GnRH. This is transported in the capillary plexus down the pituitary stalk to the anterior part of pituitary, where it stimulates the synthesis of LH and FSH.

Primary hypothalamic failure

This occurs in various conditions and presents with clinical evidence of GnRH deficiency. Any CNS tumor, e.g. glioma, can be associated with amenorrhea, but the latter is of little consequence and often occurs with other anterior pituitary hormone deficiencies. More important from the endocrine viewpoint is congenital GnRH deficiency, which results in poorly developed females with absence of menarche (isolated gonadotropin deficiency). This can occur in association with anosmia due to a coexisting congenital abnormality of the olfactory bulb and is typically X-linked (Kallman's syndrome).

Hypothalamic functional disorders

These are the most common causes of secondary amenorrhea. The majority of causes are related to emotional/psychological stress, weight loss, or excessive physical exercise. They are most common in teenagers.

With loss of body mass, the onset of amenorrhea is often abrupt and cycles do not return immediately after the weight is regained. Severe gonadotropin deficiency is seen in anorexia nervosa. Estrogen HRT must be considered in the management of such patients.

Table 12.1 Causes of amenorrhea and their frequency

Cause	Frequency (%)
Polycystic ovarian disease	33
Hypothalamic disorders	35
Hyperprolactinemia (prolactinoma in 50%)	20
Primary ovarian failure	12
Thyroid disease	1
Adrenal causes	<1
Anatomical causes	<1

Pituitary dysfunction

- *Primary failure* Sheehan's syndrome, which is due to postpartum hypotension with subsequent anterior pituitary gland necrosis, is now rare. Tumors causing compression of the pituitary stalk or lesions causing damage to the pituitary gland (empty sella syndrome) lead to amenorrhea either by destruction of the gonadotrophes and gonadotropin deficiency or by causing hyperprolactinemia by interfering with the negative feedback effect of dopamine secretion and transport along the pituitary stalk.
- *Pituitary functional disorders* Hyperprolactinemia is by far the most common pituitary disorder causing amenorrhea. Prolactin secretion from the pituitary lactotrophes is inhibited by dopamine transported down the pituitary stalk from the hypothalamus.

Causes of hyperprolactinemia

Physiological causes

Pregnancy and lactation are by far the most common causes of hyperprolactinemia, followed by *stress* and *exercise.* Some women find initial hospital visits very stressful. Therefore estimation of prolactin levels needs to be repeated after subsequent visits.

Nipple stimulation at times of sexual foreplay can cause both increased prolactin levels and subsequent galactorrhea. A detailed and cautious history is essential.

Pharmacological causes

Any drug that antagonizes dopamine receptors or acts as a neurotransmitter can cause hyperprolactinemia. Phenothiazines and other drugs used to treat psychiatric conditions have been implicated, together with methyldopa, opiates, and estrogens.

Pathological causes

- Moderate hyperprolactinemia (serum levels <1750 mU/L) occurs in patients with hypothyroidism and similarly in association with polycystic ovarian syndrome, possibly caused by increased unopposed estrogen in the latter.
- A *primary* pituitary neoplasm may produce excessive prolactin.
  - *Macroprolactinoma* (diameter >10 mm) is associated with very high levels of prolactin (serum levels of 8000 mU/L or more).
  - *Microprolactinomas* usually have lower levels of circulating prolactin (<3000 mU/L) and do not always require ongoing treatment with dopamine agonists.

Diagnosis and management

For diagnosis, repeat serum prolactin estimates and thyroid function tests must be performed. Pituitary imaging by CT or MRI and formal visual field evaluation are essential to reach a diagnosis, but also as part of ongoing surveillance of primary hyperprolactinemia.

Treatment is for subfertility or symptomatic galactorrhea or estrogen replacement to avert long-term complications of hypogonadism.

- *Bromocriptine* is effective in over 90% of patients with a prolactinoma. Galactorrhea also decreases in the vast majority of patients. Side effects include nausea, dizziness, and postural hypotension. These can be reduced by incremental and split dosage regimes, starting with a 1.25 mg dose taken before bedtime with the aim of increasing to a target dose of 7.5 mg.
- *Carbegoline*, a potent and long-acting dopamine agonist, is an alternative therapeutic option. The recommended initial dose is 0.25 mg twice weekly, aiming for a maximum of 1 mg twice weekly. Carbegoline is better tolerated than bromocriptine.
- *Transphenoidal surgery* as part of the management of prolactinomas is now mostly limited to patients with dopamine agonist resistance or marked intolerance.

Hyperprolactinemia and fertility

There is no benefit in performing serum prolactin levels with ongoing subfertility in women who have regular menstrual cycles. Confusion can arise in the rare event of finding high levels of nonbioactive macro (large) prolactin levels. Not much is known about this condition, which does not appear to affect fertility.

Unless there is a coexisting problem, regular menstrual cycles return and so does fertility in the majority of women with prolactinomas once the prolactin levels are normalized with dopamine agonists.

Treatment during pregnancy

During pregnancy, the normal pituitary gland is known to enlarge.

- The risk of a treated microprolactinoma enlarging significantly during pregnancy is extremely low. Therefore treatment can be stopped once pregnancy is diagnosed.
- A macroprolactinoma must be treated and tumor shrinkage to within the sella and normal fields confirmed prior to considering a pregnancy. Treatment can be stopped once pregnancy is diagnosed. There is controversy about the need for surveillance during pregnancy.
    - Visual fields during the second and third trimester are often performed, although sudden and unpredictable acute suprasellar extension rarely occurs. If suspected, therapy with a dopamine agonist is resumed after confirmation by MRI.

Gonadal failures

The primary ovarian disorders include the following:
- Premature ovarian failure
- Autoimmune disease
- Destruction
- Sex chromosomal abnormalities.

Premature ovarian failure

The menopause occurs before the age of 40 in 1% of women and, in more than two-thirds of such cases, the etiology remains unknown. This is termed *premature ovarian failure* and accounts for approximately 10% of amenorrheic women. This can occur at any age and may even present with absence of menarche (primary amenorrhea). The main candidate gene for premature ovarian failure (hypergonadotropic hypogonadism) is the FSH receptor gene.

Autoimmunity

Based on the presence of autoantibodies (thyroid and, less frequently, ovarian antibodies), autoimmunity has been estimated to be the cause of ovarian damage in 20–30% of women with primary ovarian failure. Treatment with glucocorticosteroids has been reported to restore fertility in this subgroup. However, spontaneous resumption of ovulation may also occur.

The resistant ovary syndrome

Another small subgroup of women with clear hypergonadotropic amenorrhea of unknown cause do, after a period of time, resume spontaneous menstrual cycles and even conceive—*the resistant ovary syndrome.* The place for exogenous gonadotropin therapy in this subgroup remains unclear.

Destruction

Radiotherapy and *chemotherapy* for neoplastic conditions are increasing causes of premature ovarian failure, e.g. treatment of lymphomas. Freezing of ovarian tissue or, more recently, oocyte cryopreservation can be offered to women prior to therapy, but future use has not as yet been clearly defined.

In the older age group, *surgery* is a common cause of premature menopause requiring hormone replacement therapy.

Sex chromosome abnormalities

Turner's syndrome (46,X; ovarian dysgenesis) is the most common sex chromosome abnormality. It presents with primary amenorrhea, short stature, and sexual infantilism. Patients with Turner's mosaics very occasionally develop secondary sexual features and menstruate. Other forms of abnormalities including 46,XY gonadal dysgenesis and testicular feminization are discussed in Chapter 11 📖 *p.440*.

The treatment of Turner's syndrome includes growth hormone and estrogens, both causing a growth spurt. The estrogen should be started from about the age of 10–11 years to stimulate normal secondary sex characteristic development (first year 5 μg/day, second year 10 μg/day, and third year 20 μg/day). A withdrawal bleed is likely to occur any time after 10 μg/day and, when it occurs, a combined estrogen–progestogen preparation should be introduced.

Investigations of amenorrhea and oligomenorrhea

- *Serum FSH* Raised in primary ovarian failure. Normal size ovaries by ultrasound scan and autoantibodies suggest autoimmune ovarian failure.
- *Serum LH* Raised in polycystic ovary syndrome (PCOS), but a normal level is of no diagnostic value.
- *Serum prolactin* Raised level is diagnostic of hyperprolactinemia.
- *Serum testosterone* Requested only if there is associated hirsutism. Significantly raised levels (>7 nmol/L (>200 ng/dL)) are suspicious of tumor.
- *Thyroid function test*
- *Progestogen challenge test* A negative test is suggestive of estrogen deficiency due to primary or secondary (hypothalamic/pituitary) ovarian failure. A positive test suggests estrogenized endometrium as in PCOS.
- *Chromosome analysis* Important in certain patients with primary amenorrhea.
- *Diagnostic imaging* Lateral X-ray, CT, or MRI of pituitary fossa in all women with suspected secondary amenorrhea of hypothalamic/pituitary origin.
- *Pelvic ultrasound* is useful to investigate the structure of ovaries and the size of the uterus, including endometrial thickness.

Dysmenorrhea

Crampy lower abdominal pain radiating to the back and legs associated with menstruation is a common symptom in women of reproductive age. Primary dysmenorrhea in adolescents usually occurs in the absence of pelvic pathology. Secondary dysmenorrhea is pain that develops later in reproductive life and is more likely to be associated with pelvic pathology, such as uterine fibroids or endometrial polyps.

Primary dysmenorrhea

This starts soon after menarche with the onset of ovular cycles. It is suprapubic, tends to be worst on the first day of menstruation, and improves thereafter. Patients with primary dysmenorrhea have been shown to have increased frequency and amplitude of myometrial contractions mediated by prostaglandins.

- *Investigations* of primary dysmenorrhea are predominantly to exclude any pelvic pathology and are similar to those for secondary dysmenorrhea (see below).
- *Treatment* Over 80% of women with this condition respond to therapy with NSAIDs started 24–48 hours before the onset of pain. Mefenamic acid 500 mg or ibuprofen 400 mg three times a day are often prescribed. Side effects are mostly gastrointestinal.
    - The use of combined oral *estrogen–progestogen* contraceptives leading to anovulatory cycles is a useful second line of management which should be continued for 9–12 months if symptoms improve. Otherwise, investigations are stepped up as for secondary dysmenorrhea.

Secondary dysmenorrhea

This exhibits various patterns depending on the underlying pathology.

- The presence of dyspareunia (pain with intercourse) is significant, and the associated pelvic/lower abdominal pain occurs either intra/postmenstrually, starts premenstrually, or only occurs on days 1 and 2 of the menstrual cycle. This is discussed in detail in Chapter 14 📖 *p.571*.
- The pattern of secondary dysmenorrhea caused by an endometrial polyp is similar to that seen with submucous fibroids and usually occurs at the beginning of menstruation.

Investigations planned are determined by the history and clinical examination findings. They may include basic hematological investigations and ESR or C-reactive protein with or without microbiological swabs from the genital tract followed by ultrasound, laparoscopy, and/or hysteroscopy.

The *treatment* of secondary dysmenorrhea is that of the underlying condition discussed in the relevant chapters.

Dysfunctional uterine bleeding: diagnosis

Dysfunctional uterine bleeding (DUB) is defined as excessively heavy (>80 mL per month) or prolonged uterine bleeding in the absence of systemic or genital tract pathology. It is a diagnosis of exclusion. Overall, it affects 10% of women, and is the most common cause of iron deficiency anemia and gynecological referrals. Although up to 30% of women report symptoms of heavy or prolonged menstrual bleeding (menorrhagia), this is confirmed on objective measurement in fewer than a third of cases. Dysfunctional uterine bleeding is divided into ovulatory, which is associated with regular painful periods, and anovulatory, which is more common in the postmenarcheal and perimenopausal age groups.

Diagnosis

History

Ask about age, parity, fertility, current contraception, and previous treatment for abnormal uterine bleeding. To assess the heaviness of bleeding, ask about the duration of the periods, amount, sanitary protection used, and whether the women passes clots during menstruation. The presence of bleeding between periods or a recent onset of pain at the time of menstruation are suggestive of pelvic pathology.

Examination

A general examination may reveal signs of thyroid disease, anemia, or clotting disorders. An abdominal examination should precede a pelvic examination. All women with abnormal genital tract bleeding must have a speculum examination to visualize the cervix and vagina to exclude any local cause. A cervical smear is taken if not recently performed. On pelvic examination, check for uterine enlargement (fibroids) or the tender fixed uterus typical of pelvic inflammatory disease or endometriosis.

Investigations

Abnormal bleeding can occur in early pregnancy. If there is any possibility of pregnancy, this should be excluded by a blood pregnancy test. A CBC to exclude anemia should be carried out for all women complaining of abnormal uterine bleeding. Thyroid function tests and a hormone profile are not usually required unless otherwise clinically indicated. Pipelle endometrial sampling, hysteroscopy (as an outpatient or day-case surgery under general anesthesia), and transvaginal ultrasound scan should be carried out to exclude endometrial pathology for patients >40 years. Below the age of 40, the risk of endometrial cancer is very low and endometrial sampling is not normally required for regular heavy periods. Irregular bleeding warrants hysteroscopy and sampling to rule out endometrial pathology.

Recommended further reading

1. Weeks AD, Duffy SRG (1996). Abnormal uterine bleeding: diagnosis and medical management. *Prog Obstet Gynecol* **12**, 309–26.

Medical management of dysfunctional uterine bleeding

The treatment of DUB should be with the simplest regimen with the fewest side effects that is effective. First-line therapy is medical, and will depend on the patient's need for contraception and on whether irregularity of the cycle is a problem. Regardless of which therapy is chosen, treatment should be reviewed after 3 months and, if there is no response, the patient should be referred for further investigation.

Patients with a regular cycle who do not require contraception

- *Tranexamic acid* (antifibrinolytic) is the most effective first-line drug. It acts by inhibiting tissue plasminogen activator (a fibrinolytic enzyme that has raised levels in women with DUB) and reduces menstrual blood loss by around 50%. The dose of tranexamic acid is 1 g three to four times a day during menstruation. The side effects are mainly gastrointestinal symptoms. It is contraindicated where there is a history of thromboembolic disease.
- *NSAIDs* such as mefenamic acid are effective, well tested, and well tolerated. They act by inhibiting cyclooxygenase which blocks myometrial prostaglandin production. NSAIDs reduce menstrual blood loss by 25% and are also analgesic drugs, so they are often used as a first-line treatment in the presence of dysmenorrhea. Mefenamic acid is commonly used at a dose of 500 mg three times a day for 5 days during menses. The main side effect is gastrointestinal irritation.

Patients with an irregular cycle or who need contraception

- *The combined oral contraceptive pill* (COCP) is commonly used, especially in the younger age group. It reduces menstrual blood loss by 20%, helps to regulate periods, and provides contraception. The mode of action is by inhibition of ovulation, production of inactive endometrium, and possibly by reduction in endometrial prostaglandin synthesis and altered fibrinolysis. See Chapter 16 📖 *p.574* for further details of side effects and contraindications.
- In the perimenopausal age group, sequential combined *hormone replacement therapy* can be used in a similar way to regulate the cycle and reduce mean blood loss.
- *Progestogens.* Synthetic progestogens (e.g. norethisterone 5 mg every 8 hours from day 12 to 26 or day 5–26) are the most popular drugs prescribed for the treatment of menorrhagia, even though they have minimal or no effect on menstrual blood loss. Progestogen therapy can be of value in regulating an irregular cycle. The main side effects are weight gain, bloating, and androgenic symptoms such as acne.

- *Levonorgestrel-releasing intrauterine contraceptive device (Mirena)* releases 20 μg of levonogestrel per 24 hours over 5 years. The modes of action of levonogestrel are a reduction in endometrial prostaglandin synthesis, the production of inactive endometrium, and a reduction in endometrial fibrinolytic activity. It reduces menstrual blood loss by 86% after 3 months.
- If a copper intrauterine contraceptive device is already *in situ*, either treat with tranexamic acid/NSAIDs or change to levonogestrel intrauterine device. Patients should be warned that irregular and heavy bleeding is common during the first 3 months after insertion.
- Depoprovera used for contraception is also associated with reduced menstrual blood loss and amenorrhea in some women.

Second-line medical treatment

- *Danazol* (100 mg 6–24 hourly) is a synthetic steroid that acts in a number of ways. It inhibits steroid synthesis, blocks androgen and progesterone receptors, and inhibits pituitary gonadotropins. These actions combine to inhibit endometrial growth. Its use is limited by androgenic side effects (acne, hirsutism, breast atrophy, and weight gain) and high cost.
- GnRH agonists downregulate the pituitary and inhibit FSH and LH production. They are highly effective in producing amenorrhea in DUB, but treatment is generally limited to 6 months because of the induced medical menopause and risk of osteoporosis.
- *Ethamsylate*, which acts by preventing the breakdown of capillaries, is ineffective in reducing menstrual blood loss.

Recommended further reading

1. Irvine GA, Cameron IT (1999). Medical management of dysfunctional uterine bleeding. *Baillière's Clin Obstet Gynecol* **13**, 189–202.
2. Prentice A (1999). Medical management of menorrhagia. *Br Med J* **319**, 1343–5.
3. Barrington JW, Bowen-Simpkins P (1997). The levonorgestrel intrauterine system in the management of menorrhagia. *Br J Obstet Gynecol* **104**, 614–16.
4. Weeks AD, Duffy SRG (1996). Abnormal uterine bleeding: diagnosis and medical management. *Prog Obstet Gynecol* **12**, 309–26.

Surgical management of dysfunctional uterine bleeding

Surgical management can be considered for patients who have completed their family and have failed medical management.

Endometrial ablation or resection (hysteroscopic procedures)

These are useful alternatives to hysterectomy in cases of DUB. Approximately 75% of women obtain a satisfactory improvement in their symptoms and the recovery time is significantly less than that for hysterectomy. About 40–50% of patients become amenorrheic after endometrial ablation, with a further 20–30% reporting reduced menstrual bleeding. About 20–30% of patients have no improvement, and up to 10% require further treatment such as hysterectomy. The procedure can be performed using laser photovaporization, electrosurgical resection or ablation by resectoscope, or intrauterine thermal coagulation (balloon procedures). These procedures are less effective in women under 35, where pain is a significant associated symptom, or when the uterus is enlarged. They are contraindicated if future fertility is desired. GnRH-analogs for 8 weeks prior to surgery are often used to thin the endometrium. These procedures can be carried out as day-case surgery, offer quick recovery, and are highly effective with significant reduction in menstrual blood loss. There is a small risk of serious complications such as uterine perforation, hemorrhage, or fluid overload.

Hysterectomy

Hysterectomy is one of the most common major operations in the developed world. It is the definitive treatment for patients with DUB, with a higher rate of patient satisfaction than in hysteroscopic endometrial ablation at 6 months. By the age of 65, 20% of all women in developed countries have had a hysterectomy. More than 40% of hysterectomies are for DUB. Hysterectomy can be performed abdominally, vaginally, or laparoscopically. Abdominal hysterectomy carries a higher risk of morbidity than vaginal hysterectomy, and so vaginal hysterectomy is the route of choice unless contraindicated. Selecting one approach over another depends on various factors, such as age, parity, history of pelvic surgery, desire for ovarian preservation, and the presence of pelvic disease (such as endometriosis or adhesions). Abdominal hysterectomy should be reserved only for a small group of patients who cannot be offered the less invasive approaches (vaginal or laparoscopic hysterectomy). Complications of hysterectomy include the following:

- *Intraoperative*: bleeding, damage to pelvic organs, and anesthetic complications.
- *Postoperative*: bleeding, wound infection and dehiscence, thromboembolism, ureteric or vesical fistula, chest and urinary tract infection.
- *Long-term complications* are urogenital prolapse and early ovarian failure.

Premenstrual syndrome

Premenstrual syndrome (PMS) is also known as premenstrual tension (PMT). It is a very common disorder affecting up to 95% of women. It is rarely life-threatening, but has been cited as a factor in poor work performance, criminal acts, suicide, and even murder.

Etiology and incidence

The etiology is unknown but it is likely to be a consequence of the hormone changes over a normal menstrual cycle.

- It has been suggested that PMS symptoms are caused by various excesses or deficiencies of estrogen or progesterone, but no consistent abnormality has been found.
- Side effects caused by the progestogen component of cyclical HRT are very similar to those with PMS, and the temporal relationship of symptoms to progesterone production in premenopausal women is strong.
- Serotonin and β-endorphins have also been implicated.
- It is likely that PMS is an exaggerated end-organ response to the normal cyclical changes in ovarian hormones.

Estimates for the incidence vary from 5% to 95% of women being affected at some point. About 20% of women will seek help for PMS symptoms. Typically, PMS is said to occur most frequently in the thirties and forties, often after childbirth. However, it may be that this group of women simply reports it most frequently.

Symptoms and diagnosis

Symptoms of PMS fall into three main groups: physical, emotional, and behavioral (Table 12.2). Most women will experience at least one symptom, but tolerate these without interference with their normal functioning.

Most women will self-diagnose PMS, but they may be mistaken in their interpretation of their symptoms. There is no objective method of measuring PMS but, for practical purposes, the diagnosis is made through the history, structured questionnaires, and the exclusion of competing diagnoses.

- Symptoms must be of sufficient severity to produce social, family, or occupational disruption, and must occur in most menstrual cycles. They occur in the premenstrual phase, resolving or markedly improving at menstruation. Ideally, the symptoms should be monitored prospectively for at least 2 months with a menstrual diary.
- Various quality of life questionnaires have been used to attempt to quantify the amount of distress (e.g. Moo's menstrual distress questionnaire).
- Blood tests are unhelpful, except to exclude other causes of symptoms. Measurements of hemoglobin and thyroid function can be useful in this respect, whilst FSH may be checked to exclude climacteric symptoms. Premenstrual symptoms may merge into climacteric symptoms in the forties.

Table 12.2 Symptoms of PMS

Physical	**Emotional**	**Behavioral**
Backache	Anxiety	Violence
Headache	Irritability	Aggression
Breast tenderness/swelling	Fatigue	Clumsiness
Bloating/fluid retention	Depression	Loss of concentration
Food craving	Anorexia	Mood swings

Treatment of premenstrual syndrome

As there is no accepted etiology for PMS, treatment remains empirical. In research studies looking at the effectiveness of treatments, there is a large placebo response. This makes it difficult to show a true effect of treatment, but treatment can be beneficial in clinical practice.

Active treatment can be chosen on the basis of treating the most severe symptoms first.

Nonhormonal therapy

- *Support and reassurance* In milder cases, listening to the patient and acknowledging the problems can be helpful. Many women simply need the reassurance that the problem is being addressed by a sympathetic practitioner. Education and explanation of the physiological basis for the condition will ease frustration and anxiety. However, for the majority of women who approach a doctor, more help may be needed.
- *Stress management and relaxation techniques.* Various techniques have been tried and are of benefit to certain women.
  - Yoga
  - Hypnosis
  - Music therapy
  - Homeopathy
  - Acupuncture
  - Self-help groups, etc.
- If any of these appeal to the patient, then they can be encouraged. Side effects are rare and avoidance of reliance on pharmacotherapy is seen as a benefit by many.
- *Exercise* Aerobic physical exercise in the latter part of the menstrual cycle can be useful. The exercise causes an increase in endorphin production and this seems to have a 'mood-elevating' effect. Improvements may also come because the exercise usually takes the woman away from the stressful home environment for a while. Many women relish this form of treatment as it is seen as 'self-help'.
- *Vitamin B_6* This is a cofactor in the synthesis of various neurotransmitters including serotonin and dopamine. This treatment may be useful for emotional and behavioral symptoms, but studies have shown only small advantages over placebo. There is some concern that overdosage may cause peripheral neuropathy.
- *Evening primrose oil* Prostaglandin precursors such as linoleic and gammalinoleic acid are contained in the oil of the evening primrose flower. It is postulated that a deficiency of E series prostaglandins allows an increased response to circulating ovarian hormones. Some benefits are seen over placebo treatments (clumsiness, depression, headache, bloatedness). Like vitamin B_6, this treatment is available 'over the counter'.
- *Diuretics* Only a few women truly experience premenstrual fluid retention and weight gain, although many think that they have this problem because of perceived bloatedness. For women where there is a measurable weight gain, spironolactone may be effective in the premenstrual phase.

- *Selective serotonin reuptake inhibitors (SSRIs)* It may be that women with serotonin deficiency are more sensitive to cyclical ovarian hormone changes and there can be dramatic relief of PMS with SSRI drugs in some women. They are usually taken throughout the cycle at a standard dose. They are most useful for psychological symptoms. Side effects can limit the usefulness of long-term treatment.

Hormone therapy

- *Progesterone supplements* Many studies have looked at progesterone supplementation because of the belief that PMS is caused by progesterone deficiency. It has been given by various routes (suppositories, pessaries, injections, oral micronized). Although there is a wealth of anecdotal evidence suggesting benefits, placebo-controlled studies have shown disappointing results. It may be that progesterone has an anxiolytic effect in higher doses.
- *Progestogens* Dydrogesterone has been used premenstrually, but studies have shown disappointing results.
- *Combined oral contraceptive pill (COCP)* The response to treatment with the COCP is unpredictable: some women will gain benefit whereas others may become worse. However, it may be worth a trial for 3 months.
- *Bromocriptine* Prolactin was at one time considered to be a potential causative agent for PMS. Treatment with bromocriptine may be useful for cyclical breast symptoms, but not for other symptoms.
- *Danazol* Low doses of danazol (100 mg daily) have been shown to be beneficial in treating breast symptoms without causing cycle suppression or severe side effects. However, other PMS symptoms are not improved.
- *Estradiol* 17β-Estradiol implants (50–100 mg pellet 6-monthly) or transdermal estradiol patch therapy (100–200 μg patch, used continuously) act by causing cycle suppression. They can be very effective but, in non-hysterectomized women, a progestogen has to be given cyclically. This can reproduce PMS-like symptoms, which limits the usefulness of this regimen. However, by using the Mirena intrauterine system (IUS) as the progestogen component of treatment, systemic absorption is minimized and the acceptability of the treatment increased. Symptoms tend to return when treatment is discontinued and cyclical ovarian hormone production restarts.
- *GnRH analogs* PMS is usually eliminated when cycles are suppressed with GnRH analogs. In severe cases, this treatment can bring prompt and welcome relief from symptoms. However, the ensuing estrogen deficiency symptoms can be equally troublesome. These can be minimized by giving add-back therapy with cyclic or continuous combined HRT. GnRH analogues are expensive for long-term treatment. If the patient has shown a good response, surgery may be the logical next step.

Surgery for premenstrual syndrome

For surgery to be effective, it is best to remove both the ovaries and uterus and then recommend estrogen-only HRT. If the uterus is left, treatment will need to include progestogens, which may give rise to the same symptoms again. Surgery is a major step to take and only justified in severe cases. It is usually best to give a trial of a GnRH analog first to ensure that PMS will resolve when the ovaries are removed.

Chapter 13

Early pregnancy problems

Termination of pregnancy

Termination of pregnancy (TOP) is defined as the removal of pregnancy from the uterus in a manner that does not anticipate subsequent survival of the fetus. The laws governing TOP vary from country to country.

In the USA, the right of a woman to electively terminate an unwanted pregnancy prior to viability was established by a landmark decision reached by the US Supreme Court on 22 January, 1973, which determined that laws against abortion violate the constitutional right to privacy. In this case, known as Roe v. Wade, a pregnant single woman (Roe) brought a class action challenging the constitutionality of the Texas criminal abortion laws, which at that time proscribed procuring or attempting an abortion except on medical advice for the purpose of saving the mother's life. That decision overturned all state laws that banned or restricted abortion.

In the UK, TOPs are performed under the legal umbrella of the 1967 Abortion Act (amended as the Human Fertilization and Embryology Act 1990). Two doctors need to decide in good faith that one or more of the following five conditions apply and complete Form HSA 1.

(a) The continuance of the pregnancy would involve risk to the life of the pregnant woman greater than if the pregnancy were terminated.
(b) The termination is necessary to prevent grave permanent injury to the physical or mental health of the pregnant woman.
(c) The pregnancy has not exceeded its 24th week and the continuance of the pregnancy would involve risk, greater than if the pregnancy were terminated, of injury to the physical or mental health of the pregnant woman.
(d) The pregnancy has not exceeded its 24th week and the continuance of the pregnancy would involve risk, greater than if the pregnancy were terminated, of injury to the physical or mental health of any existing child(ren) of the family of the pregnant woman.
(e) There is substantial risk that if the child were born it would suffer from such physical or mental abnormalities as to be seriously handicapped.

When it comes to the ethics and practicalities of elective termination of pregnancy, a number of points should be clarified:

- No practitioners are under any duty to participate in abortion procedures if they have a conscientious objection provided that this does not involve risk of grave permanent injury or death to their patient.
- Clinics and operating lists dedicated to such procedures will likely achieve better counseling and lower operative complication rates.
- It is advisable to care for TOP patients separate from other gynecological cases, especially those with infertility and spontaneous miscarriage.
- Confidentiality is essential in the management of women seeking termination and it may be necessary to make it clear to patients that it is always maintained, especially for teenagers seeking TOP without parental awareness.

Management prior to termination of pregnancy

- A full clinical history and examination should be carried out, especially menstrual history and gestational age.
- Arrange an ultrasound scan if there is any doubt about gestational age.
- Check hemoglobin and blood group. (Cross-match is not routinely indicated. May need anti-(Rh)D immunoglobulin if the mother is Rh-negative).
- Genital tract swabs should be taken to check for chlamydia, gonorrhea, and bacterial vaginosis. Any infection should be treated preoperatively. If swab results are not available, antibiotic prophylaxis should be used.
- Take a cervical smear, if due.
- Counsel on the procedure and complications. Obtain written consent.
- Discuss and arrange future contraception, but, in general, avoid sterilization at the time of TOP. The unplanned pregnancy is often a result of inadequate or total lack of contraception, and the consultation provides a valuable opportunity to address this.

Consent

Valid written consent is necessary, and should be secured after full counseling. Although parental involvement is ideal, girls under age 18 may sign consent for TOP if they decline parental involvement and doctors feel they are 'mature' enough (Gillick competent) to comprehend their circumstances. In the USA, certain states mandate parental consent for girls under age 18 years.

Methods

First trimester

- *Vacuum aspiration* This is usually a day-case procedure under paracervical block, but may be performed under general anesthesia. Vacuum aspiration is the conventional method used from 7 to 12 weeks' gestation. The cervix may be primed with vaginal prostaglandin preoperatively and dilated to 8–12 mm at surgery. A plastic aspiration cannula is used with a vacuum device to empty the uterus, and an oxytocic may be administered to reduce blood loss.
- *Medical TOP* Up to 7 weeks' gestation, oral mifepristone (RU 486) 600 mg followed 48 hours later by vaginal prostaglandin, e.g. misoprostol 600 μg or a PGE_2 preparation 1 mg, will produce complete abortion in 95%, incomplete abortion in 4%, and failure in <1%. Using such an approach, a surgical procedure can be avoided in 95% of cases. Unfortunately, many women present too late for this option.

Second trimester

- *Dilatation and evacuation (D&E)* This is a similar procedure to first-trimester vacuum aspiration, but needs further cervical dilatation and may require removal of fetal parts with forceps. It also needs considerable skill to minimize complications.
  - There is a higher risk of major complications with D&E, e.g. uterine perforation and visceral damage.

    - There is also some evidence that forced dilatation of the cervix at the time of D&E may predispose to cervical incompetence in a subsequent pregnancy.
    - It is not suitable for cases of fetal abnormality when post-mortem examination is recommended.
- *Hysterotomy*. This is now very rarely used for TOP. It may be appropriate in extremely rare cases, e.g. conjoined twins in mid-trimester when vaginal expulsion may not be feasible.
- *Medical TOP*
    - *Medication by oral route* Oral mifepristone 600 mg followed 36–48 hours later by PGE_2 1 mg vaginally. Administration of PGE_2 1 mg 3 hourly, to a maximum of five pessaries is recommended for mid-trimester TOP. Other published regimens include 200 mg oral mifepristone followed by vaginal misoprostol 400 µg, and 200 mg oral mifepristone followed by PGE_2 1 mg 6 hourly.
    - *Medication by vaginal route* Vaginal PGE_2 1 mg 3 hourly (maximum five pessaries in 24 hours) or misoprostol (200–600 µg) 4–6 hourly results in abortion within 24 hours in 85% of cases. The fetus, although non-viable, may be born alive (with a heartbeat), causing undue distress to staff and patients. The advantage of this method is that surgery is avoided and the fetus is delivered intact for post-mortem examination in cases of fetal anomaly.
    - *Medication by extra-amniotic route* A self-retaining catheter is passed through the cervix into the extra-amniotic space and a continuous infusion of PGE_2 is given until the cervix is sufficiently dilated to allow the catheter balloon to be expelled, followed by an oxytocic infusion.
    - *Medication by intra-amniotic route* This is currently the recommended method after 20 weeks' gestation. Amniocentesis is performed, and 100–200 mL of amniotic fluid is removed and replaced with 80–120 mL of 20% urea and up to 5 µg of PGE_2.This usually produces fetal death before expulsion, thereby reducing the distress to patients and staff. Continuous ultrasound scanning is essential for the procedure to prevent intravascular injection leading to coagulopathy and cardiogenic collapse.

Fetal demise can also be achieved by intracardiac potassium chloride (KCl) injection under ultrasound guidance.

Recommended further reading

1. MacKenzie IZ (1992). Pregnancy termination. In: Brock DJH, Rodeck CH, Ferguson-Smith, eds. *Prenatal Diagnosis and Screening*, pp. 675–87. Churchill Livingstone, New York.
2. Say L, Kulier R, Gulmezoglu M, Campana A (2005). Medical versus surgical methods for first trimester termination of pregnancy. *Cochrane Database Syst Rev* **1**, CD003037.
3. Kulier R, Gulmezoglu AM, Hofmeyr GJ, Cheng LN, Campana A (2004). Medical methods for first trimester abortion. *Cochrane Database Syst Rev* **2**, CD002855.

Complications I

The majority (>95%) of TOPs are undertaken on otherwise healthy young women for personal and social reasons. Complaints and litigation are not that uncommon when complications occur. Complication rates depend on stage of gestation, method of termination, skill of operator, and coexisting conditions, e.g. uterine abnormalities.

Hemorrhage

The incidence of excessive hemorrhage at the time of TOP is 1.5 in 1000 under 13 weeks' gestation and 8.5 in 1000 over 20 weeks' gestation. Significant hemorrhage (needing blood transfusion) at the time of TOP or soon after is rare in the first trimester. It is more likely with a retained placenta in the second trimester. Secondary hemorrhage, usually from infection, can result in significant blood loss if not promptly treated.

Infection

In the presence of chlamydia, gonorrhea, and bacterial vaginosis, there is a high risk of postoperative pelvic inflammatory disease (PID), which may result in infertility. This risk is minimized by taking swabs preoperatively and by using prophylactic antibiotics at the time of TOP. Preoperative metronidazole 1 g rectally and erythromycin 1 g orally, or postoperative doxycycline 100 mg twice daily for 7 days will provide sufficient cover. A single dose of azithromycin is also effective. Uncomplicated TOP does not impair fertility but, if other problems occur, it may result in subfertility and the patient is likely to reflect adversely on the TOP.

Major complications leading to hysterectomy, although rare, imply loss of fertility. These aspects should be discussed during preoperative counseling.

Retained products of conception (RPOC)

This has an incidence of 1–2%. It may sometimes necessitate repeat uterine evacuation. Antibiotic cover should be given if repeat evacuation is being considered. The risks of infection and perforation are higher than at the first procedure.

Ultrasound is sometimes useful in diagnosis, but blood clots are commonly seen within the uterine cavity making diagnosis difficult. Therefore clinical features must be foremost in the diagnostic process.

Uterine perforation

The incidence is 1–4 in 1000. This may go unnoticed at the time of TOP and present later as abdominal pain and tenderness or shock. When suspected at TOP, a laparoscopy is indicated. If bleeding from the perforation is significant, laparotomy and primary repair may be required. Otherwise, it may be possible to manage the patient expectantly, including antibiotic cover. It is still necessary to complete the TOP, and this should be done under laparoscopic control or at the laparotomy.

During mid-trimester D&E, bony fetal parts may lacerate or perforate the uterus. When a suction cannula has been inserted into a perforated uterus, visceral damage should be considered. A laparoscopy should be performed and, if an injury is identified, it should be repaired, usually by laparotomy. A bowel surgeon or other appropriate surgeon should be involved or be closely at hand. If perforation has occurred into the broad ligament, the damage to blood vessels may be such that hysterectomy may be required to control the hemorrhage.

Failure to abort

The overall incidence of failure to achieve pregnancy termination is 2.3 in 1000 for surgical TOP and 6 in 1000 for medical TOP.

- Failure to abort is more likely at early gestations, especially less than 6 weeks. Skilled operators can usually recognize that less tissue has been obtained by suction than expected.
- Unknown multiple pregnancy or bicornuate uterus may lead to failure to abort as one fetus may be completely spared or the suction cannula introduced only into the empty horn.
- Ectopic pregnancy may also be missed, especially when coexisting with an intrauterine pregnancy (so-called heterotopic pregnancy). If ectopic pregnancy is suspected during a TOP procedure, a diagnostic laparoscopy is indicated.

Products of conception are not routinely sent for histological examination after TOP performed for 'social' indications. Unlike medical TOP, follow-up is not usually arranged for surgical TOP and thus there may be a delay in diagnosing failure to abort. The risk may be reduced by giving verbal and written instructions on what to expect after TOP, e.g. rapid cessation of pregnancy symptoms and return of menstruation in about 4 weeks. If in doubt, follow-up with ultrasound scan and serum β-hCG is prudent.

Recommended further reading

1. MacKenzie IZ (1992). Pregnancy termination. In: Brock DJH, Rodeck CH, Ferguson-Smith M, eds. *Prenatal Diagnosis and Screening*, pp. 675–87. Churchill Livingstone, New York.

Complications II

Cervical trauma

Incidence is <1%. Cervical trauma is usually minor in form, e.g. lacerations from forceps used in holding the cervix and creation of a false passage. If a false passage is created, it is extremely difficult to find the cervical canal. Postponement, with cervical priming at a later date, may be necessary.

- Damage to the circular fibers of the cervix may result in cervical incompetence.
- Dilatation beyond 10 mm is usually necessary for D&E, and this is more likely to cause cervical incompetence. Cervical priming with misoprostol 400 μg or PGE_2 1 mg reduces the risk of trauma to the cervix.

Rhesus isoimmunization

Anti-Rh(D) immunoglobulin should be given in appropriate dosage to prevent Rh isoimmunization of Rh-negative women.

Hysterectomy

Rarely, hemorrhage is uncontrollable and hysterectomy unavoidable. Every effort should be made to discuss this with the patient or to contact the patient's family to discuss the problem while she is under anesthesia. A full explanation should be given to patient and family as soon as possible after the procedure.

Psychological sequelae

Because TOP is often sought because of personal and social difficulties, feelings of guilt are common after the procedure. Preoperative counseling should ensure that patients have given careful thought to their options. Further postoperative counseling should be arranged, when indicated. This may include social services input if appropriate. If a patient has doubts about undergoing the procedure preoperatively, it is best to allow some time for her to reach a definite decision before committing to TOP. A small number of women may appear unable to decide for themselves. It is advisable that a medical practitioner does not decide what is best for them.

Recommended further reading

1. MacKenzie IZ (1992). Pregnancy termination. In: Brock DJH, Rodeck CH, Ferguson-Smith M, eds. pp. 675–87. Churchill Livingstone, New York.

Ectopic pregnancy

Introduction

Ectopic pregnancy refers to implantation occurring outside the uterine cavity. It affects 11.5 in 1000 pregnancies. The number of cases has doubled over the last 10 years, although this may be in part due to better methods of diagnosis. It is the major cause of maternal mortality in the first trimester of pregnancy (4% of maternal deaths, 4 deaths in 10 000 ectopic pregnancies).

Etiology

Tubal transit of the fertilized ovum takes approximately 3–4 days and depends on the patency of the fallopian tube, the action of the ciliated epithelium lining of the tube, tubal peristalsis, and relaxation of the tubal isthmus. If tubal transit is delayed, implantation occurs on the papillary fronds, leading to obliteration of the tubal epithelium, invasion of the muscularis layer of the tube, and often perforation into the retroperitoneal space. If rupture does not occur, the blood and embryo are either expelled from the tube (tubal abortion) or reabsorbed.

- Factors associated with an increased risk of ectopic implantation include previous tubal surgery and ectopic pregnancy, failed sterilization or intrauterine contraceptive device (IUCD), PID, and assisted reproductive techniques.

Presentation

Of all ectopic pregnancies, 97% occur in the fallopian tubes, the most common site being in the ampullary region; 25% of cases occur in the narrower tubal isthmus where rupture and early presentation are more likely, and 3% implant on the cervix, ovary, or peritoneum. Simultaneous intrauterine and tubal ectopic pregnancies (heterotopic pregnancies) occur in 1 in 3000–30 000 pregnancies.

- Fifteen percent of cases present acutely with abdominal pain, amenorrhea, and hemodynamic compromise (shock).
- Patients may complain of shoulder tip discomfort bilaterally because of referred pain as a result of irritation of the diaphragm from intraperitoneal hemorrhage.
- There may be a history of syncope or feeling faint.
- Irritation of the pelvic peritoneum causes pain on defecation and diarrhea or pain on micturition.
- In most cases, the history will be more chronic.
- Typically, ectopics present after 6–8 weeks of amenorrhea but they can present at any stage of pregnancy (or even when there is no history of a missed period).
- There may be associated vaginal bleeding. This is due to shedding of the decidual lining of the uterus rather than bleeding from the ectopic itself and is usually lighter than that seen with miscarriage. Classically, it occurs after the onset of symptoms of abdominal pain, whereas that from miscarriage tends to precede abdominal pain. The abdominal pain tends to be more unilateral than that seen with miscarriage.

- Ectopic pregnancies may also be identified incidentally at the time of early ultrasound, and should be suspected following a uterine evacuation for suspected miscarriage when the histology report fails to show any evidence of chorionic villi but a decidual reaction (Arias–Stella reaction) is evident.

Diagnosis of ectopic pregnancy

Clinical

Ectopic pregnancy should be excluded in any woman with pain or irregular bleeding in early pregnancy. There may be a history of risk factors. On examination, look for signs of intraperitoneal hemorrhage including abdominal tenderness (95%), peritonism, abdominal distension, or pain on movement of the cervix (cervical excitation, 50%). If there is pelvic tenderness, it will tend to be localized more to one adnexum and there may be an adnexal mass (63%). The cervical os will be closed.

Ultrasound

The presence of an intrauterine gestational sac will usually exclude ectopic pregnancy, but can be mimicked by the decidual reaction (decidual ring) associated with ectopic pregnancy (look for a yolk sac or fetal pole). An intrauterine gestational sac should be identified in an ongoing viable intrauterine pregnancy by 6 weeks or where the serum β-hCG level is >1000 IU/L by transvaginal scan or >6000 IU/L on abdominal ultrasound.

- The presence of free fluid within the peritoneal cavity or of an adnexal mass in the absence of an intrauterine pregnancy is highly suggestive of an ectopic pregnancy. Rarely, it may be possible to identify an extrauterine fetal heartbeat.

NB: The primary goal of ultrasound in this setting is to exclude an intrauterine pregnancy and not to look for evidence of an adnexal mass.

hCG measurement

Following conception, hCG can be detected in the maternal serum within 7 days and in maternal urine by the time the first period would have been due had conception not occurred.

- A negative urinary pregnancy test will exclude all but 3% of pregnancies, and a negative serum hCG effectively excludes the possibility of ectopic pregnancy.
- Quantitative serum hCG measurement is also of value in determining whether an intrauterine pregnancy should be seen on ultrasound (see above).
- At lower levels of hCG, serial measurements 48 hours apart will show an increase of more than 66% in 85% of normal pregnancies and a suboptimal rise in more than 80% of ectopic pregnancies.

Laparoscopy

This remains the definitive method of diagnosis, but is associated with a 1 in 500 risk of injury to the bowel or abdominal blood vessels. False-negative results occur in 4–5% of cases.

Management and prognosis of ectopic pregnancy

Patients with suspected ectopic pregnancy should be referred for urgent hospital assessment.

- Pelvic examination should be delayed until facilities for resuscitation and surgical treatment are available.
- IV access should be secured and blood sent for group and cross-matching, CBC, and hCG measurement.
- If the patient is in shock, site two 14G cannulas and give colloid as fast as possible pending immediate transfer to the operating room. Notify anesthesia immediately.
- In the acutely compromised patient, surgery should not be delayed to allow full preoperative transfusion.
- Rh(D)-negative women should be given anti-Rh(D) immunoglobulin.

Surgical treatment

If there is evidence of acute intraperitoneal hemorrhage with hemodynamic compromise, arrangements should be made for immediate laparotomy and ligation of the bleeding point. This may involve removal of the tube containing the ectopic pregnancy. On no account should patients be transferred between hospitals in this condition. If no gynecological team is available at the referring hospital, the help of a general surgical team should be sought. Where the patient is hemodynamically stable, surgical treatment can usually be deferred until normal working hours and time allowed for the results of ultrasound and hCG evaluation.

- Surgical treatment may be carried out laparoscopically or through a mini-laparotomy incision.
- Laparoscopic treatment is associated with lower postoperative morbidity and quicker recovery, but requires the availability of suitably trained staff and appropriate operating equipment.
- In either case, treatment may be by removal of the fallopian tube (salpingectomy) or by aspiration of the ectopic through an incision in the wall of the fallopian tube (salpingotomy).
- If the contralateral tube is healthy, both procedures are associated with similar intrauterine pregnancy rates in subsequent pregnancies, but conservative surgery is associated with a higher risk of recurrence of ectopic pregnancy.
- Of cases treated by conservative surgery, 5–10% will be complicated by the presence of persistent trophoblastic tissue requiring further surgical or medical treatment. Therefore follow-up with serial hCG measurements is required.

Medical treatment

Suitable patients are those who are hemodynamically stable, have a serum hCG of <10 000 IU/L, have no evidence of extrauterine fetal heart activity on ultrasound, and are able to comply with the need for protracted follow-up.

- Systemic methotrexate at a dose of 50 mg/m^2 is given as an IM injection and the patient followed with serial hCG measurements until these become negative.
- An initial rise in hCG levels within the first 3–4 days following treatment and some abdominal discomfort are common.
- Tubal rupture may still occur, and a falling hCG level does not definitively exclude this possibility.
- Surgery will be required in 5–10% of cases.
- Patients must avoid alcohol and excessive exposure to sunlight following treatment, and should be advised to avoid becoming pregnant again for at least 6 months.

Prognosis

Following a single ectopic pregnancy, 60–70% of women wishing to have further pregnancies will have an intrauterine pregnancy. Of all subsequent pregnancies, 10–15% will be ectopic. The likelihood of recurrence is determined principally by the condition of the remaining fallopian tube and the rest of the pelvis at the time of treatment, although recurrence is slightly more common following conservative surgery. Patients should be advised about the need to seek medical advice and to have an early ultrasound scan in subsequent pregnancies to confirm an intrauterine pregnancy, even if they are asymptomatic.

Recurrent miscarriage: causes I

A miscarriage is loss of a pregnancy before viability. Recurrent miscarriage is defined as three pregnancies ending spontaneously before the 20th week of gestation in the USA (before the 24th week of gestation in the UK). These pregnancy losses need not be consecutive. This is a rare condition, with an expected chance of three consecutive pregnancy losses of 0.4%, and an observed risk of 1% of couples suffering from recurrent miscarriage. Overall, over 15% of diagnosed pregnancies will miscarry.

Couples who have recurrent early pregnancy losses are usually extremely distressed and hope for a diagnosis and therefore preventive measures for the future. Identification of a specific cause for the miscarriages is rarely possible, and very few specific effective therapies exist. Some have been discredited, and studies of new modalities of treatment must take into account the overall spontaneous 'cure rates' of over 50%.

Causes

More than one factor may exist within one individual, but couples must be warned prior to the onset of investigations that a cause is rarely identified. Only in special circumstances should women be investigated after two or fewer losses.

Anatomical causes

Prior to performing corrective surgery, which carries inherent potential postoperative infertility risks, the causal relationship between the anatomical abnormality and recent pregnancy losses must be very clear.

- *Uterine retroversion* as an etiological factor leading to recurrent miscarriage is now thought not to be relevant.
- *Intrauterine adhesions and submucous fibroids* are unlikely to cause infertility, although the latter could cause very early miscarriage if implantation occurs on the fibroid. Myomectomy or endoscopic resection of fibroids carry the risk of adhesion formation.
- *Cervical incompetence* causes mid-trimester pregnancy loss, with typical spontaneous rupture of membranes and painless cervical dilatation. Cervical incompetence is overdiagnosed. The use of cervical cerclage in suspected cases leads to a modest reduction in the incidence of preterm deliveries, but no significant improvement in fetal survival.
- *Congenital malformation* of the uterus, usually caused by abnormal fusion of the Müllerian ducts, is rare. The reported incidence varies between 0.1% and 3%. Implantation problems are thought to be more frequent in women with a single uterine horn or a bicornuate uterus. Restoring the uterine cavity to normal should only be considered as a last resort, and is best performed by experienced surgeons.

Infections

Many organisms have been put forward as causing recurrent miscarriages. Severe infection causing a high fever, e.g. malaria, can lead to a *sporadic* pregnancy loss. The TORCH group of organisms (toxoplasmosis, rubella, cytomegalovirus, and herpes) are now thought to be unlikely causes of recurrent miscarriage. The same applies to bacterial vaginosis.

Genetic causes

A high percentage of sporadic spontaneous miscarriages are chromosomally abnormal and, in a few cases, this may be the cause of the recurrent condition. However, it is important to evaluate the chromosome complement of both partners. An abnormal karyotype will be diagnosed in one of the partners in 3–5% of couples with recurrent miscarriage. The most common abnormality (over 60%) is a balanced reciprocal translocation, with 30% being a Robertsonian translocation. All such couples should be referred for formal genetic counseling.

Hormonal causes

It is clear that estrogen and progesterone are important in the support of early pregnancy, but deficiencies of either have never been clearly identified as a cause of miscarriage. Moreover, the use of exogenous progesterone and hCG after the onset of pregnancy does not reduce the risk of recurrent losses. Despite the lack of clear benefit, both are started at the time of conception in assisted reproduction pregnancies.

Polycystic ovarian syndrome (PCOS) is seen more frequently in patients with recurrent miscarriage (58%) compared with the general population (20%). This is possibly caused by the high LH levels seen in PCOS, but downregulation and lowering LH levels does not improve the pregnancy outcome. Women with PCOS should be informed of the higher early pregnancy losses when embarking on an ovulation induction program.

Poorly controlled hyper- or hypothyroidism and hyperprolactinemia have also been associated with recurrent pregnancy loss.

Recommended further reading

1. Stirrat GM (1990). Recurrent miscarriage I: definitions and epidemiology. *Lancet* **336**, 673–5.
2. Mowbray JF (1994). Genetic and immunological factors in human recurrent abortion. *Am J Reprod Immunol* **15**, 261–74.

Recurrent miscarriage: causes II

Immune causes

The mechanisms that stop fetal rejection by the mother remain unidentified. This may reflect either active maternal immunosuppression or a failure of maternal immune system response. The theory that women who have recurrent miscarriages share a higher proportion of HLA antigens with their partners and hence are unable to initiate the above mechanisms leading to fetal rejection has now been discredited. Similarly, studies using infusions of a partner's lymphocytes to induce immune tolerance, although initially promising, have been shown not to improve pregnancy outcome.

Autoimmune factors

Thrombophilic defects are now known to be an important cause of recurrent miscarriage. The initial association between recurrent miscarriage and antiphospholipid antibody syndrome has now been extended to include inherited thrombophilias, such as activated protein C resistance and antithrombin III and factor XII deficiencies. Low levels of the naturally occurring anticoagulants protein C and protein S have also been associated with this problem.

The common mechanism leading to pregnancy loss and other pregnancy problems is likely to be uteroplacental microthrombosis.

- Low-dose aspirin, heparin, and steroids (prednisolone/dexamethazone) have been used either in combination or singly to treat women with autoimmune thrombophilic defects and associated recurrent miscarriage. Cyclosporin, a drug that decreases the development of stem cells in the bone marrow and is used for transplant patients, has been proposed for use in early pregnancy (up to 10 weeks' gestation). Controlled data are awaited.
  - Treatment with corticosteroid is associated with significant maternal and fetal morbidity, and does not seem to improve the live birth rate.
  - The treatment of choice is low-dose aspirin alone (60–100 mg daily) or with added low-dose heparin 5000–10 000 IU SC every 12 hours).

Unexplained cause

This is a significant group who require explanation, support, and reassurance. The prognosis for future successful pregnancy is good—over 75% in the future. It is important to resist empirical treatment of this group.

Recommended further reading

1. Stirrat GM (1990). Recurrent miscarriage I: definitions and epidemiology. *Lancet* **336**, 673–5.
2. Mowbray JF (1994). Genetic and immunological factors in human recurrent abortion. *Am J Reprod Immunol* **15**, 261–74.

Investigation and treatment of miscarriage

Investigation

History, examination, and investigations may help to identify a possible etiological factor. Investigations include the following:

- Karyotyping for both partners
- Pelvic ultrasound
- Day 2 LH/FSH
- Antiphospholipid antibodies (including lupus anticoagulant and anticardiolipin antibodies)
- Activated protein C resistance and/or genetic testing for factor V Leiden mutation
- Genetic testing for prothrombin (factor II) gene mutation
- Circulating levels of antithrombin III
- Circulating levels of protein C and S
- Thyroid function test
- Circulating level of prolactin

Treatment

Couples who have a first or second miscarriage should be reassured and not investigated unless there is a specific reason to do so. Couples with three or more miscarriages should be fully investigated according to a protocol and, ideally, managed in a dedicated miscarriage clinic. Such couples should be warned at the outset that, in the majority of couples, no explanation will be found. Empirical treatment in this large group must be resisted. In situations when surgical treatment is available, the benefits must be thoroughly weighed against the drawbacks with the couple. Similarly, treatment of thrombophilic defects can be associated with maternal and fetal morbidity, but remains promising with increasing live birth rates with combination heparin and low-dose aspirin treatment.

Recommended further reading

1. American College of Obstetricians and Gynecologists (2002). ACOG Practice Bulletin No. 24. Management of recurrent pregnancy loss. *Int J Gynaecol Obstet* **78**, 179–90.
2. MRC/RCOG Working Party on Cervical Cerclage (1993). Final report of the Medical Research Council/Royal College of Obstetricians and Gynaecologists multicentred randomized trial of cervical cerclage. *Br J Obstet Gynaecol* **100**, 516–23.
3. Li TC (1998). Guides for practitioners. Recurrent miscarriage: principles of management. *Human Reproduction* **13**, 478–82.

Chapter 14

Genital tract infections, vaginal discharge, and pelvic pain

Lower genital tract infections: introduction

Introduction

Most women experience lower genital tract infections at some time. Not all are sexually transmitted. Vaginal discharge may also be physiological or due to a retained foreign body. If one sexually transmitted disease (STD) is diagnosed, there is an increased likelihood of others being present. Therefore patients should be treated in a genitourinary clinic where full bacteriological and serological screening can be carried out. Treatment of women with STDs should be done in conjunction with screening and treatment of partners and follow-up tests of cure where possible.

Risk factors for STDs include multiple partners, pregnancies before the age of 20, being in the age group 15–34, previous TOP, other or previous STD, abnormal cervical cytology, and prostitution.

A *sexual history* should include the following:
- Time since last intercourse
- Type of intercourse (oral, vaginal, or anal)
- Contraception used
- Number of previous partners
- Menstrual history
- Previous pregnancies
- Previous treatment for STD in patient or her partner
- History of travel abroad
- History of IV drug use by patient or her partners

Lower genital tract infections I

Bacterial vaginosis

This is due to an overgrowth of anaerobic organisms such as *Gardnerella vaginalis, Bacteriodes, Mycoplasma hominis, and Mobiluncus* spp. that are normally present in the vagina. It may occur in women who are not sexually active. It is more common in women undergoing termination of pregnancy and those with an IUCD *in situ* or with PID. It is associated with an increased risk of second trimester miscarriage, preterm delivery, and pelvic infection after surgery.

- *Presentation* may be asymptomatic. The symptom is usually a white or pale yellow vaginal discharge with an offensive fishy odor.
- *Diagnosis* Characteristic vaginal discharge on examination. An increase in vaginal pH (use pH strips) to >5.5. If a few drops of 10% potassium hydroxide are added to the discharge, it produces a characteristic fishy smell. Microscopic examination may show 'clue cells' (squamous epithelial cells with small bacteria adherent to the wall). There will be large numbers of cocci and relatively few gram-positive bacilli (*Lactobacilli*). The presence of the above anaerobes on culture from high vaginal swab is not diagnostic by itself, as these can be isolated from normal vaginal flora.
- *Management* Bacterial vaginosis may resolve spontaneously. Treatment is indicated if symptomatic, prior to termination of pregnancy, and in women with a previous history of second-trimester miscarriage or unexplained preterm delivery. Metronidazole 400 mg (200 mg if pregnant) twice daily for 5 days or 2 g as a single dose. Clindamycin 2% cream (one applicator full at night vaginally for 7 days) is a suitable topical alternative. Recurrence after treatment is common.

Candida (thrush)

There are several species of this yeast, the most common being *Candida albicans*. It affects 75% of women at some time and an estimated 20% are carriers (in the gut). Predisposing factors include the following:

- Conditions or drugs that impair immunity
- Antibiotics
- Pregnancy or high-dose combined oral contraceptive pill (COCP)
- Diabetes or thyroid, parathyroid, or adrenal disease

Presentation Symptoms include vulval itching and soreness (worse at night), 'curdy' white discharge (may also be thin and watery), dysuria, and dyspareunia. On examination, look for an erythematous vulva with fissuring and white plaques in the vagina that are adherent.

Diagnosis can be confirmed by culture or by the presence of gram-positive spores and long pseudohyphae on wet preparation microscopic examination. The vaginal pH is usually normal. In recurrent infections, look for anemia, thyroid disease, and diabetes, and consider acquired immunodeficiency.

Treatment Asymptomatic women do not require treatment.

- Topical preparations such as clotrimazole 500 mg either as a single-dose pessary or as a cream for 14 days are usually effective.
- Recurrent or persistent infection can be treated by systemic antifungal agents such as fluconazole 150 mg (avoid in pregnancy; only effective against *C. albicans* strains).
- Treatment of the partner is usually recommended, although reinfection may occur from the gut.
- Acetic acid jelly may prevent or relieve mild attacks.
- Advice about simple hygiene measure may help, such as wiping the vulva from front to back, avoiding chemical irritants on the vulva such as bath salts, and the use of cotton underwear.

Gonorrhea

Neisseria gonorrheae is an intracellular gram-negative diplococcus which grows in columnar epithelium (incubation period 2–5 days).

- *Presentation* Fifty percent of women are asymptomatic but 15% present as acute-onset PID with abdominal pain that may be associated with pronounced vaginal bleeding. May also cause bartholinitis/skeinitis, vaginal discharge, perihepatitis, septicemia, arthritis, or a rash.
- *Diagnosis* is made by culture or the presence of intracellular gram-negative diplococci on gram-stained preparations from cervical, urethral, or rectal swabs.
- *Treatment* Amoxycillin 3 g with probenicid 2 g, ciprofloxacin 500 mg, or azithromycin 1 g all given as a single dose. Treatment should also be given empirically for chlamydia. Contact tracing and treatment of partners is essential prior to resuming intercourse. Confirmation of cure should be obtained by repeat cultures following treatment.

Herpes

Herpes is caused by DNA viruses: herpes simplex (HSV) types 2 (genital) and 1 (oral, cold sores). Fifty percent of genital lesions are due to HSV1.

- *Presentation* Incubation period of 21 days. The first attack is the most severe, with pain, vulvitis (may be severe enough to cause urinary retention), ulceration, lymphadenopathy, and discharge. It resolves after 3–4 weeks, but may cause a secondary sacral radiculomyelopathy or meningitis. Recurrence can be triggered by stress, sex, or menstruation, but subsequent attacks are normally shorter and less severe. There may be prodromal symptoms. Asymptomatic shedding of the virus may occur.
- *Diagnosis* Culture of serum collected from vesicles by aspiration or by swabbing the base of the ulcers. Serum anti-HSV antibody levels are increased with both types of infection, and are not generally useful in making the diagnosis.
- *Treatment* is largely supportive, with analgesia and treatment of any secondary infections. Acyclovir 200 mg five times a day for 5 days if given within 5 days of onset of symptoms shortens the duration of the primary attack and may abort recurrent episodes if taken when prodromal symptoms occur. Condoms should be used.

Lower genital tract infections II

Chlamydia

Chlamydia trachomatis, an obligate intracellular bacterium, is the most common cause of salpingitis and is present in up to 50% of genital infections in developed countries.

- *Presentation* is as vaginal discharge (cervicitis), urethritis, PID, perihepatitis (Fitz-Hugh–Curtis syndrome), or Reiter's syndrome (arthropathy, rash, and conjunctivitis). It is commonly asymptomatic (80% of women), and so patients undergoing procedures such as TOP should be screened for infection.
- *Diagnosis Chlamydia* can be cultured, but requires special medium. The diagnosis is usually made by ELISA detection of antigen obtained by swabbing the endocervix. PCR or ligase chain reaction tests to detect bacterial DNA are more sensitive and can be performed on urine samples and vaginal swabs, but are more expensive. Perihepatic adhesions may be seen at laparoscopy.
- *Treatment* If untreated, there is a significant risk of tubal damage and subsequent infertility.
  - Doxycycline 100 mg twice daily for 10 days (avoid during pregnancy and lactation; use erythromycin 500 mg four times daily for 10 days).
  - Azithromycin 1 g is effective as a single-dose treatment.
  - Contact tracing of partners and treatment is essential to prevent reinfection.
  - Confirmation of cure should be obtained after treatment by repeat swabs.

Molluscum contagiosum, pubic lice, and scabies

- *Molluscum contagiosum* is a member of the poxvirus group.
  - *Presentation* Papules up to 5 mm in diameter with central umbilication usually in the pubic area.
  - *Treatment* is by topical application of phenol or by cryotherapy.
- The pubic louse is a sexually transmitted parasite that lays its eggs on pubic hair.
  - *Presentation* Itch secondary to reaction to its bite.
  - *Treatment* Topical aqueous malathion (30–60 g) applied as a single application to all parts of the body for 12 hours or overnight and repeated after 7 days.
- *Scabies* is caused by *Sarcoptes scabiei*, a mite that burrows into the skin and lays eggs. There is both sexual and non-sexual transmission.
  - *Presentation* Itch, rash over trunks and limbs.
  - *Treatment* Topical aqueous malathion (30–60 g) applied as a single application to all parts of the body for 12 hours or overnight.

Syphilis

Treponemum pallidum is a treponemal infection (others include yaws and pinta). There is both sexual and vertical transmission. The incubation period is 9–90 days.

- Presentation.
  - Primary infection usually presents 3–6 weeks after infection with chancre (painless genital ulceration) and inguinal lymphadenopathy.

The most common site for chancre in women is the cervix, and therefore it may be relatively asymptomatic. The primary infection will resolve after a few weeks, even if untreated.
  - Secondary syphilis may arise immediately after the primary disease or up to 6 months later. Signs include rash, fever, joint pains, condylomata lata (wart-like lesions), iritis, and hepatitis.
- *Diagnosis* The organism can be identified in exudate obtained from the primary lesion mixed with saline using dark field microscopy. The most sensitive serological test is the fluorescent treponemal antibody test (FTA). In primary disease, initial serology may be negative.
- *Treatment* IM penicillin 1.2×10^6 U for 12 days is the treatment of choice. Doxycycline 100 mg twice a day for 14 days or erythromycin 500 mg four times a day for 14 days are suitable alternatives in nonpregnant patients. In pregnancy, penicillin is the treatment of choice. Women with a significant penicillin allergy should undergo penicillin desensitization prior to treatment. Contact tracing may need to involve partners from several years previously.

Trichomonas

Trichomonas vaginalis is a protozoan with four flagellae. It is sexually transmitted.

- *Presentation* It may be asymptomatic. Symptoms are a mucopurulent yellow or green offensive vaginal discharge associated with vulvovaginitis. The cervix may have a 'strawberry' appearance because of the presence of punctate hemorrhages.
- *Diagnosis* Viable flagellate organisms can be seen on wet slide preparation or can be cultured.
- *Management* Metronidazole 400 mg twice daily for 7 days (200 mg three times a day in pregnancy) or 2 g as a single dose. Treat partner and check for other STDs (gonorrhea).

Warts (human papillomavirus)

The most important serotypes are 6, 11, 16, 18, and 31 of which 6 and 11 are the most common. Serotypes 16, 18, and 31 have been linked to the development of cervical cancer. There is an incubation period of weeks to months. The virus may be carried (and shed) without any visible lesions being present. Infection is sexually acquired.

- *Presentation* The lesions are usually asymptomatic (any itch is usually due to secondary infection). The appearance depends on the site. They are associated with other STDs (25%).
- *Treatment*
  - Visible lesions are treated with cryotherapy or topical application of podophyllin once or twice a week for 6 weeks. Surgical excision or ablation by laser or diathermy are alternatives.
  - Relapse is common whatever the method of treatment used, especially in immunocompromised patients.
  - Sexual partners should be examined for warts and other STDs. Barrier contraception is usually advised during treatment.
  - There is no need for women with warts to have more frequent cervical screening, although patients with cervical warts should be referred for colposcopic assessment.

Causes and diagnosis of vaginal discharge

Introduction

Vaginal discharge may be physiological or pathological. It is likely to be physiological if associated with menstruation, mid-cycle ovulation, and sexual excitement. It is often pathological when associated with blood, pruritus, foul odor, vulvitis, ulcers, and soreness.

Causes

Physiological causes

The discharge is mucoid or white (leukorrhea). Quantity and quality vary throughout the menstrual cycle.

- Discharge is maximal at mid-cycle (ovulation), premenstrually, and with the use of IUCDs or during sexual excitement.
- Coitus produces an increase in cervical and vaginal discharge, together with semen.
- In pregnancy, estrogen causes mucus-secreting columnar epithelium to evert into the ectocervix causing an increase in vaginal discharge.
- Maternal estrogen may cause a self-limiting vaginal discharge in neonates.

Pathological causes

These vary in the premenarcheal, reproductive, and peri/postmenopausal years with some degree of overlap. Premenarcheal causes include poor hygiene, foreign bodies (organic or inorganic), threadworms, sexual interference, and sarcoma botryoides (rare and usually associated with a bloodstained discharge). Vaginal discharge during the reproductive years may be due to the following.

- *Infections: Candida albicans, Chlamydia trachomatis, Neisseria gonorrhoeae, Trichomonas vaginalis, Gardnerella vaginalis,* herpes genitalis, syphilitic chancre, or nonspecific agents, e.g. streptococci.
- *Neoplasms* Benign or malignant and usually bloodstained.
- *Trauma or iatrogenic* Sensitivity/allergy to contraceptive rubber, spermicidal creams, douching chemicals, retained products such as tampons, post-abortum, or puerperal.
- *Local causes* Examples include cervical ectropion, polyp, or fistulas (urinary or fecal). Peri/postmenopausal vaginal discharge is often due to a low estrogen state resulting in atrophic vaginitis. The discharge is quite often bloodstained.

It is important to exclude the above infective causes as well as any unrevealed genital tract malignancy.

Diagnosis

Take a good history to include the following:

- Features of the discharge:
  - nature (mucoid, serous, purulent, bloody)
  - color (clear, white, yellow-green, bloodstained)
  - consistency (watery, viscid, curd-like)

  - duration (continuous, intermittent)
  - amount (the need for added protection such as pads)
- Associated symptoms: irritation, itching, burning
- Frequency of attacks
- Relationship to menstrual cycle, sexual intercourse, pregnancy
- Hygiene practices: douching, use of tampons
- Risk factors and likelihood of sexually transmitted diseases
- Associated urinary tract infection
- Associated medical conditions, e.g. diabetes mellitus
- History of allergy to rubber/spermicides
- Drug history, especially antibiotics
- Last cervical smear

Physical examination includes general and abdominal as well as pelvic examination. The objective here is to establish the diagnosis (usually infective), determine the extent of morbidity (any associated vulvitis or pelvic inflammatory disease), and exclude a malignancy.

Investigations include cervical cytology, vaginal pH, saline wet mount, wet mount on 10% potassium hydroxide solution (10% KOH), gram stain of vaginal discharge, specimen for culture (high vaginal and endocervical swabs), and colposcopy if indicated.

Diagnostic features of some common conditions

- *Candidiasis* Whitish to yellowish discharge with plaques at times; pH slightly more acidic than normal (4.5–4.8); hyphae/pseudohyphae on saline/10% KOH wet mount; gram stain; culture (Nickerson's medium), especially in recurrent cases (for *Candida glabrata*).
- *Trichomoniasis* Watery grey-green frothy discharge; pH usually 5.0–6.0, motile trichomonads visible on saline mount; culture (Stuart's medium).
- *Gardnerella vaginalis vaginitis* Watery grey offensive discharge; pH 5.0–5.5, saline wet smear—demonstration of 'clue cells'. Application of 10% KOH produces a fishy odor ('whiff test').
- *Mucopurulent cervicitis* (*Chlamydia trachomatis*) Endocervical scrapings should be taken. A direct immunofluorescent test using tagged monoclonal antibodies against chlamydial surface antigens is a quick diagnostic test. Culture in McCoy cell lines is possible.
- *Mucopurulent cervicitis* (*Neisseria gonorrheae*) Demonstration of intracellular gram-negative diplococci; culture on Thayer–Martin medium.
- *Syphilis* Primary syphilis presents with painless indurated ulcers. Demonstration of treponeme by dark field microscopy of a slide with exudate from ulcer. Serologic tests: nonspecific reagin type antibody tests (rapid plasma reagin (RPR), the Venereal Disease Research Laboratory (VDRL) test for syphilis) and specific antitreponemal antibody tests (*Treponema pallidum* immobilization (TPI), fluorescent treponemal antibody absorption (FTA-ABS), and *Treponema pallidum* hemagglutination (TPHA)).
- *Herpes genitalis* Tzank test to demonstrate multinucleate giant cells; cultures of vesicular fluid.

Other diagnoses are unusual but they must be kept in mind. Make use of clinical examination, colposcopy, and biopsy if indicated.

Treatment of the common conditions

- *Candidiasis*
  - Polynes: pessaries containing nystatin.
  - Imidazoles: clotrimazole, miconaxole.
  - Triazoles: fluconaxole, itraconazole.
  - In recurrent infections, predisposing factors must be sought and treated.
  - The concomitant use of oral agents such as triazoles helps eradicate gastrointestinal and subepithelial reservoirs, but liver function tests must be monitored.
- *Trichomoniasis* Metronidazole 200 mg three times daily for 5–7 days. Metronidazole 2 g single dose. Treatment should be undertaken concurrently by both partners.
- *Gardnerella vaginalis vaginitis* Oral or topical metronidazole or topical clindamycin.
- *Mucopurulent cervicitis*
  - *Chlamydia trachomatis* Doxycycline 100 mg twice daily for 10–14 days. Erythromycin 500 mg four times daily for 10–14 days.
- *Neisseria gonorrheae* Treatment should aim at the penicillinase-producing strain. Ceftriaxone 250 mg IM as a single dose.
- *Syphilis* 2.4×10^6 U benzathine penicillin. Erythromycin 500 mg four times daily for 15 days.
- *Herpes genitalis* Local symptomatic relief with lidocaine jelly. Systemic therapy with oral acyclovir.
- *Atrophic vaginitis* A diagnosis of exclusion after other infective and possible neoplastic causes have been excluded. Topical estrogen creams cause a reversal of symptoms within a week. Maintenance therapy with local application one to three times a week helps maintain a healthy vaginal epithelium. HRT should be considered.
- *Other conditions* Treatment will depend on the cause identified.

Principles to remember

- Neoplasia, though not common, must be looked for.
- If one STD is identified, other STDs must be looked for and contact tracing and treatment of partners should be carried out.
- Refractory cases may need frequent intermittent therapy and are best dealt with by a specialist. Reinfection should be considered.
- Predisposing factors must be identified.

Vaginal discharge in obstetrics

Principles of management

- An understanding of the management of vaginal discharge outside of pregnancy in the reproductive years.
- Remember that vaginal discharge may be physiological in pregnancy. A history of associated pruritus, bloodstaining, purulent nature, vulvitis, ulceration, soreness, or foul odor would indicate a pathological cause.
- Identification of the organism.
- Modification or delay of treatment for fetal reasons.
- Exclusion of leaking amniotic fluid in later pregnancy.

Treatment for infective causes

- Candidiasis
  - Nystatin pessaries: one tablet (100 000 IU) twice daily for 10–14 days.
  - Clotrimazole: 500 mg (Canestin 1, Bayer) single pessary.
  - Local antifungal cream (Canesten/Gyno-Travogen, Daktarin).
- Trichomoniasis
  - Topical povidone–iodine
  - Metronidazole is relatively contraindicated in the first trimester, and treatment can be delayed in asymptomatic pregnant women. In cases that need treatment, use metronidazole 200 mg three times daily for 7 days (consider treating couple simultaneously).
- *Gardnerella vaginalis* vaginitis.
  - Oral ampicillin 500 mg 6-hourly for 1 week.
  - Oral metronidazole 200 mg three times daily for 7 days. Local metronidazole may also be effective.
- *Chlamydia trachomatis* cervicitis.
  - Erythromycin 500 mg four times daily for 14 days.
- *Neisseria gonorrhoea* cervicitis
  - Ceftriaxone 250 mg IM as a single dose.
- Syphilis
  - 2.4×10^6 U benzathine penicillin.
  - Erythromycin and clindamycin do not adequately cross the placenta and therefore are not recommended in pregnancy. In women with a significant penicillin allergy, inpatient desensitization followed by penicillin therapy is recommended.
- *Herpes genitalis*
  - The risk to the fetus must be kept in mind, and third-trimester management must be tailored to expose the fetus to minimum risk.
  - Topical acyclovir and lidocaine jelly for relief of symptoms.

Causes, presentation, and diagnosis of pelvic inflammatory disease

Introduction

PID is a common diagnosis for women presenting with lower abdominal pain. Although only a small proportion actually have pelvic infection, it is important to confirm the diagnosis because of the serious sequelae and associated problems of contact tracing.

PID is defined as an acute clinical syndrome associated with ascending spread of microorganisms, usually unrelated to pregnancy or surgery, from the vaginal cervix to the endometrium, fallopian tubes, and/or contiguous structures. PID may affect the pelvic peritoneum (pelvic peritonitis), the ovaries (oophoritis), the fallopian tubes (salpingitis), or the uterus (endometritis).

Causal organisms

- *Chlamydia trachomatis* is the major pathogen in PID in developed countries, although it may not be the same throughout the world. *Chlamydia* is an obligate intracellular 'parasitic bacterium'. The extent of damage caused by *Chlamydia* is variable, from being asymptomatic to causing severe pelvic infection.
- *Neisseria gonorrheae*. Gonococcal infections appear to be decreasing in frequency whilst chlamydial infections have increased. It is estimated that 15–20% of pelvic infection may be due to gonococci. Gonococci selectively invade the nonciliated cells in the mucosa of the fallopian tube, although it is the ciliated cells that are damaged.
- It is uncertain what role *Mycoplasma* play in PID as they may be found in the flora of the genital tract of healthy women.
- *Bacterial vaginosis* (BV) causes a disturbance in the vaginal flora with an increase in the amount of anaerobic organisms. However, it is uncertain whether BV plays a role in the etiology of PID.

Presentation

The spectrum of clinical presentation for PID is very wide ranging from asymptomatic to severe.

- *Asymptomatic* There may be no history at all of symptoms and the disease may be picked up incidentally at laparoscopy.
- *Mild* Some women present with a vague lower abdominal pain with no vaginal discharge.
- *Moderate* Moderate pain associated with dyspareunia and a vaginal discharge.
- *Severe* In severe cases, there may be evidence of high fever, rigors, peritonism, and a mass suggesting abscess formation.

Diagnosis

History

Because the spectrum of disease is so wide, the following features that raise the possibility of PID should be looked for in the history:

- Constant lower abdominal pain
- Purulent vaginal discharge, sometimes offensive, sometimes irritating
- Deep dyspareunia
- Dysmenorrhea
- Menstrual irregularities
- Current or previous IUCD use
- History of infertility or ectopic pregnancy

Examination

The following features are associated with PID:

- Pyrexia
- Lower abdominal pain
- Cervical excitation pain
- Tenderness on pelvic examination with a tender uterus and adnexae and reduced mobility of the pelvic organs
- Adnexal enlargement (abscess or hydrosalpinges or tubo-ovarian mass)

Criteria for diagnosis

There is no proven ideal way to diagnose PID, but various criteria may be taken into account. Rolf's criteria for diagnosis of PID are the following:

- Lower abdominal tenderness
- Bilateral adnexal tenderness
- Cervical motion tenderness
- No evidence of a competing diagnosis

With these criteria, antibiotic treatment should be started for probable PID. In more severe cases, hospitalization will be necessary and further investigations may be required.

Investigations

If the history and examination are suggestive of PID, the following investigations should be considered:

- CBC and differential white count
- β-hCG (in appropriate patients)
- Midstream urine for microscopy, culture, and sensitivity
- High vaginal swab
- Endocervical swabs for *Chlamydia* and gonococci
- Blood cultures in patients with severe symptoms
- Pelvic ultrasound scan
- Laparoscopy

Sequelae, treatment, and prevention of pelvic inflammatory disease

If it is treated inadequately or the diagnosis is unrecognized, PID may result in the following:

- Infertility: following one episode of PID, 8% of women will have tubal factor infertility, 20% will be affected after two infections, and 40% after three or more infections.
- Recurrent PID: after initial PID, 25% of women will develop a second infection.
- Ectopic pregnancy: there is a sixfold increase in the risk of an ectopic pregnancy after pelvic infection.
- Chronic pelvic pain and dyspareunia.
- Tubo-ovarian abscess.

Treatment

Treatment depends on the severity of the disease. Patients with severe disease (e.g. pyrexia, pelvic peritonitis, severe pain and unable to do normal work, tender adnexal masses) should be admitted to hospital, whereas milder infections may be treated in the community.

- Antibiotic treatment should involve broad-spectrum antibiotics, initiated before the pathogens have been identified. A useful combination for treatment will include a second- or third-generation cephalosporin or amoxycillin with probenecid, a tetracycline, and metronidazole.
  - In severe cases, treatment is usually IV initially and should continue for up to 14 days.
- In severely ill patients, analgesia and IV fluid replacement should be given.
- Laparoscopy is indicated if symptoms do not improve within 24–48 hours, and laparotomy and surgical drainage are usually necessary for pelvic abscesses.

Prevention

Successful strategies have been employed in many developed countries to control genital chlamydia and gonorrhea, and this has led to a significant reduction in the occurrence of symptomatic pelvic infection. Education is important, particularly for the young. This needs to be culturally sensitive, and local cultural practices will determine the age at which it should be started. Contact tracing should be rigorous for all patients with proven genital tract infection, with treatment and eradication of disease in sexual partners.

Acute pelvic pain

The common causes of acute pelvic pain are as follows:

- Early pregnancy complications such as ectopic pregnancy and miscarriage
- Pelvic inflammatory disease (PID)
- Appendicitis
- Ovarian cyst 'accidents' or Mittelschmerz

Other causes of acute pelvic pain include the following:

- Ovarian hyperstimulation syndrome
- Hematometra and hematocolpos
- Necrosis of uterine fibroids
- Other nongynecological causes such as bowel or urinary disease

Early pregnancy complications are discussed in Chapters 2 and 13 📖 *p.55* and *p.477* respectively and PID is discussed earlier in this chapter.

Ovarian cyst accidents

These include the pain produced as a result of torsion (leading to occlusion of the blood supply with ischemic pain and necrosis) as well as bleeding into or from a cyst. This may be the presenting symptom of ovarian neoplasia, but is more commonly associated with functional ovarian cysts in younger women. Ovarian cysts may rupture causing an acute chemical peritonitis if they contain irritant material (such as endometriotic or dermoid cysts). Torsion presents with sudden onset of colicky pelvic pain, often located to one or other of the iliac fossae. The pain may become more constant after several hours or even disappear. During the first few hours, the patient is usually afebrile, but later on necrosis can cause fever. Dermoid cysts, teratomas, or simple cysts are more common causes of torsion.

Mittelschmerz

Mittelschmerz (from the German *mittel* = middle and *Schmerz* = pain) is mid-cycle pain occurring at the time of ovulation, more commonly in teenagers and older women.

Recommended further reading

1. Economy KE, Laufer MR (1999). Pelvic pain. *Adolesc Med* **10**, 291–304.

Chronic pelvic pain

Pelvic pain is deemed chronic when it is of more than 6 months duration. Chronic pelvic pain is the most common gynecological problem affecting women of reproductive age.

Endometriosis and chronic PID are discussed in this chapter and Chapter 15 📖 *p.546*, respectively.

Pelvic adhesions

It remains unclear whether adhesions cause chronic pelvic pain. Adhesiolysis results in pain relief in 60–90% of cases in uncontrolled studies. However, in a randomized controlled trial of adhesiolysis, only patients with severe, vascularized, and dense adhesions involving bowel benefited from surgery. There appears to be little benefit from adhesiolysis for simple pelvic adhesions.

- *Ovarian remnant syndrome* or the trapped ovary syndrome refers to chronic pelvic pain caused by dense fibrous adhesions around the ovarian tissue. This can be relieved by ovarian suppression or removal.

Pelvic congestion

Pelvic congestion is characterized by dilatation of pelvic veins, which leads to cyclical 'dragging' pelvic pain. The pain usually occurs during the premenstrual phase of the cycle and is worse on standing or walking. It varies in site and intensity and may be associated with deep dyspareunia after intercourse. The dilated pelvic veins may be demonstrated by laparoscopy and sometimes by ultrasound scan.

- *Treatment* is by using medroxyprogesterone acetate (MPA) 30–50 mg daily for 3 months. Side effects include weight gain, amenorrhea, and bloating.
  - Suppression of ovarian activity with GnRH analogs has been used to treat pelvic pain.
  - In severe cases, hysterectomy with bilateral oophorectomy (with HRT afterwards) is curative.

Bowel-related pain

- *Irritable bowel syndrome* (IBS) is the most common bowel-related cause of chronic pelvic pain. It affects around 10–20% of the general population and is common in women of reproductive age. It is a functional disease. The diagnosis of IBS is based on the history of pain and bowel symptoms. Treatment is with high-fiber diet and antispasmodic drugs.
- *Constipation* is a common cause of bowel distension and chronic pelvic pain. Other conditions such as *inflammatory bowel disease* may present with pain, but other symptoms, such as bloody diarrhea, are usually present.

Urological causes

- *Interstitial cystitis* (IC) is an inflammatory condition of unknown cause, which may cause pain and urinary symptoms such as urgency, frequency, and nocturia. The pain increases as the bladder fills and is relieved by passing urine. The diagnosis is made by cystoscopy with the characteristic appearance of submucosal edema and petechiae. Dyspareunia is more common among women with IC.

- *Chronic urethral syndrome* is characterized by symptoms of irritation, postvoiding fullness, and incontinence.
- Other conditions such as urethral diverticulae, urinary calculi, bladder neoplasia, or radiation cystitis may also cause chronic pain.

Musculoskeletal pain

- In *sacroiliac dysfunction,* pain may arise from the joints themselves or from the associated muscle spasm. The pain is typically worse with movement.
- Some patients with chronic pelvic pain have an *abnormal posture,* which may cause chronic muscle tension and strain on joints and ligaments, which then becomes a source of chronic pelvic pain.
- *Tension myalgia* of the pelvic floor itself may be a cause of pelvic pain.

Neuropathic pain

Neuropathic pain arises from a damaged nerve rather than tissue damage. Nerve entrapment in scar tissue or fascia may give rise to pain. The pain may be sharp or stabbing in nature, or may be a constant dull ache. The diagnosis can be confirmed by injecting a local anesthetic at the site of maximal tenderness. Presacral neurectomy has been used for patients with endometriosis with mixed results.

Psychosocial factors

Chronic pelvic pain may have a number of contributory factors: psychological, physical, and social. The balance between the factors will vary from patient to patient and at different times for each individual's disease. The presence of chronic pelvic pain may exacerbate or provoke difficulties in sleeping or depression. Psychological morbidity is more likely to be a consequence than a cause of chronic pelvic pain. However, chronic pelvic pain is often associated with negative findings at clinical examination and laparoscopy, and more than 50% of patients have evidence of significant emotional disturbance. Pelvic pain may improve after reassurance following a negative laparoscopy. Women with chronic pelvic pain have a higher incidence of past sexual abuse than those with other types of pain or no pain.

Recommended further reading

1. Carey MP, Slack MC (1996). GnRH analogue in assessing chronic pelvic pain in women with residual ovaries. *Br J Obstet Gynaecol* **103**, 150–3.
2. Collett BJ *et al.* (1998). A comparative study of women with chronic pelvic pain, chronic non-pelvic pain, and those with no history of pain attending general practitioners. *Br J Obstet Gynaecol* **105**, 87–92.
3. Prentice A (2000). Medical management of chronic pelvic pain. *Best Practice Res Clin Obstet Gynaecol* **14**, 495–9.

Diagnosis of pelvic pain

History

- Ask about the location of the pain, mode of onset, whether it is constant or colicky in nature, radiation, and relation to the menstrual cycle.
- When was the last menstrual period?
- What contraception is she using?
- Is there any associated vaginal discharge or bleeding?
- Are there any bowel or urinary symptoms?

Physical examination

- Is the patient able to move or is she curled up in bed?
- Check blood pressure, temperature, and pulse.
- On abdominal examination, look for the location of the pain, rebound tenderness or guarding, and any mass or hernia.
- Carry out a pelvic examination (including speculum) to look for vaginal discharge or a pelvic mass and to assess pelvic tenderness.
  - If movement of the cervix elicits increased pain (cervical excitation), this may indicate the presence of blood in the peritoneal cavity (ectopic pregnancy) or inflammation of the peritoneum (PID).
  - Pelvic examination should not be done in ovarian hyperstimulation syndrome (risk of rupture of ovarian cysts) and is only carried out when a diagnosis of ectopic pregnancy is suspected if facilities are available for immediate laparotomy.

Investigations

- Triple swabs (high vaginal, cervical, and endocervical) should be obtained to exclude STDs such as chlamydia and gonorrhea.
- Send a midstream urine specimen to exclude urinary tract infection.
- Take blood samples for CBC, group and save, and C-reactive protein.
- A urinary or serum β-hCG should be checked to exclude pregnancy.
- Pelvic ultrasound scan: vaginal/abdominal to exclude pelvic pathology.
- Laparoscopy has an important place in the management of conditions that cause pelvic pain in women of reproductive age. It is the 'gold standard' investigation for the diagnosis of ectopic pregnancy, endometriosis, and PID.

Recommended further reading

1. Economy KE, Laufer MR (1999). Pelvic pain. *Adolesc Med* **10**, 291–304.
2. Porpora MG, Gomel V (1997). The role of laparoscopy in the management of pelvic pain in women of reproductive age. *Fertili Steril* **68**, 765–79.

Chapter 15

Subfertility and reproductive medicine

Primary care management of female subfertility

Introduction

A woman who has had over a year of unprotected sexual intercourse and has never conceived in the past is described as having *primary subfertility*. Early referral and investigations should be encouraged if there are clear problems, e.g. amenorrhea or in a couple where the female partner is over 35 years of age. Fertility decreases with increasing maternal age, and this decrease becomes much steeper as one approaches the age of 40.

Over 90% of healthy couples will conceive within 12 months of unprotected sexual intercourse, but 5–10% will seek specialist help. This is likely to increase with social changes in lifestyle; in developed countries, over 50% of women presenting with primary subfertility are over the age of 35.

The purpose of subfertility investigations is to identify a cause and treat accordingly to improve fertility and achieve a pregnancy. In practice, it is rarely that simple, and it is of utmost importance that the interest and welfare of the unborn child be constantly considered. Therefore primary care providers, who have in-depth information about their patients, are in a privileged position to initiate subfertility investigations and also to help them prepare for pregnancy, both physically and mentally. Subfertility can be very stressful to both partners. Therefore sympathetic management starting in primary care is essential.

Primary care management

The use of a local protocol should be agreed for general practice management and the referral of subfertile couples. This improves quality of care, avoids delays and repetition of investigations, and should be encouraged.

- Both partners should be involved in the management of their subfertility. A full history and examination of both partners should be performed early in the primary care management, and advice given about regular intercourse two or three times a week.
- *Rubella status* should be checked and immunization administered if seronegative. Ideally, adequate contraceptive cover should be used to avoid conception within 1 month of receiving a live attenuated vaccine.
- *Folic acid* 0.4 mg daily should be started and continued until 12 weeks of gestation. This is to reduce the incidence of neural tube defects (NTDs). Women with a past history of NTDs or on anticonvulsant medications should be given folic acid 4 mg daily instead of 0.4 mg.
- General advice should cover stopping smoking, reducing excessive alcohol use, and diet. There is also a need to control ongoing medical conditions prepregnancy (especially diabetes and hypertension).
- Early referral of the female partner should take place in the following circumstances:
  - Aged over 35 years
  - Amenorrhea/oligomenorrhea
  - Previous abdominal/pelvic surgery
  - Past history of STD
  - Abnormal findings at examination

Initial laboratory investigations

- Semen analysis (discussed later in this chapter).
- Consider measuring mid-luteal phase progesterone levels. If cycles are longer than 28 days, the serum progesterone level should be estimated 7 days before the onset of menstruation.
  - If >30 nmol/L, there is adequate ovulation.
  - If <30 nmol/L, repeat in another cycle.
  - If level is consistently low, couple should be referred to a gynecologist for further evaluation of luteal phase deficiency.
- Check rubella status.
- LH/FSH, prolactin, and thyroid function test prior to early referral in women with oligo/amenorrhea.

Management in secondary care I

- All the information accrued during the couple's primary care management must be communicated to the secondary care team. This will greatly hasten the subsequent investigations and management of the couple.
- The secondary management of infertility should preferably take place in a dedicated clinic run by trained staff who are readily accessible to help couples make their choices and orientate the management of their subfertility.
- Both partners should be seen together, but care is required to maintain individual's confidentiality if prompted by the referral letter.
- Full histories and examinations of both partners are performed if this has not been done previously.
- The initial set of investigations requested will be dependent on those already performed and issues raised from the history and examination. If no abnormalities are identified after the initial investigations, tubal function is investigated with the purpose of achieving a diagnosis prior to treatment and to avoid empirical non-evidence-based treatments. Table 15.1 lists the diagnostic groups and the estimated prevalence of each diagnosis. Many couples have more than one problem leading to their joint subfertility.

Male factors and endometriosis are discussed later in this chapter. Ovulation disorder will only be briefly discussed here. (see Chapter 12 📖 *p.462* and later in this chapter).

Ovulation disorder

Anovulation may present with amenorrhea, oligomenorrhea, or rarely with regular menstrual cycles but low serum progesterone in previously investigated cycles. Some causes of anovulation are listed in Table 15.2.

- Investigations to be performed, if not already available, should be serum FSH (high in primary ovarian failure) and serum LH (high in polycystic ovarian syndrome (PCOS)) in the early 'follicular' phase of a menstrual cycle.
  - Serum prolactin and thyroid function tests (TFTs) are mandatory in women with secondary amenorrhea (for further investigations see Chapter 12 📖 *p.462*).
  - Serum estradiol concentration varies widely and a single measurement is rarely of value. Assessment of endogenous estrogen production can be performed using a *progestogen challenge test* after a negative pregnancy test (medroxyprogesterone acetate (MPA) 10 mg three times a day for 1 week, which will induce a withdrawal bleed in women with adequate estrogen levels).
- Ultrasound scan of the pelvis is helpful to identify polycystic ovaries and exclude large endometriomas. As part of later investigations, tracking of follicular growth and rupture using serial ultrasound scans is used for the rare diagnosis of the *lutenized unruptured follicle syndrome,* where a preovulatory follicle fails to rupture.

Table 15.1 The diagnostic groups and the estimated prevalence of each diagnosis

Diagnostic groups	Estimated prevalence (%)
Ovulation disorders	20–30
Endometriosis	5–15
Tubal factor	20–35
Cervical factor	5
Male factor	25
Unexplained	27
Sexual dysfunction	5

Table 15.2 Causes of anovulation

Primary ovarian failure
Autoimmune
Genetic, e.g. Turner's syndrome
Secondary ovarian disorders
Polycystic ovarian syndrome
Abnormal gonadotropin regulation
  Specific
    Hyperprolactinemia
    Kallman's syndrome
Functional
    Weight problems
    Excessive exercise
    Idiopathic
Gonadotropin deficiency
    Pituitary tumor
    Previous pituitary surgery

Management in secondary care II

Induction of ovulation

Induction of ovulation regimes are chosen based on a diagnosis of the cause of the anovulation. All patients must be given clear information about the risks of multiple pregnancy and ovarian hyperstimulation (see later in this chapter). The aim of an ovulation induction program is to achieve a unifollicular ovulation.

- The dopamine agonist, bromocriptine, is effective treatment for women with hyperprolactinemia (normal or low FSH and raised prolactin). Those patients should ideally be managed in a multispecialty clinic run by an endocrinologist and a gynecologist. The same applies to women with co-existing thyroid dysfunction.
- In anovular women with normal FSH and normal endogenous estrogen levels, the first-line management to induce ovulation should be an anti-estrogen such as clomiphene citrate starting at 50 mg on days 2–6 of the menstrual cycle. This should only be performed if monitoring of response to therapy using endocrine and ultrasound means is readily available. Treatment is changed thereafter according to the monitored response, and up to 12 cycles of treatment should be considered after informed counseling of couples.
- Women with low estrogen levels and normal/low FSH can have ovulation successfully induced with exogenous gonadotropins or pulsatile gonadotropin-releasing hormone (GnRH). A regular or low-dose gonadotropin regime is used in PCOS.
- There is no evidence that ovulation induction is effective in women with primary ovarian failure or with persistently raised FSH levels in the early follicular phase. Assisted reproduction with egg donation is an effective option in such women.

Tubal factor

The gold standard investigation remains a diagnostic laparoscopy and dye insufflation, but a hysterosalpingogram (HSG) is an effective initial screening investigation for women without significant past history and ongoing symptoms.

- HSG provides an outline of both the uterine cavity and the fallopian tubes. This investigation can occasionally produce abdominal pain and antibiotic cover should be used where there is a past history of pelvic inflammatory disease (PID).
- Tubal factor subfertility suggested at HSG can be corrected by subsequent laparoscopy, which is indicated whenever the HSG is abnormal.
- HSG using ultrasound and a galactose-containing contrast medium (HyCoSy) is now available and yields similar information to a conventional HSG, but avoids radiation exposure.
- *Laparoscopy and dye* is also commonly recommended prior to a diagnosis of unexplained infertility, despite a normal HSG. The pelvis should be systematically examined prior to methylene blue being injected transcervically.

- The findings and extent of pelvic pathology should lead to a management plan. The options are selective salpingorrhaphy/tubal catheterization (only available in a few centers), surgery, or assisted reproduction in the form of *in vitro* fertilization (IVF).
- Peritubular adhesions interfere with ovulation and ovum pick-up, and so laparoscopic adhesiolysis when tubes are patent results in good cumulative conception rates. A microsurgical approach for women with tubal proximal disease is appropriate for mild tubal disease (grade I or II). If pregnancy has not occurred within 12 months of surgery, IVF should be considered. The latter should be considered as first-line treatment for all other women with tubal disease.

Unexplained infertility

This is a diagnosis of exclusion reached when investigations have been completed and no clear explanation reached for the couple's ongoing inability to conceive after 2 years of unprotected sexual intercourse.

- Cervical factor subfertility is first excluded by an *in vivo* postcoital test (PCT) with or without further *in vitro* sperm–mucus interaction studies.
- Without an underlying diagnosis, treatment is empirical and careful counseling of couples is essential before starting treatment. Continued expectant management after counseling depends on the duration of subfertility and the age of the women. Spontaneous pregnancy is still common for couples with 2 years of unexplained infertility.
- Ovarian stimulation with intrauterine insemination is an effective form of treatment (monthly fertility of 9.5% versus 3.3% in controls) but treatment with ovulation induction alone is of limited benefit. Gamete intrafallopian transfer (GIFT) carries similar outcome results when compared with intrauterine insemination with ovulation induction (IUI + OI). IVF provides further therapeutic options for this group of couples, and is now the next step after failed IUI cycles.

Counseling in subfertility

This should be available to all couples and backed up by detailed and regularly reviewed information leaflets. Counseling, although part of general clinical management, should be provided by an independent qualified counselor. This takes the form of information, discussion of implications, support, and therapeutic counseling.

Male subfertility

Introduction

Male infertility affects about 25% of subfertile couples. In the majority of these, the male partner is subfertile and, in a small number, infertile.

Andrology is the branch of science and medicine that deals with the reproductive functions of the male of which subfertility and hypogonadism with desired paternity are central topics. At the core of andrology is semen analysis (seminology).

The organs of reproduction

These consist of two testes, in which normal spermatogenesis takes place in the seminferous tubules and efferent duct system, and a number of accessory glands. The duct starts as an extremely coiled tube lying on the surface of the testis (the epididymis) which then straightens out to become the ductus deferens or 'vas'. The vas empties into the prostatic urethra, which is continuous with the penile urethra. The accessory glands, of which the epididymis acts as one, are the seminal vesicles, the prostate, and the urethral glands, all of which empty into the prostatic urethra. The penis has tubes of erectile tissue—corpora cavernosum and spongiosum.

Sperm production and control

The testes have two functions—production of spermatozoa and production of male sex hormones. Each function is complementary to the other, and the two functions take place in different compartments. Some 2×10^{12} spermatozoa are produced in a lifetime, and the main regulators of spermatogenesis, FSH and testosterone, act on the Sertoli cells and spermatogenic (germ) cells, both being within the tubular compartments of the testes.

In the absence of these hormones, spermatogenesis eventually stops. Sertoli cells are thought to control the proliferation and development of spermatogonia, leading to spermatozoa. This process takes 74 days.

In the intertubular compartment of the testes, testosterone is synthesized from cholesterol within the Leydig cells. This is regulated by LH. There are known to be specific receptors to LH and FSH in the Leydig and Sertoli cells, respectively.

Similarly to other endocrine control mechanisms, testosterone and inhibin, produced from Leydig cells, exert negative feedback regulation on the release of pulsatile pituitary LH and FSH. The end-product of this process, a spermatozoon, has four features which make it unique when compared with other body cells. It is devoid of cytoplasm, has a mobile tail, functions independently of other spermatozoa, and is haploid. Spermatozoa form 10% or less of the volume of seminal fluid ejaculated.

Sperm transport

Penile erection and ejaculation are under the control of the autonomic nervous system. During sexual arousal, parasympathetic impulses cause vasodilatation of the pudendal arteries. The distal branches of the pudendal arteries are coiled in the corpora cavernosum and, with vasodilatation, these penile arteries straighten out and fill the sinus of erectile tissues with blood. This compresses venous outflow and leads to erection.

Ejaculation or delivery of the seminal fluid into the prostatic urethra is under sympathetic control. Epinephrine causes contractions of local smooth muscles. Coagulated semen is then released.

In the female, millions of sperm are deposited around the external cervical os. Sperm penetration and passage through the cervical mucus is dependent on sperm motility and the quality of the mucus. Myometrial contractions transport the sperm from the cervix to the uterotubal junction. In the human female, orgasm is thought to aid this process. In the fallopian tube, cilial activity and sperm motility lead to progress toward the middle third of the tube where fertilization usually occurs.

Recommended further reading

1. Abshagen K, Behre HM, Cooper TG, Nieschlag E (1998). Influence of sperm surface antibodies on spontaneous pregnancy rates. *Fertili Sterili* **70**, 355–6.

Diagnosis of male infertility

Ideally, history taking and examination should precede semen analysis. However, in clinical practice, this often only takes place if the initial analysis is not entirely normal. A thorough case history and examination can yield important information and allow meaningful interpretation of the analysis.

History

- A medical history must include details about onset of puberty, any testicular maldescent and timing of surgery, hernia repair, and ongoing general medical conditions (diabetes mellitus). Past history of mumps and other causes of orchitis (recurrent trauma) or STD is also important.
- Family history should include enquiries about cystic fibrosis and other possible genetic causes of hypogonadism.
- Many drugs can affect spermatogenesis and sexual function, including the use of anabolic steroids.
- Certain occupations with inherent exposure to heat, chemical, dyes, and toxins can cause infertility.
- Finally, smoking, excessive alcohol intake, and excessive athletic activities are also important.

Examination

- Physical examination should include body proportions and fat distribution, as well as other clinical features of androgenicity (voice, hair, and skin). Anosmia is diagnostic of Kallmann's syndrome.
- Testicular size is then determined by palpation with or without the use of a Prader orchidometer. The normal range is 12–30 mL (average volume 18 mL). Normal volume with azoospermia is suggestive of an obstruction, and small soft testicles are indicative of low gonadotropins.
- Undescended or maldescended testis, swelling of the epididymis (spermatocele), and distension of the pampiniform plexus (varicocele) must be looked for. Congenital absence of the vas deferens is seen in about 2% of patients. The urethral opening should be at the end of the penis.

Semen analysis

Semen analysis forms the cornerstone of the assessment of the subfertile couple.

Collection of the sample

An instruction sheet should be given to the patient. The specimen should be produced by masturbation. Condoms should not be used as they contain spermicides. Abstinence from coitus for 48–72 hours is suggested. This improves the standardization of the test and may increase the total count. Prolonged abstinence beyond 5 days is associated with a decrease in motility.

Wide-mouth sterile plastic containers should be used and labeled with the date and time of production. Most fertility units have a dedicated room for production on site; this allows optimum analysis once liquefaction has taken place. Otherwise, the sample should be delivered to the laboratory within 30 minutes of production.

Normal values for semen analysis

Laboratories reporting semen analysis results should establish normal ranges for their own population, and indicate these on the report. Table 15.3 gives the WHO standards for 'normal' semen samples.

Recently ejaculated spermatozoa are actively motile and normally are able to swim with a forward progressive motion (grade I, fast; grade II, slow). Low motility and minimal forward progression (grade III) and no motility (grade IV) in a freshly ejaculated sample might indicate the presence of autoantibodies to the sperm. Further specific investigations are then indicated. Samples with high white cell count should be screened for infection.

Further investigations

- The evaluation of serum levels of LH, FSH, testosterone, and prolactin provides important information for specifying the cause of subfertility and hypogonadism.
- High gonadotropin levels with low testosterone indicate a testicular origin of hypogonadism—primary testicular failure.
- Chromosome analysis should be performed if testicles are also small and firm—Klinefelter's syndrome.
- Low gonadotropin and testosterone levels usually indicate a central cause.
- Other investigations occasionally needed to complete the investigation of the male factor are ultrasound of the scrotum, MRI of the pituitary gland, and pituitary stimulation tests.
- Azoospermia with a normal endocrine profile raises the possibility of an obstruction. Vasogram and testicular biopsy are then best performed in units where there are facilities for sperm recovery and cryostorage.

Table 15.3 WHO standards for 'normal' semen samples

Parameter	Normal range
Volume	2–5 mL
Liquefaction time	Within 30 minutes
Concentration	20–200 million/mL
Motility	Greater than 40% motile (grades I and II)
Morphology	Greater than 40% normal forms
White blood cells	Less than 1 million/mL

Treatment of male subfertility

Concern has been expressed that, with assisted reproduction techniques (ART), most treatments are now designed to enhance sperm quality *in vitro* rather than to treat the underlying problem. These techniques, including gamete donation, are discussed later in this chapter.

Specific dysfunctions can be treated successfully.

- Infection in the male genital tract should be treated if present, although there is no evidence that fertility is improved.
- Where a diagnosis of hypogonadotropic hypogonadism is made in the male partner, the use of gonadotropin may be effective.
- Similarly, the use of bromocriptine is effective if hyperprolactinemia is diagnosed.
- The use of systemic corticosteroids for the treatment of antisperm antibodies and the surgical correction of varicocele remain controversial.
- The use of antioxidants, mast cell blockers, zinc, and certain vitamins (for the treatment of men with abnormalities of semen quality) needs further evaluation before they can be used in clinical practice.

Recommended further reading

1. Nieschlag E (1998). Update on treatment of varicocele: counselling as effective as occlusion of the vena spermatica. *Hum Reprod* **13**, 2147–50.
2. World Health Organization (1992). WHO *Laboratory Manual for the Examination of Human Semen and Sperm–Cervical Mucus Interactions* (3rd edn). Cambridge University Press, Cambridge.
3. Buchter D, Behre HM, Kliesch S, Nieschlag E (1998). Pulsatile GnRH or human chorionic gonadotrophin/human menopausal gonadotrophin as effective treatment for men with hypogonadotrophic hypogonadism: a review of 42 cases. *Eur J Endocrinol* **139**, 298–303.
4. Abshagen K, Behre HM, Cooper TG, Nieschlag E (1998). Influence of sperm surface antibodies on spontaneous pregnancy rates. *Fertili Sterili* **70**, 355–6.

Polycystic ovarian syndrome

Introduction

PCOS is one of the most common endocrine disorders, although its etiology remains unknown. It was originally described as a clinical diagnosis based on the presence of oligomenorrhea, hirsutism, and obesity—the classical Stein–Leventhal syndrome. This is now thought to be the extreme end of a spectrum. PCOS in modern practice applies to women who have classical ultrasound evidence of polycystic ovarian changes (enlarged ovaries with multiple cysts, 2–8 mm in diameter, scattered around an echodense thickened central stroma) and symptoms of oligomenorrhea, obesity, and hyperandrogenism, all of varying degrees. Biochemical abnormalities—elevated LH-to-FSH ratio, raised androgens, and reduced sex-hormone-binding globulin (SHBG) are also often seen, but ovarian morphology remains the most sensitive marker for PCOS. Because of the heterogeneous nature of this condition, a universally accepted definition remains elusive.

However, PCOS is not only an ovarian disease. Adrenal hyperactivity, abnormal pituitary hormone secretion, and changes in hepatic and adipose tissue functions are increasingly described in women with PCOS.

Features and prevalence of PCOS

PCOS is easy to recognize in its classical form, but only one or two of the three main components (anovulation, obesity, and hyperandrogenic features) are expressed in many women. For example, hyperandrogenic women with PCOS can ovulate spontaneously and, conversely, anovulation in PCOS can occur in the absence of clinical or biochemical features of hyperandrogenic activity.

In the absence of a gold standard for diagnosis, the prevalence of PCOS in the general population cannot be precisely determined. An estimate of over 5% (documented range varies from 3 to 22%) makes PCOS the most common endocrine disorder, depending on the criteria used. The symptoms of obesity, hyperandrogenism, and menstrual cycle disturbance are reported to occur in 38%, 70%, and 66%, respectively, of patients with an ultrasound diagnosis of PCOS.

Ultrasound measurements

Laparoscopy with ovarian biopsy is too invasive and does not form part of the diagnosis of PCOS. Transvaginal ultrasound is used instead.

- Ultrasound criteria
  - Increased ovarian area/volume
  - 10 to 15 microcysts (<10 mm diameter) organized in a peripheral rosary pattern
  - Increased echogenicity of ovarian stroma

Endocrine measurements

LH stimulates androgen secretion from theca cells of the ovary, while FSH regulates the function of the granulosa cells that convert androgens to estrogens through the aromatase system—the pivot of mammalian female reproduction.

- In PCOS, *LH hypersecretion*, which is particularly associated with menstrual disturbance and subfertility, occurs as measured by mean LH levels, peak frequency, and amplitude of LH pulses. In the early follicular phase, the LH-to-FSH ratio is normally 1. In PCOS, the persistently raised LH concentration (>10 IU/L) leads to an increased LH-to-FSH ratio (>3:1 in severe cases). This endocrine feature appears to cause reduced fertility and increased rates of pregnancy losses.
- Disturbed intraovarian regulation of ovarian androgen in PCOS leads to increased *testosterone* and *androstenedione* with subsequent reduction of *SHBG*.
- Moderate *hyperprolactinemia* is sometimes seen with PCOS. This requires careful consideration and exclusion of other causes of hyperprolactinemia.
- In women who present predominantly with hirsutism, acne, and alopecia, adrenal androgens must be evaluated and congenital adrenal hyperplasia excluded. In PCOS, *17-α hydroxyprogesterone* is normal and *dehydroepiandrosterone sulfate* (DHEAS) levels are variable, but only moderately raised.

Obesity

Obesity, especially of the abdominal–visceral phenotype, is a common problem in PCOS. Thirty-eight percent of women with PCOS have a BMI >25 kg/m^2. The BMI correlates with an increase in hirsutism, cycle disturbance, and subfertility.

Weight gain starts in adolescence, when there is a normal degree of insulin resistance. Probably inherited insulin resistance in PCOS, with a tendency to obesity, leads to further weight gain. This provokes further resistance and hypersecretion of insulin, and a vicious cycle is established. Eleven percent of women with PCOS have impaired glucose tolerance. Insulin also stimulates ovarian secretion of androgens, thereby worsening the hyperandrogenic status. Weight reduction in obese women with PCOS (BMI >30 kg/m^2) is an essential part of the management of this condition, which appears to have a strong genetic component. This is most likely to be by dominant inheritance as suggested by family studies.

Recommended further reading

1. Stein FI, Leventhal ML (1935). Amenorrhea associated with bilateral polycystic ovaries. *Am J Obstet Gynecol* **29**, 181–91.
2. Adams J, Franks S, Polson DW, *et al.* (1985). Multifocal ovaries: clinical and endocrine features and response to pulsatile gonadotrophin releasing hormone. *Lancet* ***ii***, 1375–8.

Management of polycystic ovarian syndrome

The therapeutic approach to individual women with PCOS is determined by the presenting problem caused by the underlying endocrinopathy. The need to lose weight in women with obesity and PCOS is common to all management strategies.

Weight loss

Even moderate obesity (BMI >27 kg/m^2) is known to be associated with a lower chance of ovulation, and women with central body fat distribution have more severe hirsutism and cycle disturbance.

In women with a BMI >30 kg/m^2, weight loss is known to have a significant beneficial effect on endocrine function and ovulation, with improved fertility. With weight reduction, serum androgen and fasting insulin concentrations fall, thus eventually improving hyperandrogenic symptoms, leading to spontaneous ovulation and increased fertility with or without therapy. Ovulation induction (often involving expensive and potentially dangerous drugs) is known to be less effective when BMI is >30 kg/m^2. Pregnancy also carries greater risks in the obese.

Therapeutic strategies

Hirsutism affects over 70% of women with PCOS. Various drugs are available, but the long-term outcome remains disappointing without weight reduction.

Cycle disturbance in women when fertility is not an issue can be treated with progestogens alone or with combined preparations of estrogen and progestogen. This will induce menstrual cycles and minimize the adverse effects of unopposed estrogen, thus reducing the risk of endometrial hyperplasia, which may lead to atypical changes and eventually to endometrial adenocarcinoma. Thickened endometrium over 10 mm on ultrasound in association with PCOS amenorrhea requires further management such as the following:

- Oligo/amenorrhea:
  - progestogens
  - combined oral progestogens and estrogen.
- Dysfunctional uterine bleeding:
  - progestogens
  - combined oral progestogens and estrogen.

The combined preparations used should not contain 17 nortestosterone progestogens, which will further lower SHBG and increase free testosterone. MPA is the ideal single progestogen to use; it also suppresses LH and ovarian androgen secretion.

Recommended further reading

1. Nahum R, Thong KJ, Hillier SG (1995). Metabolic regulation of androgen production by human cells *in vitro*. *Hum Reprod* **10**, 75–81.

Subfertility therapies I

In women with regular cycles, anovulation must first be confirmed. In the majority of women with cycle disturbance, it is helpful to assess estrogen production prior to ovulation induction. A *progestogen challenge test* (MPA 30 mg daily for 1 week) performed after a negative pregnancy test is a simple way of investigating endogenous estrogen, but it also facilitates onset of ovulation induction treatment.

Clomiphene citrate ovulation induction therapy

Clomiphene citrate and other forms of ovulation induction (unless the patient has longstanding amenorrhea) should only be used after thorough subfertility investigations, including hysterosalpingogram or laparoscopy, confirming tubal patency.

In well-estrogenized PCOS patients (with normal FSH and prolactin levels), the first treatment of choice for induction of ovulation is the use of clomiphene—an antiestrogen. This is an oral therapy using 50 mg per day for 5 days starting on day 2 of a spontaneous or progestogen-induced bleed. Antiestrogens block the negative feedback of estradiol on the hypothalamus and pituitary. This increases endogenous FSH levels, which promote follicular growth leading to ovulation. Clomiphene citrate also has a direct effect on the ovary's FSH-induced aromatase activity.

Clomiphene is an effective treatment for anovulation in appropriately selected women—obesity being the major correctable adverse factor. Although clomiphene is reported to induce ovulation in over 70% of patients, only 40% conceive. Up to 10 cycles of treatment can be considered after full discussion and counseling of the patients about the possible link between continued ovulation induction and ovarian cancer. This is imperative if more than six cycles are to be used. A subsequent pregnancy is reported to abrogate this putative risk.

Ovulation induction with clomiphene should only be performed in circumstances that allow access to ovarian ultrasound and endocrine monitoring. If ovulation does not occur using 50 mg daily, the dose should be increased to 100 mg daily. There is probably no benefit to increasing the dose of clomiphene once ovulation is achieved. A further increase, in 50 mg increments up to 200 mg, is advocated by some if the initial response is inadequate, but a daily dose of more than 100 mg rarely confers any benefit. When a dose of over 50 mg is used, the antiestrogenic possible adverse effect of clomiphene on the mid-cycle cervical mucus changes must be investigated by a mid-cycle postcoital test.

Gonadotropin ovulation induction therapy

An injection of 5000 IU of hCG, timed by the use of ultrasound to assess follicular growth, can be used to mimic the LH surge and trigger ovulation. Ovulation occurs 24–36 hours later, and intercourse can be precisely timed.

Gonadotropin ovulation induction therapy is indicated for women with PCOS who are resistant to clomiphene. Women who ovulate with clomiphene, but fail to conceive, are probably best served by moving to assisted conception (e.g. IVF) as opposed to an alternative method of ovulation induction.

Two regimens of gonadotropins are widely used: daily or alternate day injections of gonadotropins, increasing the dose every 5–7 days based on closely monitored follicular response. The usual starting dose is 75 units of gonadotropin. There is no advantage in using GnRH analogs in conjunction with gonadotropins for ovulation induction in women with clomiphene-resistant PCOS as there is no increase in the pregnancy rate.

The aim of monitoring by using ultrasound and serum estradiol levels is to allow timing of the hCG injection to induce ovulation without causing hazardous ovarian hyperstimulation.

Subfertility therapies II

Ovarian hyperstimulation syndrome (OHSS)

Some patients undergoing gonadotropin stimulation show a marked response to the drugs with multiple follicular development believed to result from an overproduction of estrogen. To minimize the occurrence and severity of OHSS, gonadotropin cycles are closely monitored. When OHSS is suspected, further stimulation is withdrawn, hCG is withheld, and the treatment cycle is postponed. The pathophysiology of OHSS is still not completely understood and so it is difficult to prevent and to treat. Although OHSS may occur after a spontaneous LH peak, this risk is much less than after the long-acting hCG preparations.

Hyperstimulation still provokes much fear because of morbidity needing intense treatment. Hyperstimulation is generally classified as mild, moderate, or severe (and in all cases there is excessive estrogen secretion, with symptoms usually appearing 3–6 days after hCG administration/ spontaneous ovulation).

- *Mild hyperstimulation* is defined as ovarian enlargement up to 5 cm diameter, accompanied by some mild abdominal swelling and pain. There is little cause for concern, and therapy should consist of rest at home, careful observation, and analgesia.
- *Moderate hyperstimulation* is defined as ovarian enlargement up to 12 cm diameter, accompanied by more pronounced symptoms including abdominal distension and pain, nausea, vomiting, and occasional diarrhea. Therapy includes bed rest and close observation to detect any progression to severe hyperstimulation in cases where conception has occurred. Hospital admission is sometimes required. Pelvic examination of the enlarged ovaries should be gentle in order to avoid rupture of the cysts. In the majority of cases, symptoms should subside spontaneously within 2–3 weeks.
- *Severe hyperstimulation* is a rare but serious complication characterized by ovarian enlargement in excess of 12 cm in diameter. Symptoms include pronounced abdominal distension and pain, ascites, pleural effusion, hemoconcentration (packed cell volume (PCV) >45%), reduced urine output, electrolyte imbalance, and, sometimes, shock. *Hospital admission is mandatory*. Treatment should concentrate on restoring fluid balance by giving IV fluids (colloids, rather than crystalloids) and heparin to prevent thromboembolism. In view of the recent concerns about its use, IV albumin is best avoided. Patients should also be given oral intake of high-protein fluids. A strict fluid balance chart should be kept as well as daily measurements of electrolytes, renal function, CBC, clotting screen, and serum albumin. Paracentesis may be indicated and performed under ultrasound guidance if the abdominal discomfort is severe. The acute symptoms subside over several days. However, symptoms may be prolonged if conception occurs.

Results of gonadotropin therapy

- Range of reported pregnancy rate per cycle, 20–30%.
- Range of reported multiple pregnancy, 10–35%.

Laparoscopic ovarian diathermy surgery

This has now replaced open ovarian wedge resection. It is also slowly replacing gonadotropin therapy as the second-line therapy for clomiphene resistance in women with PCOS, and is thought to be equally effective. The risk of ovarian hyperstimulation and multiple pregnancy with gonadotropin is replaced by the risk of periovarian adhesions. The potential risk of ovarian destruction causing subsequent ovarian failure still remains a theoretical concern.

Insulin-lowering medications

These are new adjuncts to the management of PCOS. Lowering insulin concentrations with metformin or other similar agents improves hyperandrogenism by reducing ovarian enzyme activity which results in androgen production.

Although side effects with these medications are rare, further evidence is awaited before widespread introduction into clinical practice.

Recommended further reading

1. Armar NA, Lachelin GCL (1993). Laparoscopic ovarian diathermy: an effective treatment for anti-oestrogen resistant anovulatory infertility in women with the polycystic ovary syndrome. *Br J Obstet Gynaecol* **100**, 161–4.
2. Velasquez EM, *et al.* (1994). Metformin therapy in women with polycystic ovary syndrome reduces hyperinsulinaemia, insulin resistance, hyperandrogenaemia, and systolic blood pressure while facilitating menstrual regularity and pregnancy. *Metabolism* **43**, 647–55.
3. Lord J, Wilkin T (2004). Metformin in polycystic ovary syndrome. *Curr Opin Obstet Gynecol* **16**, 481–6.

Hirsutism and virilization

Introduction

- *Hirsutism* in females is the growth of pigmented terminal hair in a typical male distribution pattern—face, chest, abdomen, and limbs. It is often associated with acne and seborrhea.
- *Virilization* is the extreme of the spectrum. It includes baldness, voice changes, and clitoromegaly. This is a rare condition, but indicates a serious cause.
- Conversely, hirsutism not associated with menstrual disturbance is unlikely to be the result of serious underlying pathology.
- Excessive hair growth in women is difficult to define precisely—the amount that causes problems varies in different ethnic cultures.
- It is generally a subjective diagnosis, with facial hair being the most unacceptable.

The pilosebaceous unit

The process that regulates the growth and differentiation of hair follicles and sebaceous glands is not fully understood. At birth, the skin is covered with short fine unpigmented vellus hair. Scalp hair and eyebrows/eyelashes are non-sexual and grow continuously thereafter.

- At puberty, androgen production results in sex-hormone-dependent hair growth in the axillae and lower pubic triangle in both sexes.
- In the female, excessive androgen exposure at any time after puberty causes hirsutism, except on the scalp, where hair loss can occur in a male pattern.
- Hair follicles within the pilosebaceous unit go through successive phases of actively producing hair and resting hair. This is termed the *hair growth cycle* and can last up to 3 years.
- Human terminal hair growth is affected by several factors, with androgens being the most obvious regulator.

Androgen action in the hair follicle

Circulating unbound androgens diffuse into dermal papilla cells at the base of the hair bulb. Intracellularly, testosterone is converted by the enzyme 5α-reductase to its active metabolite, dihydrotestosterone (DHT). This and other less bioactive androgens then bind to specific nuclear receptor proteins leading to the regulation of target genes.

The follicle increases in size and is transformed from a small vellus follicle into a terminal hair-producing follicle. Men with 5α-reductase deficiency have a female hair growth pattern.

Circulating androgens

The major androgens are testosterone, DHT, DHEAS, and androstenedione. These are produced by the ovaries (25%), adrenals (25%), and peripheral conversion (50%).

- Androgens have different potencies and binding affinities. Therefore they determine the onset, severity, and progression of symptoms.
- LH and insulin control ovarian androgen production via LH and insulin receptors found in the theca interstitial ovarian cells. ACTH from the anterior pituitary controls adrenal androgen production.

- In women, circulating testosterone is highly bound to SHBG. Free testosterone is biologically active, and small changes in SHBG can have marked effect on the biologically active free fraction available. *Hyperandrogenism* and *obesity* lower SHBG levels, leading to higher levels of free active testosterone with 'normal' total testosterone levels. Androstenedione and DHEAS are not bound to SHBG in significant amounts.

Recommended further reading

1. Hamada K *et al.* (1996). The metabolism of testosterone by dermal papilla cells cultured from human pubic and axillary hair follicles concurs with hair growth in 5-α-reductase deficiency. *J Invest Dermatol* **106**, 1017–22.

Clinical evaluation of hirsutism

History

A detailed history, including age of onset and speed of progression of hirsutism, and details of menstrual cycles may reveal the more common causes of hirsutism.

- Regular menstrual cycles and excessive hair on limbs and around lips only usually indicate *familial idiopathic hirsutism.*
- PCOS is the most common cause of oligomenorrheic anovular hirsutism, starting in the late teenage years.
- Fast-progressing hirsutism of sudden onset leading to virilization is more likely to be associated with serious disease, including androgen producing tumors.

Examination

During examination, the severity of the hirsutism can be graded using general descriptive terms or, more precisely, using the Ferriman and Galloway score (Table 15.4). Other signs of androgen production must be looked for; these will indicate the severity of androgen production. Hirsutism tends to be followed in order by acne, oily skin, male hair pattern, breast atrophy, and clitoromegaly with deepening of the voice.

Acanthosis nigricans, which are velvety pigmented changes in the skin and indicate insulin resistance in women with PCOS, can be seen around the neck and armpits.

Recommended further reading

1. American College of Obstetricians and Gynecologists (1995). ACOG Technical Bulletin No. 203. Evaluation and treatment of hirsute women. *Int J Gynaecol Obstet* **49**, 341–6.

Table 15.4 The Ferriman and Galloway scoring system (a score of 0 indicates absence of terminal hair)

Score	Criteria
Upper lip	
1	A few hairs at outer margin
2	A small mustache at outer margin
3	A mustache extending from outer margin
4	A mustache extending to midline
Chin	
1	A few scattered hairs
2	Scattered hairs with small concentrations
3 & 4	Complete cover, light and heavy
Chest	
1	Circumareolar hairs
2	With midline hair in addition
3	Fusion of these areas, with three-quarter cover
4	Complete cover
Upper back	
1	A few scattered hairs
2	Rather more, still scattered
3 & 4	Complete cover, light and heavy
Lower back	
1	Sacral tuft of hair
2	With some lateral extension
3	Three-quarter cover
4	Complete cover
Upper abdomen	
1	A few midline hairs
2	Rather more, still midline
3 & 4	Half and full cover
Lower abdomen	
1	A few midline hairs
2	A midline streak of hair
3	A midline band of hair
4	An inverted V-shaped growth
Arm	
1	Sparse growth occupying not more than a quarter of the limb surface
2	More than this; cover still incomplete
3 & 4	Complete cover, light and heavy

Forearm, thigh, and *leg* are scored as for the arm

Causes of hirsutism

- Idiopathic (familial) hirsutism
- Ovarian
    - PCOS
    - Neoplasms
    - Arrhenoblastoma
    - Gonadoblastoma
    - Hilus cell tumors
    - Pregnancy luteoma
- Adrenal
    - Congenital adrenal hyperplasia (CAH)
    - Cushing's syndrome
    - Neoplasms
- Iatrogenic/drugs
    - Anabolic steroids
    - Danazol
    - Phenytoin
    - Androgenic progestogens (high doses)

Idiopathic (familial) hirsutism

This usually presents with excessive hair on the limbs and around the lips of mild to moderate severity. Androgen levels are normal and menstrual cycles are regular. It affects 5–15% of women, and is defined by some as the presence of hirsutism in the absence of ovulatory dysfunction as determined by luteal progesterone if required.

Up to 30% of women with idiopathic hirsutism are satisfied to learn that they are healthy and are happy to continue with mechanical hair removal. The rest need medical therapy.

Ovarian causes of hirsutism

The clinical and hormone profile of PCOS, the most common cause of oligomenorrheic anovular hirsutism, is described earlier in this chapter. There is now a clear link between genetic insulin resistance and ovarian hyperandrogenism. At the extreme end of the PCOS spectrum, acanthosis nigricans (a manifestation of insulin resistance) and marked hyperandrogenism with virilization occur. These usually coexist with abdominal obesity, which itself correlates with the presence of significant insulin resistance. Insulin also reduces production of SHBG in the liver, thus magnifying the effects of androgens.

- *Ovarian neoplasms* producing androgens are extremely rare. Serum testosterone levels are extremely high and often within the male biochemical range. Hirsutism rapidly progresses to frank virilization.
- Luteoma of pregnancy are benign hCG-driven tumors which can cause significant androgenic symptoms. Luteomas regress spontaneously after pregnancy.
- Occasional ovarian stromal hyperplasia seen in parallel with serous cystadenoma, teratomas, and other neoplasms can produce high levels of androstenedione causing androgenic symptoms.

Adrenal causes of hirsutism

- In CAH, a partial block (enzyme defect) of cortisol synthesis results in increased levels of ACTH with subsequent increased androgen secretion. There are three such enzyme defects that lead to hyperandrogenism, the most common being 21-hydroxylase deficiency. Premature puberty is discussed elsewhere.
- A milder form of 21-hydroxylase deficiency can become apparent in early adult life, causing amenorrhea, hirsutism, and virilization—hence the term late-onset or incomplete CAH. PCOS can occur in association with this form of CAH.
- Adrenal tumors resulting in hyperandrogenism without evidence of glucocorticosteroid excess are extremely rare. DHEAS levels are extremely high.
- Similarly, in Cushing's syndrome, the well-described features are predominantly caused by excess glucocorticoid, and only extremely rarely present to a gynecologist.

Recommended further reading

1. Hamada K *et al.* (1996). The metabolism of testosterone by dermal papilla cells cultured from human pubic and axillary hair follicles concurs with hair growth in 5-alpha-reductase deficiency. *J Invest Dermatol* **106**, 1017–22.

Investigations and treatment of hirsutism

Laboratory evaluation

The serum hormone evaluations of excessive androgen production are testosterone (total), androstenedione, DHEAS, 17-hydroxyprogesterone, LH/FSH, SHBG with or without prolactin, and thyroid function tests. In women with regular menstrual cycles, the levels are best performed in the morning in the early follicular phase. Tests showing high levels should be repeated. High testosterone levels (>5 nmol/L (>200 ng/dL)), although sometimes seen in PCOS, warrant further ovarian imaging investigations, as a very high DHEAS level necessitates exclusion of an adrenal neoplasm.

Adult-onset CAH is *not* always associated with a raised random 17-hydroxyprogesterone level. If suspicious or when the level is mildly elevated, measurement should be repeated after an ACTH stimulation test.

Further investigations

- A 9 a.m. serum and 24 hour urinary cortisol should be estimated if Cushing's syndrome is suspected, and followed by a dexamethazone suppression test.
- Ultrasound and MRI/CT are the imaging investigations used if ovarian and adrenal neoplasms are suspected.

Treatment

Non-medical

- *Weight loss* remains an integral part of management, and enhances other treatment modalities.
- *Destructive methods* can be used alone or in parallel with medical therapy. These methods either disguise or remove terminal hair (waxing, bleaching, shaving, electrolysis, or laser therapy).

Medical

- *Combined oral contraceptive pills* (COCPs) are most widely used and must be a combination that does not contain androgenic progestogen. COCPs will stimulate SHBG production, thereby reducing free testosterone levels; gonadotropins will also be suppressed with a further reduction of adrenal androgen production. With combined preparations, as with other medical treatments, improvement in hirsutism is slow and no benefit is likely be seen for at least 6 months. Treatment must be continued for 18 months.
- The *antiandrogen* cyproterone acetate (CPA) is now often effectively used. This compound binds to the androgen receptor and also has progestogenic activity. CPA further reduces serum androgen levels by hepatic enzyme induction, thereby increasing metabolic clearance of androgens.
- CPA is prescribed in a combination with ethinyl estradiol (EE) (Table 15.5). Both regimes in Table 15.5 provide good cycle control and contraception, but the reverse sequential regime is best reserved

for severe hirsutism because of side effects. These are more frequently seen with higher doses, and include loss of libido, weight gain, and, less frequently, headache and mood changes. If taken in early pregnancy, feminization of a male fetus is a risk.

- *Flutamide* is another antiandrogen, but is less commonly used.
- *Spironolactone*, an aldosterone antagonist, has a similar mode of action to that of CPA. Doses of spironolactone range from 50 to 200 mg daily, but it is rarely used long term.

CAH is treated with glucorticoids, and surgery may be needed for other rare causes of androgen excess when specifically indicated.

Table 15.5 Combined regimen of cyproterone acetate and ethinyl estradiol

	CPA (mg)	**EE (μg)**
Dianette	2	35
Reverse sequential regime	5–15 (100 days)	5–26 (30 days)

Recommended further reading

1. American College of Obstetricians and Gynecologists (1995). ACOG Technical Bulletin No. 203. Evaluation and treatment of hirsute women. *Int J Gynaecol Obstet* **49**, 341–6.
2. Lord J, Wilkin T (2004). Metformin in polycystic ovary syndrome. *Curr Opin Obstet Gynecol* **16**, 481–6.
3. Van der Spuy ZM, le Roux PA (2003). Cyproterone acetate for hirsutism. *Cochrane Database Syst Rev* **4**, CD001125.
4. Farquhar C, Lee O, Toomath R, Jepson R (2003). Spironolactone versus placebo or in combination with steroids for hirsutism and/or acne. *Cochrane Database Syst Rev* **4**, CD000194.

Endometriosis

Introduction

This painful inflammatory condition is characterized by the presence of benign *endometrial tissue at ectopic sites.* Endometriosis is diagnosed at laparoscopy, and should then be classified using the American Fertility Society (AFS) system of classification. It is highly likely that women with this condition have a genetic predisposition to both implantation of the ectopic endometrium and, more importantly, to the inflammatory response that occurs with cyclical endometrial changes.

Prevalence is estimated as 1–20% during reproductive years. Up to 25% of women presenting with gynecological symptoms are found to have endometriotic lesions at thorough laparoscopic assessment.

Pathogenesis

A number of theories have been proposed—the 'disease of theories'. Retrograde menstruation, although probably universal, is the most likely cause. Endometriosis is certainly estrogen dependent and regresses after bilateral oophorectomy. Distant sites can be explained by celomic metaplasia, but in all cases a genetic and immunologic basis is emerging from immunohistochemical studies. There is now extensive evidence of altered immune function in endometriosis. A large proportion of women have retrograde menstruation, but only a minority of those develop endometriosis. In this condition, peritoneal cell populations are increased and activated. This, in turn, leads to a chronic inflammatory response also seen in other autoimmune disorders with local release of prostanoids and cytokines, and subsequent peritoneal scarring.

Clinical presentation

The classic form of pelvic pain in endometriosis usually takes the form of secondary dysmenorrhea (32% of women), becoming apparent after a lapse of years following menarche and starting before the onset of a period and continuing throughout. With increasing tissue damage and scarring, the duration of the chronic pelvic pain (16%) increases to occur outside and seemingly with less relation to menstruation.

The uterosacral ligaments and ovaries are a very common site for endometriotic deposits leading to deep dyspareunia, which is a complaint in 26% of women with endometriosis.

Pain in endometriosis is caused by the following:

- Local peritoneal inflammation
- Deeply infiltrating deposits
- Formation of adhesions and fibrosis limiting movements
- Traction on tissues

In this enigmatic condition, severe pelvic pathology is often seen in women with no symptoms and, overall, studies have not detected any correlation between severity of endometriosis and pelvic pain symptoms. The role of endometriosis in the pathogenesis of infertility remains unclear. It is easy to see how *severe* endometriosis can affect fertility by mechanical distortion of the tubes and ovaries and the formation of adhesions. It is uncertain to what extent *minimal* to *mild* endometriosis affects fertility, and medical treatment of these women does not enhance their fertility if they are clearly subfertile.

Possible mechanisms of endometriosis associated with subfertility include the following:

- Tubal dysfunction
- Failure of oocyte collection
- Ovulation dysfunction
- Luteinized unruptured follicle syndrome
- Peritoneal inflammation with local immune activation
- Dyspareunia, if present, often as part of pelvic pain, can also affect fertility by reducing sexual activity

Diagnosis

This depends on the sites involved. Endometriosis can be detected on clinical examination. Commonly, involved ovaries enlarge with endometrioma or uterosacral ligaments become nodular and tender and can be felt on bimanual pelvic examination. A fixed retroverted tender uterus indicates disease in the pouch of Douglas.

- *Ultrasound* is useful for distinguishing between different adnexal enlargements. Endometriomas are highly echogenic and cystic as opposed to a tubular hydrosalpinx.
- *Adenomyosis* (myometrial endometriosis) causes uniform enlargement of the uterus, unlike uterine fibroids.
- *Tumor markers* CA-125 (carcinoma antigen-125) can be used as a marker for extensive disease, but is also found to be elevated in 2.6% of healthy women and up to 20% of those with other benign gynecological conditions. CA-125 is not very helpful in monitoring results of medical treatment. Other markers, such as placental protein 14, are less helpful.
- *Laparoscopy* is essential to confirm the diagnosis suspected on clinical grounds or to exclude the diagnosis in women with pelvic pain or subfertility. This invasive diagnostic tool enables description and staging of the disease by visual inspection.
- *Ovarian endometrioma* is seen on the ovarian surface as pigmented and retracted areas, often with adhesions to the ovarian fossa. Small endometriomas can easily be missed unless the full ovarian surface is inspected.
- *Peritoneal lesions* are seen to be papular or vesicular, containing red hemorrhagic fluid in the early stages and becoming more puckered black 'powder-burn' lesions or whitish scar tissue, which probably indicates old deposits. Nodular lesions are more often seen on the uterosacral ligaments.

The AFS 1985 revised system of classification is currently used to stage pelvic endometriosis. This involves an estimation of the size and depth of peritoneal and ovarian lesions, the extent and type of adhesions, and the degree of obliteration of the pouch of Douglas with surrounding tissue scarring.

Treatment of endometriosis

Many aspects remain unclear, but in all cases treatment must be individualized based on the following:

- Age
- Presenting symptoms
- Desire for future fertility
- Severity of condition based on the AFS classification

Ongoing subfertility

Minimal to mild endometriosis

- There is no evidence to show that the successful medical treatment of minimal to mild endometriosis without mechanical distortion of tubes and ovaries enhances fertility in subfertile women.
- Surgical ablation, best performed at the time of the initial laparoscopy, does improve fertility. This might also slow the progress of the condition, subsequently causing pain. If pregnancy then fails to occur and the patient remains asymptomatic after expectant management, resumption of treatment should proceed along the lines of 'unexplained infertility'.
- Ovarian stimulation with IUI is more effective than either no treatment or IUI alone.
- The presence of minimal to mild endometriosis does not adversely affect pregnancy rates in IVF/GIFT.

Medical therapy is to inhibit endometrial growth, e.g. with the use of continuous hormonal contraceptives. However, evidence suggests that the effect of medical therapy on the appearance of the disease may be temporary.

Moderate to severe endometriosis

Moderate to severe endometriosis with coexisting mechanical pelvic subfertility should have further surgery if the anatomical problems can be corrected. This can be done after an episode of medical treatment, and can be performed with either open surgical techniques or better approached endoscopically. There are *no* controlled studies and *no* comparison of the success of this treatment with assisted reproduction techniques. Iatrogenic postsurgical adhesions remain a problem, and assisted reproduction techniques should be considered as an alternative to or following unsuccessful surgery. Large ovarian endometriomas are best treated surgically prior to assisted reproduction to facilitate egg collection and, subsequently, to improve pregnancy rate. Presurgery medical treatment can be considered, but will further delay treatment cycles.

Recommended further reading

1. Thomas EJ (1993). Endometriosis. *BMJ* **306**, 158–9.
2. Brosens I, Puttemans P, Deprest J (1993). Appearances of endometriosis. *Baillière's Clini Obstet Gynaecol* **7**, 741–57.
3. Hornstein MD, Gleason RE, Barbieri RL (1990). A randomized double-blind prospective trial of two doses of gestrinone in the treatment of endometriosis. *Fertili Sterili* **53**, 237–41.

4. Shaw RW and Zoladex Endometriosis Study Team (1992). An open randomized comparative study of the effect of goserelin depot and danazol in the treatment of endometriosis. *Fertili Sterili* **58**, 265–72.
5. American College of Obstetricians and Gynecologists (2000). ACOG Practice Bulletin No. 11. Medical management of endometriosis. *Int J Gynaecol Obstet* **71**, 183–96.
6. Hart R, Hickey M, Maouris P, Buckett W, Garry R (2005). Excisional surgery versus ablative surgery for ovarian endometriomata: a Cochrane Review. *Hum Reprod* **20**, 3000–7.
7. Allen C, Hopewell S, Prentice A, Allen C (2005). Non-steroidal anti-inflammatory drugs for pain in women with endometriosis. *Cochrane Database Syst Rev* **4**, CD004753.
8. Hughes E, Ferdorkow D, Collins J, Vandeherckhove P (2003). Ovulation suppression for endometriosis. *Cochrane Database Syst Rev* **3**, CD000155.

Treatment of symptomatic endometriosis

Definitive surgery in the form of a hysterectomy and bilateral salpingo-oophorectomy for pain can only be considered after completion of family or if pregnancy is not a requisite. Otherwise, surgery is conservative and used in tandem with or as a supplement to medical treatment.

- *Danazol*, an androgenic steroid, is used in increasing doses to achieve amenorrhea, starting with 200 mg daily and increasing to 800 mg. The treatment is continued for 6 months. Long-term follow-up studies have shown a recurrence of 37% for minimal and over 60% for severe disease. The side effects are mostly androgenic, such as acne, seborrhea, hirsutism, and weight gain. All these side effects are reversible on cessation of therapy, apart from reported voice changes as recorded by audiology measurements. Compliance can be poor because of side effects.
- *Gestrinone*, an antiestrogen, is used orally twice a week in doses of 2.5 or 1.25 mg. This is also continued for 3–6 months, and the side effects are similar to those of danazol. There is no adverse effect on bone density, but gestrinone significantly increases the low-density to high-density lipid (LDL/HDL) ratio. This returns to normal within 6 months.
- *Progestogens* in the form of MPA 10 mg three times a day can be associated with troublesome spotting.
- *COCPs* used continuously for 6 months are associated with less breakthrough bleeding, and the estrogen dose can be increased to minimize this problem at the expense of weight gain and breast symptoms. This treatment is as effective as that with GnRH agonists.

GnRH agonists

There are four agonists available, of which the intranasal spray buserelin 150 μg per dose three times a day or goserelin 3.6 mg SC every 28 days are the most widely used. This treatment is continued for 6 months and is associated with minimal bone loss. To alleviate the hypoestrogenic vasomotor symptoms and to prevent bone loss, add-back estrogen is now available. This is essential if downregulation is to continue beyond 6 months.

Three months of treatment with a GnRH agonist can be used to prepare patients for planned surgery and allow more extensive ablation to be performed. However, the disease often recurs. Unless a successful pregnancy occurs with the help of fertility treatment, more radical and definitive surgery is often performed, followed by estrogen replacement therapy.

Recommended further reading

1. Thomas EJ (1993). Endometriosis. *BMJ* **306**, 158–9.
2. Brosens I, Puttemans P, Deprest J (1993). Appearances of endometriosis. *Baillière's Clini Obstet Gynaecol* **7**, 741–57.
3. Hornstein MD, Gleason RE, Barbieri RL (1990). A randomized double-blind prospective trial of two doses of gestrinone in the treatment of endometriosis. *Fertili Sterili* **53**, 237–41.

4. Shaw RW and Zoladex Endometriosis Study Team (1992). An open randomized comparative study of the effect of goserelin depot and danazol in the treatment of endometriosis. *Fertili Sterili* **58**, 265–72.
5. American College of Obstetricians and Gynecologists (2000). ACOG Practice Bulletin No. 11. Medical management of endometriosis. *Int J Gynaecol Obstet* **71**, 183–96.
6. Hart R, Hickey M, Maouris P, Buckett W, Garry R (2005). Excisional surgery versus ablative surgery for ovarian endometriomata: a Cochrane Review. *Hum Reprod* **20**, 3000–7.
7. Allen C, Hopewell S, Prentice A, Allen C (2005). Non-steroidal anti-inflammatory drugs for pain in women with endometriosis. *Cochrane Database Syst Rev* **4**, CD004753.
8. Hughes E, Ferdorkow D, Collins J, Vandeherckhove P (2003). Ovulation suppression for endometriosis. *Cochrane Database Syst Rev* **3**, CD000155.

Assisted reproductive techniques I

Introduction

The first 'test-tube baby' was born in the UK in 1978. Since then, IVF has been 'fine tuned' and many other forms of ART have been developed for specific clinical indications. IVF remains the most widely used ART to treat all categories of subfertility, and the number of IVF cycles has increased tenfold over the last 10 years. The success of ART is dependent on the skill and expertise of the staff in individual units, as shown by wide variations between institutions (the take-home baby rate per IVF/intracytoplasmic sperm injection (ICSI) cycle ranges from 11% to 36% for all ages).

Overall, only about one in six IVF cycles is successful. On average, 76% of IVF cycles are unsuccessful, 12% result in singleton births, 7% result in multiple births, and 5% experienced one or more adverse pregnancy outcomes (ectopic pregnancies, spontaneous miscarriages, stillbirths, and neonatal deaths).

Features affecting outcome

- *Maternal age*. Female fertility reduces with advancing maternal age. Similarly, IVF outcome is affected by age. IVF pregnancy rates are highest between the ages of 25 and 35, with a steep decline thereafter. Predicted live birth rate for a 30-year-old is 16.1% and it is down to 7.3% at 40. Outcome is not affected by paternal age.
- *Duration of subfertility*. This has a major effect on the outcome of ART treatment cycles. At under 3 years of subfertility, the live birth rate per cycle is 15% compared with 8% after 12 years of subfertility.
- *Previous cycles of treatment*. The best chances of conceiving are in the first ART cycle (14% live birth rate), with reduced outcome for each subsequent cycle (8.9% with four cycles of treatment).
- *Previous pregnancies*. Women who have had a previous successful pregnancy, either spontaneous or following an ART cycle, have a higher chance of conceiving with IVF treatment.

In vitro fertilization

The recommendation for IVF now includes a wide range of indications.

- *Tubal disease* if not amenable to surgery or if pregnancy fails 12 months after successful surgery.
- *Unexplained infertility* after failed IUI + OI using partner's sperm.
- *Male factor* with satisfactory sperm function. The chance of fertilization can be improved using a high insemination concentration (IVF-HIC), but this is now being replaced by ICSI.
- *Endometriosis*: moderate and severe disease.
- *Ovulation disorders*: If conception fails to occur after 6–12 cycles of successful ovulation induction.
- *Donor insemination*: failure to conceive after 10–12 cycles of donor insemination with or without ovulation induction.

- *Egg donation* for women with premature ovarian failure, gonadal dysgenesis, iatrogenic menopause, carriers of a genetic condition, and raised FSH levels in older women.
- *Surrogacy* for women with absent uterus, but with functional ovaries.

Steps of IVF cycle

- Downregulation of ovaries for 10–14 days started during the luteal phase of the previous cycle.
- Gonadotropins (FSH or human menopausal gonadotropin) generally in higher doses than those used in patients undergoing ovulation induction to cause superovulation. Short or long treatment protocols are widely used.
- Monitor treatment (serum estradiol) and measure follicular response and growth by ultrasound. This is essential to prevent serious side effects (ovarian hyperstimulation syndrome).
- Oocyte collection is carried out under ultrasound guidance through the vaginal wall. The follicles are aspirated by gentle suction from a vacuum pump. Up to 90% of follicles yield an oocyte. In a minority of women, collection is performed at laparoscopy.
- Sperm sample is provided on the same day as oocyte collection.
- Oocyte and sperm are cultured overnight and, if fertilization has occurred, the embryos are further cultured. In some centers, ICSI is performed as a routine to assist fertilization.
- Embryo transfer performed using a fine catheter through the cervix and into the uterine cavity 2–3 days postfertilization. Between one and three embryos are typically returned to the uterus. The rest are cryopreserved for use in future cycles.
- Luteal support using progesterone is followed by pregnancy testing.

Recommended further reading

1. Templeton A, Morris JK, Parslow W (1996). Factors that affect outcome of *in vitro* fertilization treatment. *Lancet* **348**, 1402–6.
2. Templeton AA, Morris JK (1998). Reducing the risk of multiple births by transfer of two embryos after IVF. *N Eng J Med* **339**, 573–7.
3. Pandian Z, Templeton A, Serour G, Bhattacharya S (2005). Number of embryos for transfer after IVF and ICSI: a Cochrane review. *Hum Reprod* **20**, 2681–7.
4. Pandian Z, Bhattacharya S, Vale L, Templeton A (2005). *In vitro* fertilisation for unexplained subfertility. *Cochrane Database Syst Rev* **2**, CD003357.

Assisted reproductive techniques II

Intracytoplasmic sperm injection (ICSI)

This is a newer technique in which a single sperm is injected directly into the oocyte. It is used for severe male-factor subfertility. It involves a conventional IVF treatment cycle and, as with IVF, a maximum of three embryos are typically transferred into the uterus. The outcome with ICSI has improved the success rate for severe male-factor subfertility, and the success rate of ICSI is now higher than that of IVF.

There are still concerns about the use of potentially abnormal sperm. Screening for cystic fibrosis is often performed pre-ICSI treatment cycles, which have now replaced SUZI (subzonal insemination) and PZD (partial zonal dissection).

Sperm can be surgically recovered from the testis (testicular/epididymal sperm aspiration (TESA)) or the epididymis (percutaneous epididymal sperm aspiration (PESA)) in men with vas deferens obstruction (past infection or after vasectomy) or congenital absence of the vas. The extracted sperm can be frozen initially and used for injection into the oocyte using ICSI.

Gamete intrafallopian transfer (GIFT)

This is only effective with functional fallopian tubes in couples with unexplained subfertility. The oocytes are collected at laparoscopy, mixed with washed and resuspended sperm, and returned into the fallopian tubes. This is now used less frequently.

Intrauterine insemination and ovulation induction (IUI + OI)

This involves replacing carefully washed sperm into the uterine cavity at the time of ovulation. IUI requires ovulation induction with follicular growth monitoring using ultrasound to determine the day of insemination. Both fallopian tubes must be patent. The main indications are unexplained male- and cervical-factor subfertility.

Donor insemination (DI)

This treatment is offered to couples when the male partner has azoospermia or the semen analysis is such that a pregnancy is unlikely: severe oligozoospermia, gross teratozoospermia, and severe asthenozoospermia. Otherwise, DI can be appropriate for couples who have a past history of severe rhesus isoimmunization with a homozygous Rh(D)-positive male partner or if genetic testing suggests a high risk of major genetic problems.

- DI requires careful consideration, and all couples are advised to have formal counseling. It should be pointed out that the male partner's name will appear on the birth certificate, but informing the child later on in life must be strongly considered.
- The female partner should be investigated prior to starting DI, including tubal investigations. To maximize outcome, accurate timing of insemination is essential. Therefore ovulation is closely monitored using ultrasound following ovulation induction.

- The frozen donor sperm is thawed and placed in the cervix or, after preparation, IUI is performed.
- Couples are offered four to six cycles, and failure must be followed by a formal review.
- *The donors* are men between 18 and 55, with a normal sperm count. After detailed family, social, and medical history, potential donors are also counseled. All donors are screened for hepatitis and STD, including HIV. The sperm straws are then frozen and quarantined for 6 months or more, after which the donors are retested for HIV before the straw is released for use. Most clinics do their best to use a donor who has physical characteristics similar to those of the male partner.
- *Outcome for women below the age of 38*: the live birth rate is currently 10% and is 6% per treatment cycle started. Chances of success decrease with increasing maternal age.

Donor oocyte within an IVF/ICSI cycle

This has been successfully used since 1984. The main indication for egg donation is women with premature ovarian failure. Women with persistently raised gonadotropin levels in the early follicular phase of the menstrual cycle are also good candidates, since success with their own eggs is extremely poor.

Recommended further reading

1. Hughes EG (1997). The effectiveness of ovulation induction and intrauterine insemination in the treatment of persistent infertility: a meta-analysis. *Hum Reprod* **12**, 1865–72.
2. Pandian Z, Templeton A, Serour G, Bhattacharya S (2005). Number of embryos for transfer after IVF and ICSI: a Cochrane review. *Hum Reprod* **20**, 2681–7.
3. van Rumste MM, Evers JL, Farquhar CM (2004). ICSI versus conventional techniques for oocyte insemination during IVF in patients with non-male factor subfertility: a Cochrane review. *Hum Reprod* **19**, 223–7.

Counseling in subfertility

Clinics offering ART to treat subfertile couples should offer independent counseling. This is because such therapy creates a great deal of stress for the majority of couples who, often as a consequence of the subfertility and failure of treatment, experience a deep bereavement. This counseling takes the form of information, implication, and support counseling. Confidentiality is paramount as part of counseling, but also in all aspects of subfertility management.

Recommended further reading

1. Templeton A, Morris JK, Parslow W (1996). Factors that affect outcome of *in vitro* fertilization treatment. *Lancet* **348**, 1402–6.

Gonadotropin-releasing hormone

Introduction

GnRH agonists available for clinical use are derived from the naturally occurring hypothalamic GnRH decapeptide, but are over 100 times more potent than the natural endogenous hormone. The molecule is altered to decrease enzyme breakdown and therefore has an increased half-life.

Mode of action

During the luteal phase, endogenous GnRH pulses are large and relatively infrequent, leading to a similar pattern of LH secretion. In the follicular phase, GnRH pulses increase in frequency, causing similar increases of LH production.

With pharmacological GnRH agonists, the majority of GnRH receptors in the pituitary glands are occupied, resulting in an initial surge of plasma gonadotropin levels. After the initial stimulation, continued receptor occupancy downregulates pituitary gonadotropin production, resulting in the suppression of gonadotropin secretion. A reversible 'menopause' is activated by prolonged GnRH agonist treatment.

Indications for GnRH agonist use

- Precocious puberty
- Endometriosis
- Fibroids
- Premenstrual syndrome
- Induction of ovulation in women with PCOS and for controlled hyperstimulation in assisted reproduction

Precocious puberty

This can be treated with a GnRH agonist when no cause can be found or when a cause cannot be removed. Pubic hair will not disappear, but further menstruation, the growth spurt leading to premature epiphyseal closure, and breast development will be inhibited. Normal adult height can be achieved by delaying bone maturation until adrenarche.

Endometriosis

Treatment with a GnRH agonist is usually limited to 6 months. The initial surge of gonadotropins can cause a transient deterioration of symptoms. To avoid disturbing hypoestrogenic symptoms and to prevent loss of bone mineral content, long-term therapy with a GnRH agonist is combined with 'add-back' therapy. The additional estrogen and progestogen can be used sequentially or continuously. Two preparations commonly used are Cyclo-Progynova and Tibolone. It is preferable to start the add-back replacement after the downregulation is well established.

The *side effects* of GnRH agonists, which include bone loss associated with prolonged use, are similar to those that occur in menopausal women, i.e. bone loss, vasomotor symptoms, reduced libido, vaginal dryness, and irritability, and are relieved by the use of add-back estrogen (and progestogen). The estrogen effect of add-back therapy is much less than that due to estrogen in the natural cycles and hence does not stimulate endometriosis.

Fibroids

Not all GnRH agonists are licensed for use to shrink fibroids, but they are widely used in clinical practice. The benefits of such therapy only last for as long as it is continued.

In cases needing myomectomy, some use GnRH analog preoperatively for the following reasons:

- Reduced intraoperative blood loss
- Relief of symptoms
- Relief of anemia and reduced need for transfusion
- May enable use of lower transverse incision if fibroids shrink
- Reduction of tissue trauma at myomectomy

Ultrasound scans should be used during therapy to measure reduction in size of uterus/fibroids. Loss of tissue planes and being unable to identify smaller fibroids at myomectomy are disadvantages that are outweighed by the benefits of such therapy. However, this is an expensive approach, and the use of add-back estrogen to relieve vasomotor symptoms and avoid bone loss remains uncertain for this indication.

Premenstrual syndrome

This has been effectively treated by GnRH agonists, but treatment should be limited to 6 months or less. Symptoms often gradually recur after cessation of therapy, which is therefore best used as a diagnostic test of the long-term benefits of bilateral salpingo-oopherectomy in severe cases of PMS.

Recommended further reading

1. West CP, Lumsden MA, Baird DT (1993). Gozerelin (Zoladex) in the treatment of fibroids. *Reprod Med Rev* **2**, 1–97.
2. Hussain SY, Massil JH, Matta WH, *et al.* (1992). Buserelin in premenstrual syndrome. *Gynecol Endocrinol* **6**, 57–64.
3. Tom SL, Maconachie M, Doyle P, *et al.* (1994). Cumulative conception and live-birth rates after *in vitro* fertilization with and without the use of long, short and ultrashort regimes of the gonadotrophin-releasing hormone agonist buserelin. *Am J Obstet Gynecol* **171**, 513–20.

Induction of ovulation

There are two areas where GnRH agonists are used in regimes to stimulate folliculogenesis.

- Ovulation induction in women with anovulatory subfertility
- Stimulation for assisted reproduction

Over 20% of anovulatory women, especially those with PCOS, do not respond to clomiphene, which is the first line of therapy. Gonadotropins are commonly used in this group. However, this approach carries a high rate of multiple pregnancy and a high risk of ovarian hyperstimulation syndrome. These are not improved by the *routine* use of GnRH agonists, and neither is the pregnancy rate improved. Downregulation in this group reduces the risk of a premature endogenous LH surge before follicular maturation is complete, and can improve hCG injection timing.

There is no one ideal regimen for ovulation stimulation in assisted reproduction, but the use of GnRH agonists together with gonadotropins prevents spontaneous endogenous LH surges and improves egg collection rate and subsequent fertilization and implantation. This leads to an improved pregnancy rate per cycle.

- A recent meta-analysis has shown that, with the use of GnRH agonists in assisted reproduction, cycle cancellation rates are reduced, oocyte recovery is increased, and the pregnancy rate per embryo transfer is improved.
- Two basic protocols are widely used.
  - In the *short* protocol, no downregulation is induced and GnRH agonist and gonadotropins are used in parallel.
  - The *long protocol*, in which stimulation of the ovary only starts after complete pituitary downregulation, results in higher pregnancy rates but is more expensive and time consuming.

Preparations

A number of GnRH agonists are now available, two as nasal sprays and two as injection/intramuscular or biodegradable implants (Table 15.6).

Table 15.6 GnRH agonist preparations currently available

Preparation	Mode of use	Dosage	Frequency
Buserelin	Nasal spray	150 μg	3 doses a day
Nafarelin	Nasal spray	200 μg	2 doses a day
Goserelin	Implant	3.6 mg	28 days
Leuprorelin	Subcutaneous	3.75 mg	28 days

Recommended further reading

1. Tom SL, Maconachie M, Doyle P, *et al.* (1994). Cumulative conception and live-birth rates after *in vitro* fertilization with and without the use of long, short and ultrashort regimes of the gonadotrophin-releasing hormone agonist buserelin. *Am J Obstet Gynecol* **171**, 513–20.
2. Griesinger G, Diedrich K, Devroey P, Kolibianakis EM (2006). GnRH agonist for triggering final oocyte maturation in the GnRH antagonist ovarian hyperstimulation protocol: a systematic review and meta-analysis. *Hum Reprod Update* **12**, 159–68.

GnRH antagonists

New analogs have been synthesized which also bind to the pituitary GnRH receptors but do not induce an initial release of gonadotropins. These analogs are much more complex than GnRH agonists. Their mode of action is different. They do not act through downregulation of receptors and desensitization of gonadotropins, but by competitive binding to the GnRH receptor leading to a reduction in the secretion of gonadotropins within hours. Suppression is then maintained by continuous treatment without initial stimulatory effect.

- Two such compounds are available (cetrorelix and ganirelix) and both have been successfully used in OI protocols in assisted reproduction.
- Cetrorelix is for use in single dose (3 mg SC injection) or multiple dose (0.25 mg SC daily injections) regimens. Limited reports suggest that it is well tolerated with reduced risks of ovarian hyperstimulation when compared with agonists.

GnRH antagonists open new treatment options that require more clinical data.

Psychosexual problems and sexual dysfunction

Sexual problems within a relationship are not uncommon, and more women and men now feel able to seek advice about them. The recognition of a problem as a psychosexual disorder will be influenced by the expectations of society and the individual or couples concerned as well as by those of their professionals. The prevalence of sexual dysfunction in a study of 4000 randomly selected patients in four general practices was reported to be 44% among men and 36% among women. The prevalence varies according to how people are surveyed and what definition of sexual dysfunction is adopted.

Physiology of human sexual function

The physiology of human sexual response was described in the 1960s by Masters and Johnson. They described the five phases of human sexual response as sexual desire, sexual arousal or excitement, plateau phase, orgasm, and resolution. The physiological changes observed during sexual response are mediated by psychic and/or physical sexual stimulation, but can be inhibited, to a greater or lesser extent, by subconscious influences.

- *Sexual desire* is stimulated by the thought, sight, smell, or touch of another person. It may be suppressed or merge into the arousal phase.
- The *arousal or excitement phase* is the initial response to sexual stimulation—physical or psychological. It is characterized by reflex vasodilatation in the genitalia. There is an associated systemic component characterized by a rise in pulse and respiratory rate and blood pressure. Arousal at this stage remains vulnerable to distracting influence (thoughts, noise) and may also be affected by fatigue, alcohol, or worry.
- *Plateau phase*. During this phase, the changes in the arousal phase are consolidated and further enhanced, as is the sexual pleasure and the partners' desire for penetrative intercourse. Lower genital tract and breast changes reach a maximum, while continuing stimulation may build up sexual excitement to the intensity required to achieve orgasm.
- *Orgasm* provides an intense feeling of pleasure associated with the discharge of sexual tension built up in the preceding phases. In both sexes, it is associated with rhythmic contractions of the genital muscles.
  - Following ejaculation, the male experiences a refractory period that may vary in length and increases from a few minutes in the teenager to several hours in the elderly.
  - Many women and a minority of men do not have a refractory period, with further stimulation leading to further orgasms in this group.
- *Resolution*. Following orgasm the body returns to the nonaroused state unless stimulation is continued. In the initial moments after orgasm the penis and clitoris are exquisitely sensitive, but this is very transient with rapid decongestion of the tissues in the lower genital tract in both sexes.

The phases of sexual response leading up to orgasm are mediated by the parasympathetic nerves and lead to vasodilatation and vasocongestion of the genital organs. Failure of sexual arousal and therefore of these changes to occur results in erectile failure in a man and general sexual dysfunction in a woman. The orgasmic phase is mediated by the sympathetic nervous system, leading to the clonic contractions of the pelvic and other muscles. Where the sympathetic component fails to occur in an orderly fashion, there is premature or retarded ejaculation as a result. The feeling of pleasure experienced by both sexes appears to have its origin in the sex centre in the thalamic and limbic areas of the cortex. Failure to achieve orgasm in women is often a result of a failure of the sensations invoked in the clitoris and vagina to be transmitted to the brain.

Assessment of the patient

Presentation

Problems may be hidden behind a variety of 'opening gambits'. Sexual difficulties underlie many cases of vague ill health in women which defy diagnosis until repeated attempts at communication are made. Lack of energy, backache, and irritability, along with anxiety and depression, may be the presenting symptoms. Similarly, patients may present in family planning clinics focusing their problems on contraception, but where the hidden agenda is 'permission' or 'approval' that sexual intercourse is respectable when the aim is pleasure and love rather than procreation. Every one of the basic gynecological symptoms may be wholly or partially determined by organic pathology or psychogenic distress.

Obtaining a sexual problem history

A good fundamental knowledge of human sexual functioning as well as experience in interviewing and counseling skills is paramount. It is essential to be guided by the patient, using the information offered to focus on establishing what the current problem is rather than taking a more general sexual history. Once the main problem has been defined, a history of its development and progression should be obtained. This information should include the duration, nature of onset, whether improving or deteriorating, whether situational (i.e. present in one relationship but not another, one position and not another, etc.), and any factors that exacerbate or ameliorate the problem. It is also helpful to explore the patient's own assessment of the cause.

The consultation has to determine whether the problem is primary or secondary by ascertaining when the problem started and whether it is causally associated with any other event occurring at the time it came to surface. It is also important to determine what prompted the patient to present at this point in time. One of the goals of the consultation is also to exclude any possible underlying organic factor.

Clinical examination

The role of clinical examination is to exclude developmental abnormalities which may interfere with sexual function. This includes detection of potential causes of dyspareunia and evidence of other medical conditions that may interfere with sexual function. Vaginal atresia and imperforate hymen in the female and undescended testes or hypospadias in the male are among causes that would be identified on clinical examination.

In cases of *dyspareunia*, a clinical assessment is imperative.

- Spasm of the pubococcygeus muscle may be detected during pelvic examination, leading to a possible diagnosis of vaginismus, while deep pelvic pain elicited on bimanual examination may be similar to discomfort experienced on intercourse.
- Acute infections such as candidiasis, herpes, and trichomoniasis along with acute or chronic inflammation of Bartholin's gland or the vestibular glands, may lead to vulvovaginal irritation and superficial dyspareunia.

- Pelvic examination may detect evidence of PID or endometriosis as a cause of deep dyspareunia. A normal anatomical variant of a retroverted uterus and ovaries prolapsing into the pouch of Douglas may be a further cause of deep dyspareunia.

Medical conditions such as respiratory or cardiac disease may interfere with sexual activity, as would osteoarthritis and limited mobility of the hips. Loss of sensation or reflexes in the perineal area, as may be associated with multiple sclerosis (MS) or damage to pelvic nerves through extensive pelvic surgery and associated scarring, are other causes that may interfere with sexual function.

Any investigations should be guided by the suspected underlying pathology, but great care should be taken not to ascribe the cause of a sexual problem to an incidentally discovered abnormality.

Sexual dysfunction in the female I

The majority of sexual dysfunctions do not have an organic basis to them. Many stem from the following:

- Poor relationship with partner
- Low or mismatched sexual drive between partners
- Ignorance about sexuality or sexual technique
- Performance anxiety
- Changing age affects sexual drive, desire, and response
- Illness or treatment side effects
- Fear that sex may aggravate an existing medical condition
- Depression
- Excess alcohol

The main sexual dysfunctions in women can be viewed under the following headings:

- Inhibited sexual desire
- Failure to achieve orgasm
- Dyspareunia
- Apareunia/vaginismus

Inhibited sexual desire (hypoactive sexual desire disorder or general sexual dysfunction)

Inhibited sexual desire may have a prevalence as high as 10% and affects women more than men. It is characterized by the absence of sexual fantasies and desire for sexual activity. It may have its onset at puberty or may occur some months or years after normal sexual activity. Inhibited sexual desire may be a manifestation of clinical depression or of a deteriorating relationship, but may present as a mismatch between the sexual desires of the partners. Although the woman may not be aroused by or reject her partner's sexual advances, she derives little or no enjoyment from them. A variety of factors may contribute to this lack or loss of desire. These include guilt about sexual activity acquired through upbringing, fear of pregnancy, or infection or injury, e.g. following surgery or a myocardial infarction. Relationship difficulties and the boredom of routine, along with pressures of life and work, may all have detrimental effects on sexual desire.

Management of inhibited sexual desire needs to involve both partners as the difficulties may arise from poor communication between the couple. Intensive therapy involves some level of compromise between the psychoanalytic and behavioral approaches, and is loosely based around the work of Masters and Johnson and Annon and Kaplan. One of the most commonly used approaches is the use of graded 'tasks' which the couple perform at home in a relaxed atmosphere.

Failure to achieve orgasm

In 90% of women, the thrusting of the penis in the vagina or digital or oral stimulation of her clitoral area directly leads to orgasm. Half of sexually active women achieve orgasm when the clitoral area is directly stimulated, while a quarter reach it during penile thrusting in the vagina. One in six women are able to achieve multiple orgasms, while one in ten is unable to achieve orgasm.

Orgasmic dysfunction may be associated with a general inability to become aroused or, alternatively, may be a failure to climax after normal arousal and plateau phases. Most experts would agree that inability to achieve orgasm by intercourse alone is sufficiently common not to constitute a dysfunction if the woman is able to achieve climax by masturbation or oral/finger stimulation by her partner. Despite this, the common but erroneous belief among the lay public is that, unless a woman reaches orgasm during penile thrusting, preferably simultaneously with the man, she is sexually dysfunctional. A number of techniques are available for a woman who wishes to achieve orgasm. The most successful of these is masturbation, and learning to achieve orgasm by masturbation supplemented by discussion and counseling from a trained practitioner often cures anorgasmia.

Sexual dysfunction in the female II

Dyspareunia

Dyspareunia is defined as recurrent or persistent pain during or after intercourse. It is traditionally divided into superficial (when the pain is solely at the vaginal introitus) or deep (when the pain is felt deep in the pelvis). There may be an organic component to the pain, and therefore organic causes need to be excluded before it can be classed as psychosomatic. It is important to elicit whether the pain is sufficient to prevent intercourse, whether it is continuous or intermittent, and whether it persists after attempts at intercourse have ceased.

It is essential to enquire about the basic features that are associated with any pain such as onset, duration, radiation, associated features, and ameliorating and exacerbating features. Organic causes of superficial dyspareunia include vulvovaginal infections, atrophic changes of the lower genital tract, and conditions such as lichen sclerosis and painful episiotomy scars, along with inadequate lubrication associated with inadequate sexual stimulation. Deep dyspareunia may be associated with PID, endometriosis, ovarian cysts, and pelvic tumors, along with a retroverted uterus and ovaries prolapsing in the pouch of Douglas. After a total hysterectomy where a vaginal cuff has been removed, deep dyspareunia is more common because of thrusting against a scarred vault that no longer has the capacity to balloon on arousal. Furthermore, in a proportion of women, hysterectomy will result in earlier than usual ovarian failure, and continued sexual enjoyment may well require estrogen replacement therapy. Vaginal repair operations for prolapse may also result in vaginal narrowing and dyspareunia.

Psychosomatic disorders are more likely to be longstanding. The causes of psychogenic dyspareunia may include lack of sexual knowledge, guilt about sexuality, childhood sexual abuse, or history of sexual assault.

Patients who have undergone gynecological cancer treatment (surgery and/or radiotherapy) may have an organic and psychosomatic component to sexual dysfunction. Thus libido may be affected by depression occurring as part of the illness process or reaction to the diagnosis, while radical surgery may be mutilating, leading to deterioration of body image and consequently of sexual relationships. Radiotherapy, especially in the setting of cervical cancer, may lead to cervical stenosis, reduced lubrication, and soreness, and therefore is best prevented by the prophylactic use of dilators.

Vaginismus/apareunia

In apareunia, the woman is unable to have penetrative intercourse. This is usually a result of involuntary spasm of the pubococcygeus muscle surrounding the introitus and lowest third of the vagina. Attempts at penetration cause pain in the clenched muscle, thus aggravating the situation. In its most severe form, the patient is not even able to tolerate the examiner's finger in the vagina because of the marked muscle spasm. Vaginismus may affect up to 3% of women of reproductive age.

In the majority of cases the problem is psychosomatic, but organic causes such as vaginal atresia, vulvovaginal infection, and erectile failure in the man need to be excluded. Occasionally, vaginismus may be traced to a sexual assault during childhood, or a painful or brutal initial experience of sexual intercourse, or simply an inadequate or faulty sex education. Primary vaginismus is usually due to fear and therefore is similar to a phobic disorder.

Management evolves around identifying and, if possible, treating any underlying physical cause. If treatment is not possible, alternative techniques may be suggested to enable her to enjoy her sexuality. A therapist may be able to 'educate' the patient to relax her perineal muscles and reinforce the idea that there is no physical abnormality and that her genital structures are normal. A series of graded exercises such as inserting a lubricated finger in the vagina, progressing gradually to two and three fingers may be helpful. Alternatively, metal or glass dilators may serve the same purpose.

Special circumstances

Sexual assault

Defined as 'carnal knowledge/intercourse/sexual contact with a woman without her consent by force, fear, or fraud', sexual assault includes rape and incest. The epidemiology of rape suggests that, while fewer than one-third of rapes are reported, in three-quarters of cases the perpetrator is known to the woman. Furthermore, about one woman in 200 has been raped or suffered attempted rape in the preceding year.

Women who have been subjected to rape need to be listened to nonjudgmentally and sympathetically, addressing both emotional and physical issues. Physical examination will need to be performed, and its significance and nature need to be discussed with the woman. During the examination, careful documentation needs to be made of all findings including scratches and bruises on the arms and legs. The vulva and vagina need to be inspected for evidence of bruising, blood, or seminal staining, while a vaginal smear is examined for spermatozoa. Screening should also be offered for STDs and postcoital contraception offered if there is a risk of pregnancy.

Pregnancy

During pregnancy, there is a wide variation between couples with regard to interest and responsiveness to sexual activity. In general, there is a trend towards reduction in frequency and satisfaction as pregnancy advances. Postnatally, dyspareunia is common but underreported, with a recent survey indicating that 58% had painful intercourse at 3 months with the problem persisting in almost 30% at 9 months. Vaginal dryness may also be a problem, especially in the breast-feeding group.

Chapter 16

Contraception

Combined oral contraceptives

The use of contraception is widespread. Over 95% of sexually active women wishing to avoid pregnancy use contraception. There has been a significant rise in the use of contraception worldwide, but contraceptive use is much lower in less developed countries, falling to less than 15% in some parts of Africa. Adolescents and women over 40 are less willing to use contraception, despite not wishing to become pregnant. This is partly responsible for the estimated 30% of babies that are delivered whose conception is unplanned. The vast majority of unplanned pregnancies end in termination. Contraceptive methods and their frequency of use are shown in Table 16.1. This chapter will deal with hormonal contraception, intrauterine contraceptive devices (IUCDs), and emergency contraception.

The combined oral contraceptive pill (COCP) was approved for use in the 1960s. The usual combination is of ethinyl estradiol and a synthetic progesterone (progestogen). Ethinyl estradiol (a highly potent estrogen compared with naturally occurring 17β-estradiol) is the usual estrogen. This is given in a dosage of 20–50 μg daily, with the most common dosage being in the 20–35 μg bracket.

Second-generation progestogens (norethisterone, levonorgestrel, ethynodiol diacetate) are most commonly used, with the third generation (gestodene, norgestimate, desogestrel) in some of the newer preparations.

The third-generation progestogens appear to have a less atherogenic lipid profile (lower low-density lipoprotein cholesterol (LDL-C) and a higher high-density lipoprotein cholesterol (HDL-C)). This lipid profile should, in theory, give rise to less myocardial infarction. However, this is a very rare complication. Recent studies suggest an increased risk of venous thromboembolism (VTE) associated with third-generation progestogens. However, the absolute risk is smaller than that associated with pregnancy. The spontaneous incidence of VTE in healthy nonpregnant women is 5 in 100 000, with second-generation pills it is 15 in 100 000, and with third-generation pills it is 25 in 100 000.

Mode of action

The COCP acts to inhibit ovulation. Ethinyl estradiol suppresses follicle stimulating hormone (FSH) whilst the progestogen suppresses the luteinizing hormone (LH) surge. There is also some effect on cervical mucus, which is thicker and less penetrable by sperm.

Dosages and regimen

The pill is usually given at a dosage of 20–35 μg daily. Better cycle control is achieved with the higher estrogen dosages, although all seem to be similarly effective. In older women, lower dosages are preferred to reduce the risk of side effects. The COCP is taken for 3 weeks with a 1 week gap when menstruation occurs. The dosage is either the same throughout the cycle (monophasic) or alters with increasing dosages mid-cycle (triphasic). If used properly, the failure rate is very low (see Table 16.2). The riskiest pills to miss are the first or last of the 3 week cycle.

Table 16.1 Contraceptive methods and their frequencies of use

Method	Frequency of use (%)
COCP	36
Barrier methods	20.8
Vasectomy	16
Female sterilization	10.1
IUCD	7.3
COCP and barrier contraception	3.3
Natural family planning (NFP)	1.5
Withdrawal (coitus interruptus)	1.1
No method	3.6

Table 16.2 Efficacy of various methods of contraception

Method	Failure rate (%)*
No contraception (young women)	80–90
Male condom	2–15
Copper IUCD	0.3–1
Mirena IUS	<0.5
POP	0.3–4
COCP	0.2–3
Injectable	0–1
Implanon/Norplant	0–1
Sterilization (female)	0–0.5
Sterilization (male)	0.02

* Failure rate per 100 women-years of use.

Contraindications and side effects of the COCP

Contraindications

- Current or past history of cardiovascular disease.
- Migraine: focal migraine, crescendo migraine, first attack of migraine on the COCP, severe migraines requiring the use of ergotamine.
- Personal history of venous thrombosis.
- Obesity.
- Heavy smoking in women over the age of 35.
- Estrogen-dependent cancer.
- Family history of venous thrombosis in women under 45. May need thrombophilia testing.
- Varicose veins, if severe.
- Various liver conditions.

Side effects

Side effects are common in the first few months of use and may lead to discontinuation of the method. However, many will settle with time. It may be worth changing the COCP after 3–4 months if side effects persist.

- *Weight gain* A weight gain of 2–3 kg is common in the early months of treatment, but this weight will often be lost later on.
- *Hypertension* Approximately 2% of women may become hypertensive after commencing the pill.
- *Headaches* are common in the early months of treatment, but will often resolve. They need to be differentiated from migraines (see 'Contraindications').
- *Breakthrough bleeding* Check compliance; try alternative progestogen or triphasic pill. If it persists, it is necessary to exclude local pathology.

Advantages

- Menstruation is regular, lighter, and less painful and there is less premenstrual syndrome.
- Reduced incidence of ovarian cysts.
- Reduced incidence of fibroids.
- Reduced incidence of pelvic infection.
- Acne and hirsutism may be improved.
- Reduced risk of endometrial and possibly ovarian cancer.
- Can be used in women over 35. Ideally, a 20 μg pill can be used in slim non-smoking women with no other contraindications.

Other contraceptives

Progestogen-only contraception

The progestogen-only pill (POP or mini-pill) is only used by about 5% of women. It is a useful alternative when the COCP is contraindicated because of estrogenic side effects. Precise explanations must be given to a woman commencing the POP. It must be taken at the same time each day, and taken continuously. If a pill is missed by more than 3 hours, a barrier method should be used for at least 7 days. If unprotected intercourse occurs after a missed pill, emergency contraception should be considered.

Mode of action

The POP acts to thicken cervical mucus and prevents sperm penetration. In 56–60% of women, ovulation may be inhibited and, in a small proportion, all follicular development may be suppressed, resulting in amenorrhea.

Indications

- During breast-feeding.
- Women at risk of cardiovascular disease: diabetic women, smokers over 35, women with hypertension, some women with hyperlipidemia.
- Migraine sufferers.
- Women at increased risk of thromboembolism.
- Side effects from COCPs.

Contraindications

- Previous ectopic pregnancy.
- Ovarian cysts.

Side effects

Erratic bleeding is common and around 20% of women will cease use because of this. The POP has a relatively short half-life and a slightly increased failure rate. However, the POP does not appear to be associated with any serious long-term risks.

Injectable contraceptives

There are two long-term injectable contraceptive progestogens: depot medroxyprogesterone acetate (DMPA, Depo-Provera) 150 mg IM every 12 weeks), and norethisterone enanthate (NET-EN) 200 mg IM every 8 weeks).

DMPA is used worldwide (9 million women). There do not appear to be any increased risks of cancer and there appears to be a powerful protective effect against endometrial cancer. Injections need to be given every 12 weeks, with the first injection during the first 5 days of menstruation. It is inexpensive, safe, and effective. It can be used for breast-feeding mothers and particularly for women with poor compliance on other methods. Dysmenorrhea, menorrhagia, pelvic inflammatory disease (PID), and premenstrual tension may all be reduced.

However, weight gain and acne can be problems in the early stages of treatment. Amenorrhea is common (over 50%). The return to fertility may be delayed after the normal 12 week duration of the injection.

Contraceptive implants

The first licensed contraceptive implant was Norplant. This consisted of six silastic rods containing levonorgestrel inserted subdermally on the inner aspect of the upper arm. Local anesthetic is needed for insertion and removal of the implants. The mode of action is similar to other progestogen-only methods, and fertility typically returns swiftly after removal of the rods. This product is now rarely prescribed since the licensing of the newer product Implanon, but there are still patients who need removal of the Norplant rods. Implanon is a single silastic rod containing 3-keto-desogestrel, lasting for 3 years. Frequent and prolonged bleeds remain a problem, affecting 17% of women. Removal and insertion times are much reduced with the single rod.

Intrauterine contraceptive devices (IUCDs)

The IUCD is a long-lasting and highly effective method of contraception. It causes local inflammatory response in the endometrium, interfering with sperm and egg function and inhibiting fertilization and implantation. The IUCD consists of copper wire wound on an inert frame. This can be inserted without anesthetic or with a local block, but is easier in women who have had a previous vaginal delivery. IUCDs last 5–8 years.

Risks of IUCDs include explusion, perforation, and pelvic infection. When fitting IUCDs, cervical swabs should be taken to establish that the woman has no pelvic infection or prophylactic antibiotics should be prescribed at the time of insertion. If the IUCD user becomes pregnant, there is a higher likelihood that the pregnancy will be ectopic. Menorrhagia and dysmenorrhea are common side effects, related to increased local production of prostaglandins. These side effects can be effectively treated with NSAIDs, but also limit the usefulness of IUCDs.

Intrauterine system (Mirena IUS)

The Mirena IUS is a levonorgestrel-releasing system similar to the copper coil in its insertion and removal. The hormone is contained in a reservoir on the stem of the device and lasts for 5 years. It releases approximately 20 µg of hormone daily locally to the endometrium, with only a small amount being absorbed into the circulation. This reduces the chance of progestogenic side effects. The contraceptive efficacy is extremely good, whilst blood loss is substantially reduced (80–95% in women with heavy periods).

Emergency contraception

Either hormonal contraception or a copper-containing IUCD can be used for emergency contraception. The Mirena IUS should not be used in these circumstances.

Levonelle (750 μg levonorgestrel given immediately and repeated 12 hours later) is a more effective emergency contraceptive than the previously marketed PC4 (ethinyl estradiol and progestogen). The failure rate is 0.4% if treatment is within 24 hours. Every 12 hour delay increases the failure rate by 50%. This may result in the treatment being available without prescription in the near future. There are fewer side effects with the newer regimen (vomiting <6%).

Absolute contraindications are:

- existing pregnancy
- known acute porphyria
- current warfarin treatment (may alter anticoagulation and monitoring is necessary).

Recommended further reading

1. Cheng L, Gulmezoglu AM, Oel CJ, Piaggio G, Ezcurra E, Look PF (2004). Interventions for emergency contraception. *Cochrane Database Syst Rev* **3**, CD001324.

Assessment and counseling with female sterilization

Sterilization is the method of contraception used by 26% of all couples and 50% of those over the age of 40.

Assessment

- Ask about the reasons for requesting sterilization, current contraception, menstrual history, and previous gynecological or abdominal surgery.
- Women under the age of 25, those without children, or those who have had recent relationship loss are more likely to regret sterilization. Try to assess whether the woman is making the decision of her own free will or being coerced by family or by social or healthcare professionals.
- Note any major medical problems, current medication, and allergies.
- Note the date and result of the last cervical smear.
- On examination, note especially the BMI and any abdominal scars and pelvic masses. Obese patients and those with a history of previous abdominal surgery are at increased risk of laparoscopic problems and may need to have an elective open rather than laparoscopic procedure.

Counseling

The following points should be covered.

- The *alternative methods* of long-term contraception should be discussed. Sterilization may be wrongly perceived as the only other solution to contraceptive needs in women who have problems with the contraceptive pill or barrier methods.
  - Injectables and the levonorgestrol intrauterine system have failure rates comparable to those of female sterilization.
  - The advantages and disadvantages of vasectomy should be discussed with couples. Vasectomy can be performed more readily under local anesthetic and has a lower failure rate of 1 in 2000 (after two azoospermic samples 2–4 weeks apart).
- *The permanence of the operation* Sterilization should only be undertaken by patients who are certain that their family is complete. Even so, 5–10% of patients will ask for reversal later. Additional care also needs to be taken when counseling women taking the decision during pregnancy. Funding for reversal operations is limited and success rates vary according to the method of sterilization used.
- *The procedure has a failure rate* There is a 1 in 200 lifetime risk of failure. Pregnancies may occur several years after the operation. Early failures may occur if the procedure was incorrectly performed or if conception had already occurred when the sterilization was carried out in the second half of the cycle (luteal phase pregnancy). Later failures may be due to recanalization of the tubes. There is an increased risk of ectopic pregnancy (10–30%) if sterilization does fail. Patients should be warned to make sure they are not pregnant if they miss a period or have unusually light periods.

- *The nature of the sterilization operation and its risks should be explained* The nature of the operation, including the proposed method of access and the proposed method of tubal occlusion, should be explained. There is a risk associated with laparoscopy of bowel and vessel injury. A laparotomy may be required to repair injury and the hospital stay may be prolonged. A mini-laparotomy may also be required if the sterilization cannot be completed laparoscopically.
  - Sterilization will not affect weight, menstruation, or the time of menopause. However, patients who are currently using contraception that might affect menstruation such as the COCP may notice a change in their period pattern when these are stopped.
- *The need for adequate contraception prior to sterilization* Effective contraception should be used until the first period following the procedure. An IUCD *in situ* can be removed at the time of operation only if this is carried out in the first half of the menstrual cycle. Otherwise, it should be left and removed at the time of the next period.

Patients should be offered printed information including the above points to take away and read prior to the operation. A record in the notes should be made that the patient has been told about the irreversibility, failure rate (and ectopic pregnancy risk), and potential complications of the operation.

Female sterilization

The operation

Prior to surgery, check the date of the last menstrual period and current contraception. Separate consent forms are no longer usually used for sterilization. It is not necessary to obtain the partner's consent for sterilization, but where there is doubt over mental capacity to consent, prior sanction by a high court judge should be obtained.

The operation itself is usually carried out under general anesthetic as a day-case procedure. It can be done at any time of the menstrual cycle, but a pregnancy test must be arranged for any woman whose period is late or who thinks she may be pregnant.

- The perineum and abdomen are cleaned, a pelvic examination performed, and the bladder emptied.
- The cervix is held with a valsellum or other forceps and the uterus instrumented to allow manipulation.
- A Veres needle (a large-bore needle with a retractable sharp tip) is inserted through a small incision, usually made below the umbilicus, and 2–3 L of CO_2 instilled into the peritoneal cavity. This displaces the anterior abdominal wall away from the abdominal contents so that a larger trochar can be introduced through the same incision. The pelvic organs are visualized through this portal using a laparoscope.
- A second incision is made in the lower abdomen for a second port through which the instrument used to perform the sterilization is inserted.
  - Sterilization is most commonly performed by applying occlusive clips or rings across the tubal isthmus 1–2 cm from the uterus.
  - Diathermy of the tubes is a suitable alternative, especially if there is technical difficulty in applying rings or clips.
  - Partial or complete salpingectomy is more commonly done when sterilization is carried out at the time of cesarean delivery or when there is preexisting tubal disease.
  - The fallopian tubes must be definitively identified by positive identification of the fimbrial ends of the tubes and by identifying adjacent structures such as the round ligaments.
- Local anesthetic injection into the tube may be used to provide additional postoperative pain relief.
- After the procedure, the gas is released from the abdomen and the abdominal incision closed with a semi-absorbable suture.
- Routine curettage of the uterus to prevent luteal phase pregnancy is not recommended.

Postoperative care

- Inform the patient of the final method used for the sterilization and if any complications occurred.
- Check pulse and blood pressure.
- Inspect the wounds for any signs of bleeding. The abdomen should be soft.
- Patients should have been able to tolerate fluids and passed urine prior to discharge.

- The patient will need to take 3–7 days off work and may notice some abdominal discomfort for 2–3 weeks. Warn her that she may have some shoulder tip pain because of diaphragmatic irritation from the CO_2.
- Warn the patient to seek medical advice if her pain is not controlled by simple analgesia or if there is increasing pain or vomiting.
- Remember that fewer than 50% of bowel injuries occurring at laparoscopy are diagnosed at the time of surgery and signs of peritonitis may not be apparent for up to 72 hours.

Sterilization at the time of pregnancy

- Where possible, sterilization procedures after pregnancy should be performed as an interval procedure 3–6 months later. This is because sterilization performed at the time of pregnancy has a higher failure rate and may be associated with an increased risk of maternal complications such as thromboembolism. If carried out at the same time as pregnancy termination, there is likely to be an increased regret rate for both procedures. These drawbacks have to be balanced against the reliability of contraception during the interval period and, in some cases, will be outweighed by the risk of further unplanned pregnancy.
- Sterilization at the time of cesarean delivery has the additional advantage of avoiding the need for a second operation. It is usually done by partial salpingectomy after the uterus has been closed. Consent should have been obtained after antepartum counseling remote from delivery.
- Sterilization at the time of pregnancy termination is normally carried out laparoscopically.

Recommended further reading

1. Nardin JM, Kulier R, Boulvain M (2003). Techniques for the interruption of tubal patency for female sterilisation. *Cochrane Database Syst Rev* **1**, CD003034.

Chapter 17

Menopause and urogynecology

Menopause

Introduction

The menopause is defined as the last menstrual period when the cessation of menstruation occurs as a result of the loss of ovarian follicular activity and a reduction of estradiol. The average age of menopause is 51–52 years. With an increasingly aging population, most women in Western countries will expect to live 30 years postmenopause. This constitutes more than one-third of their lives.

The climacteric is the time around the menopause when the menopausal transition takes place and symptoms begin. This is due to declining estrogen and progesterone production from the failing ovary. The menopause transition starts on average 4 years before the menopause, although menstruation can cease abruptly. Bleeding more than 12 months after the last menstrual period is considered abnormal.

Causes

The menopause occurs when the store of oocytes is exhausted. Follicle-stimulating hormone (FSH) levels rise (FSH >30 IU/L) but the ovary fails to respond adequately. Once estradiol production falls below a critical threshold, endometrial stimulation does not occur and bleeding ceases. FSH and luteinizing hormone (LH) levels then remain permanently elevated.

Other causes for the menopause include surgery (bilateral oophorectomy), radiation, or chemotherapy used to treat malignancies such as Hodgkin's disease. A premature menopause is defined as menopause at less than 40 years of age, although, for practical clinical reasons, 45 years may be a more appropriate definition.

Short-term effects

Symptoms begin during the climacteric, before the last menstrual period.

- *Menstrual symptoms* As the ovaries fail to respond, ovulation may not occur despite some estradiol production. The ensuing anovulatory cycles may be erratic and heavy, initially more frequent and then becoming less frequent.
- *Vasomotor symptoms* Hot flushes and sweats are the most common symptoms occurring in up to 80% of perimenopausal women. The frequency can vary from many episodes each hour to only a few episodes during the week. The underlying pathophysiology is uncertain. Flushes are often associated with shivering, tachycardia, and sweating. They are associated with frequent wakening at night. These symptoms do not seem to occur in young women with hypoestrogenemia, and priming with estrogen before the eventual hypoestrogenism appears to be an important factor.

- *Urogenital aging* The vagina and the trigone of the bladder share a common embryological origin. Both are sensitive to changes in estradiol levels. In the vagina, hypoestrogenism causes atrophy with thinning of the vaginal epithelium, loss of rugae, and dryness. Gram-positive Doderlein's bacilli are lost, with a resultant fall in lactic-acid production. The pH of the vaginal secretions rises and this gives decreased resistance to infections with bacteria and yeast. There is a loss of elasticity in the underlying tissues and this, associated with the dryness, may cause dyspareunia. The overall size of the vagina decreases, and it becomes shorter and narrower.
- *Urinary tract effects* Because the trigone and urethra are estrogen-sensitive, atrophic changes may lead to the urethral syndrome: urinary frequency, urgency, and dysuria in the absence of infection.
  - Stress incontinence is more common in older women, particularly around the time of the menopause. However, the association between low estradiol levels and stress incontinence is much weaker than that with the urethral syndrome.
- *Psychological problems* Although there may be an increase in psychological problems around the time of the menopause, the association between these and low plasma estradiol levels is weak. However, psychological problems may well occur secondarily to other effects of the menopause (poor sleep, urogenital problems, sexual problems, poor concentration, etc.). Libido certainly appears to be reduced. There are cultural differences between attitudes to the menopause and these may have a strong underlying influence. For example, Japanese women report far fewer complaints about menopausal symptoms than women from the USA.
- *Sexual problems* are common complaints during the climacteric and postmenopause. About a third of women will complain of a loss of libido. However, there is a complex relationship between sexuality and the menopause.

Recommended further reading

1. American College of Obstetricians and Gynecologists (1995). Health maintenance for perimenopausal women. ACOG Technical Bulletin No. 210. *Int J Gynecol Obstet* **51**, 171–81.

Long-term effects of menopause

Cardiovascular disease

Coronary heart disease is a leading cause of death in women and the incidence increases with age. Compared with that in men, the onset of cardiovascular disease tends to be later and women have a relative protection premenopausally. After the menopause, there is a two- to threefold increase in risk. There is uncertainty as to the relative influence of low estradiol levels and aging, and various mechanisms have been postulated for this increase in risk. These include adverse changes to lipids and lipoproteins, insulin resistance, and changes in clotting. There are also direct effects of estrogen on the cardiovascular system, and estrogen receptors have been found throughout the cardiovascular system. A typical estrogenic effect is a relaxation in arterial tone and a decrease in resistance.

Osteoporosis

This is a systemic skeletal disease leading to increased fragility and more susceptibility to fracture. Bone mass in women rises during childhood and reaches a peak during the third decade. It remains relatively stable until the menopausal transition when loss of bone density occurs. There is an accelerated rate of bone loss following the menopause but the rate gradually slows into old age. Table 17.1 lists the risk factors for developing osteoporosis.

- *Prevalence of osteoporosis* The WHO has defined *osteoporosis* as a bone mineral density more than 2.5 standard deviations below the young adult mean (T-score). A reduction of 1.0–2.5 standard deviations represents *osteopenia*. Densitometry-defined osteoporosis associated with fragility fractures is called severe or established osteoporosis. The prevalence of osteoporosis increases with age, with less than 1% of young women having osteoporosis but 70% of women aged over 80 being affected.
- Typical osteoporotic fractures occur in the femural neck, vertebral body, or distal forearm (Colles' fracture). Many vertebral fractures go unnoticed. Hip fractures carry a much greater risk to significant morbidity, with up to 50% of patients losing their independence following a hip fracture.
- DEXA (dual-energy X-ray absorptiometry) bone density scanning is the gold standard for estimating bone density and risk of fracture. X-ray radiography is too imprecise to be useful. Quantitated CT scanning is accurate but involves a high radiation dose per scan. Biochemical markers will give a measure of bone turnover but not of overall bone density.

Alzheimer's disease

Like osteoporosis, the increasing age of the female population is leading to an increase in dementia. Alzheimer's disease is more common in women than in men, and there are observational data to suggest that estrogen deficiency plays a role. The condition is more common in those with previous hip fracture, infarction, or low BMI. Alzheimer's disease tends to occur later in women who take estrogen.

Treatment for the consequences of the menopause is dealt with in later in this chapter.

Table 17.1 Risk factors for developing osteoporosis

Modifiable risk factors
Estrogen deficiency (menopause, premature menopause, prolonged amenorrhea)
Low BMI
Prolonged immobility
Smoking
Alcohol abuse
Nutritional factors
Susceptibility to falls
Secondary causes, e.g. celiac disease
Nonmodifiable risk factors
Age
Race
Positive family history
Prior fragile fracture

Recommended further reading

1. American College of Obstetricians and Gynecologists (1995). Health maintenance for perimenopausal women. ACOG Technical Bulletin No. 210. *Int J Gynecol Obstet* **51**, 171–81.

Hormone replacement therapy

Introduction

Hormone replacement therapy (HRT) constitutes treatment with estrogen or combined estrogen and progestogen to treat or prevent symptoms associated with the menopause. The aim of treatment is to increase circulating estrogens to a level similar to that of the premenopause. Current evidence suggests that, in hysterectomized women, estrogen-only treatment is needed, whereas in women with an intact uterus progesterone needs to be given cyclically or continuously.

Regimens

- *Estrogen-only treatment* For hysterectomized women, estrogen-only treatment is satisfactory. Treatment is given continuously (rather than cyclically as with the combined oral contraceptive).
- *Combined sequential (standard) HRT* This is the standard regimen of HRT: continuous estrogen with progestogen given cyclically for 10–14 days each 28 day cycle.
- *Continuous combined (period-free) HRT* In older women, where cyclical bleeding may be less acceptable, the continuous combined regimen can be used. Estrogen and progestogen are given continuously in an attempt to induce an atrophic endometrium and 'no bleeding'. This regimen can only be used in women who are at least 1–2 years postmenopausal when the chance of endogenous estrogen production is reduced.
- *Long-cycle HRT* This regimen is used to give a 3-monthly withdrawal bleed rather than the standard monthly bleed. Estrogen is given continuously for 3 months with a higher dose of progestogen for the last 14 days of the 3 month cycle. This is followed by 1 week without treatment and then the cycle restarts. This regimen can be used in a woman who is virtually or actually postmenopausal. If it is used too soon, breakthrough bleeding is common.

Drugs

- *Estrogens* Conjugated equine estrogens (Premarin) have been used for over 50 years to treat menopausal symptoms. Once absorbed and metabolized, the major circulating product is estrone. Many different estrogens have been identified from the preparation and it has a proven 'track record'.
- *Estradiol* The ovary produces predominantly 17β-estradiol. Treatment can be given as 17β-estradiol, but this is best given nonorally. Estradiol valerate and micronized estradiol are also used. All appear to be similarly effective in symptom relief and prevention.
- *Progestogens* Synthetic progestogens are more potent than natural progesterone and therefore can be given in smaller quantities. The 19-nortestosterone derivatives (norethisterone, norgestrel) and the C21 derivatives (medroxyprogesterone acetate, dydrogesterone) are effective in endometrial protection. Natural progesterone can be used, but is poorly absorbed orally or transdermally. However, it is available as pessaries or vaginal gels.

Routes of administration

For most women, there are no definite advantages of one route of administration over another and therefore it is often left to the patient to decide which route suits her best.

- Oral administration of estrogens and progestogens has been used the longest and is simple to use. Most estrogen tends to be absorbed and metabolized to estrone even if administered as estradiol. However, this is equally effective in symptom relief.
- Transdermal patches are highly effective and suit most women, although a proportion can get skin irritation. The new generation matrix patches are easier to use than the older reservoir patches.
- Estradiol can be given as a subdermal hormone implant lasting 6–12 months. Testosterone implants can be useful in hysterectomized women who have poor libido, and these can be inserted at the same time.
- 17β-estradiol can be given as a percutaneous gel, although progesterone creams, while widely advertised as useful for menopausal symptoms, are actually very poorly absorbed. Progesterone creams are unlikely to provide adequate endometrial protection.
- Progesterone can be given as pessaries or vaginal gel or by using a levonorgestrel intrauterine device. These will adequately protect the endometrium.
- Estrogen can be given locally to the vagina and lower urogenital tract by creams, pessaries, or as an estrogen-impregnated soft vaginal ring pessary which lasts for 3 months.

Dosages

The dosage necessary for symptom relief tends to vary with the individual. In general, younger women require higher doses for symptom relief than older women. The bone-sparing doses shown in Table 17.2 are useful starting dosages, although a high dose may be given in young patients. In women more than 10 years past the menopause, lower dosages may be adequate, and starting at half the dosages in the table is also adequate.

Dosage should be altered after 3 months according to symptoms or side effects.

Table 17.2 The bone-sparing dosages of HRT

Drug	Dose
Oral estradiol	1–2 mg daily
Transdermal estradiol	50 mg daily
Oral conjugated equine estrogens	0.625 mg daily
Estradiol implants	50 mg implant 6 to 12-monthly

Indications and contraindications for HRT

There is still controversy as to the indications for HRT. Some enthusiasts advocate widespread use for almost every woman whilst others urge caution in view of side effects. The generally agreed indications for treatment are the following:

- *The symptomatic patient* In the absence of any contraindications, there is very little reason not to treat a woman if symptoms are affecting her quality of life.
- *Premature menopause* In a woman who has a menopause, either natural or iatrogenic, before 45 years, there is abundant evidence that treatment with HRT is beneficial. Thus treatment for such women is routine.
- *Treatment of prevention of osteoporosis* HRT is still the gold standard treatment for osteoporosis in postmenopausal women. However, in the older age group, it can be difficult to start women on HRT without side effects.
- *Prevention of cardiovascular disease* Although previous observational studies had suggested a protective effect against heart disease, the results of the largest prospective controlled study have in fact shown an increase in the incidence of heart attacks on combined HRT. Until further studies are done, HRT is no longer indicated for the sole purpose of prevention of cardiovascular disease.

Contraindications are as follows.

- HRT should not be given to women with an estrogen-dependent malignant tumor.
- Postmenopausal bleeding or abnormal perimenopausal bleeding should be investigated before starting HRT.
- A history of recent or active thrombosis contraindicates HRT.

Precautions

- In view of the increased risk of thrombosis (see below), any woman with a past history of thrombosis or a strong family history should have a thrombophilia screen before starting HRT.
- Fibroids are likely to grow under the influence of HRT and, if present, patients should be warned that this may be the case. However, they will normally regress once HRT is stopped.
- With all HRT, there is an increased risk of gallstones, and endometriosis may be reactivated by combined sequential HRT.
- The risk of breast cancer is discussed below.

These risks should be discussed and documented prior to starting HRT. It is wise to check blood pressure prior to starting HRT as a small proportion (possibly 1%) may experience an increase in blood pressure with estrogens. However, the majority will notice a small decrease in blood pressure. If there is chronic hypertension, this is best treated before starting HRT.

Recommended further reading

1. American College of Obstetricians and Gynecologists (1993). Hormone replacement therapy. ACOG Technical Bulletin No. 166. *Int J Gynaecol Obstet* **41**, 194–202.
2. Magliano DJ, Rogers SL, Abramson MJ, Tonkin AM (2006). Hormone therapy and cardiovascular disease: a systematic review and meta-analysis. *Br Obstet Gynecol* **113**, 5–14.
3. Howard BV, Kuller L, Langer R, *et al.* for the Women's Health Initiative (2005). Risk of cardiovascular disease by hysterectomy status, with and without oophorectomy: the Women's Health Initiative Observational Study. *Circulation* **111**, 1462–70.
4. Manson JE, Hsia J, Johnson KC, *et al.* for the the Women's Health Initiative Investigators (2003). Estrogen plus progestin and the risk of coronary heart disease. *N Engl J Med* **349**, 523–34.
5. Hulley S, Grady D, Bush T, *et al.* (1998). Randomized trial of estrogen plus progestin for secondary prevention of coronary heart disease in postmenopausal women. Heart and Estrogen/progestin Replacement Study (HERS) Research Group. *JAMA* **280**, 605–13.

Benefits and risks of HRT

Benefits

- There is abundant evidence to show good symptom relief with HRT. As a general rule, if symptom relief does not occur, it is because the dosage is too low, absorption poor, or the symptom is not due to estrogen deficiency.
- The risk of osteoporotic fracture is roughly halved for women taking HRT.
- Women with a premature menopause given HRT have a much reduced risk of osteoporosis or symptoms in later life.
- It is uncertain how much protection from Alzheimer's disease women receive, but recent studies suggest that the incidence is reduced by approximately a third in women taking HRT.
- There is a reduction in risk of colon cancer (relative risk 0.58 among HRT users compared with nonusers), but no difference in rectal cancer.

Risks

- *Thromboembolism* Oral HRT confers an increased risk of 1–2 in 5000 of venous thrombosis in HRT users. The increased risk of thrombosis mainly occurs in the first year of treatment. The risk appears to be smaller in nonoral estrogen preparations (patches, gels, or implants).
- *Breast cancer* The main concern for women on HRT is the risk of breast cancer. The study by the Collaborative Group on Hormonal Factors in Breast Cancer reported an analysis of 51 studies comprising 52 705 breast cancer patients and 108 411 control women. For each year of use, the risk of breast cancer increased by 1.023, a similar relative risk for nonusers for each extra year before the menopause (1.028). This translates into an increased risk of 2 per 1000 cases of breast cancer for 5 years of HRT treatment and 7 per 1000 for 10 years of HRT treatment. However, breast cancers in women on HRT appear to be at an earlier stage and at a lower grade than those in women not on HRT. Therefore the prognosis for women on HRT at the time of diagnosis is better, and it appears that HRT does not cause any increase in mortality from breast cancer.
- *Vascular disease* The relative risk of heart attacks and stroke are increased (1.29 and 1.41, respectively) in women taking combined HRT for 5 years. It is not clear whether this is related to the type of progestogen used.

Each individual woman must weigh up the risks and benefits for her of taking HRT. The most common indication for use is still symptom relief.

Recommended further reading

1. Rossouw JE, Anderson GL, Prentice RL, *et al.* and the Writing Group for the Women's Health Initiative Investigators (2002). Risks and benefits of estrogen plus progestin in healthy postmenopausal women: principal results From the Women's Health Initiative randomized controlled trial. *JAMA* **288**, 321–33.

Uterovaginal prolapse

Introduction

Prolapse is the protrusion of an organ or structure beyond the normal anatomical confines. Approximately 20% of all gynecological operations are for prolapse repair.

- *Normal pelvic anatomy* The uterus, bladder, and rectum are supported by the pelvic floor, which includes the levator ani, the coccygeal, internal obturator, and piriformis muscles, and the two transverse perineal muscles and pelvic fascia. Within the pelvis, the transverse cervical ligaments (cardinal ligaments), uterosacral ligaments, and pubocervical and pubourethral ligaments support the uterus. The round ligaments and broad ligaments do not contribute significantly to the support of the uterus.
- *Vaginal prolapse* is classified according to its contents.
    - *Urethrocele* involves the lower part of the anterior vaginal wall containing the urethra.
    - *Cystocele* is prolapse of the upper anterior wall and bladder.
    - *Rectocele* describes prolapse of the middle part of the posterior vaginal wall containing the rectum.
    - *Enterocele* involves the upper part of the posterior wall and may contain loops of small bowel from the pouch of Douglas.
    - After hysterectomy, the vaginal vault may prolapse and usually contains small bowel as well as omentum (vault prolapse).
    - Several types of prolapse may occur in the same patient.
- *Uterine prolapse* is divided into the following.
    - First-degree uterine prolapse when the uterus is within the vagina.
    - Second-degree prolapse when the cervix protrudes through the introitus.
    - Third-degree prolapse (procidentia) when the entire uterus has come outside the vagina.

Etiology

Congenital weakness of pelvic floor ligaments and fascia, and congenital shortness of the vagina and deep uterovesical or uterorectal peritoneal pouches, may be found with spina bifida or bladder exstrophy. Far more common are acquired causes of pelvic floor damage such as pregnancy, prolonged or difficult labor, and multiparity. These cause denervation of the pelvic floor muscles. A gradual increase in denervation of the striated muscle of pelvic floor with age and estrogen deficiency at the menopause can also occur in nulliparous women. Prolapse may also be a sign of increased intraabdominal pressure due to pulmonary disease, heavy lifting, chronic straining (constipation), ascites, or a pelvic mass. Prolapse may occur after surgery such as hysterectomy or Burch colposuspension.

Symptoms

- Minor degrees may be asymptomatic.
- Patients with significant uterovaginal prolapse complain of a feeling of 'something coming down'.

- Cystocele and cystourethrocele lead to dragging discomfort and the sensation of a lump in the vagina. There may be associated urinary symptoms of incontinence and recurrent urinary tract infections. Voiding difficulties can occur if a large cystocele is present and the bladder neck is anchored normally. This can lead to overflow incontinence or incomplete emptying.
- Uterine descent may cause low backache, which is relieved by lying flat or temporarily using a pessary to support the prolapse.
- A patient with procidentia may present with protrusion of cervix and a bloodstained, sometimes purulent, vaginal discharge due to decubitus ulceration of the vaginal skin.
- Rectocele may cause difficulty with defecation or a sensation of incomplete defecation, which is relieved by digital reduction of the prolapse.

Diagnosis

Predisposing factors such as chronic cough or constipation may be present, but the diagnosis is usually made by clinical examination.

- A speculum examination in the left lateral (Sim's) position is required to diagnose the type of vaginal prolapse.
- A bimanual pelvic examination should be performed to exclude any pelvic mass.
- When urinary symptoms are present, stress incontinence may be demonstrated by asking the patient to cough with a full bladder.
- A midstream specimen of urine must be sent for culture and sensitivity testing.
- Cystometry and uroflowmetry may be necessary to differentiate detrusor instability from genuine stress incontinence.
- Renal function should be checked in patients with third-degree uterine prolapse.

Recommended further reading

1. Stanton SL (1998). Vaginal prolapse. In: Shaw RW, Soutter WP, Stanton SL, eds. *Gynecology*, pp. 759–70. Churchill Livingstone, Edinburgh.

Prolapse management

Prolapse carries no risk to life unless it causes urinary obstruction. Asymptomatic patients do not require any treatment. Obese patients should be referred to a dietitian for dietary control and advised to reduce weight. Chronic cough and constipation should be corrected.

Prevention

- Minimize pelvic floor trauma during childbirth by avoiding prolonged pushing or difficult instrumental deliveries.
- Encourage the use of postnatal pelvic floor exercises.
- Ensure adequate support of the vaginal vault at hysterectomy by securing the vault to the uterosacral ligaments.
- Use of HRT may reduce the rate of denervation of the pelvic floor after the menopause.

Medical management

Minor degrees of prolapse should be treated conservatively.

Physiotherapy

Pelvic floor exercises and electrical stimulation of the pelvic floor muscles may lessen the prolapse.

Hormone replacement therapy

HRT increases vaginal blood supply and collagen turnover.

Ring pessaries

Surgery is the treatment of choice for significant symptomatic prolapse but ring pessaries are indicated:

- during and after pregnancy if further pregnancies are planned
- as a therapeutic test to confirm that surgery might help
- when the patient is medically unfit for surgery
- patient's request
- for relief of symptoms while the patient is awaiting surgery.

The ring is inserted between the posterior fornix and the pubic bone. Use the smallest diameter that keeps the prolapse reduced and does not fall out. Insertion is easier if the ring is softened in warm water first and lubricated with topical estrogen cream.

The main complication of ring pessaries is vaginal ulceration, leading to vaginal discharge and bleeding. Ulceration of the cervix may be managed by reducing the uterine prolapse and applying estrogen cream. Shelf pessaries may be helpful in cases of failure of ring pessary and when there is no pelvic support.

Surgical management

Surgical management is carried out to correct prolapse, to maintain continence, and to preserve coital function. Sexual activity should be taken into account before surgical procedure to avoid overdoing the repair, which may lead to narrowing of the vagina and dyspareunia.

- *Urethrocele/cystocele* Anterior repair (anterior colporrhaphy) is the operation of choice. A longitudinal incision is made on the anterior vaginal wall and the vaginal skin separated by dissection from the vesical fascia. One or more deep (buttressing) sutures are placed on either side of the vagina to support the bladder neck. The redundant vaginal skin is excised and the skin is closed. Approximately 50% of patients will suffer postoperative urinary retention following an anterior repair. Colposuspension may be necessary to correct stress incontinence associated with cystocele.
- *Uterine prolapse* Vaginal hysterectomy can be combined with an anterior or posterior colporrhaphy and correction of enterocele by coaptation (plication) of the uterosacral ligaments. The ovaries are inspected, and if there is ovarian pathology or the woman is over 50 years of age, vaginal oophorectomy can be accomplished at the same time. Uterine prolapse can also be treated by amputation of the cervix and suturing the cardinal (transverse cervical) ligaments in front of the shortened cervix (Manchester repair).
- *Enterocele* The technique is similar to that used for hernia repair. The vaginal skin is incised and mobilized and the peritoneum opened. The neck of the sac of the prolapse is identified and closed with a purse-string suture.
- *Vault repair* This may be done vaginally or abdominally depending on the patient's general condition and whether or not she wishes to continue intercourse. The vaginal route is simpler and provides a relatively pain-free postoperative recovery.
  - *Sacrospinous* fixation is the most common operation done vaginally, although it carries a risk of damage to the pudendal vessels and nerves. There is a significant risk of cystocele and stress incontinence.
  - The abdominal approach includes the *sacrocolpopexy* where the vault is attached to the sacrum using a nonabsorbable mesh. This area can be very vascular. Laparoscopic sacrocolpopexy has been described, but is currently performed in only a small number of centers.
- *Rectocele* Posterior colporrhaphy is the operation for rectocele. Care must be taken when removing the redundant vaginal skin as vaginal narrowing can result in severe dyspareunia. A double plication of the vesicovaginal and rectovaginal tissues may prevent the recurrence of prolapse.

Recommended further reading

1. Jackson S, Smith P (1997). Diagnosing and managing genitourinary prolapse. *BMJ* **314**, 875–80.
2. Porges RF, Smiler JW (1994). Long-term analysis of the surgical management of pelvic support defects. *Ame J Obstet Gynecol* **171**, 1518–26.

Urinary stress incontinence

Introduction

Urinary stress incontinence is the involuntary loss of urine through an increase in intraabdominal pressure (coughing, sneezing, laughing, etc.). Occasionally, this may be provoked by a detrusor contraction. However, genuine stress incontinence excludes this detrusor instability by defining it as 'involuntary' urethral loss of urine when the intravesical pressure exceeds the maximum urethral pressure in the absence of detrusor activity. Stress incontinence is usually due to urethral sphincter incompetence. However, because this loss of urine is so common, some judgment needs to be made as to whether this is a social or hygienic problem to the patient.

Etiology

Stress incontinence occurs when the intravesical pressure exceeds the closing pressure on the urethra. Childbirth is the most common causative factor leading to denervation of the pelvic floor, usually during the trauma of delivery. Occasionally, there can be congenital weakness of the bladder neck or trauma from other causes. Estrogen deficiency at the time of the menopause leads to weakening of the pelvic supports and thinning of the urothelium. After pelvic surgery or radiotherapy, there may be fibrosis of the urethra precluding efficient closure.

Symptoms and signs

- *Symptoms* Typically, a woman will complain of leakage of urine when she coughs, sneezes, runs, jumps, carries heavy loads, etc. Patients are typically multiparous, and the problem is more common in older than in younger patients. There may be associated frequency or urgency, but these symptoms can be due to detrusor instability.
- *Signs* It may be helpful to demonstrate stress incontinence by asking the patient to cough with a fairly full bladder. The presence of a leak indicates incontinence, usually stress incontinence. Prolapse of the urethra and anterior vaginal wall may be present in 50% of women.

Investigations

Because the bladder is not a reliable witness, further investigations need to be performed.

- A midstream urine (MSU) sample should be taken to exclude infection or glycosuria.
- *Uroflowmetry* is a simple noninvasive test that will exclude voiding difficulties. The patient simply urinates into a toilet with a flow-measuring device in the pan. The normal flow rate is above 15 mL/second. Bladder outflow obstruction is rare in women, but much more common in men (enlarged prostate).

- *Cystometry and videocystourethrography* are used to assess leakage and exclude detrusor instability. The bladder is filled with radioopaque fluid via a urethral catheter. Fine-pressure catheters in the bladder and rectum measure pressure rises. By subtracting the rectal pressure from the bladder pressure, detrusor pressure can be estimated. Leakage on coughing, estimated either by eye or by X-ray, should be assessed. If this occurs in the absence of a detrusor contraction, then genuine stress incontinence is confirmed. Detrusor pressure can be estimated during the voiding phase.
- If there is still doubt about the extent of leakage, a 'pad test' can be performed. A dry pad is weighed and the patient asked to wear this for an hour whilst exercising normally. The pad is reweighed and the change in weight relates to the amount of urine lost. Whilst this gives an estimate of the loss, it does not indicate the cause of loss.

Conservative treatment of urinary stress incontinence

Treatment can be either conservative or surgical. Almost all patients with genuine stress incontinence will undergo a course of conservative treatment before considering surgery.

Conservative treatment is carried out by either physiotherapists or continence nurses. General measures include the following:

- Treatment of obesity
- Treatment of chronic cough
- Treatment of chronic constipation
- Treatment of urogenital estrogen deficiency.

Specific training

Pelvic floor muscle exercise training can be taught to most patients. Patients need to understand why and how the training takes place. Feedback machines can be very helpful in this respect, giving patients an idea of their progress (which will often precede symptomatic improvement). Electrical stimulation is helpful in women who have a denervated pelvic floor. Vaginal cones are a useful method of actively and passively exercising the pelvic floor. The patient starts by keeping an unweighted cone in the vagina whilst walking round for 15 minutes. Once this is achieved, increasing weights can be added. Pelvic floor tone increases.

On average, over 50% of patients will see objective benefit from pelvic floor muscle exercises. Hospital-based treatment is superior to home treatment. The success rate appears to depend very much on the enthusiasm of the patient and the continence advisor. Patients with milder symptoms seem more likely to achieve a cure than those with severe stress incontinence.

Surgical treatment of urinary stress incontinence

There are many operations to cure genuine stress incontinence, but none is universally successful or without side effects. The choice of operation depends on the type of incontinence, associated features (such as prolapse), and the personal experience of the operator. Patients will usually be offered a choice of operation because of the different success rates, complication rates, and recovery time.

- *Anterior colporrhaphy* Vaginal repair with anterior colporrhaphy and suburethral buttressing can be useful in women with combined stress incontinence and vaginal prolapse. It has a lower success rate for curing stress incontinence than suprapubic operations, but is less likely to be associated with complications such as detrusor instability.
- *Endoscopic bladder neck suspension* Techniques such as the Stamey or Ras procedures have been used. In these techniques, a needle is used to insert a suture on either side of the bladder neck, anchoring it with a buffer for sutures in the pubocervical fascia and tying the upper end of each suture to the rectus sheath. The principle is that a cough or strain of the intraabdominal muscles will pull up on the suture and 'tighten' the bladder neck. Whilst the short-term success may be useful, the long-term success is disappointing. However, this operation may be useful in elderly patients or in selected cases.
- *Tension-free vaginal tape* This is a relatively new operation, usually performed under local or spinal anesthetic. A proline mesh is inserted on either side of the urethra with two needles. The needles emerge through the abdominal wall. The mesh is tightened with the patient being asked to cough and adjusted until there is only a minimal leak. Care must be taken not to overtighten the tape, which would lead to voiding difficulties. The tape remains in place permanently and sits suburethrally. The short-term success rate appears good (85%) with a low complication rate, but the long-term results are as yet uncertain.
- *Burch colposuspension* The approach to the bladder neck is through a transverse abdominal incision. Dissection is made in the retropubic space and the bladder neck is identified. Two or three sutures are placed in the vaginal tissue and fascia on either side of the bladder neck and tied to the iliopectineal ligament. When tightened, these create a shelf on the bladder neck. The short-term success rate is again about 85%, but with well-proven long-term success. The procedure can cure anterior vaginal wall prolapse at the same time. Complications include urinary retention, voiding difficulties, and the occurrence of detrusor instability. Posterior vaginal wall prolapse or enterocele may occur as a late complication.

- *Marshall–Marchetti–Krantz procedure* This operation is a widely used suprapubic procedure. As in the Burch procedure, the retropubic space is dissected. The sutures are inserted between periurethral tissues along the proximal half of the urethra, and are then attached to the periosteum or perichondrium of the symphysis pubis. One major complication is that of osteitis pubis (up to 5% of cases). Unlike colposuspension, this operation is unlikely to cure a cystocele.
- *Sling procedures* There are many different types of slings using either organic or inorganic materials. Commonly, the patient's rectus fascia is used, but tissues such as porcine dermis can also be used. Inorganic materials such as meshes are stronger, but if they become infected they can be very difficult to remove. Cure rates for stress incontinence are again around 80–90%. Complications include voiding difficulties, detrusor instability, and sling erosion.
- *Periurethral injections* Injections of substances such as collagen are made either transurethrally or periurethrally. These form a cushion of tissue that reduces the caliber of the bladder neck and thus the chance of urinary incontinence. The injections are expensive, but have the advantage of being simple to insert with small risk of complications. However, some patients develop urinary retention. The success rate of periurethral injections is less than that of other types of surgery (approximately 50% continence rate). The injections can be repeated with a small improvement in continence rate.

Failed continence surgery

Second or third operations may be successful for those patients with failed surgery. However, the success rate appears to be about 10% less than for a primary operation. The risk of developing problems such as bladder instability is greater for each subsequent operation. As a last resort, an artificial sphincter can be inserted, but there is a significant risk of infection or mechanical failure. Long-term catheterization may be an option for women who are unfit for surgery.

Micturition: frequency and urgency

Frequency of micturition is common and has many causes. Normally, women should not empty their bladder more than seven times a day or once at night. Voiding in excess of this is defined as frequency or nocturia. Urgency is the strong and sudden desire to void urine, and may often be followed by urge incontinence. It tends to be due to an involuntary detrusor contraction, but some women may be unaware of this.

Causes

- *Gynecological* Pregnancy or pelvic mass can press on the bladder giving symptoms. A prolapse, particularly a cystocele, will often cause these symptoms, as will postmenopausal urogenital atrophy.
- *Urological* A urinary tract infection typically gives such symptoms. Detrusor instability will commonly present with multiple symptoms, including urgency and frequency. Bladder pathology, such as interstitial cystitis, bladder calculus, mucosal lesions, or urethral problems, may present in such a way.
- *Medical problems* Treatment with diuretics causes frequency, mainly limited to the few hours following treatment.
- *Endocrine* Diabetes mellitus, diabetes insipidus, and hypothyroidism can all cause frequency and urgency.
- *Psychological* Some patients habitually have frequency, often in an attempt to prevent leakage of urine. Excessive fluid intake must also be looked for.

Investigation

The etiology may be obvious from the history, but usually is not.

- The history should include information about the length of time for which the patient has had symptoms, fluid intake, associated diseases, previous surgery, and a history of childhood enuresis. Many women will have associated problems during sexual intercourse and may not complain of these unless asked directly.
- Investigations should include urine culture and an intake–output fluid volume chart.
- Urodynamic investigations, including uroflowmetry and urodynamic assessment by cystometrogram, may be helpful. These will help identify an unstable bladder (defined as one shown objectively to contract during the filling phase, either spontaneously or on provocation, while the patient is attempting to inhibit micturition).
- Cystoscopy may be useful if intravesical pathology is suspected.

Treatment

Treatment depends on the cause. Excessive fluid intake can be curbed and infections treated. It is helpful for a patient to avoid bladder stimulants such as tea, coffee, and alcohol. Ideally, they should limit their fluid intake to 1–1.5 L/day. Diuretic therapy may be changed or stopped.

- *Medication* In postmenopausal women, local estrogen treatment to the vagina can be helpful, particularly in those with sensory symptoms. A glass of cranberry juice each day appears to relieve some women's symptoms. Musculotropic relaxants such as oxybutynin or tolterodine will help the unstable bladder, although side effects (dry mouth, blurred vision) limit their effectiveness. Tricyclic antidepressants can be useful, particularly for the treatment of nocturia and nocturnal enuresis.
- *Behavioral therapy* In bladder drill (bladder training), the patient is instructed to void by the clock commencing initially at 90 minute intervals and then gradually increasing the time interval. Concurrent treatment with musculotropic relaxants can increase the success rate, but relapse is common. Biofeedback techniques can be helpful, as can hypnotherapy. Electrical stimulation may also inhibit spontaneous detrusor contractions and can be performed by specialist nurses.
- Very rarely is *surgery* indicated, but the 'clam' enterocystoplasty has been used with some success in severe cases. Conventional bladder neck surgery is not useful in the treatment of detrusor instability.

Chapter 18

Benign and malignant gynecological conditions

Benign neoplasms of the genital tract and vulva

The genital tract can be the seat of various benign tumors which may be clinically significant and require intervention, but are often asymptomatic. Benign neoplastic lesions arising from different parts of the genital tract are described below.

Clinically significant diseases of the vulva are rare in gynecological practice. Inflammatory disorders (vulvitis) are far more common than benign neoplasms and are described in Chapter 14 📖 *p.498*. Benign neoplasms can be categorized as solid lesions and cystic lesions.

Solid lesions

- *Lipoma/fibroma* Fibrofatty and muscular tissues of the labia and mons pubis or ischiorectal fascia may give rise to benign fibromas, lipomas, and leiomyomas. These tumors are relatively infrequent and histologically may contain a mixture of both elements. Clinically, they may cause discomfort or interfere with sexual intercourse. These growths should be excised.
- *Granular myoblastoma* is a benign lesion arising from the nerve sheath. Myoblastoma is not a well-localized tumor and may locally recur. Treatment is local resection of the lesion.
- *Hemangiomas* Different varieties of these can occur. Pyogenic granuloma is a type of hemangioma characterized by the proliferation of capillaries of labia. It usually occurs during pregnancy. These lesions are the largest and most symptomatic of adult vulvar hemangiomas. Bleeding and infection are common and can often give rise to purulent discharge. Treatment is by deep excision.
- *Endometrioma* Ectopic endometrium may arise by metaplasia or by implantation of viable endometrium at the time of surgery or delivery in a genetically susceptible individual. A history of cyclical enlargement of nodule and pain with menses is highly suggestive. Local excision is diagnostic and curative.
- *Hidradenoma* This tumor usually occurs in the vulva of sexually active Caucasian women. It arises from the sweat gland. These tumors are rare, and excisional biopsies are both diagnostic and curative.

Cystic lesions

- *Inclusion cysts* are also known as epidermal cysts. They are lined by a smooth layer of keratinizing squamous epithelium, and the contents of the cysts are largely keratin and cellular debris. They have a sebaceous appearance and odor. Acutely inflamed cysts should be treated with a warm pack and incision and drainage. Excision may become necessary to prevent recurrence.

- *Bartholin's cyst* Dilatation of Bartholin's duct is the most common cystic swelling of the vulva. Most of these cysts occur because of a purely mechanical problem, i.e. a blockage of outflow of the mucus. Rapid enlargement and pain can be secondary to abscess formation. Marsupialization is the treatment of choice, i.e. the inner cyst wall is folded back and stitched to the skin. Gonococcal infection should be excluded. Persistent episodes of abscess formation may require excision of the gland.
- *Hydrocele of the canal of Nuck* Cysts of the canal of Nuck are not true hernias, but are analogous to hydrocele in men. Treatment is often not indicated unless cysts become symptomatic, at which point excision is indicated.

Vagina and cervix

Vagina

Neoplasms of the vagina can present with a sensation of fullness in the vagina. Benign neoplasms can be either solid or cystic.

- *Inclusion cysts* arise from inclusion of the vaginal skin underneath the surface resulting from perineal lacerations or from imperfect surgical repair of the perineum. Treatment is surgical removal and is only indicated when the cysts cause symptoms such as discomfort, dyspareunia, or infection.
- *Gartner duct cysts* arise from vestigial remnants of the Wolffian or mesonephric system. They are generally located on the anterolateral aspect of the vagina and are usually small. Occasionally, they may be large and bulge from the introitus. No treatment is necessary if the cysts are small and asymptomatic, but surgical excision may be required if they are large and obstruct the outlet.
- *Condyloma acuminatum* is a viral disease caused by human papillomavirus. It is multifocal in character and is associated with vulvar and cervical lesions. It is mostly benign, but specific subtypes may give rise to cervical or vaginal cancers. This disease is considered to be sexually transmitted. Rarely, lesions are passed to the offspring of infected mothers and may be found in the mucous membrane of the newborn as well as in the larynx. Lesions have a flowery appearance, classically known as wart. Biopsies are recommended to rule out verrucous carcinoma. Laser vaporization or cryotherapy may be used to treat the lesions. Medical treatment with 5-fluorouracil or podophyllin is also effective. Lesions in pregnant women can hypertrophy and proliferate, and may develop to the degree that they obstruct the outlet of the vagina necessitating cesarean delivery. However, this is extremely rare.
- *Endometriosis* Endometriotic implants in the vagina are rare. They are generally seen on the top of the vagina. They usually respond to medical therapy.
- *Leiomyoma* is very rarely seen in the vagina. It may be locally excised.
- *Adenosis vaginae* is found in female offspring of women who were exposed to diethylstilbestrol (DES) during pregnancy. Adenosis is a benign lesion and requires no treatment. However, it should be carefully observed for malignant transformation.

Cervix

- *Cervical polyps* are the most common benign growth of the cervix. They are usually pedunculated, arising from the endocervical mucosa, but they occasionally arise from the external or vaginal surface of the cervix. Clinically, they present as small bright-red growths that protrude from the cervical canal. They may be inflammatory in origin and range up to few centimeters in diameter. Polyps can be asymptomatic and are discovered as an incidental finding during routine smear test. They can produce intermenstrual spotting or contact bleeding after coitus. When polyps are identified, removal is indicated because of the risk of malignancy, although this risk is low (said to be 1 in 6000). Sometimes (e.g. in the presence of irregular bleeding) this may need to be combined with hysteroscopy and curettage of the endometrial cavity to rule out any polyps in the uterus. Recurrence is not uncommon.

- *Nabothian cysts* are mucus-retention cysts caused by blockage of the openings of the endocervical mucous glands. They are usually seen on the surface of the cervix and may be associated with chronic cervicitis and chronic infection of the endocervical canal. Normally no treatment is required unless they are infected, at which point cryotherapy or cautery to the cervix may be indicated.

Uterus and endometrial polyps

Uterus

Leiomyomas are the most common benign tumor of the uterus, occurring in an estimated 25–30% of women of reproductive age. They arise from the smooth muscle cells of the myometrium (hence the name) but, perhaps because they are firm or for some illogical reason, they are more often referred to as fibroids. They have not been reported before menarche and rarely develop after menopause. Genetic influences are involved, because these tumors are considerably more frequent in African Caribbean than in other ethnic groups. Estrogens probably stimulate their growth. Conversely, they shrink in size after menopause. Leiomyomas can be single but are usually multiple. They may be entirely asymptomatic and be discovered only on routine pelvic examination or post-mortem. The most frequent manifestation when present is menorrhagia with or without intermenstrual bleeding. Large masses may present with lower abdominal swelling, dragging sensation, or urinary symptoms. Whether these benign tumors ever become transformed into sarcomas is highly questionable, and indeed this may never occur.

Leiomyomas are classified by their location in the myometrium and their proximity to endometrial and serosal surfaces. Submucous, intramural, and subserous are the three most common types.

Treatment

Leiomyomas can be treated conservatively or with surgery. Radiation therapy was used in the past for patients considered poor surgical risks and those with excessive bleeding to induce menopause, but this management is now rare. Shrinkage of fibroids by embolization of feeding vessel may be possible but is still under investigation.

Conservative treatment

Leiomyomas discovered during routine pelvic examination in a patient without any symptoms usually require no active treatment, but pelvic examinations should be done to monitor the growth at intervals of 6–12 months. Closer observation is indicated if rapid growth or symptoms are reported.

Surgical treatment

Surgical treatment is usually indicated in patients with large leiomyomas and for those associated with heavy periods or other symptoms. Occasionally, the position of the tumor within the uterine cavity may be the cause of repeated miscarriages or even subfertility.

- *Myomectomy* can be used to remove symptomatic single or multiple leiomyomas. It is indicated when fertility is a concern or if the patient does not wish to part with her uterus for social or religious reasons. Excessive bleeding during operation is a significant risk factor and may even necessitate a hysterectomy. Patients should be appropriately counseled.

- *Hysterectomy* is indicated when there are large leiomyomas and the possibility of preserving the uterus by myomectomy is minimal or nonexistent. The risk of recurrence is high, and so hysterectomy is the treatment of choice for those patients who do not intend further childbearing. In younger patients, the ovaries are generally conserved.

Endometrial polyps

Endometrial polyps are the result of focal overgrowth of endometrial glands and stroma. Recent cytogenetic studies confirm that most endometrial polyps are monoclonal and that stromal cells are the neoplastic component. Although endometrial polyps may occur at any age, they develop more commonly at the time of menopause. Their clinical significance lies in the production of abnormal uterine bleeding and, more importantly, the risk of giving rise to cancer. Approximately 1% of endometrial polyps are malignant.

Ovary

Neoplasms of the ovary make up an amazing diversity of pathological entities. This is because of the presence of three cell types in the normal ovary: the multipotential surface (celomic) epithelium, the totipotential germ cells, and the sex cord stromal cells. Each of these cell types can give rise to a variety of tumors:

- Cystadenoma (serous or mucinous)
- Brenner tumor (rarely malignant)
- Neoplastic tumors arising from germ cells
- Dermoid (benign cystic teratoma)
- Neoplasms arising from ovarian stroma
- Fibroma
- Adenofibroma
- Thecoma
- Physiological cysts
- Follicular cysts
- Luteal cysts

Overall, 90% of ovarian tumors are benign, although they are more likely to be malignant in the older women. The most common solid tumor in younger women is the cystic teratoma, also commonly known as a dermoid. Epithelial cell tumors are more common among older women. Benign ovarian tumors are often asymptomatic, but they can present with pain, abdominal swelling, pressure effects, menstrual disturbances, or hormonal effects. Pain may be due to torsion or bleeding inside the cyst. Masses that are 12 cm or more in diameter may be palpable abdominally above the symphysis pubis. Bimanual examination usually reveals a mass in the pelvis, and it may be possible to assess the mobility, consistency, and tenderness of the mass and the presence of nodules in the pouch of Douglas. The presence of ascites and a hard irregular fixed mass suggests malignancy.

Pelvic ultrasound, CT scan, and measurement of tumor markers (CA-125) are useful adjuncts for diagnostic evaluation of ovarian cysts.

Treatment

- Even when asymptomatic, older women gain little from conservative treatment. As the risk of malignancy is high, detailed evaluation of the cysts and removal is usually indicated. Often this involves hysterectomy and bilateral salpingo-oophorectomy.
- Women under 35 are less likely to have malignancy and may also wish to have children. Ovarian cysts more than 10 cm in diameter are unlikely to be physiological or to resolve spontaneously, and therefore should be surgically removed. Smaller cysts can be followed up with ultrasound. If the cyst does not regress or becomes symptomatic, laparoscopy or laparotomy is indicated. Ovarian cystectomy or oophorectomy is usually carried out provided that the clinical appearance of the cyst is entirely benign. Frozen section (histology report intraoperatively) should be arranged, where possible, to guide therapy.

- Ovarian cysts detected during pregnancy are mostly benign. The conservative approach of monitoring cyst size with ultrasound is often adequate. In the presence of acute symptoms or if the cyst is large or is growing rapidly, laparotomy may well be required regardless of gestation.

Cancer screening

Screening is the process of identifying those asymptomatic individuals in the population who are at sufficiently increased risk of a condition to justify referral for further investigation and treatment. Therefore a screening test does not necessarily diagnose the condition. The ultimate aim of screening programs in cancer is to reduce deaths and morbidity from the disease.

Conditions suitable for screening should ideally satisfy a number of criteria:
- The condition should represent an important public health problem.
- The natural history of the condition should be known.
- There should be a recognizable early stage of the condition.
- An effective intervention should be available.
- A suitable screening test should be available.
- The benefits should be greater than the harm caused by screening.

A suitable screening test should:
- have a high sensitivity and specificity
- be acceptable to patients
- be cost effective
- be reproducible.

Here are some useful definitions.
- *Sensitivity* is the proportion of subjects tested who have the disease who have a positive screening test.
- *Specificity* is the proportion of people who do not have the disease and who have a negative test.
- The *positive predictive value* of a test is the chance that, given a positive result, the individual tested has the condition and the *negative predictive value* is the probability that the individual tested does not have the disease if the test is negative.
- The *odds ratio* of a test is the number of individuals with a positive screening result for each person with confirmed disease.

Although, clearly, a test must have sufficient sensitivity to be able to detect cases of the disease, it is the specificity of the test that is most important in screening. This is especially true when an invasive and potentially dangerous procedure is required to confirm the diagnosis, as would be the case in, for example, ovarian cancer (laparoscopy, laparotomy). In these circumstances, a screening test with an odds ratio >10:1 is unlikely to be acceptable. In order to have an odds ratio of 10, a screening test for ovarian cancer in women over the age of 40 needs to have a specificity of 99.6%.

Recommended further reading

1. Stone EG, Morton SC, Hulscher ME, *et al.* (2002). Interventions that increase use of adult immunization and cancer screening services: a meta-analysis. *Ann Intern Med* **136**, 641–51.

Cervical carcinoma

Rationale

Invasive disease is preceded by cervical intraepithelial neoplasia (CIN). Effective treatment of CIN prevents progression. Women at risk of having CIN can be identified by exfoliative cytology.

Methods

Papanicolau smear

Screening is by cervical cytology (Papanicolaou smear). In most developed countries, this is carried out every 3–5 years from the age of 20 to 65. Testing every 3 years identifies more than 95% of abnormalities detected by annual screening and so is more cost-effective than annual screening in a low-risk population. Interpretation of smears in postmenopausal women may be difficult, and cervical neoplasia is unlikely if smears prior to this have been normal.

- A pelvic examination is performed using a speculum. A suitable spatula inserted into the external cervical os is rotated through 360°, smeared evenly over a glass slide, and fixed immediately with an acetic acid/alcohol mixture. After staining, the slide is examined by a technician or cytopathologist for the presence of epithelial cells with neoplastic changes (increased nuclear to cytoplasmic ratio, mitotic figures).
- Alternatively, the epithelial cells attached to the spatula can be eluted into a solution and the cells examined using the thin-prep technique either by a cytopathologist or, more recently, by a computer.
- The presence of cells from the endocervix is used as an indication that the sample has been taken across the squamocolumnar junction and has included the transformation zone.

Smears are reported as: normal; unsatisfactory; inflammatory; borderline; mild, moderate, or severe dyskaryosis; suspicious of malignancy; or showing abnormal glandular cells.

- *Unsatisfactory smears* occur in 10–15% of cases and can be due to insufficient cells, inflammatory cells, or red blood cells obscuring the epithelial cells. A repeat after 3–6 months is recommended and, if a second repeat is unsatisfactory, referral for colposcopy.
- Patients with *borderline nuclear abnormalities* (also known as *abnormal squamous cells of undetermined significance* (ASCUS)) and *mild dyskaryosis* should have a repeat smear after 6 months and are referred if successive smears are abnormal.
- All other women are referred for colposcopy.

Note that the diagnosis of CIN itself requires a tissue sample from biopsy, and the correlation between the degree of abnormality on cytology and histology is poor. False-negative results (i.e. women with CIN who are reported as having a normal smear) occur in up to 20% of cases. Reasons include errors in sampling technique, distortion of the cervix from previous surgery, and laboratory error. Ten to fifteen percent of all women will have an abnormal smear and 5–10% will be referred for colposcopy. Premalignant changes in the endocervical epithelium (cervical glandular intraepithelial neoplasia (CGIN)) cannot be reliably detected by cervical screening. The introduction of cervical screening has been associated with a 40% fall in deaths from cervical cancer over the last 20 years. Regular cervical screening reduces (but does not eliminate) the risk of death from cervical carcinoma by 75%.

Other methods of screening

Cervical carcinoma is the second most common cause of female cancer-related deaths worldwide. Using cervical smears for screening requires a sophisticated infrastructure, laboratories, and trained staff. These are expensive and therefore are not available in many developing countries where mortality rates from cervical carcinoma are higher. Other alternative approaches to screening in developing countries are visual inspection of the cervix by trained nonmedical health workers looking for early-stage disease and photographing the cervix after staining with acetic acid (cervicography).

Testing for the human papillomavirus (HPV)

Infection with HPV is common in sexually active women. However, certain serotypes (16, 18, 31, and 33) are more commonly found in the presence of invasive disease. Routine testing for a limited range of HPV types using samples taken from the cervix at the time of cervical smear testing identifies a higher proportion of women with CIN than conventional cytology. HPV testing may also be of value in predicting whether or not low-grade changes will progress. However, the routine use of HPV testing in addition to conventional cytology would significantly increase the cost per case detected. The role of HPV testing is currently under evaluation. Possible strategies might include the following:

- Using HPV testing to determine whether patients with low-grade CIN or borderline changes require treatment or referral for colposcopy.
- Only screening women who are positive for certain HPV types by cytology.
- Referring women with high-risk HPV disease for colposcopy.

Recommended further reading

1. American College of Obstetricians and Gynecologists (2003). ACOG Committee Opinion No. 247. Routine cancer screening. *Int J Gynaecol Obstet* **82**, 241–5.
2. American College of Obstetricians and Gynecologists (2001). ACOG Committee Opinion No. 239. Breast–ovarian cancer screening. *Int J Gynaecol Obstet* **75**, 339–40.

Ovarian and endometrial carcinoma

Ovarian

Rationale

Seventy-five percent of cases present with advanced disease. The prognosis for early-stage disease is better than that for advanced disease. If the disease could be diagnosed earlier in asymptomatic women, overall survival might be improved.

Methods

- Ultrasound examination to look for ovarian cysts. As many cysts in premenopausal women are functional (follicular or corpus luteum), more than one measurement may be required. Suspicious features are increasing size, internal septa, solid areas within the cyst, and increased blood flow (Doppler). False-positive results may be due to benign ovarian tumors (which might need to be removed in any case), endometriosis, and inflammatory masses. Screening needs to be done centrally and requires some operator expertise. There have been significant improvements in odds ratio for both ovarian malignancy (7:1) and all abnormalities (2:1).
- CA-125 is a glycoprotein shed by 85% of epithelial tumors. Cut-off levels of between 30 and 65 IU/L have been used for screening. CA-125 lacks sufficient specificity if used alone, but can be used as a primary screen to identify candidates for ultrasound. It does not require specialist expertise or equipment at point of collection. False-positive results occur in other malignancies (liver, pancreas), endometriosis, pelvic inflammatory disease (PID), and early pregnancy. Sensitivity can be improved by looking at serial measurements in women with borderline values. Up to 50% of stage 1 tumors will have a value of less than 35 IU/L.

The current situation

Ultrasound, either used alone or in combination with CA-125, may have sufficient sensitivity and specificity, but most studies to date have not compared long-term death rates in screened and unscreened populations. Large multicenter studies randomizing women into screened and unscreened controls are in progress, but at the moment the value of screening the general population remains unproven. Women with hereditary disease should be offered testing, where possible, to see if they are carriers of an abnormal *BRCA* gene. Carriers may be offered annual screening with ultrasound sonography and CA-125, and prophylactic oophorectomy when their family is complete. Even in these groups, the value of such an approach in increased survival is unproven.

Endometrial carcinoma

There is no screening program for endometrial carcinoma. Possible methods of screening would be the use of ultrasound to detect increases in endometrial thickness in postmenopausal women or the routine use of endometrial sampling. The value of doing this even in high-risk groups is unproven.

Recommended further reading

1. American College of Obstetricians and Gynecologists (2003). ACOG Committee Opinion No. 247. Routine cancer screening. *Int J Gynaecol Obstet* **82**, 241–5.
2. American College of Obstetricians and Gynecologists (2001). ACOG Committee Opinion No. 239. Breast-ovarian cancer screening. *Int J Gynaecol Obstet* **75**, 339–40.

Cervical intraepithelial neoplasia

The cervical canal is lined by endocervical glandular epithelium. The vaginal portion of the cervix is covered by squamous epithelium. The junction between these two epithelia is called the squamocolumnar junction (SCJ). From late fetal life to the menopause, the position of this junction changes. When columnar epithelium is exposed to the acid vaginal pH, transformation occurs. Although in most cases physiological squamous metaplasia occurs, the transformation zone (TZ) is where cervical intraepithelial neoplasia (CIN) develops.

Early intercourse, multiple sexual partners, smoking, HPV infection, and immunocompromise are associated with an increased risk of CIN.

Pathology

- CIN is a single continuous disease process with disordered growth and development of the epithelial lining of the TZ of the cervix, with varying degrees of nuclear enlargement and pleomorphism.
- CIN1 is defined as disordered growth of the lower third of the epithelial lining.
- In CIN2, there is failure of the cells to mature in the lower one- to two-thirds of the epithelium with a greater degree of nuclear atypia.
- In CIN3, undifferentiated cells extend into the upper third of the epithelium.

Cytologically, the dyskaryotic cell is characterized by anaplasia, increased nuclear-to-cytoplasmic ratio (the nucleus is larger), hyperchromatism with changes in nuclear chromatin, multinucleation, and abnormalities in differentiation. CIN is a precursor of squamous cell carcinoma. Possibly only 30% of untreated CIN3 cases will progress to invasive squamous cell carcinoma within 20 years, with spontaneous regression in one-third of cases.

Screening for CIN

National cervical screening programs generally recommend that all women aged 20–64 should be screened by cervical cytology at least once every 5 years. The following patients should be referred for colposcopy:

- Suspected carcinoma of the cervix
- One smear showing moderate or severe dyskaryosis
- Two successive smears showing mild dyskaryosis
- Persistent smears showing borderline nuclear abnormalities or being unsatisfactory for reporting
- Glandular changes

Colposcopy

- At colposcopy, the cervix is examined under low power (6–20×) binocular magnification and an intense light source.
- After application of 3–5% acetic acid to the cervix, a transient coagulation of the protein of the superficial cells occurs and atypical areas stand out from normal epithelium.

- The major abnormal patterns at colposcopy are aceto-white epithelium, punctation, mosaicism, and atypical vessels.
  - Aceto-white epithelium is related to the abnormal nuclear-to-cytoplasmic ratio which occurs in dysplastic or neoplastic cells.
- After application of acetic acid, addition of Schiller's or Lugol's iodine (a weak aqueous solution) may enhance the definition of the outer limit of the TZ and enable detection of any abnormal areas of vaginal epithelium.
- The Schiller test is based on the principle that normal squamous epithelium of the cervix contains glycogen, which combines with iodine to produce a deep mahogany-brown color. Nonstaining indicates abnormal squamous (or columnar) epithelium. The test is not specific for dysplasia, but merely reveals non-glycogen-containing epithelium. Immature metaplasia may be nonstaining.

At colposcopy one must assess:
- whether the SCJ can completely be seen
- the area of aceto-white epithelium and any atypical vessel patterns
- the outer limit of the TZ including any evidence of extension on to the vaginal wall.

A diagnostic biopsy for histological assessment must be taken from abnormal areas if treatment by a local ablation technique is contemplated.

Recommended further reading

1. Fraser A, Hellmann S, Leibovici L, Levavi H (2005). Screening for cervical cancer: an evidence-based approach. *Eur J Gynaecol Oncol* **26**, 372–5.

Treatment of cervical intraepithelial neoplasia

It is customary to recommend treatment for all patients with higher-grade lesions (CIN2 and CIN3).

The following therapies are used for the treatment of CIN:

- *Local ablation methods:* cryocautery, cold coagulator, electro-diathermy, and CO_2 laser vaporization.
- *Excision methods:* large loop excision of the transformation zone (LLETZ), knife cone biopsy, laser cut cone (CO_2), hysterectomy.

Local ablation should only be used when:

- the SCJ can be seen completely
- there is no cytological, histological, or colposcopic suggestion of microinvasive or frankly invasive disease
- there is no suggestion of glandular abnormality
- the patient is considered reliable and will attend for regular follow-up.

If the SCJ is not completely seen or the patient has previously been treated, local ablation is contraindicated. Excision of the abnormal epithelium, enabling histological assessment of the total abnormal area, should be undertaken.

Knife cone biopsy and hysterectomy will usually be performed under general anesthesia, but most other treatments are suitable for outpatient management. Hysterectomy is rarely required for the management of CIN. However, it may be indicated in those who have completed their childbearing and have coexisting gynecological problems or in postmenopausal women where cone biopsy may be technically difficult. Where the lesion involves the upper vagina, a combination of local ablative or excisional treatment with laser vaporization of the vaginal part of the lesion may be appropriate.

Management of minor changes (CIN1) is controversial. Low-grade changes can be treated immediately or kept under surveillance by a combination of cytology and colposcopy. It is likely that a significant proportion may regress. Unfortunately, we are as yet unable to identify those patients whose CIN is likely to progress. It is possible that HPV testing may identify those patients in whom progression of CIN might be more likely to occur, and hence identify those to treat rather than observe. Prospective randomized trials are required to validate this possibility.

Follow-up

All patients treated for CIN require follow-up. Routinely, all patients should have two cervical smears within the first year and then annual smears for at least 5 years. Thereafter, smears every 3 years may be appropriate. It is recommended that patients treated by hysterectomy without vaginal extension of their intraepithelial neoplasia should have a vaginal vault smear at 6 and 12 months. They may then discontinue follow-up. If the histological report of the removed cervical tissue suggests incomplete excision or that there has been a wide lesion extending beyond the cervix, follow-up by colposcopy and smears is indicated.

Special situations

- *Pregnancy* Abnormal cervical smears in pregnancy may be assessed by colposcopy to rule out an invasive lesion. Although the gravid cervix is more vascular, directed biopsies can be performed. If CIN is confirmed, serial colposcopic examinations can be performed and treatment undertaken postpartum. Pregnancy does not appear to cause abnormal progression.
- *Immunosuppression* Women who are immunosuppressed, such as those on immunosuppressive agents following organ transplant or those with autoimmune diseases, have an increased incidence of lower genital tract dysplasia. If the smear is abnormal, an annual cervical smear with colposcopic surveillance is recommended.

Cervical glandular intraepithelial neoplasia

There is probably a continuum of glandular change ranging from normality to adenocarcinoma *in situ* (AIS). Histological diagnosis of AIS is based on changes suggesting malignancy without evidence of penetration of the basement membrane. It is recognized in the mucin-secreting columnar epithelium by stratification of the epithelial cells, loss of nuclear polarity; loss of mucin-secreting capacity; increase in the nucleocytoplasmic ratios; cellular pleomorphism and nuclear hyperchromatism, and the presence of numerous, sometimes atypical, mitoses. Because of the difficulties of distinguishing glandular abnormalities, it has been suggested that the spectrum is divided into two grades: low- and high-grade CGIN or glandular atypia and AIS.

Colposcopy should be undertaken in all cases of glandular anomalies noted on cervical smear. A squamous lesion may be identified in the absence of other anomaly.

- If the smear shows high-grade anomalies, a cone biopsy with uterine curettage should be performed.
  - AIS may be multifocal. Even if the surgical margins of the cone biopsy are clear of abnormal epithelium, follow-up with careful sampling with an endocervical brush is essential.

Recommended further reading

1. Martin-Hirsch PL, Paraskevaidis E, Kitchener H (2000). Surgery for cervical intraepithelial neoplasia. *Cochrane Database Syst Rev* **2**, CD001318.
2. American College of Obstetricians and Gynecologists (2005). ACOG Practice Bulletin No. 66. Management of abnormal cervical cytology and histology. *Obstet Gynecol* **106**, 645–64.

Malignant disease of the cervix

Introduction

Carcinoma of the cervix is the second most common female cancer worldwide. In developed countries, it constitutes around 4% of female malignancies with an annual incidence of 9.5 in 100 000 women. The overall incidence of cervical cancer and death rate from it (approximately 3.1 in 100 000 per annum) have declined recently because of aggressive screening programs.

Etiology

Sexual activity has been correlated with the disease, especially age at first intercourse and number of sexual partners. Cancer of the cervix is four times as frequent in prostitutes as in other women. A strong link between smoking and cervical cancer has been noted. Smoking reduces the number of Langerhans cells, which are involved in local immune surveillance. HPV types 16, 18, and 33 are associated with invasive tumors. HPV 16 and 18 produce E6 and E7 proteins, which alter normal cell function by forming complexes with cell proteins involved in cell cycle regulation. Other factors associated with the disease include immunocompromised host, oral contraceptive use, and a high-risk male sexual partner.

Pathogenesis

The columnar epithelium of the uterine cervix meets the stratified squamous epithelium of the vagina and cervix at the squamocolumnar junction (transformation zone). Most of the cases of preinvasive and invasive disease occur at this site. Most cervical cancers probably begin as dysplastic changes with gradual progression over a period of several years. Cervical cancers spread mainly by direct local invasion and by the lymphatics and blood vessels in very advanced cases. Lymphatic spread occurs via parametrial lymphatics to the internal and external iliac nodes and from there to lymph plexuses surrounding the aorta and vena cava. Blood-borne spread to distant organs is noted in advanced cases. The age distribution of the tumor is bimodal with peaks at 35–44 years and 75–85 years.

Pathology

Most cervical tumors are squamous (70%), followed by adenocarcinoma and adenosquamous carcinoma, which make up 25% in roughly equal proportions. The rest involves rarer types such as small cell, transitional cell, lymphomas, and sarcomas.

FIGO has dropped the term 'early stromal invasion' and uses the terms microinvasive and invasive carcinoma of cervix (detailed in Table 18.1).

Table 18.1 Staging of cervical carcinoma

Stage	Features
0	Preinvasive carcinoma (carcinoma *in situ* (CIN))
I	Carcinoma confined to the cervix (extension to the corpus should be disregarded)
Ia	Invasive cancer identified only microscopically. All gross lesions even with superficial invasion are stage Ib cancers. Measured stromal depth should not be more than 5 mm and no wider than 7 mm*
Ia1	Measured invasion no greater than 3 mm in depth and no wider than 7 mm
Ia2	Measured depth of invasion >3 mm but no >5 mm and no wider than 7 mm
Ib	Clinical lesions confined to cervix or preclincal lesions greater than Ia
Ib1	Clinical lesions <4 cm in diameter
Ib2	Clinical lesions >4 cm in diameter
II	Carcinoma extending beyond the cervix but not on to the pelvic wall. The carcinoma involves the vagina but not as far as the lower third
IIa	No obvious parametrial involvement
IIb	Obvious parametrial involvement
III	The carcinoma has extended on to the pelvic wall. On rectal examination there is no cancer-free space between the tumor and the pelvic wall. The tumor involves the lower third of vagina. All cases with hydronephrosis or nonfunctioning kidney should be included unless they are known to be due to another cause
IIIa	No extension to pelvic wall but involvement of lower third of vagina
IIIb	Extension to the pelvic wall or hydronephrosis or nonfunctioning kidney
IV	The carcinoma has extended beyond the true pelvis or has clinically involved the mucosa of the bladder or rectum
IVa	Spread of the growth to adjacent organs
IVb	Spread to distant organs

* The depth of invasion should not be more than 5 mm from the base of the epithelium, either surface or glandular, from which it originates. Vascular space involvement, either venous or lymphatic, should not alter the staging.

Clinical features and investigations of cervical carcinoma

- The common presenting features are postcoital bleeding, foul-smelling bloodstained discharge, postmenopausal bleeding, and irregular vaginal bleeding. In abnormal bleeding in pregnancy cervical pathology needs to be ruled out.
- In very early cases, the disease may be asymptomatic and detected by abnormal cervical cytology.
- Late cases present with pelvic/leg pain, backache, hematuria, edema of the lower legs, malaise, and weight loss.
- Invasion of the parametrium may involve the ureters leading to ureteric obstruction and renal failure.
- Bone and nerve involvement causes severe pain. Involvement of the lymphatics causes intractable edema of the legs.
- Involvement of the bladder causes dysuria, frequency, and hematuria.
- Involvement of the bowels causes tenesmus, diarrhea, and rectal bleeding.
- Fistula formation may occur between the bladder or bowel and the vagina.
- Death occurs from uremia following ureteric obstruction or from hemorrhage and sepsis.

Examinations and investigations

Physical examination includes checking the supraclavicular glands, inguinal glands, and palpation of the abdomen to detect any organomegaly (liver/kidney). In early cases, colposcopic examination is required to visualize suspicious features such as atypical vessels, intense aceto-whiteness, and/or raised/ulcerated surfaces. Diagnosis is based on histology. Sufficient material for histological assessment should be obtained by cone/wedge biopsy. Bimanual examination may reveal a hard irregular friable cervix. The cervix becomes fixed as tumor invades the parametrium. Rectal examination has to be done to assess parametrial and posterior spread. The tumor may grow within the endocervix, producing barrel-shaped cylindrical enlargement of the cervix.

Routine examination includes CBC, urea and electrolytes, liver function tests, chest X-ray, and intravenous pyelogram (IVP).

Examination under anesthesia, including rectal examination, should be done for proper staging. Cystoscopy and proctoscopy/sigmoidoscopy should be done in cases that are suspected to have locally advanced disease. In selected cases, lymphangiography may be needed. In all cases, diagnosis is established histologically by biopsy of the tumor.

Recommended further reading

1. FIGO (International Federation of Gynecology and Obstetrics) (1994). *FIGO Annual Report on the Results of Treatment in Gynecologic Cancer*, Vol. 24. FIGO, London.

Treatment of cervical carcinoma

Microinvasive disease

For stage Ia1 disease, local excisions by cone biopsy may be done, especially in young women who want to preserve fertility. In older women who have completed their family, a total hysterectomy is performed. Treatment of stage Ia2 with marked lymphatic space involvement includes radical hysterectomy or hysterectomy with lympadenectomy or hysterectomy with radiotherapy.

Invasive disease

Treatment of invasive disease involves surgery or radiotherapy or a combination of both. Surgery is preferred in younger patients with stage Ib with low-volume tumors as it allows conservation of ovaries, fewer bowel and bladder problems than with radiotherapy, and preservation of a more normal vagina. Radiotherapy is used for bulky stage Ib and IIa, advanced cases, and also in older and surgically unfit patients.

- *Surgery*. Radical hysterectomy and pelvic node dissection (Wertheim's hysterectomy) include removal of the uterus, upper third of the vagina, and internal and external iliac and obturator lymph nodes. In older women, bilateral salpingo-oophorectomy is done, but the ovaries may be conserved and may be placed outside the field of radiotherapy, should it be needed. Complications include hemorrhage, infection, damage to urinary or intestinal tracts, and, postoperatively, pulmonary embolism, atonic bladder, and fistula of the urinary tract.
- *Radiotherapy* is given by intracavity and external beam irradiation. Intracavity irradiation gives effective treatment to the cervix and surrounding tissues, and external beam irradiation is used to control spread within the pelvis, especially to lymph nodes. Complications of radiotherapy include diarrhea, colicky abdominal pain, and urinary symptoms. Late complications include subacute obstruction, diarrhea due to radiation colitis, hematuria due to radiation cystitis, and, rarely, vesicovaginal fistula.
- *Chemotherapy* as single-agent (cisplatin, bleomycin, methotrexate) and combination regimens with either radiotherapy or surgery has been used. The use of neoadjuvant chemotherapy and radiotherapy has not resulted in improved survival.
- *Combination of surgery and radiotherapy*. Postoperative radiotherapy is considered if multiple lymph nodes are involved or the resection margin was inadequate or in cases of large tumor volume. This reduces the incidence of pelvic recurrence. Preoperative intracavity radiotherapy followed by surgery has not shown improved survival.

Special cases

- The management of cancer of the cervix in pregnancy depends on the stage of the disease, gestational age, and the patient's wishes. Before 24 weeks, treatment is the same as that for nonpregnant women and after that treatment may be delayed to allow fetal maturity. Treatment of carcinoma of the cervix after simple hysterectomy depends on the stage. Usually pelvic irradiation followed by vault irradiation is given. Alternatively, the parametrium, upper vagina, and pelvic lymph nodes are removed surgically.
- Treatment of cancer of the cervix in cervical stump is by radiotherapy.
- Recurrent cervical cancer following surgery is managed by radiotherapy.
- In postradiation failures or in local recurrence involving bladder or rectum, pelvic exenteration is offered to suitable surgical candidates.
- New procedures such as radical trachylectomy (removing cervix and paracervical tissue) after a meticulous lymph node dissection are being evaluated. This procedure is for women with early ectocervical disease so that they have a chance to have children.

Results of treatment

- The overall 5 year survival rate in stage Ib following surgery is around 82%.
- In good radiotherapy centers, the figures are 80% (stage I), 61% (stage II), 32% (stage III), and 15% (stage IV).

Follow-up

All patients need follow-up for reassurance, symptomatic relief, psychosexual counseling, hormone replacement therapy in younger patients, evaluation of treatment, and early detection of recurrence.

Ovarian cancer

In developed countries, there is an incidence of 18 in 100 000 women per year. There is a 1.3% risk of developing the disease by the age of 74. Ovarian carcinoma is the fifth most common cause of cancer in women in developed countries, but the fourth most common cause of death from cancer. It is rare under the age of 30. The incidence increases with age, but reaches a plateau of 60 in 100 000 women per year after the age of 65. About 6% of all ovarian cysts are malignant.

Etiology

- One percent of cases of ovarian cancer occur in women with a family history of two or more affected first-degree relatives (mother or sister). In most of these families, a predisposition to breast and ovarian cancer is inherited in an autosomal dominant manner by an abnormal tumor suppressor gene (*BRCA1*) located on chromosome 17.
- Carriers of the abnormal gene have an up to 70% lifetime risk of developing cancer. Other family members can be tested once the site of the defect has been determined. Women with a single affected relative have a two- to threefold increased risk.
- The majority of cases are sporadic and the cause is unknown.
- The relative risk of epithelial tumors is increased in nulliparous women and those with infertility, late menopause, and early menarche. There may be an increased risk after treatment for infertility using drugs to induce ovulation if pregnancy does not occur. The risk is reduced by use of the combined oral contraceptive pill (up to 60%) and having children (up to 40%).
- Abnormal ovarian development, such as the streak gonads seen in Turner's syndrome, is associated with an increased risk of dysgerminomas.

Pathology

Epithelial tumours

Epithelial ovarian cancer (EOC) accounts for 85% of all ovarian cancers. The tumors may be undifferentiated or lined by epithelium which resembles that seen elsewhere in the female genitourinary tract. The most common types are the following:

- *Serous cystadenocarcinomas* (40%) are usually unilocular cysts containing serous fluid lined by ciliated columnar epithelium in papillary fronds with solid areas. They are bilateral in 30% of cases.
- *Mucinous cystadenocarciomas* (10%) are more often multilocular, mucin-filled, and lined by columnar glandular cells. They are associated with tumors of the appendix and gall-bladder. Rupture of a mucinous cyst may disseminate mucin-secreting cells, leading to a build-up of mucinous fluid in the abdomen (pseudomyxoma peritonei) requiring interval laparotomy to clear.
- *Endometrioid cystadenocarcinomas* (20%) resemble endometrial adenocarcinoma (associated in 15% of cases).

- *Clear cell (mesonephroid) cystadenocarcinomas* (5%) are thin-walled unilocular tumors with cells characterized by clear cytoplasm. These are the most common tumors found in association with endometriosis.
- *Borderline tumors or tumors of low malignant potential* comprise 10% of EOC and can occur in any of the above epithelial types, although mucinous borderline tumors are the most common. They are characterized by cellular atypia with increased mitosis and multilayering without invasion. The prognosis is much better than that for invasive carcinomas, although late recurrence (>10 years) may occur.

Other tumors

- *Sex cord stromal tumors* (6%) are usually of low-grade malignancy.
  - They include granulosa cell tumors, the most common estrogen-producing tumors (menstrual problems, postmenopausal bleeding, precocious puberty), and Sertoli–Leydig cell tumors, the most common androgen-producing lesions (amenorrhea, hirsutism, virilization).
- Fibromas are solid fibrous tissue tumors that may be associated with pleural effusions (Meig's syndrome) and ascites, but are benign.
- *Germ cell tumors* (2–3%). Teratomas contain multiple tissue types including hair, teeth, and skin. Mature cystic teratomas or dermoid cysts are more common and benign. Teratomas may be hormonally active (hCG, AFP, thyroxine). Immature teratomas are solid, malignant, unilateral, and heterogeneous. The prognosis depends on the amount of embryonal tissue present and degrees of atypia. Other malignant tumors are rare and include dysgerminomas, which are solid nodular tumors similar to seminomas of the testis, ectodermal sinus tumors (yolk sac tumours), which may produce AFP, and nongestational choriocarcinomas, which secrete hCG. They usually occur in women under 30.
- *Secondary tumors* comprise 6% of presentations. The most common primary sites are breast, stomach (Krukenberg), and colon.

Recommended further reading

1. FIGO (International Federation of Gynecology and Obstetrics) (1994). *FIGO Annual Report on the Results of Treatment in Gynecologic Cancer*, Vol. 24. FIGO, London.

Presentation, management, and prognosis of ovarian cancer

Ovarian carcinoma commonly remains asymptomatic until late in the course of the disease and is detected as a mass on pelvic examination. Where symptoms do occur, these are due to distension, torsion or bleeding (causing pain), pressure effects on adjacent structures, and hormone effects (postmenopausal bleeding, virilization). The staging of ovarian cancer is given in Table 18.2.

Screening and diagnosis

Pelvic examination is of no proven value as a method of screening for ovarian carcinoma. Transvaginal ultrasound with or without tumor marker measurement (CA-125) can be used to detect early-stage asymptomatic disease. However, the value of routine screening in reducing mortality from ovarian carcinoma remains unproven.

Diagnosis is on the basis of the clinical findings of a solid or cystic mass arising from the pelvis. The uterus is felt separately. There may be associated ascites. Arrange an ultrasound to exclude other causes of pelvic mass such as fibroids and to look for suspicious features such as solid areas within the cyst or free fluid. A chest X-ray should be done to look for pleural effusions. CT or MRI scans may give an indication of spread, but will not usually alter management. Ovarian carcinoma is associated with increased serum levels of a number of oncofetal proteins of which CA-125 is the most important. However, 15% of EOCs will have normal levels. Blood should be taken for tumor markers, complete blood count, liver function tests, and electrolytes.

Management

Where possible, patients with suspected ovarian cancer should be managed in a specialist gynecological cancer center.

- *Surgery* is the primary method of treatment as well as the method of obtaining histological confirmation of the diagnosis and staging the disease. A laparotomy is performed through a midline incision with careful inspection of the liver and peritoneal surfaces. Washings from the peritoneal cavity or any ascites are sent for cytology. Where possible, a total abdominal hysterectomy and bilateral salpingo-oophorectomy and infracolic omentectomy are performed. The aim is to remove all macroscopic disease, if possible, as this outcome is associated with a better prognosis. If this is not possible, the aim should be to remove as much tumor >2 cm in size as possible. The retroperitoneal lymph nodes are biopsied in women with clinically less than stage IIIc disease. This is controversial, but is performed because up to 20% of clinically 'stage I + II' disease will have positive nodes.

Table 18.2 Staging of ovarian carcinoma

Stage	Description
I	Disease confined to the ovaries (25% of presentations)
Ia	Involving only one ovary
Ib	Involving both ovaries
Ic	Positive cytology or ascites or breaching the capsule of either ovary
II	Confined to pelvis (5–10% presentations)
III	Confined to peritoneal cavity (45% presentations)
IIIa	Micronodular disease outside the pelvis
IIIb	Macroscopic tumor deposits <2 cm
IIIc	Tumor >2 cm or retroperitoneal node involvement
IV	Distant metastases (20% of presentations)

- *Chemotherapy* is given to all patients after surgery, now including those with stage I tumors. The overall response rate is 70–80%. Chemotherapy has improved median survival, but has had minimal effect on overall mortality rates from the disease. Platinum-based drugs (cisplatin/carboplatin 50–100 mg/m^2) give the highest response rates. Addition of other agents in primary chemotherapy does not appear to give better results, although it does increase morbidity. Treatment is given at intervals of 3–4 weeks for 6 months (but stop if no response after 3 months). Side effects are nausea, bone marrow suppression, neurotoxicity, renal toxicity (with cisplatin to reduce risks, prehydrate), and neuropathy. Carboplatin is less toxic and is less likely to require hospital admission. Leukopenia and thrombocytopenia are the dose-limiting side-effects.
- Radiotherapy is used in some centers.

Follow-up/recurrence

The routine use of second-look operations does not improve survival. Follow-up is usually for 5 years at intervals of 3–12 months. A rising serum CA-125 has high predictive value for recurrence with a 3–6 month lead-time over clinical signs. CT/ultrasound scanning is of value in assessing response to treatment and identifying localized recurrence. The prognosis for recurrent disease is poor, although it is more likely to respond to further chemotherapy if it occurs more than 3 years after original diagnosis or if the previous treatment did not include platinum. Better response rates in recurrent disease may be obtained with other drugs such as paclitaxel. Surgery may be palliative for obstruction or isolated recurrences.

Prognosis

Prognosis depends on stage, differentiation, residual tumor bulk, and chemosensitivity. The 5 year survival for EOC is 30–35% overall with 67% for stage I disease, 51% for stage IIa, 20% for stage III, and 5% for stage IV. The overall survival for germ cell tumors is 77%.

Recommended further reading

1. FIGO (International Federation of Gynecology and Obstetrics) (1994). *FIGO Annual Report on the Results of Treatment in Gynecologic Cancer*, Vol. 24. FIGO, London.

Endometrial cancer

Introduction

Endometrial cancer, or cancer of the body of the uterus, is the second most common gynecological cancer (approximately 14 in 100 000 cases per year). The incidence of endometrial cancer worldwide is on the increase, which reflects the impact of the age structure of the Western population as it is four to five times more common in Western industrialized countries than in the developing countries of Southeast Asia. Furthermore, the reduction in the incidence of cervical cancer has also contributed to the prominence of endometrial cancer. Endometrial cancer is predominantly a disease of postmenopausal women; most cases occurr in the sixth and seventh decades, with less than 5% of cases in women under 40 years of age. The lifetime risk of developing endometrial cancer is 1.1%, while the lifetime risk of dying of endometrial cancer is 0.4%, reflecting the good prognosis of the condition with early diagnosis.

Risk factors

- *Age* This is principally a disease of postmenopausal women with peak incidence in the age group 65–75 years, with less than 5% of cases occurring in women under 40 years of age.
- *Excessive endogenous estrogens* This is the common pathway shared by most of the common risk factors such as early menarche (before age 12), late menopause (after age 52), obesity, nulliparity, and/or continuous anovulation associated with polycystic ovarian syndrome.
    - An important source of extra-ovarian estrogens in postmenopausal women is the aromatization of adrenal androgens in fat tissue. Thus it is not surprising that endometrial cancer is more common in obese postmenopausal women.
    - A rare sex cord stromal tumor of the ovary, a granulosa-theca cell tumor, also produces endogenous estrogens and is associated with endometrial hyperplasia and endometrial carcinoma in 10% of cases.
    - There may also be an increased risk in women with cirrhosis of the liver due to decreased degradation of estrogens.
    - Endometrial hyperplasia, excessive proliferation of the endometrial glands and to a lesser extent of the endometrial stroma, is thought to be due to excessive endometrial estrogen stimulation. The severity of endometrial hyperplasia is divided into simple, complex, or atypical and may progress to well-differentiated endometrial carcinoma. The risks associated with simple and complex hyperplasia are in the region of 1–3%, while hyperplasia with cytological and architectural atypia is associated with a 23% risk of endometrial carcinoma over 10 years.
- *Unopposed estrogen therapy* in postmenopausal women increases the risk of endometrial carcinoma six- to eight fold as first observed in the 1970s. The addition of 10–14 days of progestogens at least every 3 months significantly reduce this risk.

- *Tamoxifen* is an antiestrogen widely used in the treatment of postmenopausal breast cancer, but it also has weak estrogenic action on the genital tract. It is associated with a twofold increase in the risk of endometrial cancer when used for 5 years or more. It is also associated with increased risks of developing other benign endometrial changes such as hyperplasia and polyps.
- *Miscellaneous.* There appears to be a higher risk of endometrial cancer in women with breast, ovarian (endometrium type), and colorectal cancers.

Presentation and investigations of endometrial cancer

Presentation

- The most common presenting symptom of endometrial cancer is postmenopausal bleeding.
- Endometrial cancer may also present with postmenopausal vaginal discharge or pyometra.
- Endometrial cancer should also be excluded in peri- or premenopausal women with persistent intermenstrual bleeding or polymenorrhea, especially if the latter fails to respond to hormonal treatments.
- It is also important to consider endometrial carcinoma as part of the differential diagnosis of asymptomatic women with glandular abnormalities on routine cervical cytology.
- Over 90% of women with endometrial cancer will present with vaginal bleeding, and 7–10% of women with postmenopausal bleeding may turn out to have the disease.
- Advanced disease may present with symptoms attributable to local and distant metastases or paraneoplastic syndromes.

Pathology

Endometrial carcinomas are predominantly (80–85%) endometrioid adenocarcinomas, which at the well-differentiated end of the spectrum may be difficult to distinguish from complex endometrial hyperplasia. Within adenocarcinomas there may be foci of squamous metaplasia, which, where benign, are known as adenoacanthomas and, where malignant, are referred to as adenosquamous carcinoma.

Approximately 10% of endometrial carcinomas are papillary serous type, and 4% are clear cell carcinomas. Both these subtypes are associated with more aggressive tumors and poorer prognosis and, despite their relative infrequency, account for 50% of treatment failures. They are both similar to tumors found in the ovaries and fallopian tubes and tend to spread in a fashion akin to that of ovarian cancer.

Spread

Endometrial cancer spreads directly through the endometrial cavity to the cervix and through the fallopian tubes to the ovaries and peritoneal cavity. The tumor invades and infiltrates the myometrium, reaching the serosal surface and parametria. Very rarely, there may be direct invasion of the pubic bones.

Lymphatic spread is to pelvic and para-aortic nodes, the former being more common. Although para-aortic node involvement may occur in the absence of pelvic node involvement, pelvic node involvement when para-aortic nodes are involved is the more likely finding. Inguinal node involvement is a rare finding.

Hematogenous spread is rare, but may occur to the lungs.

Investigations

All women with symptoms and signs suggestive of or suspicious of endometrial carcinoma should be investigated. In the past, the gold standard was a dilatation and curettage (D&C) to obtain an endometrial sample for histopathological assessment. This has the shortfall that it is performed 'blindly' and therefore randomly samples a proportion of the uterine cavity, potentially missing isolated foci of disease.

- The current gold standard is a combination of visualization of the cavity by hysteroscopy combined with targeted endometrial biopsy either as an outpatient/local anesthetic procedure or under a general anesthesia.
- Alternatives to hysteroscopy and directed biopsy include a combination of outpatient endometrial sampling with a pipelle (randomly samples a small proportion of the cavity) in combination with assessment of the uterine cavity by means of transvaginal ultrasound to assess endometrial thickness, homogeneity, and the presence of fluid or polyps within the cavity as well as presence of ovarian masses. A transvaginal ultrasound indicating a thin midline homogeneous endometrium less than 5 mm in thickness has a high negative predictive value.
- Ultrasound also has a role in assessing the depth of endometrial invasion in cases of confirmed endometrial cancer, but MRI is superior in this respect as it assesses cervical involvement and metastases to pelvic and para-aortic nodes.
- In confirmed cases of endometrial cancer, a chest radiograph is essential to exclude pulmonary spread.

Treatment of endometrial cancer

Surgery

The treatment of choice for patients with early (stages I and II) disease is a total abdominal hysterectomy and bilateral salpingo-oophorectomy (TAH + BSO). The exceptions to this are patients who are medically unfit or a very high surgical risk, in whom radical radiotherapy may be the chosen mode of treatment accepting that surgery with or without radiotherapy offers a better prognosis than radiotherapy alone. For patients with clinical stage III or IV disease, radical radiotherapy with or without hormonal manipulation and/or chemotherapy is the standard mode of therapy. Patients with stage III disease may sometimes be suitable for radical surgery, and therefore treatment should be individualized aiming to perform TAH + BSO and maximally debulk the disease followed by radiotherapy.

Lymphadenectomy is not typically performed at the time of TAH + BSO for endometrial cancer. This is because the extent of optimum lymph node dissection remains unclear and this procedure significantly increases the morbidity in a generally unfit group of patients. The morbidity and effectiveness of complete pelvic lymphadenectomy in women with endometrial cancer is currently being evaluated.

Radiotherapy

In practice, most patients with early disease receive a combination of surgery and radiotherapy after review of any adverse features of the operative and histopathological findings. Patients who are treated by surgery alone are limited to those where the carcinoma is of endometrioid type, confined to less than 50% of the myometrial thickness, and is grade 1 or 2 (well or moderately differentiated). The widely used radiotherapy regime involves a combination of high-dose intracavitary brachytherapy to reduce risk of vault recurrence and 25 fractions of low-dose external beam radiotherapy to reduce the risk of pelvic recurrence. Radiotherapy may also be used in the palliative setting with advanced disease to control vaginal bleeding and bone pain.

Hormone therapy

Progestogens are the most commonly used form of hormonal therapy in endometrial cancer. They have no role in the prevention of recurrence, but their main contribution is to the management of recurrent disease with a response rate of up to 30% (higher in estrogen and progesterone receptor positive tumors) reported using medroxyprogesterone acetate (MPA) in doses of 200–400 mg daily. Other hormonal agents which have been reported to have limited roles in achieving a response include gonadotrophin-releasing hormone (GnRH) analogs and tamoxifen.

Chemotherapy

The use of chemotherapy in endometrial cancer is uncommon, but should be considered in fit patients with systemic disease. Drugs with response rates of 25–30% include epirubicin and doxorubicin (anthracyclines) and cisplatin or carboplatin (platinum drugs), either alone or in combination, but their responses are partial and short-lived and their use may be limited by a patient's advanced age and poor performance status.

Recommended further reading

1. Green JA, Kirwan JM, Tierney JF, *et al.* (2001). Survival and recurrence after concomitant chemotherapy and radiotherapy for cancer of the uterine cervix: a systematic review and meta-analysis. *Lancet* **358**, 781–6.
2. Humber C, Tierney J, Symonds P, *et al.* (2005). Chemotherapy for advanced, recurrent or metastatic endometrial carcinoma. *Cochrane Database Syst Rev* **3**, CD003915.

Prognosis of endometrial cancer

Prognostic factors

- *Stage* The overall survival is affected by stage at diagnosis. Stage I disease is associated with a 72% overall survival, dropping to 56%, 32%, and 11% moving up from stages II, III, and IV, respectively. Table 18.3 gives the staging of endometrial cancer.
- *Depth of myometrium invasion* The depth of myometrial involvement is reflected in the subclassification of stage I disease (see Table 18.3). The depth of myometrial invasion correlates well with pelvic and para-aortic lymph node involvement in early disease. There is also a close correlation between tumor grade and depth of myometrial invasion.
- *Tumor grade* As tumor grade increases (the tumor becoming less differentiated), the risk of associated myometrial invasion and lymph node involvement increases. Thus 90% of grade 1 tumors will be limited to the endometrium or inner half of the myometrium, while almost half of the grade 3 tumors will be found invading the outer half of the myometrium. Tumors are graded as follows:
  - Grade 1. Well differentiated tumors have less than 5% squamous solid growth pattern.
  - Grade 2. Moderately differentiated tumors have 6–50% solid squamous growth pattern.
  - Grade 3. Poorly differentiated tumors have >50% solid squamous growth pattern.

The presence of nuclear atypia in addition to the growth pattern raises grade 1 and 2 tumours to the next grade.

- *Histological type* Endometrioid adenocarcinomas have the best prognosis, while clear cell and papillary cell tumors are associated with a poorer prognosis. Over 70% of endometrial cancers are positive for estrogen and progesterone receptors. Absence of receptors is associated with a poorer prognosis.
- *Lymphovascular space involvement* appears to be an important prognostic factor in terms of survival and disease recurrence for stage I disease.

Table 18.3 Staging of endometrial cancer

Stage	Description
I	Disease confined to the body of the uterus
Ia	Carcinoma confined to the endometrium
Ib	Myometrial invasion <50%
Ic	Myometrial invasion >50%
II	Cervix involved
IIa	Endocervical gland involvement only
IIb	Cervical stromal invasion but does not extend beyond the uterus
III	Spread to serosa of uterus, peritoneal cavity, or lymph nodes
IIIa	Carcinoma involving serosa of uterus or adnexae, positive ascites, or positive peritoneal washings
IIIb	Vaginal involvement either direct or metastatic
IIIc	Para-aortic or pelvic node involvement
IV	Local or distant metastases
IVa	Carcinoma involving the mucosa of the bladder or rectum
IVb	Distant metastases and involvement of other abdominal or inguinal lymph nodes

Prognosis

The 5 year survival rates for endometrial cancer by stage are as follows:

- Stage I, 75%
- Stage II, 58%
- Stage III, 30%
- Stage IV, 10%

The overall 5 year survival for the disease is around 70%, reflecting the fact that the majority of endometrial cancers present early because of abnormal vaginal bleeding.

Premalignant disease of the vulva

Introduction

Although premalignant lesions of the vulva (vulval intraepithelial neoplasia (VIN)) are seen most commonly in postmenopausal women, about 40% of cases are seen in premenopausal women. The vulval skin is part of the anogenital epithelium which extends from the perianal skin and perineum to the cervix. Multiple foci of dysplasia are seen when there are neoplastic changes of the vulval skin. Viral etiological factors such as human papillomavirus (HPV) are thought to be involved, but their role is uncertain at present.

Pathology

The International Society for the Study of Vulvar Diseases have standardized the reporting of vulval dysplastic lesions as VIN1, 2, or 3 depending on the degree of loss of cellular maturation. This has replaced older and more confusing terminology such as Bowen's disease, Bowenoid papulosis, and erythroplasia of Queyrat. Dysplasia of the vulva is multicentric. Vulval dysplasia is usually squamous VIN, although adenocarcinoma *in situ* (Paget's disease) can rarely occur on the vulva. The histological features and terminology of VIN are the same as those of cervical intraepithelial neoplasia (CIN), and the histology of Paget's disease is similar to that of the lesions seen in the breast.

Presenting features

The most common presenting symptom is pruritus. However, VIN may be asymptomatic and detected only during treatment of the preinvasive/invasive lesions of the cervix/lower genital tract. The lesions may be raised or flat, single or multiple, and diffuse or discrete. They may form papules. The color is variable: white in cases of hyperkeratinization, red due to thinness of the epithelium, or dark brown due to increased melanin deposition in epithelial cells.

Diagnosis

Careful inspection of the local area is needed to identify the full extent of the disease. This is helped by application of 5% acetic acid. The changes may be seen by naked eye, but it becomes easier if a colposcope is used. VIN lesions turn white, and mosaicism or punctation may be visible. An abnormal vascular pattern is associated with a severe degree of VIN/invasive disease. Toluidine blue is sometimes used as a nuclear stain. As mentioned earlier, because of VIN's developmental origin, a thorough colposcopic evaluation of the cervix and upper vagina needs to be done. Frequently, condyloma of the genital tract is associated with these lesions.

Adequate biopsies must be taken from abnormal areas to rule out invasive disease. This can usually be done in an outpatient clinic with a Keyes or 4 mm Stiefel punch biopsy. Microscopic appearances are characterized by cellular disorganization and loss of stratification depending on the grade of the lesion. Cellular changes involve size variability, multinucleated and giant cells, numerous mitotic figures, and hyperchromatinism.

Treatment

The treatment of VIN poses some problems such as the multifocal nature of the disease and the discomfort and mutilation from the therapy, especially in young patients. However, it must be remembered that VIN 3 may progress to vulvar cancer if not treated. The incidence of unifocal lesions is higher in older women, whereas multifocal lesions are more common in younger women.

- Excision of a small lesion may be both diagnostic and therapeutic.
- Multifocal lesions and lesions covering wide areas may need skinning vulvectomy with or without skin grafting or simple vulvectomy.
- Carbon dioxide laser treatment is an alternative to surgical excision, but careful control of the depth of destruction is essential for a good cosmetic result. The depth of treatment required in VIN is not clear, and hair follicle involvement makes this treatment unsuitable. In some cases, treatment of the whole vulva to such a depth will cause third-degree burns.
- The purpose of medical treatment is to relieve the symptoms. If invasion has been excluded, topical fluorodinated steroids are used, but not for more than 6 months.
  - Topical 5-fluorouracil (5-FU) therapy is painful and hyperkeratotic lesions do not respond.
  - Topical α-interferon therapy has also been tried.

VIN is becoming more common in younger women. Careful observation and treatment should be tailored to suit individual cases.

Follow-up

Recurrence has been noted in both surgical and laser-treated cases and thus follow-up is needed. Regular follow-ups with colposcopy every 6 months are needed until the patient is disease free for 2 years.

Vulval cancer

Carcinoma of the vulva is a relatively uncommon gynecological cancer. Its annual incidence is around 3 in 100 000 women per year. It is common in the elderly, with a peak incidence at around 65 and one-third of all patients are more than 70 years old. Eighty-five to ninety percent of these cancers are squamous and less common lesions are melanoma, basal cell carcinoma, carcinoma of the Bartholin gland, Paget's disease, sarcoma, and metastatic carcinoma.

Not much is known about its etiology, but viral factors have been suggested (HPV 16/18 and herpes simplex virus 2 (HSV2)). However, this cancer has been associated with smoking, immunosuppression, and a history of cervical neoplasia.

Clinical presentation

The most common symptom is longstanding vulval pruritus. Vulval pain, discharge, and bleeding are less frequently reported. Most commonly (66%), the tumor involves the labia majora and in the rest of the cases it involves the clitoris, labia minora, posterior fourchette, and perineum. The lesions may be exophytic, ulcerated, or flat. The incidence of complicating medical disease (diabetes, obesity, hypertension) is greater in the older age group. Younger patients have more chance of having multicentric disease. Frequently, patients delay reporting the symptoms or any abnormality they have seen. Sometimes physicians delay in referring cases. Performing vulval biopsy in suspected lesions is important for appropriate management.

Route of spread

The tumor spreads by the lymphatic system to the regional lymph nodes and locally to involve the adjoining organs (vagina, urethra, anal canal, clitoris, etc.). Blood spread occurs if the tumor involves blood vessels. The lymph drains from the vulva to the superficial inguinal nodes initially and then to the inguinofemoral chain and on to the pelvic nodes. In general, central vulvar structures drain bilaterally, whereas lateral structures drain to nodes on the same side. Deep pelvic nodes may be involved from the clitoris and central vulvar structures, but involvement of the deep glands in the absence of inguinal node disease is very rare.

Differential diagnosis

Ulcerative lesions on the vulva may be due to sexually transmitted diseases, benign or malignant tumors, or viral infections. Tumors of the vulva are diagnosed by biopsy and excision. The groin nodes may require fine-needle aspiration biopsy or preferably excision biopsy to establish a histological diagnosis. Usually this is done after establishing the diagnosis of the primary lesion.

Assessment and staging

As this tumor is multicentric in nature, a thorough inspection of the cervix, vagina, and adjoining organs should be made. Cervical cytology and chest X-ray are required and, at times, an IVP, lymphangiography, ultrasonography (including Doppler studies), and MRI may be used. Examination under anesthesia including the groin nodes and a full-thickness generous biopsy of the primary lesion are the most important diagnostic measures. Cystoscopy and barium enema may be needed in some cases. Apart from review by an anesthesiologist, examination by an internal medicine specialist is required if there are concomitant medical problems. The FIGO staging of vulval cancer is given in Table 18.4.

Table 18.4 FIGO staging of vulval cancer

Stage	Description
0	Carcinoma *in situ* intraepithelial cancers
I	Tumor confined to vulva or perineum or both; 2 cm or less in greatest diameter (no nodal metastasis)
Ia	Stromal invasion no greater than 1.0 mm
Ib	Stromal invasion greater than 1.0 mm
II	Tumor confined to vulva or perineum or both; more than 2 cm in greatest diameter (no nodal metastasis)
III	Tumor of any size with one or both of the following: (1) adjacent spread to the lower urethra, the vagina, and the anus; (2) unilateral regional lymph node metastasis
IVa	Tumor invading any of the upper urethra, bladder mucosa, rectal mucosa, or pelvic bones, or bilateral regional node metastasis
IVb	Any distant metastasis including pelvic lymph nodes

Treatment and prognosis of vulval cancer

Prognostic factors

The main prognostic factor is the condition of the inguinofemoral nodes. Five year survival declines with positive nodes (from 90% in node-negative to 58% in node-positive cases). Other factors include depth of invasion, tumor diameter, tumor differentiation, lymph–vascular space involvement, margin status, and the number of nodes involved.

Treatment

- *Surgery* is the primary treatment of cancer of vulva. The principle is wide excision (healthy margin) of the tumor and extirpation of the potential route of spread (radical vulvectomy and regional lymphadenectomy). This involves a large area of skin. Modifications to this include doing simple vulvectomy and vertical groin incision to reduce morbidity rather than butterfly incisions where lymph-bearing tissues and vulva are removed in continuity.
  - Regional lymphadenectomy involves bilateral superficial and deep inguinal lymph nodes.
  - Ipsilateral lymphadenectomy may be considered in a relatively small lesion in the midportion of the labia and when all nodes examined are negative.
  - If superficial lymphadenectomy of inguinal nodes is negative by thorough sampling, deep inguinal lymphadenectomy may be avoided to reduce the morbidity of the operation.
  - However, cases must be selected very thoroughly whenever modifications to radical vulvectomy and regional lymphadenectomy are made as reports of recurrence have been noted with devastating results.
- *Radiotherapy* Improvements in radiotherapy technique with the use of megavoltage external beam therapy and the judicious use of electrons and brachytherapy have now resulted in its use in vulval cancer. Radiotherapy has been used preoperatively when the tumor is large and in advanced cases where the tumor involves or is very close to the vagina, urethra, or anus. Postoperatively, it is used for groin node diseases after inguinofemoral lymphadenectomy and to prevent vulval local recurrence in cases with insufficient tumor-free margin.
- *Chemotherapy* 5-FU and mitomycin-C have produced encouraging results. They are used as radiosensitizers.

Morbidities

The most frequent complication of radical surgical treatment is wound breakdown (50%). Other complications include lymphedema of the lower extremities, lymphocyst formation in the groin, development of rectocele and cystocele due to lack of pelvic ligament support, and loss of body image and impaired sexual function.

Recurrent disease

The outcome of recurrent disease is poor. Treatment is usually palliative in the form of radiotherapy or combined with chemotherapy. In selected cases, surgical excision of the recurrence can be done. Both single-agent and combined therapy have been used.

Follow-up

All patients need follow-up, though prognosis depends on the adverse prognostic factors present in the case. A 5 year survival of 75% should be expected after surgical treatment of invasive squamous cancer. Five year survival rates are as follows: stage I, 97%; stage II, 85%; stage III, 74%; stage IV, 30%.

Paget's disease of the vulva

Paget's disease of the vulva is of apocrine origin and is confined to the epithelium in most cases. Invasive disease is present in 15–25% of cases either as underlying apocrine gland adenocarcinoma or breach of the basement membrane. It is not a common tumor. Pruritus is the most common presenting complaint. Velvety-red discoloration with development of eczemoid changes and white plaques is usually seen. Diagnosis is made by biopsy. Histology shows large pale cells, often in nests, infiltrating upward in the hyperkeratotic epithelium. It occurs with other malignancies (15–25%), and the most common organs involved are breast, genitalia, and underlying adnexae. Treatment involves wide local excision in intraepithelial cases, but in invasive cases radical surgery like that for squamous cell carcinoma is needed.

Other tumors of the vulva

The other vulval tumors include melanoma, basal cell carcinoma, Bartholin gland carcinoma, verrucous carcinoma, Merkel cell cancer, and, very rarely, sarcoma and metastatic tumors. The mainstay of the treatment is wide local excision and lymphadenectomy, depending on the type of the cancer. Bartholin gland tumours are radiosensitive. Sarcomas are treated by vulvectomy and groin node dissection.

Conclusion

Vulval cancers are more common in elderly people. Surgery is the cornerstone of the treatment, and efforts are made to reduce the morbidity from surgery and to improve the modalities of chemo/radiotherapy.

Recommended further reading

1. van der Welden K, Ansink A (2001). Primary groin irradiation vs primary groin surgery for early vulvar cancer. *Cochrane Database Syst Rev* **4**, CD002224.

Vulval pain

Introduction

The moist hair-bearing and delicate skin of the vulva is vulnerable to many nonspecific microbe-induced inflammations and dermatological disorders. The vulva has a rich somatic nerve supply and responds to acute stimuli, which are well perceived with exquisite sensitivity. The sensations experienced vary from the pain of trauma to the itching and irritation due to inflammatory or infective causes. The majority of women presenting with vulval symptoms will complain of pruritus, but a significant number will complain of burning pain of the vulva or rawness. Often, no obvious cause is demonstrated and this can be a perplexing problem for both the patient and clinician.

Causes of vulval pain

- Infection
- Dermatoses (discussed below under the heading 'Causes of pruritus')
- Vulvodynia
- Urinary tract disorders
- Malignant disease

Infections

Herpes simplex virus

The primary attack usually presents with an extremely painful vulval ulceration together with generalized malaise, fever, and inguinal lymphadenopathy. Intact vesicles may be visible. Recurrences are not uncommon and can be of variable severity. Sometimes the patient only complains of mild vulval itching and soreness which is dismissed and treated as thrush, particularly if the primary attack was missed. An acute attack should be treated with oral and topical acyclovir (oral dose of 200 mg five times daily for 5 days). Acyclovir may be used on a long-term basis to prevent recurrences.

Other causes

Other causes such as candidiasis, syphilis, gonococcal vulvovaginitis, tropical infections such as lymphogranuloma venereum caused by certain subtypes of *Chlamydia trachomatis*, and chancroid caused by *Haemophilus ducreyi* can all give rise to vulval ulceration and pain (see Chapter 14 📖 *p.500*).

Vulvodynia

Vulvodynia is a syndrome of unexplained vulval pain often coupled with sexual dysfunction and psychological disability. The pain is often described by the patient as a burning, stinging irritation and/or rawness. The pain characteristically occurs in response to stretching or pressure. The following types or subsets of vulvodynia can occur alone, simultaneously, or sequentially.

Cyclic vulvodynia

Vulval symptoms which recur in association with menstruation or coitus may be due to changes in vaginal pH. This creates an environment susceptible to infection, e.g. candidosis, bacterial vaginosis, or genital herpes. The clinical features are vulval itching and soreness that is sometimes cyclical, being worse in the luteal phase. Sexual intercourse may be uncomfortable at this time or may be associated with pain on the following day. Diagnosis is confirmed by the finding of fungal hyphae. Treatment is usually local clotrimazole or econazole pessary and/or topical application of 2% clotrimazole cream.

Vestibular papillomatosis

Vulvar squamous papillomatosis describes the appearance of multiple tiny filamentous papillae occurring on the vulva in women of all ages. They are usually found in the vestibule and posterior aspect of the introitus, but sometimes cover the entire surface of the labia minora. This is now considered to be a normal variation and of uncertain clinical significance. Most of the women with vulval papillae are asymptomatic. Symptomatic women may require colposcopy to exclude other lesions. They do not themselves require treatment and, in fact, treatment with laser or 5-FU has sometimes led to a new set of painful symptoms.

Vulvar vestibulitis

The criteria for diagnosis are:

- pain on entry or touch
- vestibular erythema
- tenderness on pressure.

This triad of dyspareunia, erythema, and tenderness to touch restricted to the vestibule distinguishes vulvar vestibulitis from vulvitis. Dyspareunia can be a minor nuisance or completely prevent sexual intercourse. The pain experienced by the patient is described as severe burning, whereas itching is not usually present.

The etiology of vulvar vestibulitis remains uncertain. Postulated causes or triggering events include infection (*Candida* in particular), bacterial vaginosis, chlamydial infection, excess urinary oxalate, HPV infection, hypersensitivity reactions, and psychosexual problems. Vulvar vestibulitis is uncommon in the African Caribbean population and is mostly found in Caucasian women aged 30–60 years.

Management depends to some extent upon its severity as many minor cases clear up spontaneously.

- Acute vestibulitis causing sufficient symptoms may be treated medically with the removal of allergen or irritant, the treatment of infection, and local corticosteroid application.
- The chronic condition is more difficult to resolve. Treatment with a topical steroid preparation containing antifungals and antibacterials may relieve symptoms.
- Dyspareunia may respond to the use of a local anesthetic gel, e.g. 5% lidocaine applied 15–30 minutes before intercourse. Surgical excision of the vestibule should be considered as the last resort for patients with significant dyspareunia. However, the results of vestibulectomy are variable and it is not without complications.

Essential vulvodynia

This is characterized by a constant diffuse unremitting burning that may extend into the thigh or buttock. Patients are usually peri- or postmenopausal and have no consistent history of previous trauma or infection. There is no cyclical pattern to the pain, and both dyspareunia and point tenderness are less marked than with vulvar vestibulitis. Essential vulvodynia is of unknown etiology, but is believed to be an altered perception of cutaneous pain rather like postherpetic neuralgia. There are no physical findings as the problem is essentially neural. Treatment is with tricyclic antidepressants such as amitryptyline 10 mg at night, increasing to 50 mg.

Idiopathic vulvodynia

There will be some patients who do not fulfil any of the diagnostic criteria discussed. There may be underlying psychological problems, and psychiatric assessment will provide patients with appropriate support and insight. Even reassurance about the normality of the anatomy can be therapeutic to some women.

Other causes of vulval pain

Urinary tract disorders

Urological disorders, such as urethral mucosa prolapse, urethral syndrome, urethral caruncle, and urogenital sinus syndrome, can give rise to vulval pain. Close cooperation between the referring doctor, the gynecologist, and the urologist is required to treat these conditions.

Malignant diseases

Carcinoma of the vulva represents about 3% of all genital tract cancers in women, occurring especially in women over the age of 60. Approximately 90% of these tumours are squamous cell carcinomas. The remainder are adenocarcinomas, melanomas, or basal cell carcinomas. HPV infection may be an etiological factor. Non-neoplastic epithelial changes, especially lichen sclerosus, can often precede invasive carcinoma of vulva.

Miscellaneous

Musculoskeletal causes of referred pain to the vulva are uncommon. Levator ani myalgia can cause vulval pain and usually responds to NSAIDs. Nerve entrapment or neuroma may result after an episiotomy or the repair of tears sustained during childbirth. It can present with superficial dyspareunia and vulval pain. Pain may be relieved by injection of 0.5% bupivacaine. Pudendal nerve neuralgia may follow an injury caused by certain activities, such as riding, or herpes simplex infection.

Causes of vulval pruritus

Dermatoses

The dermatoses are classified as non-neoplastic epithelial disorders (vulval dystrophies) of the skin and mucosa.

Eczema

Eczema can be considered as synonymous with dermatitis and therefore can have different causes. It may occur elsewhere in the body. Allergic responses to substances such as washing powders, deodorant, or perfume can result in an acutely swollen well-defined area which can be extremely itchy with a burning sensation. Secondary infection can occur, giving rise to offensive discharge. Acute moniliasis is the common differential diagnosis. Referral to a dermatologist is advised for patch-testing. Treatment is by removal of the offending agent(s), and symptom control may be achieved by using soothing applications, emollients, or local corticosteroids.

Lichen sclerosus

Lichen sclerosus is one of the skin conditions of the vulva that causes intense itching and inflammation with secondary excoriation. Characteristically, the skin is white, thin, and wrinkled, and the condition may involve the whole vulva, perineum, and perianal region. Atrophy of the labia minora occurs, often associated with labial fusion, clitoral edema, and introital narrowing. Microscopially, the epithelium is thin with disappearance of rete pegs. This is accompanied by superficial hyperkeratosis and dermal fibrosis with scant perivascular mononuclear infiltrate. It occurs in all age groups, but is most common in postmenopausal women. The pathogenesis is uncertain, but autoimmune reaction is suspected. About 1–4% of cases undergo malignant change, and so regular follow-up with particular attention to the periclitoral area is essential. Diagnosis is made on the basis of the patient's history, physical signs, and, finally, by biopsy. The treatment is with potent topical steroids initially, reducing to a maintenance regimen with moderately potent steroids.

Squamous cell hyperplasia

Previously called hyperplastic dystrophy, this disorder is marked by epithelial thickening and significant surface hyperkeratosis. It presents with itching or vulval pain and appears clinically as an area of leukoplakia. The hyperplastic epithelial changes show no atypia. No increased predisposition to cancer is generally held to be the case but, suspiciously, squamous hyperplasia is often present at the margins of established cancer of the vulva. Treatment is by local application of fluorinated corticosteroids for 4–6 weeks or until symptoms resolve.

Trophoblastic disease

Introduction

This is a group of disorders characterized by abnormal placental development. The chorionic villi are hydropic with vacuolation of the placenta and destruction of the normal stroma. Trophoblastic disorders affect 1.5 in 1000 pregnancies. However, there is considerable geographical variation in incidence, with the highest incidence being in countries of the Far East.

Etiology

Trophoblastic disease is thought to arise by fertilization of the oocyte by a diploid spermatozoon or by two haploid sperm. If this occurs in the absence of any female nuclear material, the resulting conceptus is diploid (46,XX in 90% of cases; 46,XY in the remaining 10%) and is a *complete mole*. If associated with female nuclear material, the conceptus will be triploid and a *partial mole* (typically 69,XXX or 69,XXY). Risk factors are advanced maternal age, a previous history of trophoblastic disease, and blood group A.

Pathology

- *Benign trophoblastic disease* is usually either a complete hydatidiform mole (where there is no evidence of an embryo) or a partial hydatidiform mole (which may be associated with an embryo that is usually abnormal). Other types of trophoblastic disease include invasive moles, placental site reaction, trophoblastic tumor, and hydropic change.
- *Malignant trophoblastic disease* (choriocarcinoma) complicates approximately 3% of complete moles. However, in 50% of cases of choriocarcinoma there is no history of immediately preceding trophoblastic disease. It may also occur following normal pregnancy.

Presentation

Trophoblastic disease typically (50% of cases) presents at about 14 weeks (range 8–24 weeks) with symptoms of vaginal bleeding. It is often diagnosed initially as a threatened miscarriage.

- The uterus is large for dates in 50% of cases.
- Enlarged ovarian theca-lutein cysts (see below) may cause abdominal pain if they rupture or undergo torsion.
- Products of conception containing small vesicles may be passed, and there may be exaggerated pregnancy symptoms such as vomiting and early-onset preeclampsia (20%).
- The high circulating levels of hCG have a TSH-like action and can cause clinical thyrotoxicosis.
- Choriocarcinomas may present with the symptoms of distant metastases (cerebral, pulmonary).

Diagnosis

- Ultrasound.
    - A 'snowstorm' appearance with multiple highly reflective echoes and areas of vacuolation within the uterine cavity suggests molar disease.
    - In a partial mole, a gestational sac with a fetus may also be present.
    - Large ovarian theca-lutein cysts may be present in the ovaries as a result of the high hCG levels and take up to 4 months to resolve after treatment.
- Other imaging such as chest X-rays, CT, or MRI may be indicated to exclude pulmonary or cerebral metastases if choriocarcinoma is suspected.
- The diagnosis of molar disease is usually confirmed by histological examination of products of conception removed at the time of uterine evacuation.
- Histological confirmation of metastatic deposits of choriocarcinoma is not usually required and may be dangerous.
- The diagnosis of metastatic disease is made by a combination of high levels of hCG in the absence of a pregnancy and the characteristic findings of secondary tumors (cannon-ball appearance) on imaging.

Recommended further reading

1. Soper JT, Mutch DG, Schink JC (2004). Diagnosis and treatment of gestational trophoblastic disease. *Gynecol Oncol* **93**, 575–85.
2. American College of Obstetricians and Gynecologists (2004). ACOG Practice Bulletin No. 53. Diagnosis and treatment of gestational trophoblastic disease. *Obstet Gynecol* **103**, 1365–77.

Management and prognosis of trophoblastic disease

Surgery

Evacuation of the uterus is carried out under general anesthesia by an experienced surgeon. Preoperatively, blood should be taken for serum hCG levels, CBC, cross-matching, and urea and electrolytes. The anesthesiologist should be warned about the possibility of thyrotoxicosis (risk of thyroid storm). There is an increased risk of uterine perforation and hemorrhage, and the uterus may be enlarged due to collection of blood. Performing the procedure with an oxytocin infusion running may reduce the risk of hemorrhage, but carries a theoretical risk of dissemination of trophoblastic material into the bloodstream.

If there is persistent bleeding after the initial evacuation or evidence of persistent trophoblast within the uterus on imaging or hCG measurement, repeat evacuation may be performed after 10–14 days. If more than one repeat evacuation is required, the patient should be referred to a specialist center for possible medical treatment.

Follow-up

The aim of follow-up is to detect persistent trophoblastic disease and choriocarcinoma.

- Because all trophoblastic tumors produce hCG, patients can be monitored by measurement of urinary or serum hCG levels.
- These are checked fortnightly until the serum level is less than 2 IU/L and then monthly for 6 months following this if the hCG is negative within 6 weeks of treatment, or for 12 months and then every 3 months for a further year if the hCG takes longer than 6 weeks to become negative.
- Patients should be advised to avoid another pregnancy until at least 6 months after the hCG level is less than 2 IU/L and to avoid using the combined oral contraceptive pill for at least 4 months.

Chemotherapy

All patients requiring chemotherapy should be referred to specialist centers. Indications for treatment are a rising hCG level in the absence of a new pregnancy, an hCG persistently more than 20 000 IU/L by 4 weeks after treatment, persistent symptoms, or evidence of metastatic disease. Methotrexate is the mainstay of treatment (with folinic acid rescue).

Prognosis

- Overall 5 year survival is more than 99%.
- There is a 0.8–2.9% risk of recurrence in subsequent pregnancies after one mole and 15–28% after two moles.
- Patients are more likely to require chemotherapy if the initial hCG level is more than 100 000 IU/L, they are aged over 40, there are associated ovarian cysts, or when early use of the oral contraceptive pill or early pregnancy follows previous trophoblastic disease.

- Subsequent fertility does not appear to be impaired by chemotherapy and there does not seem to be an increased incidence of other chromosomal abnormalities.

Recommended further reading

1. Soper JT, Mutch DG, Schink JC (2004). Diagnosis and treatment of gestational trophoblastic disease. *Gynecol Oncol* **93**, 575–85.
2. American College of Obstetricians and Gynecologists (2004). ACOG Practice Bulletin No. 53. Diagnosis and treatment of gestational trophoblastic disease. *Obstet Gynecol* **103**, 1365–77.

Ovarian cancer chemotherapy

Most chemotherapy is given every 3 weeks, but some types may be given more or less frequently depending upon the nature of the drugs being used. Side effects are common and potentially serious, but may be prevented by a variety of measures.

Side effects

- Leukopenia and thrombocytopenia are common for most regimens and treatment should not be given unless the white cell count is ≥3.0 × 103/mL, the absolute neutrophil count is ≥1.5 × 103/mL, and the platelet count is ≥100 × 103/mL. The nadir count is normally 7–14 days after giving treatment, and it is essential to be aware of the possibility of neutropenic sepsis at this time as this is potentially fatal unless treated very rapidly with IV antibiotics. Granulocyte colony-stimulating factor (GCSF) may prevent leukopenia, but it is expensive.
- Nausea and vomiting can be very distressing, but can generally be controlled with the use of modern antiemetics, such as ondansetron and granisetron, coupled with high-dose dexamethazone and other more conventional oral antiemetics.
- Hair loss is common with many drugs. A hairpiece should be provided for the patient before she loses her hair, which is usually 3 weeks after the start of treatment. Hair grows back in again after 6 months. It usually grows back curly, but reverts to normal after 6 months. Hair loss may be prevented for some drugs by the use of scalp cooling, but this is not effective for doxorubicin and taxol. Cisplatin and carboplatin do not normally give rise to hair loss.
- Anemia: platinum compounds frequently give rise to anemia after three or four cycles and, if symptomatic, the patient can be transfused. Erythropoietin may be used instead of a blood transfusion, but it is expensive.
- Renal toxicity is a potential problem with cisplatin, but can be minimized by hydration before and during therapy and by ensuring an adequate urine flow of at least 100 mL/hour whilst having treatment and for a minimum of 4 hours afterwards. Mannitol may be used to produce this diuresis. Methotrexate is excreted unchanged in the urine, and the dose must be reduced in patients with poor renal function.
- Neurotoxicity is exhibited by those receiving cisplatin and the taxanes, with taxol giving rise to 18% grade 2 or 3 neurotoxicity lasting for up to 2 years. The main effect is peripheral neuropathy, which gives tingling initially in some cases and may progress to loss of sensation and difficulty in walking. Vincristine can also give rise to neurotoxicity, and the total dose should not exceed 12 mg (1–2 mg/week).
- Doxorubicin and to a lesser extent epirubicin can give rise to cardiomyopathy in a high cumulative dose. A total dose of 500 mg/m^2 should not be exceeded. Concurrent use of cyclophosphamide potentiates the cardiomyopathic effect of doxorubicin and, in this case, a total dose of 450 mg/m^2 of doxorubicin should not be exceeded.

- Palmar–plantar erythrodysesthesia is a side effect of Caelyx® (pegylated liposomal doxorubicin) and further treatment should not be given until all evidence of this side effect has gone. Patients should be advised to wear loose clothing to minimize this problem.
- Cyclophosphamide and ifosfamide can give rise to cystitis, which is due to toxic breakdown products. In the case of cyclophosphamide, this may be prevented by adequate daily fluid intake. However, for ifosfamide, routine use of mesna is required.
- Methotrexate is bound to albumin and only the unbound drug is available for cytotoxic action. Drugs such as sulfonamides and aspirin can increase the dissociation of methotrexate from its bound form and hence increase its toxicity. Methotrexate also accumulates in ascites and pleural effusions, and caution is required in such patients as the effusions and ascites can act as a reservoir for methotrexate giving rise to prolonged exposure. Folinic acid is an effective 'antidote' to methotrexate.
- Bleomycin can give rise to lung fibrosis, and lung function tests are required in patients receiving this drug. Bleomycin also accumulates in skin and will produce excess sensitivity to sunlight within approximately 30 minutes of being given. More commonly, it will give rise to dark skin markings at pressure areas such as elbows and knuckles and may give rise to permanent black marks where there has been local trauma, e.g. scratching.

Ovarian cancer: tumor-specific chemotherapy

Germ cell tumors

Intensive treatment with bleomycin, etoposide, and cisplatin with monitoring of markers is curative in more than 95% of such patients.

Tumors of stromal origin

This very rare variant of anaplastic granulosa cell tumor can be cured in approximately two-thirds of patients with the same combination of bleomycin, etoposide, and cisplatin.

Tumors of epithelial origin

Stage I disease

Until recently there was no evidence that adjuvant chemotherapy was of any value in these patients after complete removal of all evidence of tumour, but results of the International Collaborative Ovarian Neoplasm (ICON) 1 and ACTION trials showed a 9% increase in survival with the use of adjuvant chemotherapy. Therefore all patients should be offered six courses of single-agent carboplatin given at 4-weekly intervals.

Stages II, III, and IV disease

A combination of doxorubicin, cyclophosphamide, and cisplatin has for many years been regarded as standard treatment for these patients, giving six courses at intervals of 3 weeks assuming that the patient has adequate renal function with a glomerular filtration rate (GFR) of more than 60 mL/minute.

- The ICON 2 trial showed that carboplatin given every 3 weeks for five cycles is equally effective and is much better tolerated, particularly by the elderly. Nausea and vomiting are relatively easily controlled with carboplatin. Leukopenia and thrombocytopenia can be a problem, but neutropenic sepsis is rare. Hair loss does not occur, but anemia is common after three or four cycles.
- The combination of doxorubicin, cyclophosphamide, and cisplatin produces nausea and vomiting, which is more difficult to control. Hair loss is inevitable, and some loss of renal function may occur even with adequate hydration. Neutropenic sepsis is much more common than with carboplatin.
- With both regimens, a combined complete and partial response of 70–80% is to be expected, with approximately 2 years median survival and 25% of patients still alive at 5 years.
- The taxanes (taxol and taxotere) are also effective in epithelial ovarian cancer and are regarded as the first-line treatment of choice in the USA. This is still debatable, but the ICON 3 trial with over 2000 patients has shown no survival advantage for a combination of taxol and carboplatin compared with carboplatin alone. This trial is the largest ever undertaken in the history of ovarian cancer. Median survival was approximately 3 years.

Second-line treatment

The longer the treatment-free interval before recurrence, the more likely it is that the patient will respond to further platinum-based chemotherapy. After a long treatment-free interval, responses can be almost as high as with first-line treatment. New drugs such as topotecan, gemcitabine, and liposomal doxorubicin are all currently being investigated as second-line treatments. The results of the recently published ICON 4 trial suggest some improvement in survival at 2 years in women treated with a combination of taxol and platinum.

Other gynecological cancers

Fallopian tube cancer

This responds to the same treatment as that for epithelial ovarian cancer.

Uterine sarcoma

A recent meta-analysis has shown that patients with poor prognosis sarcomas should receive adjuvant chemotherapy based on doxorubicin, as this will markedly improve their chances of survival. A combination of doxorubicin and ifosfamide is the most commonly used combination.

Carcinoma of the endometrium

Cytotoxic chemotherapy should only be used in patients with advanced disease that is not amenable to other forms of treatment such as surgery, radiotherapy, and hormonal manipulation. A combination of cyclophosphamide, doxorubicin, and cisplatin can be effective in up to 60% of patients. Carboplatin has also been used and, more recently, taxol is being investigated.

Carcinoma of the cervix

Any chemotherapy should be based on cisplatin and common regimens involve combining one or more of the following drugs with cisplatin: 5-FU, ifosfamide, bleomycin, vindesine, mitomycin-C, vinblastine, methotrexate. The most common regimen is a combination of cisplatin and methotrexate with folinic acid rescue given every 2 weeks. It would seem that, the more frequently the chemotherapy is given in carcinoma of the cervix, the more likely it is to be effective in view of the very rapid turnover of the cells in this condition.

- Adjuvant chemotherapy is not established in the management of cervical cancer, but is being investigated.
- Neo-adjuvant chemotherapy has been used in many trials, but it is not as yet clear whether this treatment is effective.
- Concurrent chemotherapy: cisplatin-based chemotherapy given at the same time as radiotherapy can markedly increase the cure rate of the radiotherapy. Despite the increased toxicity, such treatment is now used routinely.
- Palliative chemotherapy: at present, chemotherapy is mainly reserved for those with advanced disease that is not amenable to radiotherapy or surgery and where palliation is required.

Carcinoma of the vagina

The chemotherapy regimens used for carcinoma of the cervix can be effective in this situation.

Carcinoma of the vulva

The use of chemotherapy in this elderly population remains controversial. Combinations of CCNU (lomustine), methotrexate, and bleomycin given in small doses over 6 weeks have been shown to shrink tumors sufficiently to make them operable and hence potentially curable, and other drugs such as the taxanes and 5-FU are currently being investigated in this disease. The concurrent use of chemotherapy and radiotherapy for those not amenable to surgery is currently being investigated and such treatment may be used for palliative purposes.

Radiotherapy in gynecological cancer I

Carcinoma of the endometrium

- Radical radiotherapy is given daily 5 days a week lasting for a few minutes per day. Once a course of treatment is started, there should not be any breaks at all.
- Before the patient undergoes treatment, she has to go through the planning process which involves measuring her body contour, noting the fields that have to be treated, making appropriate marks on her body for later setting up, and feeding all this information into a computer to determine the dose distribution within the treatment volume and adjustment of the various beams to ensure an even distribution of no more than 5% variation throughout the treatment volume.
- Most patients receiving gynecological external beam radiotherapy are treated with a 10 MV or higher energy linear accelerator using three or four fields to the pelvis. Standard fields cover from the L5–S1 junction down to the bottom of the obturator fossa and out laterally to 1 cm outside the pelvic sidewall. Posteriorly, they cover the cervix and part of the adjacent rectum and anteriorly halfway through the pubic bone.
- Most pelvic gynecological treatments are within the range 44–50 Gy in 4–5 weeks with or without brachytherapy and/or para-aortic irradiation where the dose does not usually exceed 40 Gy.

Brachytherapy

Brachytherapy in gynecological cancer involves the placing of applicators in the vagina or the uterus or both. Radioactive sources (usually cesium) are placed inside these applicators by a remote technique, hence avoiding irradiation to anyone other than the patient. If intrauterine treatment is required, the patient will be anesthetized in the operating room.

- If vaginal treatment alone is required, an anesthetic is not usually necessary.
- Various dose schedules exist, but commonly the patient has a single application of brachytherapy which involves staying in hospital for 1, 2, or even 3 nights depending on the dose rate for the particular machine.
- High-dose-rate brachytherapy machines are available where the dose is given over a very short period of time and may be repeated on a weekly basis with up to four insertions, depending upon dose schedule.
- The total dose of irradiation is reduced in patients treated with high-dose-rate brachytherapy, but with the intention that they receive a dose that is radiobiologically equivalent.

Side effects

These are common to all forms of pelvic radiotherapy. The short-term side effects normally subside by 6 weeks after completion of radiotherapy. Late side effects are possible. Lethargy is common to all patients.

- Diarrhea may occur during the last 7–10 days of treatment, but is easily dealt with using simple medication such as codeine phosphate.

- Frequency of micturition may also occur in the last 7–10 days and urinary tract infection should be excluded as a cause of this. If it is due to radiation, it is not as easy to alleviate this symptom in the short term.
- Vaginal stenosis will be common to all patients unless they are sexually active, but a suitable stent that should be used for 1 year after completion of treatment eliminates this problem.
- Fistulas in the bladder, rectum, or small bowel are all very rare.
- Skin changes are very uncommon with modern high-energy radiotherapy .

Radiotherapy in ovarian cancer and uterine sarcomas

- There is little place for the use of radiotherapy in ovarian cancer, although it was common practice as an adjuvant treatment 20 years ago. The current use of radiotherapy is mainly for palliative treatment of solitary metastases, either in the abdominal wall or in the vaginal vault, when such lesions do not respond to chemotherapy and give rise to symptoms sufficient to warrant radiotherapy.
- There is no evidence to support the routine use of adjuvant radiotherapy after complete surgical removal of uterine sarcoma. Large trials are in progress to assess whether adjuvant radiotherapy has any part to play.

Carcinoma of the endometrium

Adjuvant radiotherapy

In patients with stage I disease, such treatment has frequently been used in the past when the patient had disease with a poor prognosis (penetration more than halfway through the myometrium, poorly differentiated tumour, or vascular invasion), but there is no evidence that such treatment is of value. Clinical trials are currently ongoing to determine whether such adjuvant radiotherapy is of value in these poor prognosis patients and to determine the value or otherwise of pelvic lymphadenectomy in this situation.

If the patient has more than stage I disease but all evidence of tumor has been removed, adjuvant pelvic radiotherapy is conventionally given.

Vaginal vault brachytherapy is widely used in stage I patients with poor prognosis disease to prevent vaginal vault recurrence. Such patients have an approximately 16% chance of vaginal vault recurrence and brachytherapy may reduce this to 2%, but such treatment has no effect on survival.

Primary treatment

Radiotherapy is inferior to surgery in the treatment of stage I endometrial cancer, with a cure rate of 20% less on average. Therefore such treatment should only be used when the risks of surgery are very high.

Radiotherapy in gynecological cancer II

Carcinoma of the cervix

Adjuvant radiotherapy

In patients who have had surgery with radical hysterectomy and node dissection and where the nodes have been found to be involved with tumor, it is standard practice to give adjuvant radiotherapy to the pelvis, but there is no good evidence that such treatment is of value with regard to survival. It is also common practice to use vaginal vault brachytherapy in addition to the external beam therapy.

Primary treatment

Stage I

Treatment with radiotherapy involving external beam radiotherapy and brachytherapy is equally as effective as radical hysterectomy and node dissection in stage I disease. With modern anesthetics and surgical techniques, the tendency is to do more in the way of surgery and reserve radiotherapy for those patients with involved nodes or inadequate excision margins. Patients with poor general health will be treated by radiotherapy alone.

Stage II/III

Radiotherapy is the treatment of choice for those with more advanced disease, using the doses given above together with intrauterine and intravaginal brachytherapy, usually giving a dose of 20 Gy to point A, which is a point 2 cm superior and lateral to the cervix.

Advanced disease

In patients in whom cure is not possible, palliative radiotherapy involving the whole of the pelvis, usually by a two-field anterior and posterior technique giving 30 Gy in a 2 week period, can be very effective in relieving the symptoms of disease such as bleeding. Pain from bone metastases can also be relieved by a single exposure of 8 Gy to the affected area.

Chemo-radiation

Cisplatin-based chemotherapy concurrent with radiotherapy would produce a higher cure rate but more side effects in patients with carcinoma of the cervix. Trials are currently being conducted to determine the ideal combination of these two modalities of treatment.

Carcinoma of the vagina

Treatment is principally by external beam radiotherapy, but the fields come down much lower in the pelvis to ensure that all disease is covered. This may give rise to radiation covering the vulva, which is very sensitive and becomes very sore. Treatment may then be followed by vaginal cesium using an appropriate applicator. In some patients with very localized disease, such brachytherapy may be used alone.

Carcinoma of the vulva

Although surgery remains the mainstay of treatment in this condition, many will give adjuvant radiotherapy to the nodal areas if they were involved, although such treatment is still debatable. Studies are currently being devised to look at the place of chemo-radiation as an adjuvant in such patients.

For patients with advanced disease, radiotherapy can be effective in shrinking the tumor prior to definitive surgery, and an improvement in long-term survival has been obtained by this method. A short course of radiotherapy can also be effective palliation in patients with recurrent disease.

Palliative care

Introduction

Palliative care describes a range of care and support provided to meet the needs of patients with progressive illness and their carers. It can be usefully subdivided into general palliative care and specialist palliative care.

- *General palliative care* This is integral to all areas of clinical practice and aims to promote physical and psychosocial wellbeing whatever the stage of the disease. Its key principles comprise the following:
  - Focus on quality of life which includes good symptom control.
  - Whole-person approach taking into account the person's past life experiences and current situation.
  - Care that encompasses both the person with the life-threatening disease and those who matter to that person.
  - Respect for patient autonomy and choice (e.g. over place of care, treatment options).
- *Specialist palliative care* This is provided by a multiprofessional team who have undergone recognized specialist palliative care training. It addresses a level of complexity of problems that cannot be managed solely by healthcare professionals providing general palliative care. It may be appropriate at various stages of a patient's illness and in a variety of settings.

Principles of symptom management

Symptoms associated with gynecological malignancy may be due to:

- the effects of treatment
- locally progressive disease
- specific metastatic disease
- general effects of advanced malignancy, e.g. weakness

The severity of symptoms perceived by patients, particularly those with advancing disease, may also be affected by psychosocial and spiritual issues, e.g. fear, anxiety, or depression may exacerbate pain.

Successful symptom management depends upon a number of key principles:

- Defining the underlying cause of the symptom.
- Consideration of any psychosocial and spiritual issues.
- Explanation of the cause of the symptom to the patient (and family where appropriate).
- Treatment of reversible causes of symptoms, e.g. anemia, hypercalcemia.
- Consideration of any appropriate disease-oriented treatment, e.g. chemotherapy in ovarian cancer, localized radiotherapy for pain from bone metastases from endometrial cancer.
- Specific drug treatments to relieve symptoms, e.g. analgesia.
- Consideration of nondrug measures.
- The use of regular medication for persistent symptoms rather than p.r.n. (*pro re nata*, whenever needed).
- Discussion of treatment options.
- The burden of treatment should not outweigh the benefits.

- Emphasis on open and sensitive communication that extends to patients, informal carers, and professional colleagues.
- Provision of information (including written information).
- Review of the response to the treatment.
- Review of treatment options if present treatment is ineffective or incompletely effective.

The detailed assessment of the patient is an essential part of managing difficult symptoms. This may include the use of investigations but, for patients with far advanced disease, the trauma of having even simple investigations such as an X-ray may outweigh the possible benefit. Therefore the patient's view on this is extremely important.

Many symptoms can be managed in a general setting using the guidelines given in the following sections. However, for complex problems and for patients who do not seem to be responding as expected, referral to a specialist in palliative medicine is advised.

Pain management

Pain is a common symptom in advanced gynecological malignancy, with over 40% of patients with advanced ovarian cancer suffering significant pain. Severe pain is also a major symptom for patients with recurrent carcinoma of the cervix.

It is estimated that cancer pain can generally be well controlled in around 80% of patients if the WHO's analgesic ladder guidelines are followed (Table 18.5). Patients are prescribed the weakest analgesic on a regular basis and, if the pain is not fully controlled on this, a stronger analgesic from the next 'rung of the ladder' is given and so on until pain relief is adequate. It may be necessary to add other drugs to achieve satisfactory pain control (see later sections).

Table 18.5 WHO analgesic ladder

Simple/non-opioid analgesic, e.g. acetaminophen 1 g qds (4 times a day)
Weak opioid, e.g. codeine 30–60 mg 4-hourly
Strong opioid, e.g. morphine

Morphine

Morphine remains the strong opioid of choice. It should be used when necessary to control severe pain regardless of the stage of a patient's illness. It should be given orally where possible and the dose titrated to achieve adequate pain relief. Initial titration is usually best achieved using a short-acting (4-hourly) preparation, e.g. morphine sulfate solution or tablets. Once the pain is under control, change to a slow-release preparation is usually more convenient for the patient.

The starting dose of morphine will depend upon previous analgesics used, e.g. taking into account that 10 mg of codeine/dihydrocodeine is approximately equivalent to 1 mg of morphine. Dose increments for titration should be in the range 25–50% such that a typical titration of 4-hourly oral morphine doses may be

5 mg → 7.5 mg → 10 mg → 15 mg → 20 mg → 30 mg → 45 mg → 60 mg, etc.

For some patients, e.g. those whose pain is almost controlled on weaker opioids, the initial use of a long-acting morphine preparation together with p.r.n. doses of a short-acting morphine preparation for breakthrough pain may be appropriate. It is recommended that the appropriate breakthrough dose should be equivalent to one-sixth of the total daily dose, e.g. for a patient taking a 12-hourly slow-release morphine preparation 30 mg twice daily, the appropriate breakthrough dose would be 10 mg 4-hourly p.r.n.

For patients who are unable to take oral morphine because of weakness, vomiting, etc., SC morphine or diamorphine can be given. Diamorphine is more soluble in water, and therefore is preferred as the volume of injection can be smaller. SC diamorphine can be given as bolus injections every 4 hours or as a continuous infusion using a battery-operated syringe driver. Approximate dose equivalents of oral and SC opioids are:

- 3 mg oral morphine = 1 mg SC diamorphine
- 2 mg oral morphine = 1 mg SC morphine.

Side effects of morphine

It is useful to discuss potential side effects with patients when morphine is first prescribed. The most common are as follows:

- *Constipation* is almost universal and is dose dependent. It can be a distressing symptom and it is important to try to prevent it by the prescription of a regular dose of oral laxative, which both softens the stool and stimulates bowel activity, whenever morphine is commenced (unless the patient has diarrhea). Dose titration is important and will often avoid the need for rectal intervention. However, if fecal impaction develops, the use of enemas may be necessary, e.g. for fecal impaction with a hard fecal mass, arachis oil enema overnight followed by a phosphate enema.
- *Nausea and vomiting* occur in a minority of patients and seem to be largely related to changes in morphine dose. Therefore they usually settle once a patient has been stabilized on a regular dose of morphine. It can be helped by haloperidol 1.5 mg at night to twice daily orally.

- *Drowsiness/lightheadedness* is quite common, particularly in the initial stages of titration, but usually resolves when the patient is on the minimum appropriate dose to control the pain.
- *Confusion* may occur, particularly in the elderly, and may be helped by dose reduction followed by more gradual titration.

Respiratory depression is not usually encountered if oral morphine doses for pain are titrated according to the above guidelines. It is extremely important that, when an increase in morphine dose has been prescribed, the patient's response to this change is assessed. If the increased dose has not brought about an increase in pain relief, then side effects such as drowsiness and confusion may be encountered. Therefore the dose should be reduced to the previous level and the cause of the pain reassessed.

Fears associated with morphine use

Patients and their families may have the following concerns:

- The use of morphine means that the patient is about to die.
- The early use of morphine means that the pain will no longer respond when it becomes worse later on.
- The patient will become addicted to morphine.

Therefore the following discussion may therefore be helpful.

- Morphine is used earlier in patients' illnesses than it was in the past and its use is determined by the severity of pain rather than the stage of disease.
- Pain does not always become worse as the disease progresses but, if it does, further adjustment of morphine dose may help. Other methods of pain relief are also available for some types of pain.
- Psychological addiction is not usually encountered in patients taking morphine for cancer pain. Physical addiction does occur but, if the patient no longer needs opioid analgesia because the cause of the pain has resolved, then the morphine dose can be reduced gradually and discontinued without withdrawal symptoms.

Other opioids and analgesics

Other strong opioids

A number of other strong opioids are becoming available as alternatives to morphine. Their exact place in the management of cancer pain is yet to be established. However, for some patients who do not seem to be able to tolerate morphine because of side effects, alternatives may be worth considering, e.g. transdermal fentanyl.

Features of transdermal fentanyl:
- applied as a skin patch that is changed every 3 days
- associated with less constipation and drowsiness than morphine
- useful when patients are unable to take oral morphine
- more expensive than oral morphine.

Opioid responsiveness of pain

Other measures are necessary for pain that does not respond fully to strong opioids. It may often be appropriate to seek the advice of specialists in palliative medicine or pain clinics for these patients.

The causes of physical pains can be broadly classified in terms of their opioid responsiveness as follows:
- Opioid-responsive, e.g. nociceptive pain from tumors.
- Partially opioid-responsive, i.e. opioid titration seems to reach a ceiling above which an increased dose causes more side effects but no improved pain relief, e.g. bone pain and nerve compression pain.
- Opioid non-responsive, where opioids seem to have little effect on the pain, e.g. neuropathic pain due to nerve damage and pain from muscle spasm.

Therefore a detailed assessment of the physical cause of pain as described above is essential in determining the best approach and likely responsiveness to the analgesic ladder. Where there are psychosocial issues that contribute to the severity of the pain perceived, opioids may not be fully effective and other ways of addressing these issues need to be considered.

Thus effective pain relief with minimized side effects from inappropriate drug doses depends upon the following:
- An understanding of the opioid responsiveness of physical pains.
- Careful assessment of the cause of pain including psychosocial issues.
- A review of the response of pain to opioids.

In advanced gynecological malignancy, pain may be complex in that there may be a number of physical components of different opioid responsiveness. For example, an expanding pelvic tumor mass may produce opioid-responsive pain but may also cause nerve compression or damage resulting in opioid nonresponsive neuropathic pain. Para-aortic node involvement, e.g. in carcinoma of the cervix, may produce back pain and associated paravertebral muscle spasm which may not respond to opioids.

Other drugs used in pain management

- NSAIDs may be helpful in pain due to bone metastases or associated with inflammatory processes.
- Muscle relaxants, e.g. diazepam, may be helpful for muscular spasm pain.
- Tricyclic antidepressants (e.g. amitriptyline) and anticonvulsants (e.g. carbamazepine) may be helpful in neuropathic pain.
- Corticosteroids (e.g. dexamethazone) may be helpful in combination with opioids in a number of pains, e.g. hepatic capsular pain from liver metastases, perineal pain resulting from pelvic tumor, and pain associated with nerve compression. It is believed that steroids work by reducing peritumor edema and thereby relieving pressure.

Intestinal obstruction and malignant ascites

Approximately 25% of patients with late-stage ovarian carcinoma develop intestinal obstruction with a median survival of 14 weeks. Surgical relief of the obstruction where possible offers approximately 2 months palliation, but there is a significant risk of reobstruction. Symptoms include the following:

- Abdominal pain from:
  - distension
  - colic
- Nausea and vomiting
- Constipation

Where surgery is not appropriate, the following medical management may relieve symptoms.

Medical management

In intestinal obstruction, oral medication is unlikely to be absorbed so the SC route is preferable and an SC infusion of drugs using a syringe driver can be extremely beneficial. Specific symptoms and their appropriate treatments include the following:

- *Pain*
  - Pain from distension: opioids.
  - Pain from colic: anticholinergic drugs, e.g. hyoscine butylbromide.
- *Nausea and vomiting*
  - If there is no colic, the first choice is metoclopramide but, if this is not successful, change to cyclizine.
  - If there is colic, use hyoscine butylbromide and consider a trial of corticosteroids.
  - If there is residual nausea, cyclizine may be added and, if there are persistent large-volume vomits, SC octreotide may reduce these or a nasogastric tube may be considered.
  - *NB*. In the presence of small intestinal obstruction with colic, metoclopramide and stimulant laxatives may exacerbate the colic and therefore should be avoided.
- *Constipation* In some situations, e.g. recurrent subacute intestinal obstruction, a stool softener (e.g. docusate) may be helpful.
- *Hydration* Depending upon the stage of disease and likelihood of reversing the obstruction, the issue of parenteral hydration should be considered, also taking into account the patient's wishes. In some situations, SC fluids may help to relieve symptoms of dehydration.

Malignant ascites

Malignant ascites is common in advanced ovarian malignancy and may be associated with leg edema, dyspnea, reduced appetite, nausea and vomiting, and uncomfortable distension. Treatment options include the following:

- Anticancer therapy
- Paracentesis
- Diuretic therapy, e.g. with spironolactone with or without furosemide
- Peritoneovenous shunt may be helpful for symptomatic relief in some situations where other therapies have failed

Renal failure and other complications

Ureteric obstruction causing renal failure is a common feature of end-stage carcinoma of the cervix. Symptoms arising from progressive renal failure can be varied but, at times, distressing. These include the following:

- Drowsiness
- Confusion and agitation
- Nausea and vomiting
- Myoclonic jerks
- Itching

It should also be remembered that renal failure may affect the metabolism of many drugs already being used (e.g. opioids) and the doses may need to be reduced.

Drug management of these symptoms includes the following:

- Confusion/agitation: haloperidol, methotrimeprazine
- Nausea and vomiting: haloperidol, methotrimeprazine
- Myoclonic jerks: diazepam (oral or rectal), midazolam (SC)

Fistulas, hemorrhage, vaginal discharge, and other symptoms

- *Fistulas.* In advanced gynecological malignancy, particularly carcinoma of the cervix, a variety of fistulas may occur, especially between rectum and genitourinary tract or bladder and vagina. Surgical management, e.g. diverting colostomy for a rectovaginal fistula, may give the best symptom relief but may not be possible in far advanced disease. Under these circumstances, simple measures such as using laxatives to keep the stool soft often reduces the flow through the fistula. A urinary catheter may help to reduce leakage from a vesicovaginal fistula.
- *Hemorrhage.* Rectal and vaginal bleeding may occur with local tumor invasion, particularly from carcinoma of the cervix, which may erode into the rectum. Palliative radiotherapy may be helpful and the use of antifibrinolytic drugs, such as tranexamic acid, may reduce bleeding.
- *Vaginal discharge.* Foul-smelling vaginal discharge may occur in patients with advanced carcinoma of the cervix. This is often due to anaerobic infection of fungating tumor. The smell can be reduced by using metronidazole either orally or vaginally.
- *Other symptoms.* Depending upon the site of metastatic disease, numerous other symptoms may be encountered, e.g. dyspnea from pleural effusions, anorexia and cachexia, lymphedema, right hypochondrial pain from liver metastases, and headache, nausea, and vomiting from cerebral metastases. Detailed discussion of the management of these is beyond the scope of this chapter.

Terminal care

In the last days of life, it is important to continue to manage distressing symptoms. This may require the use of SC medication by bolus injection or SC infusion. Support of both the patient and family is particularly important at this stage, and explanation of symptoms, such as Cheyne–Stokes breathing, is helpful.

In general, unnecessary medication should be withdrawn but additional medication may be necessary for particular problems.

- *Retained bronchial secretions* can cause a rattling sound which is particularly distressing for those sitting by the bedside. Helpful measures include changing the patient's position, use of anticholinergics such as hyoscine butylbromide SC, and, occasionally, suction.
- *Terminal restlessness* may be caused by distended bladder or rectum, cerebral hypoxia, pain, dyspnea drugs (e.g. steroids), metabolic factors, anxiety, or fear. It is important to determine any reversible causes, e.g. distended bladder (in which case, consider catheterization). In the absence of reversible causes, drug treatment by midazolam by SC infusion is helpful.

Chapter 19

Miscellaneous gynecology

Ultrasound

Ultrasound is the most widely used method of imaging in gynecology. As in obstetrics, it has revolutionized the management of some clinical problems, such as the complications of early pregnancy. Ultrasound is based on the transmission of sound frequencies between 3 and 8 MHz and the detection of the echoes that this generates in tissue when it meets interfaces of different densities. Transvaginal scanning gives better imaging of the pelvic organs and avoids the need for a full bladder. Doppler ultrasound gives information about the blood flow around the pelvic organs.

Estimation of gestational age

This is made by measurement of the crown–rump length in the first 90 days of pregnancy or biparietal diameters in the second trimester. Observer error as a proportion of the total distance measured decreases with increasing gestation, but variation about the mean in the normal population increases. The optimum gestation for estimating gestational age is between 8 and 12 weeks.

Early pregnancy assessment

- In normal pregnancy, an intrauterine gestation sac should be visible on transvaginal ultrasound by 6 weeks' gestation or when the circulating level of hCG is >1000 IU/L.
- Ectopic pregnancy may occasionally be seen as fetal heart activity outside the uterus, but is more commonly suggested by an empty uterus, a nonspecific adnexal mass, or the presence of free fluid in the pouch of Douglas.
- Ultrasound can be invaluable in the diagnosis of miscarriage, especially early embryonic demise or anembryonic pregnancy.
- Fetal heart pulsation can normally be seen from 6 weeks. The absence of detectable fetal heart activity in a fetal pole of more than 7 mm or in a gestation sac >20 mm is diagnostic of pregnancy failure, but a repeat scan should be performed in early pregnancy after 7–10 days to confirm the diagnosis.
- Trophoblastic disease is associated with multiple echoes within the uterus giving a 'snowstorm' appearance.
- Retained products of conception in incomplete miscarriage may be suspected from the presence of echogenic material within the cavity, but this may be difficult to distinguish from blood and the diagnosis should be made on clinical grounds.

Assessment of a pelvic mass

Ultrasound is used to distinguish cysts (usually ovarian) from solid pelvic tumors such as fibroids. Occasionally, a pedunculated fibroid may be mistaken for an ovarian tumor. Functional ovarian cysts (follicular cysts, corpus luteum) are usually simple unilocular areas less than 5 cm in size which disappear when the scan is repeated after 6 weeks. The internal morphology of ovarian cysts can be used to give an indication of the likelihood of malignancy, although surgical removal is required for confirmation. Malignant change is also associated with changes in blood flow (angiogenesis) around ovarian cysts. Transvaginal scanning can be used for the detection of asymptomatic early-stage ovarian cancer.

Postmenopausal bleeding

Endometrial thickness is increased in postmenopausal women with endometrial carcinoma. Using a cut-off of 5 mm, 96% of such carcinomas can be identified by transvaginal ultrasound, although up to 55% of women with no disease will also have a positive result. Benign endometrial lesions such as polyps can be detected as localized thickenings of the endometrium. Instillation of saline into the endometrial cavity (sonohysterography) increases the sensitivity for local pathology, but is more invasive.

Infertility

In addition to its role in the diagnosis of conditions such as polycystic ovarian disease and hydrosalpinx, ultrasound is used to track follicular growth and rupture during normal and stimulated cycles in infertility treatment. It is used to determine the timing of hCG administration and whether hCG should be withheld to avoid high-order multiple gestation. Oocyte retrieval for assisted conception can be performed under ultrasound guidance. Ovarian hyperstimulation syndrome is assessed by ultrasound.

Pelvic pain

Ultrasound examination is unlikely to be informative in nonpregnant women with normal pelvic examination findings who present with pain. However, a diagnosis of endometriosis may be suggested by the presence of characteristic hemorrhagic cysts (endometrioma) on the ovaries. Adenomyosis is associated with a thickening of the myometrium with areas of reduced and increased echogeneicity. In patients with acute symptoms, ultrasound may be of value in the detection of tubo-ovarian masses in pelvic inflammatory disease or the diagnosis of hemorrhage into a functional ovarian cyst.

Recommended further reading

1. American College of Obstetricians and Gynecologists (1996). ACOG Technical Bulletin No. 215. Gynecologic ultrasonography. *Int J Gynaecol Obstet* **52**, 293–304.

Radiological imaging

Radiological imaging in gynecology has been largely replaced by ultrasound, but still has a role in the diagnosis and assessment of malignancy and infertility.

Plain radiography

- Plain radiography of the abdomen may occasionally give additional information about a pelvic tumor. Dermoid cysts often contain radio-opaque material such as teeth or bone that distinguishes them from other ovarian tumors.
- Fibroids may be detected on abdominal X-rays if they become calcified.
- Erect and supine abdominal films are indicated in the assessment of suspected ileus or bowel obstruction.
- Lost intrauterine contraceptive devices that have perforated the wall of the uterus can be located on X-ray.
- Metal clips used for sterilization are occasionally seen outside the pelvis. This does not indicate failure of the procedure as it is not uncommon for the clips to cause necrosis of the underlying tube and then become detached, but leave the tube occluded.
- Chest X-rays form part of the routine assessment of patients with suspected malignancy.
  - The presence of pleural effusions suggests stage IV ovarian carcinoma, but pleural effusions also occur in ovarian hyperstimulation and occasionally with ovarian fibromas (Meig's syndrome).
  - Choriocarcinoma is associated with cannon-ball metastases in the lungs.

Intravenous urography

Renal colic is one of the causes of acute abdominal pain. Ureteric obstruction in a patient with cervical carcinoma indicates stage III disease. Continuous urinary incontinence following childbirth, radiotherapy, or gynecological surgery may be due to fistula formation between the ureters or bladder and genital tract. Contrast studies of the renal tract should be considered when congenital malformations of the reproductive tract are diagnosed, as approximately 15% of cases are associated with abnormalities of the urinary tract. Contrast imaging of the bladder neck is used in the assessment of stress incontinence.

Hysterosalpingography

Hysterosalpingography is the injection of water-soluble contrast medium through the cervix into the uterine cavity. It is used to visualize the uterine cavity and fallopian tubes in the investigation of patients with infertility or recurrent miscarriage. The dye (2–3 mL) is injected using a Leech–Wilkinson cannula.

- Polyps or submucous fibroids produce rounded filling defects.

- The presence of intrauterine synechiae and congenital abnormalities of the uterine cavity (septate or bicornuate uterus) can also be identified.
- If the fallopian tubes are patent, dye will be seen spilling into the peritoneal cavity. The site of tubal obstruction can be identified and this is important in determining the feasibility of tubal surgery. If dye remains localized at the end of the tube, this suggests peritubal adhesions.

Hysterosalpingography is an alternative to laparoscopy for assessing tubal patency. It avoids the risks associated with the latter, but gives more limited information about pelvic pathology. Tubal spasm may cause artefactual obstruction of the tubes.

Computed tomography (CT scan)

CT scans of the pelvis are used mainly in the assessment of malignancy. The role of CT scan in diagnosis is limited in primary ovarian tumors as laparotomy is usually required to establish the diagnosis. Its value is mainly in the postoperative identification of residual disease and as a method to assess response to treatment. In patients with recurrent disease, it may be used to localize the site of disease when palliative or second-look surgery is being considered. In patients with carcinoma of the cervix, it can be used in disease staging and planning radiotherapy, although MRI is now probably the method of choice for imaging the disease.

Magnetic resonance imaging and immunoscintigraphy

MRI

MRI is an alternative method of soft-tissue imaging which avoids the need for ionizing radiation. A strong magnetic field is used to polarize the hydrogen ions in tissue so that they emit radiofrequency energy of an appropriate frequency. In gynecology, MRI is of particular value in the imaging and staging of pelvic tumors and is the method of choice for identification of local spread of cervical and endometrial carcinoma when surgery is being contemplated.

Immunoscintigraphy

This involves the injection of radiolabeled monoclonal antibody or fragments. The antibody binds to antigens that are expressed preferentially by tumor, and the site of the disease is then identified as a hot spot on external gamma camera imaging. Although its sensitivity and specificity are comparable to those of conventional imaging, it has failed to become established in routine clinical care and its main value is the detection of distant metastases and localized recurrence in ovarian cancer.

Urinary tract injuries

The close anatomical relationship between the urinary tract and the internal genital organs and lower genital tract predisposes the distal ureter and bladder to iatrogenic injury during pelvic and gynecological surgery.

Incidence and risk factors

The incidence of ureteric injuries at the time of major gynecological surgery has been reported to be 0.4–2.5%. The incidence of ureteric injury during hysterectomy for benign causes is reported at 1 in 500 cases, rising to 1% in cases of malignancy, and even higher where preoperative radiotherapy has been used. Damage to the bladder occurs in 1 in 200 cases, being more common after previous cesarean delivery. The risk of ureteric injury is higher during abdominal than vaginal hysterectomies especially when the former is associated with pelvic and para-aortic lymphadenectomy. Obstetric procedures such as repeat cesarean deliveries and puerperal hysterectomies are also associated with increased risks of injury to the lower urinary tract.

Conditions that directly or indirectly distort, scar, or infiltrate pelvic tissues and thus predispose to injury of the lower urinary tract include the following:

- Large pelvic masses
- Cervical fibroids
- Widespread endometriosis
- Oophorectomy after previous total abdominal hysterectomy
- Chronic pelvic inflammatory disease
- Pelvic abscess/pelvic hematomas, lymphocyst
- Gynecological/lower gastrointestinal cancer
- Prolapse—procidentia
- Prior pelvic surgery/radiotherapy
- Placenta accreta in the lower segment
- Congenital abnormalities of the urinary tract.

Ureteral injury

The majority of ureteric injuries in gynecological surgery occur in the lower third of the ureter. Thus the most common sites of such injury at the time of abdominal hysterectomy are:

- at the pelvic brim where the ureter lies beneath the infundibulo-pelvic ligament overlying the bifurcation of the common iliac artery
- lateral to the cervix where the ureter crosses under the uterine artery
- lateral to the vaginal fornix as the ureter passes lateral to the cervix and upper vagina on its course to enter the bladder.

Ureteric damage in the form of 'kinking', perforation, or ligation may also occur during reperitonealization of the pelvis or during retropubic urethropexy procedures. In the obstetric setting, ureteral injury may occur as a result of extension of the uterine incision or during suturing of the uterine incision or an attempt to control hemorrhage within the broad ligament. The increased vascularity of the pelvis, distortion of anatomy, and total hysterectomy when the cervix is not palpable because of effacement all contribute to the increased risk of ureteric injuries during cesarean deliveries and puerperal hysterectomies.

Bladder injury

Injury to the bladder may be an immediate result of sharp or blunt dissection during hysterectomy or repeat cesarean delivery or a result of later avascular necrosis. The bladder may also be accidentally opened during entry into the peritoneal cavity at the time of hysterectomy or, more commonly, cesarean delivery where the bladder is 'hitched up' from previous surgery.

Prevention, detection, and repair of urological injuries

Prevention

In selected cases, a preoperative IV urogram may assist in the detection of congenital abnormalities of the urinary tract as well as identify any distortion due to involvement by pelvic tumours, pelvic inflammatory disease, endometriosis, or cancer. Perioperative insertion of ureteric catheters or stents may assist in identification and dissection of ureters, but does little to reduce the overall incidence of urological injuries as most cases occur in patients where there was no indication for use of such stents.

Intraoperatively, the basic principles of safety for all pelvic procedures should be adopted, including adequate exposure of the surgical field, adequate light and assistance, restoration of normal anatomic relationships, traction and countertraction to expose adjacent structures, and dissection along tissue planes. Furthermore, it is important to avoid mass ligation of tissues. Clamping, cutting, and suturing of tissues should take place under direct vision at all times. During complex pelvic surgery, the most effective way of preventing ureteral injury is to identify the ureters as they enter the pelvis over the bifurcation of the common iliac arteries and trace each ureter through its pelvic course in the retroperitoneal space, preserving its pelvic peritoneal attachment and thus the blood supply within the adventitial sheath.

Detection

If there is a suspicion of urological injury intraoperatively, this needs to be investigated to confirm or refute such a possibility. If a cystotomy is suspected, the bladder can be backfilled with indigo carmine or methylene blue dye (or sterile milk) per urethra, and leakage of dye will confirm inadvertent cystotomy. If injury to the ureter is suspected, a number of options are available. Dissection of the ureter throughout its course in the retroperitoneal space and observing 'peristalsis' is the gold standard. Other options include intraoperative ureteral catheterization, IV dye injection to detect leakage of colored urine, and intraoperative intravenous pyelogram (IVP).

Unrecognized ureteric or bladder injuries may present with symptoms and signs of intraperitoneal or retroperitoneal leakage of urine causing abdominal distension, ileus, and urinoma. There may also be symptoms of oliguria or anuria, fever, chills, and flank pain, especially with ureteric obstruction. An abdominal ultrasound, IVP, or retrograde cystogram may be required depending on the working diagnosis.

Repair

A cystotomy can usually be repaired at the time of initial injury. It is essential to identify the ureteric orifices if the cystotomy is proximal to the point of entry of the ureters to the bladder to avoid causing a ureteric obstruction as a result of the repair. If there is difficulty in identifying the ureteric orifices, IV furosemide will increase the urine output allowing easier identification of the ureteric orifices. The bladder should be repaired in two layers with a fine absorbable suture and its water tightness tested post-repair by filling it with methylene blue. Postoperatively the bladder should be drained for 7–10 days.

Ureteric injuries may take the form of angulation (kinking), crushing, ligation, transection (complete or partial), and devascularization. The general principles of successful ureteric repair include meticulous ureteric dissection with atraumatic instruments, while preserving the ureteric blood supply by maintaining the peritoneal attachment.

- A tension-free anastomosis needs to be performed using the minimum of absorbable suture to maintain a watertight anastomosis and surrounding it with retroperitoneal fat or omentum to help healing.
- Draining the site to prevent accumulation of urine, lymph, or blood is important. A proximal urinary diversion or urinary stenting may be required. Prophylactic antibiotics are recommended until all stents and drains are removed.
- Any significant angulation or kinking of the ureter should be released to prevent obstruction.
- Minor devascularization, crush injuries, or ligated ureters after release of the suture may require no other treatment, but sometimes stenting the damaged ureter may help recovery.
- Lacerations of the ureter are dealt with using fine absorbable sutures to close the defect after insertion of stents.
- Where the ureter has been transected, repair depends on the nature and location of the injury and may include uretero-neocystostomy (ureteric reimplantation) with or without bladder flap, end-to-end uretero-ureterostomy, uretero-ureterostomy to contralateral ureter, and creation of a cutaneous ureterostomy, to name just a few.

In general, when a urological complication has occurred, the assistance and advice of a urological surgeon should be sought, given that the best results are obtained when the complication is appropriately dealt with in the first instance.

Communication and record keeping

History taking

Start by introducing yourself and explaining who you are. Establish and maintain eye contact. Try to adopt an open and conducive posture and avoid sitting with a desk or other object between yourself and the patient. Indicate that you are interested in what the patient is saying by sitting forward, asking questions, and using nonverbal encouragement such as nodding. Avoid rustling through papers, looking at the time, or concentrating on writing in the notes or on to a computer. Try to ensure that you are not interrupted during the interview by telephone calls or other people entering the room. During the interview note the patient's appearance and manner.

- *Introduction* Check the patient's name and whether she prefers to be addressed as Mrs or Miss if you are unsure about her marital status. Ask about age and occupation. Occupation may be relevant both to the level of understanding that can be assumed and the impact of different gynecological problems on the patient's life.
- *Presenting complaint* Start with open questions and allow the patient to describe her own symptoms without interruption. Use more specific closed questions to fill in additional details if necessary. Establish the effect of the problem on the patient's life and family. Use the history-taking process to explore the patient's own concerns about her condition.
- *Previous gynecological history* Ask about any previous gynecological problems and treatments. For all women of reproductive age, ask about contraception if sexually active. If appropriate, ask about the date and results of the last cervical smear. Unless it has already been covered in the presenting complaint, ask about the date of the last menstrual period (LMP) and whether it was normal and occurred at the expected time. If the menstrual cycle varies, note the minimum and maximum length.
- *Previous pregnancies* Ask about the number of previous pregnancies and their outcome (miscarriage, ectopic, abortion, or delivery after 20 weeks). Ask about the mode of delivery and if there were any antenatal problems.
- *Previous medical history* Ask about previous medical problems, especially any endocrine disease and major cardiovascular/respiratory disease and venous thromboembolism. Ask about previous operations, especially abdominal surgery, and any anesthetic problems. Ask about current medication, especially sex steroids and their antagonists and anticoagulants. Check for any allergies.
- *Social and family history* A strong family history of ovarian cancer is associated with an increased risk of developing the disease. Ask about what support the patient has at home and work. This will have a bearing on the arrangements she will need to make to come into hospital and the support she will require after discharge. Ask about smoking and consumption of alcohol or illicit drugs.

During an examination

Before any examination, explain to the patient what is involved and why the examination needs to be performed, and obtain her permission. Allow the patient to undress in privacy. Expose only those areas of the body that are needed at that time to carry out the examination. During the examination itself, restrict your comments to an explanation of what is being done and relevant questions about any symptoms. Avoid unnecessary personal comments. After the examination, explain your findings and encourage questions and discussion. Avoid giving advice or discussing management during the examination itself.

Presenting a history

Being able to summarize the history and examination findings accurately and concisely is essential when communicating with other health professionals.

Start the history by introducing the patient by name and giving a clear indication of the presenting complaint or the reason why she is in the ward or clinic. If there are several problems, say so and deal with each in turn. If the history consists of a long narrative of events, try to summarize these rather than recapitulate each event in chronological sequence. Present the remainder of the history in a logical structured way, not skipping back and forward between items. Always include the dates of the LMP and cervical smear. Include details of the social history.

- Do not appear disorganized or waffle.
- Do not simply read back your notes.
- Do not reprise past history or systems review if not relevant.
- Do not use abbreviations or medical terms you cannot define.

At the end of your history, give a summary in no more than one or two sentences.

Patients and record keeping

Giving patients information

This includes counseling about the results of tests or the implications of a particular diagnosis as well as counseling about a particular procedure.

- Use appropriate (simple) language and avoid medical jargon.
- Give information at an appropriate rate, pausing where necessary. This may involve making an assessment of the patient's level of understanding and medical knowledge.
- Start with the most important items of information first.
- If giving advice, make this specific and detailed.
- Use short sentences and use more than one way of giving information such as repetition, diagrams, or written summaries.
- Pausing to summarize can also be a useful way to check the patient's understanding of the information given.
- At the end of the interview, try to summarize what has been said and give the patient enough time to ask any questions.
- Make an accurate record in the case notes of what has been said to the patient and/or her relatives.
- Provide appropriate information leaflets for the patient to take away or write to the patient after the interview.

Breaking bad news

- Ensure that adequate time is set aside free from interruptions for the interview.
- Read through the notes, especially the results of recent investigations, before speaking to the patient.
- Encourage the patient to have a friend or relative present during the discussion. They are more likely to remember information than a patient who is trying to come to terms with what she has been told.
- Avoid medical jargon and euphemisms for conditions such as cancer.
- Encourage the patient and/or her family to ask questions and check their understanding of what has been said.
- Make sure that the patient knows what will happen next.
- Offer a further appointment or give a contact number for an appropriate team member (such as a nurse specialist) to follow up with further information.
- Make a record in the case notes of what has been said and, where possible, comment on the patient's and/or her relatives' reactions.

Dealing with an angry patient or relative

If the patient or her relatives become angry or abusive during the interview, stay calm. Remain seated and invite the patient to sit down. Keep talking in a normal tone of voice whilst acknowledging the patient's anger and inviting her to talk about the reasons for her reaction. Try to convey an impression of remaining professional and in control without appearing dismissive of the patient's concerns.

Record keeping: essential elements

- Write legibly in black ink.
- Be clear and unambiguous.
- Be accurate in each entry as to date and time. Use the same clock.
- Sign each entry: print name and grade on first entry.
- Should be contemporaneous. If written in retrospect, state this and add date and time the entry was made.
- Do not use abbreviations, meaningless phrases, or offensive subjective statements.
- Ensure that wrong entries are scored out with a single line and initialed.
- Record any warnings given to women about the risks of a particular treatment.
- Record all decisions made even if the decision is only to observe closely.
- If a woman refuses treatment, record anything said about the possible consequences of ignoring advice given. Patient should ideally countersign such an entry.

With specific reference to intrapartum record keeping:

- Note any cardiotocograph (CTG) abnormality in the case notes and the action taken.
- Meconium: record presence, thick or thin, and amount of amniotic fluid.
- CTG trace: patient details, date and time of commencement, and maternal pulse rate should be recorded.
- Check that the fetal monitor clock displays/records the correct time.
- Record on CTG when the trace ends (it may be alleged that part is missing).

Medicolegal issues in obstetrics and gynecology

Introduction

Throughout the Western world there has been a significant increase in medicolegal claims in obstetrics and gynecology over the past decade. Few clinical practitioners in the speciality have not experienced allegations of medical negligence against them, and such claims cause considerable personal anxiety and stress. However, those receiving such claims should remember that the vast majority of allegations of medical negligence eventually are not proven and, furthermore, because of the high level of claims, the receipt of such a claim is not the medical disgrace that it may have been 50 years ago.

It is the nature of obstetrics and gynecology that things can go wrong quickly, sometimes without warning, and yet a perfect outcome is expected by everybody. Equally, because in gynecology our patients are often very fit preoperatively, a perfect outcome is expected. It is for this reason that the speciality of obstetrics and gynecology was historically one of the first specialities to be hit by medical negligence claims, although other specialities are now equally affected. Because of its nature, it is difficult to avoid the risk of a claim. However, the fundamentals of good medical practice will go a long way to diminishing the risk. These are as follows:

- Be courteous to patients and relatives at all times.
- Pay careful attention to the detail of the management of a case.
- Maintain a high standard of note-keeping in medical records.

What is negligence?

To a medical layman the expression 'negligence' carries the connotation of a wilful act on behalf of the individual practitioner. Apart from a very small number of notorious individuals, the concept of a willful misdeed is horrific to most.

- However, the term negligence in law means that a duty of care owed by the practitioner (then becoming a defendant) to the patient (who has become the claimant) has been breached. Such a breach may be caused by omission rather than commission.
- In simple terms, the claimant alleges that the defendant has been careless.
- In determining the degree of carelessness, particularly in surgical procedures, recognition is made of the level of skill an individual practitioner may have.
  - For example, if a senior obstetrician–gynecologist instructs a first-year trainee to carry out a hysterectomy alone and both ureters are damaged, this outcome may have been expected. The senior obstetrician–gynecologist could be deemed to be negligent for inappropriate delegation of the task and, equally, the trainee could be deemed negligent for taking it on. This could also apply in other instances where a trainee undertook a difficult emergency case without discussing it with the attending practitioner.

- In another example, where the rectal mucosa was breached by a suture during the repair of a second-degree tear after childbirth, whether it was caused by the trainee or the attending practitioner, both could be equally liable if they had not carried out a rectal examination at the completion of the procedure to check that this had not happened. In other words, this would be exercise of a skill that all levels of practitioner should possess.

At the present time, patients and politicians expect all non-attending-level doctors to be supervised. Unfortunately, the term 'supervision' means different things to different people.

- To most, supervision of a surgical procedure by an attending surgeon means that he/she is scrubbed and taking part in the operation.
- However, it is possible to supervise an operation while standing in the operating room unscrubbed, by being on Labor & Delivery but not necessarily in the operating room, by being in the hospital, or even by not necessarily being in the hospital at all.
- In all situations, it would have to be demonstrated that the operating trainee had been adequately trained and was adequately experienced to operate on the patient at that level of supervision, and, where the case had been specifically chosen by the attending surgeon, that the case was matched to the surgeon's known level of skill and ability.
- Furthermore, if the attending surgeon is not present in the hospital, then proper arrangements have to be made for assisting the operating practitioner in the event of unexpected difficulties.

If it can be demonstrated that the duty of care had been breached by the above means, a causal connection between such a breach and the alleged damage suffered by the patient has to be demonstrated.

- This process is called determination of causation.
- In many cases this is straightforward. For example:
  - 'Surgeon operates on wrong leg.'
  - 'Failure to remove intrauterine contraceptive device (IUCD) at time of sterilization resulting in long-term pelvic pain.'
- Furthermore, how much of the damage resulting from such incidents is attributable to the negligence and how much is attributable to other causes needs to be determined.

Finally, a monetary value of such damage needs to be determined. The legal term for this is 'quantum'.

Recommended further reading

1. Chamberlain GVP (ed) (1992). *How to Avoid Medico-legal Problems in Obstetrics and Gynaecology* (2nd edn). Royal College of Obstetricians and Gynaecologists, London.
2. American College of Obstetricians and Gynecologists (2005). ACOG Committee Opinion No. 321. Maternal decision making, ethics, and the law. *Obstet Gynecol* **106**, 1127–37.
3. American College of Obstetricians and Gynecologists (2004). ACOG Committee Opinion No. 286. Patient safety in obstetrics and gynecology. *Int J Gynaecol Obstet* **86**, 121–3.

Consent for operative procedures

It is important that adequate signed consent has been obtained from the patient before any operative procedure. It is also important to check that the planned procedure matches that which is written on the consent form.

- There can be very little defence if tubes and ovaries are removed at the time of hysterectomy when the patient only consented to the hysterectomy itself.
- Similarly, if it has been agreed that something be done, e.g. removal of an IUCD at sterilization, and this is not carried out (and the patient not advised), again there is little defence.

A view is currently being put forward that consent should only be taken from patients by practitioners who are capable of performing the operation on the grounds that such a practitioner can adequately brief the patient on the procedure and any complications.

- Usually, this means that the consent should be taken by the surgeon concerned.
- In practice, this may be difficult to achieve for all situations. Provided that a practitioner is familiar with the procedure, whilst not necessarily being able to perform it, this could be considered as sufficient.
  - This could mean that junior members of the team could readily take consent for hysteroscopy and perhaps even for straightforward hysterectomy.
- However, in more complex cases, such as minimal access surgery or radical oncology procedures, the attending practitioner should ensure (and be capable of demonstrating by the medical record) that the patient has been adequately briefed on the procedure and complications at the very least even if he/she is not necessarily the signatory of the consent form.

Recommended further reading

1. Chamberlain GVP (ed) (1992). *How to Avoid Medico-legal Problems in Obstetrics and Gynaecology* (2nd edn). Royal College of Obstetricians and Gynaecologists, London.
2. American College of Obstetricians and Gynecologists (2005). ACOG Committee Opinion No. 321. Maternal decision making, ethics, and the law. *Obstet Gynecol* **106**,1127–37.
3. American College of Obstetricians and Gynecologists (2004). ACOG Committee Opinion No. 286. Patient safety in obstetrics and gynecology. *Int J Gynaecol Obstet* **86**, 121–3.

Common obstetric and gynecological medicolegal problems

Obstetric

Most medicolegal problems revolve around very consistent themes even if the details of individual cases vary. Problems invariably arise because of failure to elucidate, disclose, or discuss information about a pregnancy with patients, failure to take or maintain adequate medical records about a case, and, in particular, failure to act appropriately in the presence of abnormalities.

All first-class obstetric units (and who would wish to be otherwise) should possess a manual of guidelines/protocol of action in the event of abnormal situations arising. If it can be demonstrated, preferably through the medical report, that these guidelines and protocols have been observed, an adequate defence can usually be achieved even in the event of an adverse outcome.

Common causes of medicolegal problems in obstetrics are the following:

- *Antenatal period*
  - Failure to explain investigations and results, scan findings, etc.
  - Failure to act on abnormal results.
  - Failure to keep good records.
  - Failure to obtain good antenatal CTG recordings or appropriately annotate them.
- *Intrapartum period.*
  - Failure to keep continuous timed and signed detailed records of the progress of labor.
  - Failure to achieve good quality CTG recordings, with event annotation.
  - Failure to act in the presence of abnormal physical signs, progress, or CTG recording.
  - Failure to make and record adequate observations on a patient in the postpartum period, particularly in the event of an operative delivery, or complications such as preeclampsia.
  - Failure to act on observations and thus avoid postoperative collapse or eclampsia, for example.
- *Complicated pregnancies* such as multiple pregnancy, breech presentation, or placenta previa, all require the presence of a senior obstetrician, pediatrician, and anesthesiologist at delivery.
- *Shoulder dystocia* is a major and often unexpected sudden complication of the second stage of labor, which can have serious long-term results for the baby, particularly in the form of brachial plexus nerve palsy. For this reason, each unit should have a distinct protocol for the management of such an emergency and the protocol should be rehearsed regularly.

Gynecology

Failure to counsel patients adequately on their condition and any proposed surgical procedure is a common cause of litigation. Sterilization procedures and termination of pregnancy are frequent cases seen in gynecology and, individually, they represent the highest risk of adverse outcome and litigation. Therefore it is prudent to ensure that patients are adequately briefed. In some centers, information leaflets are issued to patients prior to operation and patients are asked to sign that they have read and understood the contents. If these are not available, record in the notes that the patients have been specifically counseled in the following areas in both topics.

- *Sterilization* The following areas must be discussed:
  - The type of operative procedure and devices used.
  - The failure rate (now usually described as 1 in 200–500 cases).
  - Potential irreversibility of the procedure.
  - Laparoscopic risks involving bowel or vessel damage that may result in laparotomy.
  - Preoperatively: the importance of determining LMP and/or excluding pregnancy.
  - Failure to remove/discuss removal of IUCD if present.
- *Termination of pregnancy* It is important to counsel concerning/discuss the following:
  - Primary or secondary hemorrhage that may lead to hysterectomy.
  - Incomplete evacuation requiring a subsequent repeat procedure.
  - Infection subsequent to procedure.
  - Infertility subsequent to procedure.
  - Uterine perforation at procedure leading to laparoscopy/laparotomy/hysterectomy.

Recommended further reading

1. Chamberlain GVP (ed) (1992). *How to Avoid Medico-legal Problems in Obstetrics and Gynaecology* (2nd edn). Royal College of Obstetricians and Gynaecologists, London.
2. American College of Obstetricians and Gynecologists (2005). ACOG Committee Opinion No. 321: Maternal decision making, ethics, and the law. *Obstet Gynecol* **106**, 1127–37.
3. American College of Obstetricians and Gynecologists (2004). ACOG Committee Opinion No. 286. Patient safety in obstetrics and gynecology. *Int J Gynaecol Obstet* **86**, 121–3.

Disclosure of operative risks

Minimal access gynecological surgery carries particular risks. Because there is very little to show on the external body surface, patients tend to think that they have had a small operation. In fact, many of them are not—they tend to be complex procedures involving high-technology equipment.

- It is important, particularly in the current climate, that anyone undertaking new operative procedures, particularly when they are complex, can demonstrate that they have been adequately trained in the procedure and the equipment to be used.
- Equally, it is very important that patients are counseled as to the expected outcomes and complications of these procedures. In particular, it must be explained that in endometrial ablation procedures there is a risk of perforation leading on to hysterectomy, and that, in laparoscopic procedures, the very nature of the surgery makes damage to collateral structures a higher risk than in open surgery even in the hands of the most experienced of laparoscopic surgeons.

In more traditional operations and those of lower medicolegal risk than sterilization and termination of pregnancy, there is a debate as to how much operative risk needs to be disclosed to the patient.

- For example, ureteric and bladder damage is a known risk of total abdominal hysterectomy. In North America, surgeons are advised to disclose such risks in detailed information sheets to patients. In Western Europe, such an approach is considered (at least at present) to be unnecessary and perhaps counterproductive in that such details would alarm patients to the point of declining the surgery when offered, even in cases where there was an overwhelming medical reason for it.
- There is also a general impression amongst gynecologists that risks only need to be disclosed to patients if they are greater than 1 in 1000 cases, 1 in 2000 cases, etc. It is by no means certain that such specificity is the case despite efforts by certain medicolegal experts to make it so.
    - For some operations, e.g. bowel/blood vessel damage at laparoscopy, an incidence of 1 in 2500, needs to be disclosed to a patient, whilst other experts maintain that an incidence of less than 1 in 1000 need not be disclosed at all.

The simple reason for this disparity is because the courts decide what the 'ordinary skilled practitioner' would do in a given set of circumstances rather than there being any set rules. Furthermore, in the case of known complications such as ureteric/bladder damage at hysterectomy, contemporary cases would suggest that, if all due care and attention has been taken at the operation and this has been properly documented in the case of complications such as significant pelvic hemorrhage during the procedure, this can be a mitigating and acceptable circumstance. However, if there is subsequently a delay at diagnosis of the resulting fistula, this could be construed as negligent. Similarly, significant wound infection with abscess formation, which certainly has a significance of greater than

1 in 1000 cases, need not specifically be counseled for preoperatively and the occurrence of such a complication would not be construed as negligent. However, if it were managed inappropriately, it could be so construed.

Special types of hysterectomy, such as radical hysterectomy where the incidence of complications is higher, do need to have particular special attention applied to the preoperative counseling. Subtotal hysterectomy, which is now becoming more popular as an elective procedure, does have particular possible problems concerning outcome, e.g. continued regular menstruation and the need for continued regular cervical cytology. These make it important that patients are counseled about the details of this particular procedure preoperatively.

Recommended further reading

1. Chamberlain GVP (ed) (1992). *How to Avoid Medico-legal Problems in Obstetrics and Gynaecology* (2nd edn). Royal College of Obstetricians and Gynaecologists, London.
2. American College of Obstetricians and Gynecologists (2005). ACOG Committee Opinion No. 321: Maternal decision making, ethics, and the law. *Obstet Gynecol* **106**, 1127–37.
3. American College of Obstetricians and Gynecologists (2004). ACOG Committee Opinion No. 286. Patient safety in obstetrics and gynecology. *Int J Gynaecol Obstet* **86**, 121–3.

Clinical risk management I

Introduction

Risk is a part of everyday life. We all seek to manage such risks, e.g. by wearing seatbelts, locking houses, and insuring property. Clinical risk management is a mechanism for dealing with risk exposure in obstetric and midwifery practice. This process enables us to recognize those events that may result in unfortunate or damaging consequences for patients, their frequency and severity, and how the risks may be controlled.

The overall objective of clinical risk management is to improve the quality of patient care by reducing or eliminating accidental harm to patients whenever possible. A review of the literature suggests that many more patients are harmed or traumatized by clinical treatment than those who consider legal action. Therefore the scale and effects of injury to patients should be the primary focus for risk management. Where quality of care is good, litigation is likely to be low.

Clinical staff involved in adverse incidents are often seriously affected by such events. Doctors involved in legal claims report great distress, worry, anger, and frustration. Loss of professional confidence and the adoption of defensive medical practice may result. Media interest in clinical negligence and professional competence issues would appear likely to increase staff stress.

Costs of clinical negligence claims in the USA are currently around $4.5 billion per year (Kaiser Family Foundation publication No. 7328 available online at www.kff.org) with obstetric practice generally being regarded as 'high risk' for legal claims. In addition, obstetric claims may involve very large financial settlements, e.g. up to $30 million damages in cerebral palsy cases. Extra costs associated with increased hospital stay and further investigation and treatment must also be considered. Equally important are the costs to the injured patient—increased pain, disability, and disruption to relationships, work, and social life.

With the possibility of litigation and/or prosecution, individual physicians and hospitals are becoming increasingly aware of the consequences of a wide range of risks that occur by accident through mischance, mishap, or mistake. Recent initiatives places a strong emphasis on risk management, clinical audit, and professional competence. The main aims of these processes are to improve standards of care and define best practice in order to improve quality.

- A proactive move towards managing clinical risk means anticipating any potential hazards that may cause harm to patients and taking steps to prevent or limit any harm that may occur.
- Reactive approaches include dealing appropriately with injured patients, learning from past mistakes, and effective claims management.
- Both approaches will require risk assessment and prioritization skills.

Risk identification

Risks to service users can be identified by a combination of methods:

- incident reporting
- analysis of complaints/legal claims/user views
- confidential enquiries and audit
- risk assessments.

Incident reporting

All grades and disciplines of staff should be encouraged to report any situation where the individual considers that a threat to patient safety may exist. This includes incidents where actual harm is caused to a patient and 'near-miss' events, i.e. where something has gone wrong but no actual harm has occurred to the patient. In order to achieve the compliance of clinical staff, it is important that organizational culture is encouraged to move from one of blame to one of openness and honesty. Assurances need to be given at board level that disciplinary action will not result against employees who commit errors, unless serious professional misconduct or a crime has been committed.

- Forms used must be 'user-friendly' in order to increase compliance—a list of specific trigger indicators is particularly useful in obstetric practice.
- Patient details, date and time of the incident, staff involved, and a brief *factual* account of the incident must be included.
- It should also be made clear that any serious outcome for a patient must be reported to appropriate persons without delay.
- Completed forms should be collated and analyzed at a central point.

Over a period of time, it may be possible to identify common factors and trends that may result in real risks to patients though they would be considered trivial when viewed in isolation.

If a legal claim is likely to result from an adverse outcome, formal statements can be collected from the staff involved in order that legal advisors can make early decisions on potential liability and prepare a defence when appropriate.

Communication with patients following adverse events

An efficient system of risk reporting also aids good communication. A senior member of the obstetric/midwifery team must be informed of adverse outcomes in order that the family are counseled appropriately and arrangements made for referral or follow-up dependent on clinical need and the patient's wishes.

Recommended further reading

1. Brennan TA, Leape LL, Laird N (1991). Incidence of adverse events and negligence in hospitalized patients: results of the Harvard medical study. *N Eng J Med* **324**, 370–7.
2. Wilson RM, Runciman WB, Gibber RW (1995). The Quality in Australian Healthcare Study. *Med J Aust* **163**, 458–71.

Clinical risk management II

Analysis of complaints/legal claims/user views

Retrospective analysis of complaints and legal claims can be used to highlight areas where improvements in care/treatment can be made. Ongoing audit of claims and complaints is an important part of clinical governance to confirm that practices are learning from previous mistakes. It may also be useful to involve consumers in the planning and development of maternity services.

Confidential enquiries and audit

Invaluable information on clinical risk can be gained from enquires into maternal and perinatal deaths. These national reports may also recommend changes to practice in order to reduce risk.

Local clinical audit processes may also highlight areas of clinical risk and can be used to monitor areas of high risk, e.g. the 'decision to delivery' interval in emergency cesarean delivery.

Risk assessments

All reported risk or near-miss situations should be formally assessed as to their frequency of occurrence and severity in order that necessary actions can be centrally prioritized. Control measures can then be identified and put into place.

Some hospitals employ specialists in risk analysis to carry out formal risk assessments, whilst others use their own staff. During the process of carrying out proactive risk assessments, widespread consultation with all grades and disciplines of staff is necessary. This encourages local ownership of problems and may well identify latent failures within the organization, i.e. the factors that contribute indirectly to medical accident and near-miss situations. Decisions can then be made on what precautions or controls are needed. These measures can be maintained whilst monitoring future risk recurrence.

Risk analysis

The risk assessment process must include analysis of the severity of effect and the likelihood of recurrence. This will include consideration of effects on the patient, service provision, and the likelihood of future legal claim. A cost-benefit analysis should also be carried out at this stage. Because of the nature of health care, it is not possible to create an environment that is entirely free of risk.

Risk control

Clinical risks can be controlled by the following:

- Avoidance—by using alternative working practices or equipment.
- Making risks less likely—e.g. by improving staff training or a review of clinical guidelines.
- Elimination—by ceasing to provide the service.
- Insuring against those the risks that cannot be reduced or eliminated so that litigation costs are reduced.

Recommended further reading

1. Pattison R, Say L, Makin J, Bastos M, Pattinson RC (2005). Critical incident audit and feedback to improve perinatal and maternal mortality and morbidity. *Cochrane Database Syst Rev* **4**, CD002961.

Risk reduction in obstetric/midwifery practice

Communication

Effective communication between health professionals and between staff and women and their families is essential to the provision of quality care. Poor communication is one of the main causes of complaint that may lead to a legal claim. Women should be encouraged to participate in decision making and in making informed choices about the care and treatments available. Written information should be available to support verbal information given to women. Provision of information in the form of audio and video tapes should also be considered. Communication in the patient's language of choice is important. Therefore effective interpreter services are an integral part of any healthcare system and should be available around the clock.

There should be a personal handover of care at shift changes for both medical and midwifery staff in order to ensure accurate sharing of information.

Policies, procedures, and guidelines

These should be based on the best available evidence and reviewed and updated regularly. Clinical audit may help to clarify that guidelines are suitable and are used by clinical staff. It is also important that out-of-date documents are correctly archived if required for future legal claims.

Valid consent arrangements

Ideally, consent for operative procedures should be obtained by a health professional capable of carrying out the procedure. If this is not possible, the health professional obtaining consent must have sufficient knowledge to inform the woman of the material risks, benefits, and alternatives to the proposed treatment. It is also essential to warn of any consequences of refusal of treatment and give the woman an opportunity to ask questions if she wishes. Again, wherever possible, counseling should occur in the patient's language of choice.

Staffing levels

Attention should be given to provision of safe levels of both obstetric and midwifery staffing levels in all areas of practice. Wherever possible, the use of locum or agency clinical staff should be minimal. When this group of staff are employed, close supervision is necessary. Handover of patient care should be by a senior member of the obstetric/midwifery team. Written information on local procedures and guidelines should also be made freely available.

Professional competence

Statutory supervision in midwifery provides an enabling and supportive framework in order that the midwife can fulfil her responsibilities. Professional guidance and advice on assessment and management of risk is also available via the supervisory relationship.

- Induction programs for all staff should be mandatory at commencement of employment.
- All clinical staff should receive additional training in CTG interpretation and the management of high-risk labor.
- Regular training of all staff in neonatal and adult basic life support should also be recommended. 'Fire drills' in the management of obstetric emergencies such as major hemorrhage and shoulder dystocia are excellent methods of maintaining professional competence.
- All staff must be familiar with equipment used in their area of work and ensure that it is regularly maintained.

Complaint management

All clinical staff should have a basic knowledge of local complaint procedures and have the necessary skills to deal with verbal complaints before a formal complaint becomes necessary.

Record keeping

Keeping and maintaining a record of care given are essential, both to aid continuity of care and to provide a defence to legal claims.

- Records must be clear, unambiguous, legible, and contemporaneous.
- It is essential that all entries are readily identifiable.
- All decisions about clinical care should be recorded.
- Local arrangements must be in place for follow-up of all clinical investigations performed.
- All test and imaging results, EKGs, and CTG tracings must be stored securely.
- Maternity records must be stored securely for future use or reference.
- Regular audit of record-keeping standards is necessary with appropriate feedback to individuals in order that standards can be improved.

Recommended further reading

1. Wilson RM, Runciman WB, Gibber RW (1995). The Quality in Australian Healthcare Study. *Medi J Aust* **163**, 458–71.
2. Pattison R, Say L, Makin J, Bastos M, Pattinson RC (2005). Critical incident audit and feedback to improve perinatal and maternal mortality and morbidity. *Cochrane Database Syst Rev* **4**, CD002961.

Index

I

Q

R

S

T

U

V

W

X

Y

Z